Amsler's Grid

The chart on the opposite page is patterned after the grid devised by Professor Marc Amsler. It can provide for the rapid detection of small irregularities in the central 20° of the field of vision. The chart is composed of a grid of lines containing a central white fixation spot. The squares on the grid are 5 mm in size and subtend a visual angle of 1° at 30 cm viewing distance.

The chart is to be viewed in modest light monocularly at a distance of 28-30 cm utilizing the correct refraction for this distance. Viewing should be accomplished without previous ophthalmoscopy and without instillation of any drugs affecting pupillary size or accommodation.

A series of questions should be asked while the patient is viewing the central white spot.

1) Is the center spot visible? The absence of the spot may indicate the presence of a central scotoma.

2) While viewing the center white spot can you see all four sides? The inability to perceive these areas may indicate the presence of an arcuate scotoma of glaucoma encroaching upon the central area or a centrocecal scotoma.

3) Do you see the entire grid intact? Are there any defects? If an area of the grid is not visible, then a paracentral scotoma is present.

4) Are the horizontal and vertical lines straight and parallel? If not, then metamorphopsia is present. The parallel lines may ''bend'' inwards giving rise to micropsia or ''bend'' outwards giving rise to macropsia.

5) Do you see any blur or distortion in the grid? Any movement? A color aberration? These changes may be present prior to the appearance of a definite scotoma.

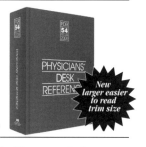

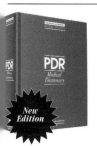

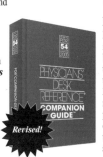

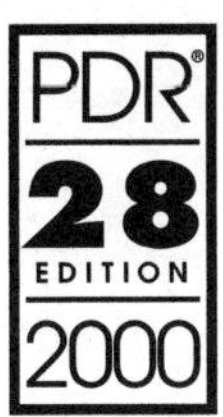

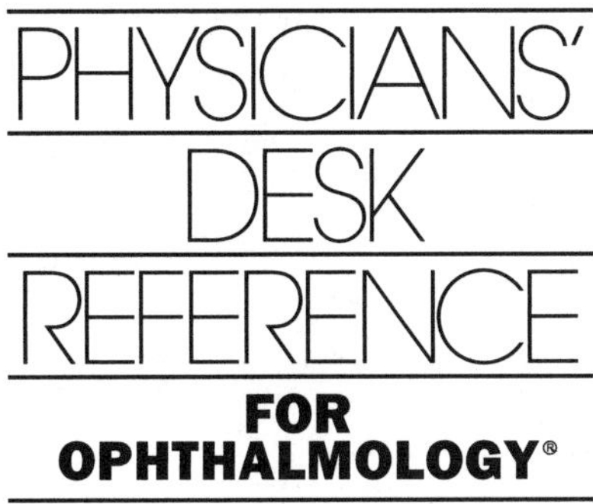

Editorial Consultants and Contributors

ISBN: 1-56363-339-6

FOREWORD TO THE TWENTY-EIGHTH EDITION

As we enter the new millennium, PDR® is pleased to present this completely revised and updated edition of *Physicians' Desk Reference For Ophthalmology*®, the profession's premier source of FDA-approved information on ophthalmological pharmaceuticals and equipment. As always, you'll find the latest guidelines for hundreds of established products, as well as full details on the many new agents released since publication of the previous edition

In addition, the book's opening sections offer you a useful set of tables summarizing the major pharmaceutical alternatives available in ophthalmology today, as well as a brief guide to suture materials and a handy bank of information on low vision. The opening sections also include an exhaustive catalog of currently available contact lenses, a variety of lens comparison and conversion tables, and the complete chapter on the visual system from the fourth edition of *Guides to the Evaluation of Permanent Impairment.* Four indices help you locate products by manufacturer, trade name, product category, and active ingredient; and there's even a full-color product identification section.

The special reference sections near the beginning of *PDR For Ophthalmology* have been prepared with the assistance of Clement A. Weisbecker, RPh, Douglas Rhee, MD, and Richard Tippermann, MD of Wills Eye Hospital in Philadelphia, Pennsylvania. Our thanks also go to F.T. Fraunfelder, MD, author of the section on ocular toxicology. The opinions expressed in these sections are those of the authors and are not necessarily endorsed by the publisher, Medical Economics Company.

If you use a computer in your practice, you can also retrieve the contents of *PDR For Ophthalmology* from the *PDR® Electronic Library*™ CD-ROM and view the data on the Internet at www.pdr.net. For personal use—on rounds or on the go—you can carry *Pocket PDR®*, a unique handheld electronic database of prescribing information that literally fits in your pocket. For more information on these or any other members of the growing family of *PDR®* products, please call, toll-free, 1-800-232-7379 or fax 201-573-4956.

Under the federal Food, Drug & Cosmetics (FD&C) Act, a drug approved for marketing may be labeled, promoted, and advertised by the manufacturer for only those uses for which the drug's safety and effectiveness have been established. The Code of Federal Regulations 201.100(d)(1) pertaining to labeling for prescription products requires that in the text of *Physicians' Desk Reference For Ophthalmology* "indications, effects, dosages, routes, methods, and frequency and duration of administration and any relevant warnings, hazards, contraindications, side effects, and precautions" must be in the *"same language and emphasis"* as the approved labeling for the products. FDA regards the words *same language and emphasis* as requiring VERBATIM use of the approved labeling providing such information. Furthermore, information in the approved labeling that is emphasized by the use of type set in a box or in capitals, boldface, or italics must be given the same emphasis in *Physicians' Desk Reference For Ophthalmology.*

The FDA has also recognized that the FD&C Act does not, however, limit the manner in which a physician may use an approved drug. Once a product has been approved for marketing, a physician may prescribe it for uses or in treatment regimens or patient populations that are not included in approved labeling. The FDA also observes that accepted medical practice often includes drug use that is not reflected in approved drug labeling. For products that do not have official package circulars, the publisher has emphasized the necessity of describing such products comprehensively, so that physicians have access to all information essential for intelligent and informed decision making.

The function of the publisher is the compilation, organization, and distribution of this information. Each product description has been prepared by the manufacturer, and edited and approved by the manufacturer's medical department, medical director, and/or medical consultant. In organizing and presenting the material in *Physicians' Desk Reference For Ophthalmology,* the publisher does not warrant or guarantee any of the products described, or perform any independent analysis in connection with any of the product information contained herein. *Physicians' Desk Reference For Ophthalmology* does not assume, and expressly disclaims, any obligation to obtain and include any information other than that provided to it by the manufacturer. It should be understood that by making this material available the publisher is not advocating the use of any product described herein, nor is the publisher responsible for misuse of a product due to typographical error. Additional information on any product may be obtained from the manufacturer.

CONTENTS

SECTION 1

INDICES

This section offers four ways to locate the product information you need:

1. Manufacturers' Index: Gives the location of each participating manufacturer's product information. If two page numbers appear, the first refers to photographs in the Product Identification Guide, the second to product information. Also listed are the addresses and telephone numbers of the company's headquarters and regional offices.

2. Product Name Index: Lists page numbers of product information alphabetically by brand name. A diamond symbol to the left of a name indicates that a photograph of the item appears in the Product Identification Guide. For these products, the first page number refers to the photograph, the second to an entry in one of the Product Information Sections. All pharmaceuticals, equipment, and intraocular products are included.

3. Product Category Index: Lists products alphabetically by type or category, such as "Contact Lenses," "Refractometers," or "Anti-Infectives." All pharmaceuticals, equipment, and intraocular products are included.

4. Active Ingredients Index: Groups products alphabetically by generic name or material, such as "Atropine Sulfate" or "Polymacon." Under each heading, all fully described products are listed first, followed by those with only partial descriptions. Equipment is not included.

PART I/MANUFACTURERS' INDEX

AKORN, INC. 103, 201
2500 Millbrook Drive
Buffalo Grove, IL 60089
Direct Inquiries to:
Customer Service
(800) 535-7155

ALCON LABORATORIES, INC. 208
and its Affiliates
Corporate Headquarters
6201 South Freeway
Fort Worth, TX 76134
Direct Inquiries to:
Pharmaceutical/Consumer Products:
(800) 451-3937
(Therapeutic Drugs/Lens Care)
Surgical: (800) 862-5266
(Instrumentation/Surgical Meds)
Systems: (800) 289-1991
(Medical Management Information Systems)

ALLERGAN 103, 224
2525 Dupont Drive
P.O. Box 19534
Irvine, CA 92623-9534
For Medical Information, Contact:
Outside CA: (800) 433-8871
CA: (714) 246-4500
Sales and Ordering:
Outside CA: (800) 377-7790
CA: (714) 246-4500

BAUSCH & LOMB, INC 104, 249
1400 North Goodman Street
Rochester, NY 14609
Direct Inquiries to:
North American Vision Care
Customer Service
(800) 553-5340

BAUSCH & LOMB .... 104, 250 PHARMACEUTICAL, INC.
8500 Hidden River Parkway
Tampa, FL 33637
Direct Inquiries to:
Customer Service Department:
(800) 323-0000
(813) 975-7700

BAUSCH & LOMB SURGICAL..... 259
555 West Arrow Highway
Claremont, CA 91711
Direct Inquiries to:
Customer Services
(800) 338-2020

CHIRON VISION
(See BAUSCH & LOMB SURGICAL)

CIBA VISION 105, 260
A Novartis Company
11460 Johns Creek Parkway
Duluth, GA 30097-1556
Direct Inquiries to:
Customer Service
(800) 845-6585
FAX: (770) 418-4000
Internet: www.cibavision.com

IOLAB CORPORATION
(See BAUSCH & LOMB SURGICAL; CIBA VISION)

LEDERLE LABORATORIES .. 105, 272
Division of American Cyanamid Co.
Pearl River, NY 10965
For Medical Information Contact:
Medical Affairs Department
P.O. Box 8299
Philadelphia, PA 19101
Day: (800) 934-5556 (8:30 AM to 4:30 PM, Eastern Standard Time, Weekdays only)
Night: (610) 688-4400 (Emergencies only; non-emergencies should wait until the next day)

MEDICAL OPHTHALMICS, INC. ... 276
40146 U.S. Hwy 19 N.
Tarpon Springs, FL 34689
Direct Inquiries to:
(800) 358-7797

MERCK & CO., INC. 105, 277
P.O. Box 4
West Point, PA 19486-0004
For Product and Service Information, and Adverse Experience Reports, call the Merck National Service Center, 8:00 AM to 7:00 PM (ET), Monday through Friday:
(800) NSC-MERCK
(800) 672-6372
FAX: (800) MERCK-68
FAX: (800) 637-2568

MERCK—*cont.*

24-Hour Emergency Product Information for Healthcare Professionals, Call:
(800) NSC-MERCK
(800) 672-6372
For Product Orders and Direct Account Inquiries Only, call the Order Management Center, 8:00 AM to 7:00 PM (ET), Monday through Friday:
(800) MERCK RX
(800) 637-2579

MONARCH PHARMACEUTICALS **106, 300**
355 Beecham Street
Bristol, TN 37620

OCUMED, INC. **308**
119 Harrison Avenue
Roseland, NJ 07068
BRANCH OFFICE:
1255 S. Commerce Blvd.
Sarasota, FL 34243
(941) 351-4631
Direct Inquiries to:
A.R. Caggia
(973) 226-2330
FAX: (973) 226-0105

PFIZER CONSUMER HEALTH CARE GROUP **107, 309**
Pfizer Inc
235 East 42nd Street
New York, NY 10017
Direct Inquiries to:
Consumer Relations Group
(212) 573-5656
FAX: (212) 973-7437
For Consumer Product Information Call:
(800) 723-7529
Internet: www.visine.com

PHARMACIA & UPJOHN **107, 311**
100 Route 206 North
Peapack, NJ 07977
For Medical and Pharmaceutical Information, Including Emergencies:
(616) 833-8244
FAX: (616) 833-8414
For Patient Information:
(800) 253-8600 ext. 3-6004
FAX: (616) 833-4551

ROSS PRODUCTS DIVISION **314**
625 Cleveland Ave.
Columbus, Ohio 43215-1724 USA
Division of Abbott Laboratories Inc.
Direct Inquiries to:
(800) 227-5767

STORZ OPHTHALMICS
(See BAUSCH & LOMB PHARMACEUTICAL, INC.; BAUSCH & LOMB SURGICAL; LEDERLE LABORATORIES; WYETH-AYERST PHARMACEUTICALS)

VISION PHARMACEUTICALS, INC. **316**
1022 North Main Street
Mitchell, SD 57301
Direct Inquiries to:
Jane Schoenfelder
(800) 325-6789
(605) 996-3356
FAX: (605) 996-7072
Internet: www.visionpharm.com

WYETH-AYERST PHARMACEUTICALS **107, 316**
Division of American Home Products Corporation
P.O. Box 8299
Philadelphia, PA 19101
For Medical Information Contact:
Medical Affairs Department
P.O. Box 8299
Philadelphia, PA 19101
Day: (800) 934-5556 (8:30 AM to 4:30 PM, Eastern Standard Time, Weekdays only)
Night: (610) 688-4400 (Emergencies only; non-emergencies should wait until the next day)

◆ **Shown in Product Identification Guide**

Italic Page Number **Indicates Brief Listing**

PART III/PRODUCT CATEGORY INDEX

A

B

Italic Page Number **Indicates Instrumentation and Equipment**

PART IV/ACTIVE INGREDIENTS INDEX

SECTION 2

PHARMACEUTICALS IN OPHTHALMOLOGY

Clement A. Weisbecker, RPh, Douglas Rhee, MD, and Richard Tippermann, MD (Wills Eye Hospital, Philadelphia, Pa), with a section on ocular toxicology by F. T. Fraunfelder, MD

Once again we are pleased to present an up-to-date overview of current pharmaceutical options in ophthalmology. This year we invite your attention in particular to new developments in the field of viscoelastic substances. You'll find them summarized in Part 11 of this section.

In all, this section offers 26 reference tables presenting therapeutic alternatives (including a number of common off-label uses) in all major categories of ophthalmic treatment, as well as a survey of recently identified adverse drug reactions encountered in ophthalmology. The material is divided into 13 parts as follows:

1. Mydriatics and Cycloplegics
2. Antimicrobial Therapy
3. Ocular Anti-inflammatory Agents
4. Anesthetic Agents
5. Agents for Treatment of Glaucoma
6. Medications for Dry Eye
7. Ocular Decongestants
8. Ophthalmic Irrigating Solutions
9. Hyperosmolar Agents
10. Diagnostic Agents
11. Viscoelastic Materials Used in Ophthalmology
12. Off-Label Drug Applications in Ophthalmology
13. Ocular Toxicology

There are a large number of excellent references related to pharmacology and treatment regimens in ophthalmology. Listed below are some of the ones we regard as particularly useful.

GENERAL REFERENCES

1. American Medical Association. *Drug Evaluations Annual.* Milwaukee, Wis: AMA Department of Drugs, Division of Toxicology.
2. Fraunfelder FT, Roy FH. *Current Ocular Therapy*, ed 5. Philadelphia, Pa: WB Saunders; 1999.
3. Fraunfelder FT. *Drug-Induced Ocular Side Effects and Drug Interactions.* Philadelphia, Pa: Lea & Febiger; 1996.
4. Reynolds L, Closson R. *Extemporaneous Ophthalmic Preparations: Applied Therapeutics,* 1993.
5. Lerman S, Tripathi R. *Ocular Toxicology.* New York, NY: Marcel Dekker, Inc; 1990.
6. Olin B (editor-in-chief). *Ophthalmic Drug Facts.* St. Louis, Mo: JB Lippincott.
7. Vaughan D, Asbury T, Riordan-Eva P. *General Ophthalmology*, ed 15. Norwalk, Conn: Appleton & Lange; 1999.
8. Mauger. *Havener's Ocular Pharmacology.* St. Louis. Mo: CB Mosby; 1994.
9. Rhee D, Deramo V. *Wills Eye Hospital Drug Manual.* JB Lippincott, Williams & Wilkins, 1998.

1. MYDRIATICS AND CYCLOPLEGICS

The autonomic drugs that produce mydriasis (pupillary dilation) and cycloplegia (paralysis of accommodation) are among the most frequently used topical medications in ophthalmic practice. The most commonly used mydriatic is the direct-acting adrenergic agent, phenylephrine hydrochloride, usually in a 2.5% concentration. The other mydriatic, an indirectly acting adrenergic hydroxyamphetamine, is available only in combination with tropicamide.

Phenylephrine is used alone or, more commonly, in combination with a cycloplegic agent for refraction or for pupillary dilation. The 2.5% concentration is favored for cases. There is a possibility of severe adverse systemic effects from the use of the 10% solution.

Anticholinergic agents have both cycloplegic and mydriatic activity. They are usually used for refraction, pupillary dilation, and relief of inflammation.

It is important to remember that the effect of these medications depends on many factors, including age, race, and eye color. For example, the mydriatics and cycloplegics tend to be less effective in dark-eyed individuals than in blue-eyed ones.

The drug dapiprazole hydrochloride (Rēv-Eyes) can be used to reverse the effects of phenylephrine and, to a lesser extent, tropicamide. Activity against phenylephrine is excellent: 88% reversal at the end of 1 hour. Against tropicamide, results are significantly lower: 38% at the end of 2 hours. It therefore remains important, when using both drugs, to instruct the patient to use sunglasses and avoid driving or operating dangerous machinery.

TABLE 1

MYDRIATICS AND CYCLOPLEGICS

GENERIC NAME	TRADE NAMES	CONCENTRATION (%)	ONSET/DURATION OF ACTION
Phenylephrine hydrochloride	AK-Dilate Mydfrin Neo-Synephrine Available generically	Soln, 2.5%, 10% Soln, 2.5% Soln, 2.5%, 10% Soln, 2.5%, 10%	30–60 min/3–5 h
Hydroxyamphetamine hydrobromide*	Paremyd	Soln, 1%	15–60 min/3–4 h
Atropine sulfate	Atropisol Atropine-Care Isopto Atropine Available generically	Soln, 1% Soln, 1% Soln, 0.5%, 1% Soln, 1% Ointment, 1%	45–120 min/7–14 days
Cyclopentolate hydrochloride	AK-Pentolate Cyclogyl Pentolair Available generically	Soln, 1% Soln, 0.5%, 1%, 2% Soln, 1% Soln, 1%	30–60 min/6–24 h
Homatropine hydrobromide	Isopto Homatropine Available generically	Soln, 2%, 5% Soln, 2%, 5%	30–60 min/3 days
Scopolamine hydrobromide	Isopto Hyoscine	Soln, 0.25%	30–60 min/4–7 days
Tropicamide	Mydriacyl AK–Tropicacyl Available generically	Soln, 0.5%, 1% Soln, 0.5%, 1% Soln, 0.5%, 1%	20–40 min/4–6 h

* In combination with Tropicamide 0.25%

2. ANTIMICROBIAL THERAPY

Antibiotics are routinely used in ophthalmology for both treatment and prophylaxis. They are used prophylactically in the management of foreign bodies and corneal abrasions and in pre- and postoperative care, administered as an ophthalmic solution, ointment, or subconjunctival injection (see **Table 2**).

Many ophthalmic institutions have been using a solution of 5% povidone-iodine (Betadine) preoperatively to "sterilize" the eye, lids, and brow. Another development is the use of collagen shields (usually 12-hour) soaked in antibiotic, with or without steroid, in place of a patch and/or subconjunctival injection.

While more expensive, the shields do have the advantage of being more comfortable for the patient and are less likely to cause tissue degeneration.

Also appearing in the literature is another prophylactic measure: the addition of antibiotics to the irrigating solution. This technique is being used in several hospitals and high-volume surgicenters throughout the country. The maximum nontoxic concentrations of antibiotics are listed in **Table 3**. For prophylaxis, however, clinicians advise using half these amounts. Note that concentrations are given in micrograms per milliliter.

When treating an active or suspected external or intraocular infection, slides for gram and Giemsa stain and aerobic and anaerobic cultures should be secured prior to initiating therapy if the severity or site of infection dictates the necessity of culturing. When fungal involvement is a possibility, additional stains to consider are: methenamine silver, acridine orange, and calcofluor white.

Corneal ulcers and intraocular infections require vigorous management. Most physicians and hospitals have protocols for their treatment. One such protocol for treating endophthalmitis, modified from Mandelbaum and Forster, is given in **Table 4**. Serious ocular infections are usually treated by the topical, subconjunctival, and intraocular routes of administration (see **Table 5**). Corneal ulcers are usually treated with one or more of the topical solutions listed in **Table 5**, usually given every $^{1}/_{2}$ to 1 hour, in alternating doses if more than one solution is used. In severe cases, such as impending or actual perforation and scleral extension, medication is given by the topical, subconjunctival, and/or intravenous route.

Fungal keratitis (keratomycosis) is relatively uncommon, but should be suspected in patients who have previously received topical steroids and/or antibiotics, and in patients whose corneal ulcer does not respond to antibiotics. Corneal scraping often permits correct clinical diagnosis. Natamycin 5% ophthalmic suspension (Natacyn) is recognized as the most potent broad-spectrum antifungal agent available for use in the eye.

Incidence of endogenous fungal endophthalmitis can be seen in intravenous drug users and patients with compromised immune systems. For these infections, amphotericin B has been used subconjunctivally, intravenously, and, where indicated, intravitreally. Sterile operating room technique and a coaxially illuminated operating microscope should be used when administering the medication intravitreally. Prior to intravitreal use, a small portion of the vitreous abscess should be aspirated for microbiologic study. Flucytosine and miconazole have also been used to treat fungal endophthalmitis. For more on treatment of fungal infections, see **Table 6**.

There has been an increase, within the last decade, in the incidence of *Acanthamoeba* keratitis. This has been linked, in many cases, to use of contaminated solutions for soft contact lenses — especially homemade saline solutions. Current therapy includes the use of polymyxin/neomycin/bacitracin ophthalmic solution.

In bacterial endophthalmitis, the use of intraocular and periocular antimicrobial therapy has significantly improved the final visual outcome. A diagnosis of bacterial endophthalmitis should be strongly suspected in a patient who is postoperative or posttraumatic, or when the intraocular inflammation is out of proportion to the situation. Ocular pain is often present before obvious inflammation. Pre- and postoperative antibiotics may decrease the incidence of postoperative endophthalmitis.

Once endophthalmitis is suspected, prompt intervention is required. Samples of the aqueous and vitreous humors must be promptly secured and treatment quickly initiated with antimicrobials appropriate to the suspected organism(s). When inflammation occurs several weeks or more after surgery or in cases of trauma or in immunosuppressed patients, fungal or anaerobic organisms should be considered.

Once the aqueous and vitreous humors have been cultured, antimicrobial agents should be directly injected into these cavities. To prevent retinal toxicity, medications should be injected slowly into the anterior vitreous cavity, with particular caution after vitrectomy. Vitrectomy and intravitreal antibiotics should always be considered when treating endophthalmitis.

In a recent study, use of intravenous antibiotics was found to make no difference in final visual acuity or media clarity. The author concluded that "omission of systemic antibiotic treatment can reduce toxic effects, costs, and length of hospital stay."

REFERENCES

Anonymous. Results of endophthalmitis vitrectomy study. *Arch. Ophthalmol.* 1995;113:1479.

Axelrod AJ, Peyman GA. Intravitreal amphotericin B treatment of experimental fungal endophthalmitis. *Am J Ophthalmol.* 1973;76:584.

Barza M. Antibacterial agents in the treatment of ocular infections. *Infect Dis Clin North Am.* 3:533-551.

Baum JL. Antibiotic use in ophthalmology. In: Tasman W, Jaeger EA, eds. *Duane's Clinical Ophthalmology.* Philadelphia, Pa: JB Lippincott; 1989; vol 4, chap 26.

Ellis P. *Ocular Therapeutics and Pharmacology.* 7th ed. St. Louis, Mo: CV Mosby; 1985.

Forster RK. Endophthalmitis. In: Tasman W, Jaeger EA, eds. *Duane's Clinical Ophthalmology.* Philadelphia, Pa: JB Lippincott; 1989, vol 4, chap 24.

Gardner S. Treatment of bacterial endophthalmitis. In: *Ocular Therapeutics and Management.* Atlanta, Ga: 1991; vol 2, no. 1.

Lamberts DW, Potter DE, eds. *Clinical Ocular Pharmacology.* Boston, Mass: Little, Brown; 1987.

Lemp MA, Blackman HJ, Koffler BH. Therapy for bacterial and fungal infections. *Int Ophthalmol Clin.* 1980; 20(no. 3):135-145.

Pavan PR, Brinser JH. Exogenous bacterial endophthalmitis treated without systemic antibiotics. *Am J Ophthalmol.* 1987; 104:121.

Peyman GA. Antibiotic administration in the treatment of bacterial endophthalmitis. II. Intravitreal injections. *Surv Ophthalmol.* 1977; 21: 332,339.

Tabbara KF, Hyndiuk RA, eds. *Infections of the Eye.* Boston, Mass: Little, Brown; 1986.

TABLE 2

COMMERCIALLY AVAILABLE OPHTHALMIC ANTIBACTERIAL AGENTS

GENERIC NAME	TRADE NAME	CONCENTRATION OPH. SOLN (%)	OPH OINT
INDIVIDUAL AGENTS			
Bacitracin	AK-Tracin	Not available	500 units/g
Chloramphenicol	AK-Chlor	0.5%	Not available
	Chloromycetin	0.16% – 0.5%	1%
	Chloroptic	0.5%	1%
	Available generically	0.5%	Not available
Ciprofloxacin hydrochloride	Ciloxan	0.3%	0.3%
Erythromycin	Ilotycin	Not available	0.5%
	Available generically	Not available	0.5%
Gentamicin sulfate	Garamycin	0.3%	0.3%
	Genoptic	0.3%	0.3%
	Gentacidin	0.3%	0.3%
	Gentak	0.3%	0.3%
	Available generically	0.3%	0.3%
Norfloxacin	Chibroxin	0.3%	Not available
Ofloxacin	Ocuflox	0.3%	Not available
Sulfacetamide sodium	AK-Sulf	10%	10%
	Bleph-10	10%	10%
	Cetamide	Not available	10%
	Isopto Cetamide	15%	Not available
	Sulamyd sodium	10%, 30%	10%
	Sulf-10	10%	Not available
	Available generically	10%, 15%, 30%	10%
Tobramycin sulfate	Tobrex	0.3%	0.3%
	Tobralcon	0.3%	0.3%
	Available generically	0.3%	Not available
MIXTURES			
Polymyxin B/Bacitracin Zinc	AK-Poly-Bac Polysporin Available generically	Not available	10,000 units - 500 units/g
Polymyxin B/Neomycin/Bacitracin	AK-Spore Neosporin Available generically	Not available	10,000 units - 3.5 mg - 400 units/g
Polymyxin B/Neomycin/Gramicidin	AK-Spore Neosporin Available generically	10,000 units - 1.75 mg - 0.025 mg/mL	Not available
Polymyxin B/Oxytetracycline	Terramycin TERAK	Not available	10,000 units - 5 mg/g
Polymyxin B/Trimethoprim	Polytrim Available generically	10,000 units - 1 mg/mL	Not available

TABLE 3

ANTIBIOTICS IN INFUSION FLUID

AGENT	MAXIMUM NONTOXIC DOSE (μg/mL)
Amikacin	10
Ceftazidime	40
Clindamycin	9
Gentamicin	8
Imipenem	16
Methicillin	20
Oxacillin	10
Tobramycin	10
Vancomycin*	30

*Usage discouraged by CDC because of increased resistant organisms.
Modified from Peyman GA, Daun M. Prophylaxis of Endophthalmitis. Ophthalmic Surg. 1994;25:673

TABLE 4

REGIMEN FOR ENDOPHTHALMITIS

1. Diagnostic anterior chamber and vitreous aspiration; diagnostic vitrectomy when liquid vitreous fails to aspirate or in cases of suspected fungal endophthalmitis.

2. Initial therapy (in operating room after diagnostic technique).
A. Intraocular: gentamicin 100 μg or amikacin 400 μg and vancomycin 1000 μg or cefazolin 2250 μg
B. Subconjunctival: gentamicin 40 mg and triamcinolone diacetate (Aristocort) 40 mg*
C. Topical: gentamicin 9.1 or 13.4 mg/mL and cefazolin 50 mg/mL and prednisolone acetate 1%
D. Systemic: cefazolin (Ancef or Kefzol) 1000 mg every 6 to 8 hours. (Ceftriaxone has good penetration of the blood ocular barrier and may be used as an alternative.) The use of systemic antibiotics is controversial; many practitioners do not employ them.

3. If cultures are positive for virulent bacteria, consider repeating the above intraocular injections at the bedside on the second and fourth postoperative days. Continue topical treatment every half hour, subconjunctival treatment daily, and systemic therapy. Consider therapeutic vitrectomy with repeat intraocular antibiotics.

4. If cultures are negative after 48 hours, do not repeat intraocular antibiotics. Consider tapering topical, subconjunctival, and systemic antibiotic therapy while continuing topical and subconjunctival corticosteroids.

5. If the endophthalmitis presents as a delayed inflammation in which a fungal etiology is considered, the vitreous sample should be obtained by a vitreous instrument using membrane filters; intraocular amphotericin B (Fungizone) at a dosage of 5 μg or miconazole at a dosage of 10 to 25 μg should be considered.

6. If the endophthalmitis presents as a delayed inflammation or chronic indolent infection, a Propionibacterium acnes infection should be considered.

Source: Mandelbaum S, Forster RK.
Anonymous. Results of Endophthalmitis Vitrectomy Study. *Arch. Ophthalmol.* 1995; 113: 1479

*Subconjunctival corticosteroids should be deferred 48 to 72 hours to await culture growth and confirmation if a fungal etiology is suspected or the inflammation is delayed.

TABLE 5

CONCENTRATIONS AND DOSAGE OF PRINCIPAL ANTIBIOTIC AGENTS

DRUG NAME*	TOPICAL	SUBCONJUNCTIVAL	INTRAVITREAL	INTRAVENOUS†
Amikacin sulfate	10 mg/mL	25 mg	400 μg	15 mg/kg daily in 2–3 doses
Ampicillin sodium	50 mg/mL	50–150 mg	500 μg	4–12 g daily in 4 doses
Bacitracin zinc	10,000 units/mL	5,000 units	. . .	. . .
Carbenicillin disodium	4–6 mg/mL	100 mg	250–2000 μg	8–24 g daily in 4–6 doses
Cefazolin sodium	50 mg/mL	100 mg	2250 μg	2–4 g daily in 3–4 doses
Ceftazidime	. . .	200 mg	2200 μg	1 g daily in 2–3 doses
Clindamycin	50 mg/mL	15–50 mg	1000 μg	900–1800 mg daily in 2–3 doses
Colistimethate sodium	10 mg/mL	15–25 mg	100 μg	2.5–5 mg/kg daily in 2–4 doses
Erythromycin	50 mg/mL	100 mg	500 μg	. . .
Gentamicin sulfate	8–15 mg/mL	10–20 mg	100–200 μg	3–5 mg/kg daily in 2–3 doses
Imipenem/Cilastatin sodium	5 mg/mL	. . .	. . .	2 g daily in 3–4 doses
Kanamycin sulfate	30–50 mg/mL	30 mg	. . .	. . .
Methicillin sodium	50 mg/mL	50–100 mg	1000–2000 μg	6–10 g daily in 4 doses
Neomycin sulfate	5–8 mg/mL	125–250 mg	. . .	. . .
Penicillin G	100,000 units/mL	0.5–1.0 million units	. . .	12–24 million units daily in 4–6 doses
Polymyxin B sulfate	10,000 units/mL	100,000 units	. . .	. . .
Ticarcillin disodium	6 mg/mL	100 mg	. . .	200–300 mg/kg daily 3 x in 4–6 doses
Tobramycin sulfate	8–15 mg/mL	10–20 mg	100–200 μg	3–5 mg/kg daily in 2–3 doses
Vancomycin hydrochloride**	20–25 mg/mL	25 mg	1000 μg	15–30 mg/kg daily in 1–2 doses

*Most penicillins and cephalosporins are physically incompatible when combined in the same bottle with aminoglycosides such as amikacin, gentamicin, or tobramycin. †Adult doses. **Usage discouraged by CDC because of increased resistant organisms.

TABLE 6

ANTIFUNGAL AGENTS

GENERIC (TRADE) NAME	ROUTE	DOSAGE	SPECTRUM
Amphotericin B (Fungizone)	Topical Subconjunctival Intravitreal Intravenous	0.1–0.5% solution; dilute with water for injection or dextrose 5% in water 0.8–1.0 mg 5 µg Because of side effects and toxicity, see main PDR for dosing instructions	Blastomyces Candida Coccidioides Histoplasma
Fluconazole (Diflucan)	Oral	800 mg on day 1, then 400 mg daily in divided doses	Candida
Flucytosine (Ancobon)	Oral Topical	50–150 mg/kg daily in 4 divided doses† 1% solution	Candida Cryptococcus
Natamycin (Natacyn)	Topical	5% suspension	Candida Aspergillus Cephalosporium Fusarium Penicillium
Miconazole nitrate (Monistat)	Topical Subconjunctival Intravitreal	1% solution 5–10 mg 10 µg	Candida Cryptococcus Aspergillus
Ketoconazole (Nizoral)	Oral	200–400 mg daily†	Candida Cryptococcus Histoplasma

†Because of potential side and toxic effects, the practitioner should consult the main PDR for possible dosage adjustments and warnings.

TABLE 7

ANTIVIRAL AGENTS

GENERIC (TRADE) NAME	TOPICAL CONC (%)	INTRAVIT DOSE	SYSTEMIC DOSAGE*
Trifluridine (Viroptic)	1.0% (oph solution)	. . .	. . .
Vidarabine monohydrate (Vira-A)	3.0% (oph ointment)	. . .	. . .
Acyclovir sodium (Zovirax)	. . .	. . .	Oral–Herpes simplex keratitis– 200 mg 5 times daily for 7–10 days. Oral–Herpes zoster ophthalmicus– 600–800 mg 5 times daily for 10 days IV†
Cidofovir (Vistide)	. . .	. . .	IV—Induction: 5 mg/kg constant infusion over 1 hour administered once weekly for 2 consecutive weeks Maintenance: 5 mg/kg constant infusion over 1 hour administered once every 2 weeks
Foscarnet sodium (Foscavir)	. . .	. . .	IV–by controlled infusion only, either by central vein or by peripheral vein–Induction: 60 mg/kg (adjusted for renal function) given over 1 h every 8 h for 14–21 days Maintenance: 90–120 mg/kg given over 2 hours once daily
Ganciclovir sodium (Cytovene)	. . .	200 µg	IV–Induction: 5 mg/kg every 12 h for 14–21 days Maintenance: 5 mg/kg daily for 7 days or 6 mg once daily for 5 days/week Oral–After IV induction, 1,000 mg 3 times daily with food or 500 mg 6 times daily every 3 h
Ganciclovir sodium (Vitrasert)	. . .	4.5 mg	Sterile intravitreal insert designed to release the drug over a 5 to 8 month period.

*Because of potential side and toxic effects, the practitioner should consult the main PDR for possible dosage adjustments and warnings.
†IV therapy should be considered if the patient is immunocompromised.

3. OCULAR ANTI-INFLAMMATORY AGENTS

A wide variety of medications are available to treat ocular inflammation. They are listed in **Table 8**. Corticosteroids are the most commonly used. Many are available in combination with antibiotics and/or other medications.

At one time, it was felt that corticosteroids were contraindicated in infectious disease states. However, it is now appreciated that steroids, when used in conjunction with appropriate antimicrobial, antifungal, or antiviral agents, may help prevent more serious ocular damage.

TABLE 8

TOPICAL ANTI-INFLAMMATORY AGENTS

NAME AND DOSAGE FORM	TRADE NAME	CONCENTRATION
Dexamethasone Ophthalmic Suspension	Maxidex	0.1%
Dexamethasone Sodium Phosphate Ophthalmic Ointment	AK-Dex Decadron Available generically	0.05% 0.05% 0.05%
Dexamethasone Sodium Phosphate Ophthalmic Solution	AK-Dex Decadron Available generically	0.1% 0.1% 0.1%
Fluorometholone Ophthalmic Ointment	FML S.O.P.	0.1%
Fluorometholone Ophthalmic Suspension	Fluor-Op FML FML Forte Available generically	0.1% 0.1% 0.25% 0.1%
Fluorometholone Acetate Ophthalmic Suspension	Flarex Eflone	0.1% 0.1%
Loteprednol etabonate	Lotemax	0.5%
Medrysone Ophthalmic Suspension	HMS	1%
Prednisolone Acetate Ophthalmic Suspension	Pred Mild Econopred Econopred Plus Pred Forte Available generically	0.12% 0.125% 1% 1% 1%
Prednisolone Sodium Phosphate Ophthalmic Solution	AK-Pred Inflamase Available generically AK-Pred Inflamase Forte Available generically	0.125% 0.125% 0.125% 1% 1% 1%
Rimexolone Ophthalmic Suspension	Vexol	1%
NONSTEROIDAL ANTI-INFLAMMATORY DRUGS		
Diclofenac Ophthalmic Solution	Voltaren	0.1%
Flurbiprofen Ophthalmic Solution*	Ocufen Available generically	0.03% 0.03%
Ketorolac Ophthalmic Solution	Acular	0.5%
Suprofen Ophthalmic Solution*	Profenal	1%

*Indicated for intraoperative miosis only.

Steroids may be administered by four different routes in the treatment of ocular inflammation. **Table 9** lists the preferred route in various conditions.

Topical corticosteroids can elevate intraocular pressure and, in susceptible individuals, can induce glaucoma. Some corticosteroids, such as fluorometholone acetate, medrysone, and loteprednol cause less elevation of intraocular pressure than others. Corticosteroids may also cause cataract formation, a complication more likely with high-dose, long-term systemic use.

There are also four nonsteroidal anti-inflammatory drugs (NSAIDs) available. They are: diclofenac (Voltaren); flurbiprofen (Ocufen); ketorolac (Acular); and suprofen (Profenal). Flurbiprofen and suprofen are indicated solely for inhibition of intraoperative miosis. They are very similar in activity and some hospitals use them interchangeably. Diclofenac has an official indication for the postoperative prophylaxis and treatment of ocular inflammation. Ketorolac is indicated for the treatment of postoperative inflammation and for relief of ocular itching due to seasonal allergic conjunctivitis. It has also shown some success in alleviating the pain associated with keratotomy, although unapproved for this use. Both diclofenac and ketorolac have also been used successfully to prevent and treat cystoid macular edema. NSAIDs cause little, if any, rise in intraocular pressure.

Other useful agents include mast-cell inhibitors, antihistamines, low concentration steroids, and decongestants to treat vernal conjunctivitis or allergic keratoconjunctivitis. Tetracycline, taken orally, in doses of 250 mg four times daily for 4 weeks, then 250 mg once daily, is useful in treating ocular rosacea.

Agents useful in treatment of seasonal allergic conjunctivitis are listed in **Table 10.**

TABLE 9

USUAL ROUTE OF STEROID ADMINISTRATION IN OCULAR INFLAMMATION

CONDITION	ROUTE
Blepharitis	Topical
Conjunctivitis	Topical
Episcleritis	Topical
Scleritis	Topical and/or systemic
Keratitis	Topical
Anterior uveitis	Topical and/or periocular
Posterior uveitis	Systemic and/or periocular
Endophthalmitis	Systemic/periocular, intravitreal
Optic neuritis	Systemic or periocular
Cranial arteritis	Systemic
Sympathetic ophthalmia	Systemic and topical

TABLE 10

AGENTS FOR RELIEF OF SEASONAL ALLERGIC CONJUNCTIVITIS

GENERIC NAME	TRADE NAME	CLASS
Cromolyn	Crolom	Mast-cell Inhibitor
Emedastine	Emadine	H_1-Antagonist
Ketorolac	Acular	N.S.A.I.D.
Levocabastin	Livostin	H_1-Antagonist
Lodoxamide	Alomide	Mast-cell Inhibitor
Loteprednol	Alrex	Corticosteroid
Naphazoline/antazoline	Vasocon-A	Antihistamine/ decongestant
Naphazoline/pheniramine	Naphcon-A Opcon-A	Antihistamine/ decongestant
Olopatadine	Patanol	H_1-Antagonist/ Mast-cell inhibitor

4. ANESTHETIC AGENTS

A. Topical anesthetics

The agents listed in **Table 11** permit the clinician to perform ocular procedures such as tonometry, removal of foreign bodies from the surface of the eye, and lacrimal canalicular manipulation and irrigation. Cocaine, the prototype topical anesthetic, is a natural compound; the others are synthetic.

Cocaine is rarely used as an anesthetic agent because it causes damage to the corneal epithelium, produces pupillary dilation, and may affect intraocular pressure. However, it is considered useful when removal of the corneal epithelium is desired, as in epithelial debridement for dendritic keratitis.

The Table lists available agents and concentrations. Most begin working within a minute and continue acting for 10 to 20 minutes. A transient, superficial punctate keratitis may develop rapidly after instillation of the agent.

B. Regional anesthetics

The actions, benefits, and drawbacks of the most common regional anesthetic agents used in ophthalmic surgery are summarized in **Table 12**.

TABLE 11

TOPICAL ANESTHETIC AGENTS

USP OR NF NAME	TRADE NAME	CONCENTRATION (%)
Cocaine hydrochloride	. . .	1% to 4%
Proparacaine hydrochloride	AK-Taine Alcaine Ophthetic	0.5% 0.5% 0.5%
Tetracaine hydrochloride	AK-T-Caine Pontocaine hydrochloride	0.5% 0.5%

TABLE 12

REGIONAL ANESTHETICS*

USP OR NF NAME	CONCENTRATION (%)/ MAXIMUM DOSE	ONSET OF ACTION	DURATION OF ACTION	MAJOR ADVANTAGES/ DISADVANTAGES
Procaine†	1%–4%/500 mg	7–8 min	30–45 min 60 min (with epinephrine)	Short duration. Poor absorption from mucous membranes
Tetracaine†	0.25%	5–9 min	120–140 min (with epinephrine)	
Bupivacaine††, **	0.25%–0.75%	5–11 min	480–720 min (with epinephrine)	
Lidocaine††	1%–2%/500 mg	4–6 min	40–60 min 120 min (with epinephrine)	Spreads readily without hyaluronidase
Mepivacaine††	1%–2%/500 mg	3–5 min	120 min	Duration of action greater without epinephrine[1]
Prilocaine††	1%–2%/600 mg	3–4 min	90–120 min (with epinephrine)	As effective as lidocaine
Etidocaine††	1%	3 min	300–600 min	

*Retrobulbar injection has been reported to cause apnea.
† Ester type compound
††Amide type compound
** A mixture of bupivacaine, lidocaine, and epinephrine has been shown to be effective in retinal detachment surgery under local anesthesia.[2]

REFERENCES:

1. Everett WG, Vey EK, Finlay JW. Duration of oculomotor akinesia of injectable anesthetics. *Trans Am Acad Ophthalmol.* 1961; 65:308.
2. Holekamp TLR, Arribas NP, Boniuk I. Bupivacaine anesthesia in retinal detachment surgery. *Arch Ophthalmol.* 1979; 97:109.

5. AGENTS FOR TREATMENT OF GLAUCOMA

A. Miotics — see **Table 13**
Parasympathomimetic agents (miotics) are used primarily as topical therapy for glaucoma. A secondary use is the control of accommodative esotropia. This class of agents mimics the effect of acetylcholine on parasympathomimetic postganglionic nerve endings within the eye. The class is subdivided into direct-acting (cholinergic) agents and indirect-acting (anticholinesterase) agents, based on their respective abilities to bind acetylcholine receptors and inhibit the enzymatic hydrolysis of acetylcholine. **Table 13** lists the parasympathomimetics approved for topical use in this country. In addition, two agents are available for intraocular use: Miochol-E, a 1% solution of acetylcholine, and Miostat or Carbastat F, a 0.01% solution of carbachol.

B. Sympathomimetics — see **Table 14**
These medications work by improving aqueous outflow and, to a lesser extent, improving uveoscleral output. The prodrug dipivefrin causes fewer systemic side effects than epinephrine and can sometimes be used in patients who have developed a sensitivity to epinephrine. A combination of epinephrine bitartrate 1% with pilocarpine 1, 2, 4, or 6% (E-Pilo, PE) is also available.

C. β-Adrenergic blocking agents — see **Table 15**
These medications work by blocking β-adrenergic receptor sites, decreasing aqueous production, and, thereby, reducing intraocular pressure. Because β-adrenergic receptors occur in a number of organ systems, systemic side effects of these drugs may include slowed heart rate, decreased blood pressure, and exacerbation of intrinsic bronchial asthma and emphysema. These agents can also enhance the effects of a number of systemic medications including β-blockers, digitalis alkaloids, and reserpine. Since betaxolol is a cardioselective β-blocker, it has significantly less effect on the respiratory system and can be used in some patients with respiratory illnesses.

D. Hyperosmotic agents — see **Table 16**
These medications decrease intraocular pressure by creating an osmotic gradient between the blood and intraocular fluid, causing fluid to move out of the aqueous and vitreous humors into the bloodstream. Though not usually used in open-angle glaucoma, these medications are employed to decrease pressure in an attack of angle-closure glaucoma, and to give a "soft" eye during surgery.

E. Carbonic anhydrase inhibitors — see **Table 17**
Used both topically and systemically, these drugs decrease the formation and secretion of aqueous humor. The systemic forms are usually used to supplement various topical agents (but not topical CAIs). Use of the systemic agents is limited by their side effects, which include paresthesias, anorexia, gastrointestinal disturbances, headaches, altered taste and smell, sodium and potassium depletion, ureteral colic, a predisposition to form renal calculi, and, rarely, bone marrow suppression. The most commonly reported adverse effects of the topical solution are superficial punctate keratitis and ocular allergic reactions. Less frequently reported are blurred vision, tearing, ocular dryness, and photophobia. Infrequent are headache, nausea, asthenia, and fatigue. Rarely, skin rashes, urolithiasis, and iridocyclitis may occur.

F. α_2 Selective agonists — see **Table 18**
There are now two medications in this class: apraclonidine and brimonidine. Apraclonidine is available as a single-dose applicator of a 1% solution for suppression of the acute intraocular pressure spikes that occur after laser treatments. A 0.5% concentration is also available, supplied in a multiple dose bottle for use with other glaucoma medications to control pressure in patients who are not responding adequately to maximally tolerated glaucoma therapy. The medication is generally useful only for short term therapy, since it has been associated with tachyphylaxis within three months in up to 48% of patients. Brimonidine, the second agent in this class, is 23 to 32 times more selective for $alpha_2$ versus $alpha_1$ adrenoreceptors than is apraclonidine. This allows the medication to be used on a chronic basis with reduced risk of tachycardia (up to 12% incidence in 12 months).

G. Prostaglandins — see **Table 19**
The new prostaglandin latanoprost was developed specifically for the treatment of glaucoma. A single daily dose has been shown to be as effective in reducing IOP as timolol 0.5% administered twice daily. Ocular side effects—hyperemia, itching, tearing, foreign-body sensation, and stinging appear to be minimal, and systemic side effects have not been observed. An increase in pigmentation in the iris occurs in 7.2% of patients with mixed-color irises. Although the exact mechanism is not understood, the change appears to be permanent. Its clinical significance is unknown.

Also available under the trade name Cosopt is a combination of the β-adrenergic blocker timolol with the carbonic anhydrase inhibitor dorzalamide.

REFERENCE

Fiscella, RG, Winarko, T. Glaucoma—New Therapeutic Options. *U.S. Pharmacist*, December, 1996.

TABLE 13

MIOTICS

GENERIC NAME	TRADE NAME	STRENGTHS (%)	SIZES
CHOLINERGIC AGENTS			
Carbachol	Isopto Carbachol	0.75%, 1.5%, 2.25%, 3%	15, 30 mL
Pilocarpine	Ocusert-Pilo	20, 40	Box of 8 inserts
Pilocarpine hydrochloride	Akarpine	1%, 2%, 4%	15 mL
	Isopto Carpine	0.25%, 0.5%, 1%, 2%, 3%, 4%, 6%, 8%, 10%	15 & 30 mL
	Pilocar	0.5%, 1%, 2%, 3%, 4%, 6%	15 & 2 x 15 mL
	Pilopine-HS gel	4%	3.5 g
	Piloptic	0.5%, 1%, 2%, 3%, 4%, 6%	15 mL
	Pilostat	0.5%, 1%, 2%, 3%, 4%, 6%	15 mL
	Available generically	0.5%, 1%, 2%, 3%, 4%, 5%, 6%	15 mL
Pilocarpine nitrate	Pilagan	2%, 4%	15 mL
CHOLINESTERASE INHIBITORS			
Physostigmine	Eserine Oph Oint Available generically	0.25%	3.5 g
Echothiophate iodide	Phospholine Iodide	0.03%, 0.06%, 0.125%, 0.25%	5 mL

TABLE 14

SYMPATHOMIMETICS

GENERIC NAME	TRADE NAME	CONCENTRATION (%)	SIZE(S) (mL)
Dipivefrin hydrochloride	Akpro	0.1%	5, 10, 15
	Propine	0.1%	5, 10, 15
	Available generically	0.1%	5, 10, 15
Epinephryl borate	Epinal	0.5%, 1%	7.5
	Eppy/N	1%	7.5
Epinephrine hydrochloride	Epifrin	0.5%, 1%, 2%	5, 10, & 15
	Glaucon	1%, 2%	10

TABLE 15

β-ADRENERGIC BLOCKING AGENTS

GENERIC NAME	TRADE NAME	CONCENTRATION (%)	SIZE(S) (mL)
Betaxolol hydrochloride	Betoptic-S	0.25%	2.5, 5, 15
	Betoptic	0.5%	2.5, 5, 10, 15
Carteolol hydrochloride	Ocupress	1%	5 & 10
Levobunolol hydrochloride	Akbeta	0.25%, 0.5%	5, 10, 15
	Betagan	0.25%, 0.5%	2, 5, 10, 15
	Available generically	0.25%, 0.5%	5, 10 & 15
Metipranolol	OptiPranolol	0.3%	5 & 10
Timolol hemihydrate	Betimol	0.25%, 0.5%	2.5, 5, 10, 15
Timolol maleate	Timoptic	0.25%, 0.5%	2.5, 5, 10, 15
	Available generically	0.25%, 0.5%	5, 10, 15
Timolol maleate (gel)	Timoptic - XE	0.25%, 0.5%	2.5, 5

TABLE 16

HYPEROSMOTIC AGENTS

USP OR NF NAME	TRADE NAME	PREPARATION	DOSE	ROUTE	ONSET/DURATION OF ACTION
Glycerin	Osmoglyn	50%	1–1.5 g/kg	Oral	. . .
Isosorbide*	Ismotic	45%	1.5 g/kg	Oral	30 min/5–6 h
Mannitol†	Osmitrol	5%–20%	0.5–2 g/kg	IV	30–60 min/6 h
Urea	Ureaphil	Powder or 30% soln	0.5–2 g/kg	IV	30–45 min/5–6 h

*Do not confuse with isosorbide dinitrate, an antianginal agent.
†Do not confuse with mannitol hexanitrate, an antianginal agent.

TABLE 17

CARBONIC ANHYDRASE INHIBITORS

USP OR NF NAME	TRADE NAME	PREPARATION	ONSET/DURATION OF ACTION
Acetazolamide	Diamox Available generically	125, 250 mg tablets 500 mg (timed-release) capsules 125, 250 mg tablets	2 h/4–6 h
Acetazolamide Sodium	Diamox Parenteral	500 mg	5–10 min/2 h
Brinzolamide	Azopt	1% ophthalmic suspension	. . .
Dichlorphenamide	Daranide	50 mg tablets	30 min/6 h
Dorzolamide HCl	Trusopt	2% ophthalmic solution	. . .
Methazolamide	Glauctabs MZM Neptazane Available generically	25, 50 mg tablets 25, 50 mg tablets 25, 50 mg tablets 25, 50 mg tablets	2 h/4–6 h

TABLE 18

α_2 SELECTIVE AGONISTS

GENERIC NAME	TRADE NAME	CONCENTRATION	SIZE(S)(mL)
Apraclonidine	Iopidine	0.5% 1.0%	5 single use bottle
Brimonidine	Alphagan	0.2%	5, 10, 15

TABLE 19

PROSTAGLANDINS

GENERIC NAME	TRADE NAME	CONCENTRATION	SIZE(S)(mL)
Latanoprost	Xalatan	0.005%	2.5

6. MEDICATIONS FOR DRY EYE

Dry eye refers to a deficiency in either the aqueous or mucin components of the precorneal tear film. The most commonly encountered aqueous-deficient dry eye in the United States is keratoconjunctivitis sicca, while mucin-deficient dry eyes may be seen in cases of hypovitaminosis A, Stevens-Johnson syndrome, ocular pemphigoid, extensive trachoma, and chemical burns.

Dry eye is treated with artificial tear preparations (see **Table 20**) and ophthalmic lubricants (see **Table 21**). The lubricants form an occlusive film over the ocular surface and protect the eye from drying. Administered as a nighttime medication, they are useful both for dry eye and in cases of recurrent corneal erosion.

TABLE 20

ARTIFICIAL TEAR PREPARATIONS

MAJOR COMPONENT(S)	CONCENTRATION (%)	TRADE NAME	PRESERVATIVE/EDTA*
Carboxymethyl cellulose	0.5%	Refresh Plus	None
	1%	Celluvisc	None
	0.25%	Theratears	None
Glycerin	3%	Dry Eye Therapy	None
Hydroxyethyl cellulose, polyvinyl alcohol		TearGard	Sorbic acid, EDTA
Hydroxypropyl cellulose		Lacrisert (biodegradable insert)	None
Hydroxypropyl methylcellulose	0.5%	Isopto Plain	Benzalkonium chloride
		Isopto Tears	Benzalkonium chloride
		Tearisol	Benzalkonium chloride, EDTA
	1%	Isopto Alkaline	Benzalkonium chloride
Hydroxypropyl methylcellulose, dextran 70		Bion Tears	None
		Ocucoat	Benzalkonium chloride, EDTA
		Ocucoat PF	None
		Tears Naturale II	Polyquad
		Tears Naturale Free	None
		Tears Renewed	Benzalkonium chloride, EDTA
Methylcellulose	1%	Murocel	Methyl-, propylparabens
Polycarbophil, PEG-400, dextran 70		AquaSite	EDTA
		AquaSite multi-dose	EDTA, Sorbic acid
Polysorbate 80		Viva Drops	EDTA
Polyvinyl alcohol	1.4%	AKWA Tears	Benzalkonium chloride, EDTA
		Dry Eyes	Chlorobutanol
	3%	Liquifilm Tears	Chlorobutanol
Polyvinyl alcohol, PEG-400, dextrose	1%	HypoTears	Benzalkonium chloride, EDTA
		HypoTears PF	EDTA
		Puralube Tears	Benzalkonium chloride, EDTA
Polyvinyl alcohol, povidone	1.4%	Murine Tears	Benzalkonium chloride, EDTA
	0.6%	Refresh	None
		Tears Plus	Chlorobutanol

*EDTA = ethylenediaminetetraacetic acid.

TABLE 21

OPHTHALMIC LUBRICANTS

TRADE NAME	COMPOSITION OF STERILE OINTMENT
AKWA Tears Ointment	White petrolatum, liquid lanolin, and mineral oil
Dry Eyes	White petrolatum, liquid lanolin, and mineral oil
Duolube	White petrolatum and mineral oil
Duratears Naturale	White petrolatum, liquid lanolin, and mineral oil
HypoTears	White petrolatum and light mineral oil
Lacri-Lube S.O.P., Lubritears	42.5% mineral oil, 55% white petrolatum, lanolin alcohol, and chlorobutanol
Puralube	White petrolatum, liquid lanolin, and mineral oil
Refresh P.M., Dry Eyes Lubricant	41.5% mineral oil, 55% white petrolatum, petrolatum, and lanolin alcohol

7. OCULAR DECONGESTANTS

These topically applied adrenergic medications are commonly used to whiten the eye. Three types are available. Those containing naphazoline and tetrahydrozoline are more stable than those with phenylephrine. Usual dosage is 1 or 2 drops no more than 4 times a day (see **Table 22**).

TABLE 22

OCULAR DECONGESTANTS

DRUG	TRADE NAME	ADDITIONAL COMPONENTS
Naphazoline hydrochloride	AK-Con* Albalon* Clear Eyes Naphcon Vasoclear Vasocon Regular*	Benzalkonium chloride, edetate disodium Benzalkonium chloride, edetate disodium Benzalkonium chloride, edetate disodium Benzalkonium chloride, edetate disodium Benzalkonium chloride, edetate disodium Phenylmercuric acetate
Oxymetazoline hydrochloride	Visine L.R. Ocuclear	Benzalkonium chloride, edetate disodium Benzalkonium chloride, edetate disodium
Phenylephrine hydrochloride	AK-Nefrin Eye Cool Prefrin Liquifilm Relief	Benzalkonium chloride, edetate disodium Thimerosal, edetate disodium Benzalkonium chloride, edetate disodium —
Tetrahydrozoline hydrochloride	Collyrium Fresh Murine Plus Visine	Benzalkonium chloride, edetate disodium Benzalkonium chloride, edetate disodium Benzalkonium chloride, edetate disodium
DECONGESTANT/ASTRINGENT COMBINATIONS		
Naphazoline hydrochloride plus zinc sulfate	Clear Eyes ACR (allergy/cold relief)	Benzalkonium chloride, edetate disodium
Phenylephrine hydrochloride plus zinc sulfate	Zincfrin	Benzalkonium chloride
Tetrahydrozoline plus zinc sulfate	Visine Allergy Relief	Benzalkonium chloride, edetate disodium

*Prescription medication.

8. OPHTHALMIC IRRIGATING SOLUTIONS

Listed in **Table 23** are sterile isotonic solutions for general ophthalmic use. They are all over-the- counter products. There are also intraocular irrigating solutions available for use during surgical procedures. They include prescription medications such as Bausch & Lomb's Balanced Salt Solution, Alcon's BSS and BSS Plus, and Iolab's Iocare Balanced Salt Solution.

TABLE 23

OPHTHALMIC IRRIGATING SOLUTIONS

TRADE NAME	COMPONENTS	ADDITIONAL COMPONENTS
AK-Rinse	Sodium, potassium, calcium, and magnesium chlorides, sodium acetate, and sodium citrate	Benzalkonium chloride
Collyrium Fresh Eyes	Antipyrine, boric acid, and borax	Benzalkonium chloride
Dacriose	Sodium and potassium chlorides, and sodium phosphate	Benzalkonium chloride, edetate disodium
Eye-Stream	Sodium, potassium, magnesium and calcium chlorides, sodium acetate, and sodium citrate	Benzalkonium chloride
Irigate	Boric acid, potassium chloride, and sodium carbonate	Benzalkonium chloride, edetate disodium
Lavoptik Eye Wash	Sodium chloride, sodium biphosphate, and sodium phosphate	Benzalkonium chloride

9. HYPEROSMOLAR AGENTS

Hyperosmolar (hypertonic) agents are used to reduce corneal edema therapeutically or for diagnostic purposes. They act through osmotic attraction of water through the semipermeable corneal epithelium.

TABLE 24

HYPEROSMOLAR AGENTS

GENERIC NAME	TRADE NAME	CONCENTRATION (%)
A. Therapeutic preparations		
Sodium chloride	Adsorbonac Ophthalmic	2% or 5% (solution)
	AK-NaCl	5% (solution and ointment)
	Muro-128	2% or 5% (solution), 5% (ointment)
B. Diagnostic preparation		
Glycerin	Ophthalgan	

10. DIAGNOSTIC AGENTS

Some of the more common diagnostic agents and tests used in ophthalmologic practice are listed below.

A. Examination of the Conjunctiva, Cornea, and Lacrimal Apparatus

Fluorescein, applied primarily as a 2% alkaline solution, and with impregnated paper strips, is used to examine the integrity of the conjunctival and corneal epithelia. Defects in the corneal epithelium will appear bright green in ordinary light and bright yellow when a cobalt blue filter is used in the light path. Similar lesions of the conjunctiva appear bright orange-yellow in ordinary illumination.

Fluorescein has also come into wide use in the fitting of rigid contact lenses, though it cannot be used for soft lenses, which absorb the dye. Proper fit is determined by examining the pattern of fluorescein beneath the contact lens.

In addition, fluorescein is used in performing applanation tonometry and one test of lacrimal apparatus patency (Jones test) uses 1 drop of 1% fluorescein instilled into the conjunctival sac. If the dye appears in the nose, drainage is normal.[1]

Rose bengal, as a 1% solution, is particularly useful for demonstrating abnormal conjunctival or corneal epithelium. Devitalized cells stain bright red, while normal cells show no change. The abnormal epithelial cells present in dry eye disorders are effectively revealed by this stain.

The Schirmer test is a valuable method of assessing tear production. It employs prepared strips of filter paper 5 by 30 mm in size. The strips are inserted into the topically anesthetized conjunctival sac at the junction of the middle and outer third of the lower lid, with approximately 25 mm of paper exposed. After 5 minutes, the strip is removed and the amount of moistening measured. The normal range is 10 to 25 mm. If inadequate production of tears is found on the initial test, a Schirmer II test can be performed by repeating the procedure while stimulating the nasal mucosa.[2] A number of variations of the Schirmer test can be found in textbooks and journals.

B. Examination of Acquired Ptosis or Extraocular Muscle Palsy

To confirm myasthenia gravis as the cause of ptosis or muscle palsy, an intravenous injection of 2 mg of *edrophonium chloride* is administered, followed 45 seconds later by an additional 8 mg if there is no response to the first dose. (In case of a severe reaction to the edrophonium, immediately give atropine sulfate, 0.6 mg intravenously.)

C. Examination of the Retina and Choroid

Sodium fluorescein solution, in concentrations of 5%, 10%, and 25%, is injected intravenously to study the retinal and choroidal circulation. It has been used primarily in examination of lesions at the posterior pole of the eye, but anterior segment fluorescein angiography (wherein the vessels of the iris, sclera, and conjunctiva are studied) is also a useful clinical tool.

Intravascular fluorescein is normally prevented from entering the retina by the intact retinal vascular endothelium (blood-retinal barrier) and the intact retinal pigment epithelium. Defects in either the retinal vessels or the pigment epithelium will allow leakage of fluorescein, which can then be studied by either direct observation or photography. For good results, appropriate filters are needed to excite the fluorescein and exclude unwanted wavelengths. The peak frequencies for excitation lie between 485 and 500 nm and, for emission, between 520 and 530 nm.

Fluorescein has proved to be a safe diagnostic agent, the most common side effects being nausea and vomiting. However, occasional allergic and vagal reactions do occur, so oxygen and emergency equipment should be readily available when angiography is performed. Patients should also be warned that the dye will temporarily stain their skin and urine; in the average patient this lasts no more than a day.

Indocyanine green (IC-Green) has been used in recent years, either alone or with fluorescein, to obtain better frames of choroid neovascularization.

D. Examination of Abnormal Pupillary Responses

Methacholine, as a 2.5% solution instilled into the conjunctival sac, will cause the tonic pupil (Adie's pupil) to contract, but will leave a normal pupil unchanged. A similar pupillary response is seen following instillation of 2.5% methacholine in patients with familial dysautonomia (Riley-Day syndrome).

Table 25 shows the effects of several drugs on miosis due to interruption of the sympathetic system (Horner's syndrome). The effect depends on the location of the lesion in the sympathetic chain.

TABLE 25

HORNER'S SYNDROME

TOPICAL DROP (CENTRAL)	NEURON III (POST-GANGLIONIC)	NEURON II (PRE-GANGLIONIC)	NEURON I
Cocaine 2%–10%	–	–	+/–
Epinephrine (Adrenalin) 1:1000	+++	+	–
Phenylephrine 1%	+++	+	+/–

Pilocarpine may be used to determine whether a fixed dilated pupil is due to an atropine-like drug or interruption of the pupil's parasympathetic innervation.[3] If an atropine-like drug is involved, the pupil will not react to pilocarpine. If dilation is due to interruption of the parasympathetic innervation (compression by aneurysm, Adie's tonic pupil) instillation of pilocarpine will cause the pupil to constrict.

REFERENCES

1. Thompson HS, Mensher JH. Adrenergic mydrisis in Homer's syndrome: hydroxyampheta mine test for diagnosis of post-ganglionic defects.*Am J Ophthalmol*. 1971;72:472.
2. Hecht SD. Evaluation of the lacrimal drainage system. *Ophthalmology*. 1978;85:1250.
3. Thompson HS, Newsome DA, Lowenfeld I E. The fixed dilated pupil. Sudden iridoplegia or mydriatic drops; a simple diagnostic test. *Arch Ophthalmol*. 1971;86:12.

11. VISCOELASTIC MATERIALS USED IN OPHTHALMALOGY

Viscoelastic substances are used in ophthalmic surgery to maintain the anterior chamber, hydraulically dissect tissues, act as a vitreous substitute/tamponade, and prevent mechanical damage to tissue, especially the corneal endothelium. The individual characteristics of the various viscoelastic materials are the result of the chain length and intra- and interchain molecular interactions of the compounds comprising the viscoelastic substance. All viscoelastic materials have the potential to produce a large postoperative increase in pressure if they are not adequately removed from the anterior chamber following surgery.

AMVISC (Chiron Vision - Bausch and Lomb) – Composed of sodium hyaluronate 1.2% in physiologic saline. The viscosity is 40,000 cSt (@25 C, 1/sec shear rate), and molecular weight is ≥ 2,000,000 daltons. Its shelf life is estimated at 2 years.

AMVISC PLUS (Chiron Vision – Bausch and Lomb) – Composed of sodium hyaluronate 1.6% in physiologic saline. The viscosity is 55,000 cSt (@25 C, 1/sec shear rate), and molecular weight is approximately 1,500,000 daltons. The greater viscosity is obtained by increasing total concentration and using sodium hyaluronate of lower molecular weight. Its shelf life is estimated at 1 year.

BIOLON (Akorn) – Composed of sodium hyaluronate 1%. The viscosity is 215,000 cps, and the molecular weight is approximately 3,000,000 daltons. The product does not require refrigeration and its shelf life is estimated to be approximately 2 years.

DUOVISC (Alcon) – Package contains two separate syringes. One syringe containing Provisc; the other containing Viscoat. Please see individual descriptions below for details of each.

HEALON (Pharmacia – UpJohn) – Composed of sodium hyaluronate 1% in physiologic saline. The viscosity is 200,000 (@ 0/sec shear rate), and the molecular weight is approximately 4,000,000 daltons.

HEALON GV (Pharmacia – UpJohn) – Composed of sodium hyaluronate 1.4% in physiologic saline. The viscosity is 2,000,000 (@ 0/sec shear rate), and the molecular weight is approximately 5,000,000 daltons. In the presence of high positive vitreous pressure, Healon GV has three times more resistance to pressure than does Healon.

OCCUCOAT (Storz – Bausch and Lomb) – Composed of hydroxypropylmethylcellulose 2% in balance salt solution (BSS). The viscosity is 4,000 cSt (@ 37 C measured on Cannon-Fenske Viscometer), and the molecular weight is approximately 80,000 daltons. Occucoat is termed a viscoadherent rather than a viscoelastic because of its coating ability, which is related to its contact angle and low surface tension.

PROVISC (Alcon) – Composed of sodium hyaluronate 1% in physiologic saline. The viscosity is 39,000 cps (@ 25 C, 2/sec shear rate) and the molecular weight is approximately 1,900,000 daltons. Clinical studies demonstrate that ProVisc functions in a similar fashion to Healon.

VISCOAT (Alcon) – Composed of a 1:3 mixture of chondroitin sulfate 4% (CS) and sodium hyaluronate 3% (SH) in physiologic saline. The viscosity is 40,000 cps (@ 25 C, 2/sec shear rate), and the molecular weight is 22,500 daltons for CS and 500,000 daltons for SH.

VITRAX (Allergan) – Composed of sodium hyaluronate 3% in balanced salt solution (BSS). The viscosity is 30,000 cps (@ 2/sec shear rate) and the molecular weight is 500,000 daltons. It is highly concentrated to produce a significantly viscous material. It does not require refrigeration and has a shelf life of 18 months.

12. OFF-LABEL DRUG APPLICATIONS IN OPHTHALMOLOGY

A. Acetylcysteine

This agent is used to treat corneal conditions such as alkali burns, corneal melts, and keratoconjunctivitis sicca. It is thought to improve healing by inhibiting the action of collagenase, which may contribute to delay in healing. The drug is available generically or under the trade name Mucomyst in 10% and 20% solutions. Though none of the commercially available solutions are approved for use in ophthalmology, they have been administered as frequently as hourly in acute cases, and up to 4 times a day in maintenance therapy.

B. Alteplase (tissue plasminogen activator)

This thrombolytic agent, trade-named Activase, is used to treat fibrin formation in postvitrectomy patients. Though initial studies were based on intraocular injections of 25 µg, more recent work has shown the drug to be effective in doses of as little as 3 to 6 µg. Because by-products of alteplase activity may mediate endothelial cell toxicity, the lower doses are preferred. This agent has also been used for submacular hemhorrage, but this use is controversial.

C. Antimetabolites

5-Fluorouracil (5-FU). This drug inhibits fibroblasts and therefore diminishes scarring after glaucoma filtering surgery. Initial recommendations called for subconjunctival injection of 5 mg twice daily for 7 days postoperatively and once daily for the succeeding 7 days. However, many physicians today are achieving positive results with as little as 4 mg administered 4 to 6 times during a 10-day period. Use of this drug is associated with a number of complications, including conjunctival wound leak, corneal epithelial defects, hypotony associated with permanently reduced vision acuity, serious corneal infections in eyes with preexistent corneal epithelial edema, and increased susceptibility to late-onset bleb infections. The drug should be considered only when there is a high risk of surgical failure.

Mitomycin. This potent chemotherapeutic agent, trade-named Mutamycin, is being used in filtering surgery for the same purpose and on the same type of patients as 5-FU. It is applied once during surgery on a small piece of Gelfilm or Weck Cell in a concentration of 0.2 to 0.4 mg/mL. Reported side effects are similar to those of 5-FU. However, some serious side effects may go unreported, since there is a possibility of delayed reactions 6 to 24 months after surgery. Mitomycin has also been administered in a 0.02% to 0.04% solution 2 to 4 times a day to prevent recurrence after pterygium surgery. Serious side effects associated with this therapy include corneal melts and scleral ulceration and calcification.

Physicians should bear in mind the possibility of major side effects from all antineoplastic agents and carefully weigh the risks and benefits of the use. Remember, too, that these agents should always be handled and discarded in accordance with OSHA, AMA, ASHP, and/or hospital policies regarding the safe use of antineoplastics.

D. Cyclosporine

This potent immunosuppressant has a high degree of selectivity for T lymphocytes. Available under the trade name Sandimmune, it has been used in a 2% topical solution as prophylaxis against rejection in high-risk, penetrating keratoplasty and for treatment of severe vernal conjunctivitis resistant to more conventional therapy, ligneous conjunctivitis unresponsive to other topical therapy, and noninfectious peripheral ulcerative keratitis associated with systemic autoimmune disorders. All contraindications for systemic use also apply to topical administration, since blood levels of up to 64 ng/mL have been observed after topical application. All patients receiving this medication should have blood work that includes cyclosporine levels, blood urea nitrogen, creatinine, lactate dehyrogenase, alkaline phosphatase, and total bilirubin.

E. Doxycycline

This derivative of tetracycline is used for the treatment of ocular rosacea and meibomianitis. The usual dose is 100 mg PO daily for a 6 to 12 week course of treatment. It has the same side effects, contraindications, and interactions as tetracycline.

F. Edetate disodium

This chelating agent plays a role in the treatment of band keratopathy. After removal of the corneal epithelium, it is used to remove calcium from Bowman's membrane.

REFERENCES

Nesburn A. Trauma topics: small corneal perforations. *Audio Digest: Ophthalmol.* 1983;12:21.

Ralph R. Chemical burns of the eye. In: Tasman W, Jaeger E, eds. *Duane's Clinical Ophthalmology.* Philadelphia, Pa: JB Lippincott; 1989 vol. 4, chap 28:14.

Jaffe G, Abrams G, et al. Tissue plasminogen activator for post vitrectomy fibrin formation. *Opthalmology.* 1990;97:189.

McDermott M, Edelhauser H, et al. Tissue plasminogen activator and corneal endothelium. *Am J Ophthalmol.* 1989;108.

Williams D, Benett S, et al. Low-dose intraocular tissue plasminogen activator for treatment of postvitrectomy firbrin formations. *Am J Opthalmol.* 1990;109:606.

Williams G, Lambrou F, et al. Treatment of postvitrectomy fibrin formation with intraocular tissue plasminogen activator. *Arch Ophthalmol.* 1988;106:1055.

Ando H, Tadayoshi I, et al. Inhibition of corneal epithelial wound healing. A comparative study of mitomycin C and 5-fluorouracil. *Ophthalmology.* 1992;99:1809.

Falck F, Skuta G, Klein T. Mitomycin versus 5-fluorouracil antimetabolite therapy for glaucoma filtration surgery. *Semin in Ophthalmol.* 1992;7:97.

Who should receive antimetabolites after filtering surgery? *Arch Ophthalmol.* 1992;110:1069. Editorial.

Welsh R, Palmer S. Mitomycin in trabeculectomy: alter your technique. *Ocular Surgery News.* May 1, 1992:67.

Dunn J, Seamone S, Ostler H. Development of scleral ulceration and calcification after pterygium excision and mitomycin therapy. *Am J Ophthalmol.* 1991;112:343.

Rubinfeld R, Pfister R, et al. Serious complications of topical mitomycin-C after pterygium surgery. *Ophthalmology.* 1992;99:1647.

Bonomi L. Medical treatment of glaucoma. *Current Science.* 1992;1040:70.

Lish A, Camras C, Podos S. Effect of apraclonidine on intraocular pressure in glaucoma patients receiving maximally tolerated medications. *Glaucoma.* 1992;1:19.

Holland E, Chan C, et al. Immunohistologic findings and results of treatment with cyclosporine in ligneous conjunctivitis. *Am J Ophthalmol.* 1989;107:160.

Bouchard C, Belin M, Letter to Editor concerning above article, with reply by author. *Am J Ophthalmol.* 1989;108:210.

Secchi A, Tognan M, Leonardi A. Topical use of cyclosporine in the treatment of vernal conjunctivitis. *Am J Ophthalmol.* 1990;110:641.

BenEzra D, Matamoros N, Cohen E. Treatment of severe vernal keratoconjunctivitis with cyclosporine A eyedrops. *Transplant Proc.* 1988;20,No.2(suppl 2):644.

Zierhut H, Thiel E, et al. Topical treatment of severe corneal ulcers with cyclosporine A. *Graefe's* Arch *Clin Exp Opthalmol.* 1989;227:30.

Hill J. The use of cyclosporin in high-risk keratoplasty. *Am J Ophthalmol.* 1989;107:506.

Belin M, Bouchard C, Frantz S, et al. Topical cyclosporine in high-risk corneal transplants. *Ophthalmology.* 1989;96:1144.

Quarterman MJ, et al. Signs, symptoms, and tear studies before and after treatment with doxycycline. *Arch Dermatol.* 1997; 133:89.

Frucht-Perry J, et al. The effect of doxycycline on ocular rosacea. *Am J Ophthalmol.* 1989;170(4):434.

13. OCULAR TOXICOLOGY — F. T. Fraunfelder, MD

The table on the following pages recounts some of the more recently published findings on ocular side effects of drugs in general, as well as systemic side effects of drugs commonly used by ophthalmologists. It is not a catalog of all such reactions, since the data would be too lengthy for this format.

The volume of ocular toxicology in the medical literature is overwhelming. However, much is based on soft data, since, in most practices, the number of patients on a particular drug falls short of providing an adequate sample. Even in a controlled experimental environment, it is often difficult to prove a cause-and-effect relationship. In clinical practice, with its multitude of variables, a definitive finding is nearly impossible. It was to alleviate this problem that the National Registry of Drug-Induced Ocular Side Effects was founded.

Established by the federal Food and Drug Administration, with endorsement of the American Academy of Ophthalmology, the National Registry works on the supposition that, if the suspicions of practicing clinicians can be pooled in a large-enough database, they can be used as a flagging system to decrease the lag time in recognizing a possible adverse ocular response.

The registry welcomes communications from all concerned clinicians. To report a suspected adverse drug response, or to obtain references for the information listed below, please contact:

F.T. Fraunfelder, MD, Director, National Registry of Drug-Induced Ocular Side Effects
Casey Eye Institute
Oregon Health Sciences/University
3375 SW Terwilliger Blvd
Portland, OR 97201-4197

REFERENCE

Fraunfelder FT. *Drug-Induced Ocular Side Effects and Drug Interactions.* 3rd ed. Philadelphia, Pa: W.B. Saunders; 1989.

TABLE 26

ADVERSE DRUG EFFECTS

GENERIC NAME	PRINCIPAL GENERAL USE	POSSIBLE ADVERSE EFFECTS
I. MEDICATION BY INJECTION		
a. Adrenal Corticosteroids		
Depo-steroids	Allergic disorders Anti-inflammatory disorders	If injected into a blood vessel, eg, the tonsillar fossa, may cause unilateral or bilateral retinal arterial occlusions due to emboli of depo-steroid. Permanent bilateral blindness may ensue.
Triamcinolone	Allergic disorders Anti-inflammatory disorders	Fatty atrophy in area of injection, ie, enophthalmus if given retrobulbar or, if given in periocular skin, some deformity can occur in area due to loss of fat.
b. Anesthetics		
Ketamine hydrochloride	Adjunct to anesthesia Short-term diagnostic or surgical procedures	Reversible nystagmus
c. Antifungals		
Amphotericin B	Aspergillosis, blastomycosis, candidiasis, coccidioidomycosis, histoplasmosis	Ischemic necrosis after subconjunctival injection Subconjunctival nodule
d. Antineoplastics		
Carmustine	Brain tumors Multiple myeloma	Optic neuritis Retinal vascular disorders
Cisplatin	Metastatic testicular or ovarian tumors. Advanced bladder carcinoma	Cortical blindness Papilledema, retrobulbar or optic neuritis
Fluorouracil	Carcinoma of the colon, rectum, breast, stomach, and pancreas	Ocular irritation with tearing, conjunctival hyperemia, canalicular fibrosis
e. Miscellaneous		
Skin Tests	Tests for allergies	Recurrence or aggravation of episcleritis or scleritis
f. Ophthalmic Dyes		
Fluorescein	Ocular diagnostic tests	Nausea, vomiting, urticaria, rhinorrhea, dizziness, hypotension, pharyngoedema, anaphylactic reaction
g. Parasympathomimetics		
Acetylcholine	Produces prompt, short-term miosis	Hypotension and bradycardia with intraocular injection
II. ORAL		
a. Amebicides		
Iodochlorhydroxyquin	Acrodermatitis enteropathica Entamoeba histolytica	Optic atrophy—may be due to a zinc deficiency of the optic nerve
b. Anthelmintics		
Levamisol hydrochloride	Connective tissue disorders Ascaris infestation	Patients with Sjögren's syndrome and possibly keratitis sicca have marked increase in systemic side effects, including pruritus and muscle weakness
c. Antianxiety Agents		
Diazepam	Acute alcohol withdrawal Preoperative medication Psychoneurotic anxiety, depression, tension, or agitation Skeletal muscle spasms	Allergic conjunctivitis Extraocular muscle paresis Nystagmus
d. Antiarrhythmics		
Amiodarone hydrochloride	Cardiac abnormalities Ventricular arrhythmias	Keratopathy Lens opacities, optic neuropathy, optic neuritis
Oxprenolol	Cardiovascular abnormalities Certain hypertensive states	Conjunctival hyperemia Decreased lacrimation, nonspecific ocular irritation, photophobia
Propranolol	Cardiovascular abnormalities Certain hypertensive states	May precipitate latent myotonia May mask hyperthyroidism; when taken off drug, thyroid stare and exophthalmos may occur

GENERIC NAME	PRINCIPAL GENERAL USE	POSSIBLE ADVERSE EFFECTS
e. Antibiotics and Antituberculars		
Chloramphenicol		Aplastic anemia
Ethambutol hydrochloride	Pulmonary tuberculosis	Optic neuropathy
Rifampin	Asymptomatic carriers of meningococcus Many gram-negative and gram-positive cocci, including Neisseria and Hemophilus influenzae Pulmonary tuberculosis	Conjunctival hyperemia Exudative conjunctivitis Increased lacrimation
Tetracycline hydrochloride	Useful against gram-negative and gram-positive bacteria Members of lymphogranuloma-psittacosis group Mycoplasma	Pseudotumor cerebri and papilledema as early as 3 days after onset of medication in infants and in young adults Transient myopia
f. Antihypertensives		
Sodium nitroprusside	Provides controlled hypertension during anesthesia Management of severe hypertension	Contraindicated in Leber's hereditary optic atrophy and tobacco amblyopia
g. Antileprotics		
Clofazimine	Dermatologic diseases—psoriasis, pyoderma gangrenosum Leprosy	Conjunctival, corneal, and macular pigmentation
h. Antimalarials and Anti-inflammatories		
Hydroxychloroquine	Malaria Lupus erythematosus Rheumatoid arthritis	Disturbance of accommodation Corneal changes Bull's-eye maculopathy—central, pericentral, or paracentral scotomas
i. Antineoplastics		
Busulfan	Chronic myelogenous leukemia	Cataracts Decreased lacrimation
Tamoxifen	Metastatic breast carcinoma	Corneal opacities Refractile retinal deposits
j. Antipsychotics		
Haloperidol	Acute and chronic schizophrenia Manic/depressive psychosis	Capsular cataracts with chronic use Cycloplegia and mydriasis
Lithium carbonate	Manic phase of manic/depressive exophthalmos psychosis	Oculogyric crisis Myoclonus
k. Antispasmodics		
Baclofen	Muscle spasms in multiple sclerosis and disorders associated with increased muscular tone	Blurred vision Hallucinations
l. Carbonic Anhydrase Inhibitors		
Acetazolamide Dichlorphenamide Ethoxzolamide	Centrencephalic epilepsies Congestive heart failure edema Drug-induced edema	Aggravation of metabolic acidosis, primarily in known CO_2-retaining diseases such as emphysema and bronchiectasis, and in patients with poor vital capacity
Methazolamide	Glaucoma	Aplastic anemia Decreased libido Impotency
m. Chelating Agents		
Penicillamine	Cystinuria Heavy metal antagonist—iron, lead, copper, mercury poisoning Wilson's disease	Facial or ocular myasthenia, including extraocular muscle paralysis, ptosis, and diplopia Ocular pemphigoid Optic neuritis and color-vision problems
n. Hormonal Agents		
Oral contraceptives	Amenorrhea Dysfunctional uterine bleeding Dysmenorrhea Hypogonadism Oral contraception Premenstrual tension	Contraindicated in patients with preexisting retinal vascular diseases Decrease in color vision with chronic use Macular edema

GENERIC NAME	PRINCIPAL GENERAL USE	POSSIBLE ADVERSE EFFECTS
o. Hydantoins		
Phenytoin	Chronic epilepsy	Optic nerve hypoplasia in infants with epileptic mothers on the drug Ocular teratogenic effects, including strabismus, ptosis, hypertelorism, epicanthus
p. Nonsteroidal Anti-inflammatory Drugs		
Ibuprofen	Rheumatoid arthritis Osteoarthritis	Decreased color vision Optic neuritis Visual field defects
Naproxen	Rheumatoid arthritis Osteoarthritis Ankylosing spondylitis	Corneal opacity Periorbital edema
Sulindac	Rheumatoid arthritis Osteoarthritis Ankylosing spondylitis	Keratitis Stevens-Johnson syndrome
q. Psychedelics		
Marijuana	Cerebral sedative or narcotic	Conjunctival hyperemia Decreased lacrimation Decreased intraocular pressure Dyschromatopsia with chronic long-term use
r. Red Blood Cell Sickling Inhibitors		
Sodium cyanate	Sickle cell hemoglobinopathy	Partially reversible posterior subcapsular cataracts
s. Sedatives and Hypnotics		
Ethanol	Antiseptic Used as a beverage	Fetal alcohol syndrome: offspring of alcoholic mothers may have epicanthus, small palpebral fissures, and microphthalmia
t. Synthetic Retinoids		
Etretinate Isotretinoin	Cystic acne and other keratinizing skin disorders	Dark eye, abnormal dark adaptation, electro-oculography (EOG) and electroretinography (ERG), cataracts, optic neuritis, pseudotumor cerebri and papilledema
III. TOPICAL		
a. Anticholinergics		
Cyclopentolate hydrochloride	Used as a cycloplegic and mydriatic	Central nervous system toxicity, including slurred speech, ataxia, hallucinations, hyperactivity, seizures, syncope, and paralytic ileus
Tropicamide	Used as a cycloplegic and mydriatic	Cyanosis, muscle rigidity, nausea, pallor, vomiting, vasomotor collapse
b. Parasympathomimetics or Anticholinesterases		
Demecarium bromide Echothiophate iodide Isofluorphate Pilocarpine	Glaucoma	Retinal detachments primarily in eyes with peripheral retinal or retinal-vitreal disease. (Patients need to be warned of this possible effect when first placed on this medication.) Miotic upper respiratory infection—rhinorrhea, sensation of chest constriction, cough, conjunctival hyperemia; seen primarily in young children on anticholinesterase agents
c. Sympathomimetics		
Dipivefrin	Open-angle glaucoma	Follicular blepharoconjunctivitis, keratitis
Epinephrine	Used as a bronchodilator Open-angle glaucoma Used as a vasoconstrictor to prolong anesthetic action	Cicatricial pemphigoid Stains soft contact lenses black Hypertension, headache
10% Phenylephrine	Used as a mydriatic and vasoconstrictor	Cardiac arrhythmias and cardiac arrests with pledget form or subconjunctival injection, possible myocardial infarcts, systemic hypertension
Betaxolol Levobunolol hydrochloride Timolol	Glaucoma	Cardiac syncope, bradycardia, light-headedness, fatigue, congestive heart failure; In diabetics—hyperglycemia; In myasthenia gravis—severe dysarthria

SECTION 3

SUTURE MATERIALS

Although the advent of sutureless cataract surgery is diminishing the need for certain sutures, there is still no other discipline that has required as many specialized needles and suture materials as ophthalmic surgery. To meet this need, manufacturers offer the ophthalmologist a comprehensive array of precisely manufactured reverse-cutting and spatula needles swaged to suture materials of collagen (plain and chromic), silk (black and white braided), virgin silk (black and white twisted), Nylon, Dacron, and synthetics.

Suture material intended for use in ophthalmic surgery can be either nonabsorbable or absorbable. Following is a list of various suture materials available for ophthalmology, with a brief description of each.

Absorbable

Plain Catgut—Prepared from the submucosal or mucosal layers of sheep or beef intestine, respectively, this material consists primarily of collagen—a fibrous protein—which is absorbed by the body. The material is chemically purified to minimize tissue reaction. Available in sizes 4–0 through 6–0.

Chromic Catgut—same as plain catgut except that it is treated with chromium salts to delay the absorption time. Available in sizes 4–0 through 7–0.

Plain Collagen—prepared from bovine deep flexor tendon. The tendon is purified and converted to a uniform suspension of collagen fibril. This fibrillar suspension is then extruded into suture strands and chemically treated to accurately control absorption rate. Available in sizes 4–0 through 7–0.

Chromic Collagen—prepared in the same way as plain collagen except that chromium salts are added during the chemical treatment to further delay absorption. Available in sizes 4–0 through 8–0.

TABLE 1

COMPARISON OF OPHTHALMIC SUTURE MATERIALS

SUTURE MATERIAL	RELATIVE TENSILE STRENGTH*	RELATIVE HOLDING DURATION†	RELATIVE TISSUE REACTION‡	EASE OF HANDLING	SPECIAL KNOT REQUIRED	BEHAVIOR OF EXPOSED ENDS	AVAILABLE SIZES§
Surgical gut or collagen							
Plain	6	1 week	4+	Fair	No	Stiff	4–0 to 6–0
Chromic	6	<2 weeks	3+	Fair	No	Stiff	4–0 to 8–0
Polyglactin 910							
Braided	9	2 weeks	2+	Good	Yes	Stiff	4–0 to 9–0
Monofilament	9	2 weeks	2+	Good	Yes	Stiff	9–0 to 10–0
Polyglycolic acid	9	2 weeks	2+	Good	Yes	Stiff	
Silk							
Virgin	7	2 months	3+	Excellent	No	Softest	8–0 to 9–0
Braided	8	2 months	3+	Good	No	Soft	4–0 to 9–0
Polyamide (Nylon)	9	6 months	1+	Fair	Yes	Stiff, sharp	8–0 to 11–0
Polypropylene	10	>12 months	1+	Fair	Yes	Stiff, sharp	4–0 to 6–0 9–0 to 10–0

Adapted from Spaeth GL. *Ophthalmic Surgery, Principles and Practice*. Philadelphia, Pa: WB Saunders; 1982:64.

*The higher the number, the greater the relative tensile strength. Strength varies with size of material; estimates apply mainly to size 8–0 sutures.

† Holding duration will vary with location and size of suture, health of patient, medications employed, etc. The time given in this table is an average of the time at which about 30% of tensile strength is lost.

‡ 1+ indicates least inflammatory response, 4+ greatest.

§ With needles appropriate for ophthalmic use. Sizes available will vary from time to time.

Synthetic Absorbable Sutures–Products include Vicryl (Polyglactin 910, a copolymer of lactide and glycolide) and Dexon (polyglycolic acid). These materials offer high tensile strength and minimal tissue reaction during the critical postoperative healing period, followed by predictable absorption. Coated Vicryl sutures are also available. Manufactured in size 4–0 through 10–0 (coated 4–0 through 8–0).

It is interesting to note that the absorption of sutures occurs in two distinct phases. After implantation, the suture's tensile strength diminishes during the early postoperative period. When most of the strength is lost, the remaining suture mass begins to decrease in what may be termed the second phase of absorption. The mass-loss phase then proceeds until the entire suture has been absorbed.

Nonabsorbable

Monofilament Nylon Sutures (Ethilon, Dermalon, and Supramid). These sutures offer high tensile strength and minimal tissue reaction. Nylon has been reported to lose tensile strength postoperatively at a rate of approximately 15% per year. Available in sizes 8–0 through 14–0.

Polypropylene Suture (Prolene)—a monofilament suture with high tensile strength and minimal tissue reaction. The material is not degraded or weakened by tissue enzymes. Available in sizes 5–0, 9–0, and 11–0.

Black Braided Silk Suture—braided under controlled conditions to maximize strength and assure resistance to breaking while knots are tied. Gums and other impurities are removed, resulting in a suture that remains tightly braided, with virtually no loose filaments and minimal tendency to broom. Available in sizes 4–0 and 6–0 through 9–0.

Virgin Silk—twisted with the individual silk filaments still embedded in their natural sericin coating, providing a smooth, uniform suture in very fine sizes. The suture is offered in black or white, permitting optimum contrast with tissues. Available in sizes 8–0 and 9–0.

Polyester Fiber Sutures–Products include Mersilene and Ti Cron. They exhibit minimal tissue reaction and are braided by a special method for tightness, uniformity, and a smooth surface that minimizes trauma. Available in sizes 4–0 through 6–0.

A variety of physical characteristics of different sutures have been published. In addition, the United States Pharmacopeia has established specifications for various suture materials. Some of the useful parameters measured have been: (1) tensile strength; (2) elasticity; (3) suture diameters; (4) weight per unit length. Data are summarized in **Tables 1** through **3.**

REFERENCE

1. Middleton DG, McCulloch C. An enquiry into characteristics of sutures, particularly fine sutures. *Adv Ophthalmol* 1970;22:35.

TABLE 2

ELASTICITY OF SUTURES

SUTURE MATERIAL	ELONGATION OF STANDARD 30.5-cm SEGMENT	INCREASE IN LENGTH	WEIGHT AT BREAKING POINT
6–0 plain gut	4.7 cm	15.4%	264 g
6–0 chromic gut	4.3 cm	14.1%	257 g
6–0 Mersilene	1.9 cm	6.3%	254 g
6–0 braided silk	1.2 cm	3.9%	237 g
7–0 chromic gut	3.6 cm	1.8%	118 g
7–0 braided silk	0.9 cm	3.0%	126 g
8–0 virgin silk	0.8 cm	2.6%	53 g
10–0 Nylon	8.7 cm	28.5%	23 g

From Middleton DG, McCulloch C. *Adv Ophthalmol.* 1970;22:35.

TABLE 3

WEIGHT OF SUTURE MATERIAL

SUTURE MATERIAL	WEIGHT/LENGTH (mg/cm)
6–0 plain gut (wet)	0.170
6–0 chromic gut (wet)	0.176
6–0 Mersilene	0.116
6–0 braided silk	0.165
7–0 chromic gut (wet)	0.062
7–0 braided silk	0.065
8–0 virgin silk	0.025
10–0 Nylon	0.007

SECTION 4

OPHTHALMIC LENSES

1. SOFT CONTACT LENSES

Information on available products is provided through the courtesy of *Contact Lenses Quarterly*, a publication of Frames Data, Inc. Drawn from the Spring 1999 issue, the table provides all pertinent physical specifications of each soft contact lens product. Also included are separate sections for the increasingly popular planned replacement systems and for disposable lenses.

TABLE 1

EXTENDED/FLEXIBLE WEAR SPHERICAL

MFR.	LENS	MATERIAL, % H_2O, PROCESS	DIAMETER (mm)	BASE CURVE (mm)	POWER (D)	CENTER THICKNESS (mm)	OPTIC ZONE (mm)	dK+ VALUE
AMERICAN BIOCURVE, INC.	Biocurve EW Spheres EW Extended Wear	methafilcon A, 55%	14.0 14.5	8.4 8.4, 8.6, 8.8, 9.0	–20.00 to +10.00 in 0.25 steps	0.06 (–), 0.15 (+)	7.8 to 8.3	18.8
BAUSCH & LOMB	Optima FW 1 Pack Visibility Tint Flexible Wear	polymacon, 38.6%, cast-mold	14.0	8.4, 8.7	+4.00 to –9.00 in 0.25 steps	0.26 to 0.035	8.0 to 10.0	9.2
	1 Pack was discontinued September 1, 1998. Will continue to sell while supplies last. Six-packs, 30-packs and single trial lenses will still be available.							
	Optima FW Vial Light Blue Visibility Tint Flexible Wear	polymacon, 38.6%, cast-mold	14.0	8.4, 8.7,*	+4.00 to –5.00 in 0.25 steps; –5.50 to –9.00 in 0.50 steps	0.26 to 0.035	8.0 to 10.0	9.2
	*9.0 BC discontinued in vial, still available in multiple blister packages. Vial discontinued September 1, 1998. Will continue to sell while supplies last. Six-packs, 30-packs and single trial lenses will still be available.							
	Soflens® 03®/04® Series* Flexible Wear –1.00 to –6.00	polymacon, 38.6%, spin-cast	03®: 13.5 04®: 14.5		–1.00 to –5.00 in 0.25 steps; –5.50 to –9.00 in 0.50 steps	0.035	12.4 (03)® 13.6 (04)®	9.2
	*04 includes therapeutic plano. 03 & 04 or daily wear only available from –6.50D to –9.00D.							
CALIFORNIA OPTICS	C.O.Soft 55 EW™	methafilcon, 55%, lathe-cut	14.2	8.4	Pl to –6.00	variable	8.0	18.8
	C.O.Soft 55 EW™	methafilcon, 55%, lathe-cut	13.0, 13.5	8.4	Pl to ±30.00	variable	7.0, 9.5	18.8
	C.O.Soft 55 EW™	methafilcon, 55%, lathe-cut	15.0	8.9	Pl to –6.00	variable	8.0	18.8
	C.O.Soft 55 EW™	methafilcon, 55%, lathe-cut	15.0	8.6	Pl to –6.00	variable	8.0	18.8
	C.O.Soft 55 EW™	methafilcon, 55%, lathe-cut	14.0, 14.5, 15.0	8.3, 8.6, 8.9, 9.2	Pl to ±30.00	variable	8.0 to 9.5	18.8
CIBA VISION CORP.	SOFTCON® EW Extended Wear	vifilcon A, 55%, cast-mold	14.0 14.5	8.1, 8.4, 8.7 8.7 in minus powers only	–8.00 to +5.00 in 0.25 steps; +5.50 to +9.50 in 0.50 steps Plano to –8.00	0.10 (–3.00), 0.16 (+3.00)	7.5	16.0
COOPERVISION INC.	CooperClear™ FW Flexible Wear	tetrafilcon A, 43%, lathe-cut	14.4	8.4 8.7	–0.25 to –10.00 in 0.50 steps above –6.50	0.03 to 0.082	13.2	9.3

EXTENDED/FLEXIBLE WEAR SPHERICAL (CONTINUED)

MFR.	LENS	MATERIAL, % H_2O, PROCESS	DIAMETER (mm)	BASE CURVE (mm)	POWER (D)	CENTER THICKNESS (mm)	OPTIC ZONE (mm)	dK+ VALUE
COOPERVISION INC.	Hydrasoft® XW Flexible Wear	methafilcon B, 55%, lathe-cut, pitch-polished	15.0	8.6, 8.9, 9.2	+10.00 to –20.00 in 0.50 steps after –10.00	0.06	8.0	18.8
			14.2	8.3, 8.6	+10.00 to –12.00 in 0.50 steps after ±8.00			
	Permaflex® Naturals Flexible Wear Flexible Wear	surfilcon A, 74%, cast-mold	14.4	8.7	–0.25 to –6.00 in 0.25 steps; –6.50 to –10.00 in 0.50 steps	0.10 to 0.18	7.0 to 8.5 AOZ	38.9
					+0.50 to +5.00 in 0.25 steps; +5.50, +6.00	0.22 to 0.41	7.9 to 8.1 AOZ	
				8.9	–1.00 to –6.00 in 0.25 steps	0.14 to 0.24	7.0 to 8.5	
	Permaflex® UV Naturals Flexible Wear Flexible Wear	surfilcon A, 74%, cast-mold	14.4	8.7	–0.25 to –6.00 in 0.25 steps; –6.50 to –10.00 in 0.50 steps;	0.10 to 0.18		38.9
					+0.50 to +5.00 in 0.25 steps; +5.50, +6.00	0.22 to 0.32		
	Permalens®	perfilcon A, 71%, lathe-cut	13.5	7.7, 8.0, 8.3	–0.25 to –20.00 in 0.50 steps above –6.00	0.10 to 0.26	7.0	34.0
			14.2	8.6	–0.25 to –10.00 in 0.50 steps above –6.00			
	Permalens® Low Plus	perfilcon A, 71%, lathe-cut	14.0	8.0, 8.3, 8.6	+0.25 to +5.00 in 0.25 steps; +5.50 to +8.00 in 0.50 steps	0.27 to 0.40	7.0	34.0
	Permalens® XL Extended Wear	perfilcon A, 71%, cast-mold	14.5	8.3	–0.25 to –6.00 in 0.25 steps; –6.50 to –10.00 in 0.50 steps	0.11 to 0.26	8.0 AOZ	34.0
	Vantage® Thin Flexible Wear	tetrafilcon A, 43%, lathe-cut	14.0	8.4	Pl to –6.50 in 0.25 steps; –6.50 to –10.00 in 0.50 steps	0.03 to 0.082	12.8	9.3
			14.4	8.7			13.2	
OCULAR SCIENCES, INC.	EDGE® III 55 Flexible Wear Extended Wear	methafilcon A, 55%, lathe-cut	14.5	8.4, 8.7	+5.00 to –10.00 in 0.50 steps above –6.00	0.09 (–3.00)	8.0 to 13.0	18.8
	Hydron Zero 4 Softblue Full Iris Visibility Tint Flexible Wear Extended Wear	polymacon, 38%, cast-molded	14.0	8.6	–0.25 to –10.00 in –0.50 steps above –6.00	0.04 (–3.00)	8.0 to 11.0	8.4
SUNSOFT	Revolution™ Light Blue Visibility Tint Extended Wear Flexible Wear	methafilcon A, 55%, patented molding process	14.0	8.5	Pl to –10.00 in 0.25 steps	varies w/ power; 0.10 (–3.00)	8.0	18.8
				8.7	+4.00 to –6.00 in 0.25 steps			
	Sunflex® Extended Wear Flexible Wear	methafilcon A, 55%, lathe-cut	15.0	8.3, 8.6, 8.9	+10.00 to –20.00 in 0.50 steps above –10.00	0.10, 0.13 (–3.00)	8.0	18.8

EXTENDED/FLEXIBLE WEAR SPHERICAL (CONTINUED)

MFR.	LENS	MATERIAL, % H_2O, PROCESS	DIAMETER (mm)	BASE CURVE (mm)	POWER (D)	CENTER THICKNESS (mm)	OPTIC ZONE (mm)	dK+ VALUE
SUNSOFT	Sunflex® Prism Ballast Extended Wear Flexible Wear	methafilcon A, 55%, lathe-cut	15.0	8.3, 8.9	+10.00 to –20.00 in 0.50 steps above –10.00	0.10, 0.13 (–3.00)	8.0	18.8
UNILENS CORP.	SOF-FORM® 55 Flexible Wear Flexible Wear	methafilcon A, 55%, lathe-cut	14.0 15.0	8.3, 8.6, 8.9	+9.75 to –10.00 in 0.25 steps	0.06 (Pl)	8.0	18.8
	SOF-FORM® 55 Custom Flexible Wear	methafilcon A, 55%, lathe-cut	any	any	any			18.8
WESLEY-JESSEN	CSI® Flexible Wear Flexible Wear	crofilcon A, 38.6%, lathe-cut	13.8 14.8	8.0, 8.3, 8.6, 8.9 8.6, 8.9, 9.35	Pl to –10.00 Pl to –7.00	0.035	10.9 to 6.5	13.0
	DuraSoft® 3 Flexiwear Flexible Wear	phemfilcon A, 55%, lathe-cut	D3-X3: 13.5 D3-X4: 14.5	8.5 median, 8.2 steep 8.6 median, 8.3 steep, 9.0 flat	±6.00 in 0.25 steps ±20.00 in 0.25 steps to ±10.00, in 0.50 steps over ±10.00	0.05 (–3.00)	8.0	16.1
	DuraSoft® 3 Lite Tint Flexible Wear	phemfilcon A, 55%, lathe-cut	14.5	8.3 steep, 8.6 median, 9.0 flat	±20.00 in 0.25 steps to ±10.00, in 0.50 steps over ±10.00	0.05 (–3.00)	8.0	16.1
	Hydrocurve II 55% Custom tint available	bufilcon A, 55%, lathe-cut	14.5 14.0	8.8 8.5	+7.00 to –12.00 in 0.50 steps above +4.00 & –6.00	0.05 to 0.10 varies w/power	8.0 to 8.5	16.0
	Soft Mate II Extended Wear Custom tint available	bufilcon A, 55%, lathe-cut	14.3 14.8	8.7 9.0	+4.00 to –8.00 in 0.50 steps above –6.00	0.05 (–3.00)	8.0 to 8.5	16.0

DAILY WEAR SPHERICAL

MFR.	LENS	MATERIAL, % H_2O, PROCESS	DIAMETER (mm)	BASE CURVE (mm)	POWER (D)	CENTER THICKNESS (mm)	OPTIC ZONE (mm)	dK+ VALUE
ACCUGEL LABS	Accugel Spherical Div. A	droxifilcon, 46.6%, lathe-cut	13.5, 14.0	8.3, 8.6, 8.9	Pl to ±10.00	all lenticular	8.0	18.7
	Accugel Spherical Div. P	droxifilcon, 46.6%, lathe-cut	13.0	7.6 to 8.6 in 0.2 steps	+20.25 to +36.00 in 1.00 steps	all lenticular	7.0	18.7
	Accugel Spherical Div. 1	droxifilcon, 46.6%, lathe-cut	13.5, 14.0	7.8 to 9.2 in 0.1 steps	Pl to ±10.00	all lenticular	8.0	18.7
	Accugel Spherical Div. 2	droxifilcon, 46.6%, lathe-cut	13.5, 14.0	7.8 to 9.2	±10.25 to ±20.00	all lenticular	8.0	18.7
	Accugel Spherical Div. 4	droxifilcon, 46.6%, lathe-cut	any	any	over ±20.00	all lenticular	8.0	18.7
ALDEN OPTICAL LABS, INC.	Alden Classic Custom lenses available upon request.	polymacon, 38%, lathe-cut	13.0, 13.5, 14.0	7.7, 7.9, 8.1, 8.3, 8.5, 8.7, 8.9	Pl ±30.00	0.12 (–3.00)	varies w/power	8.4

DAILY WEAR SPHERICAL (CONTINUED)

MFR.	LENS	MATERIAL, % H_2O, PROCESS	DIAMETER (mm)	BASE CURVE (mm)	POWER (D)	CENTER THICKNESS (mm)	OPTIC ZONE (mm)	dK+ VALUE
AMERICAN BIOCURVE, INC.	Biocurve Aphakic Spheres Handling tint available	methafilcon A, 55%	14.0 14.5 15.0	8.4 8.4, 8.6, 8.8, 9.0 8.9	+10.50 to +20.00 in 0.50 steps	0.27 to 0.42	7.8 to 8.3	18.8
	Biocurve Custom Handling tint available	methafilcon A, 55%	any	any	any			18.8
	Biocurve Spheres Handling tint available	methafilcon A, 55%	14.0 14.5 15.0	8.4 8.4, 8.6, 8.8, 9.0 8.9	–20.00 to +10.00 in 0.25 steps	0.06 to 0.26	7.8 to 8.3	18.8
AQUA-SITE	Aqua-Sphere 53	ocufilcon B, 53%, lathe-cut	14.5 or custom	8.6, 8.8, 9.0, or custom	–25.00 to +10.00 or custom	varies w/power	minus lenses 8.6, plus lenses 7.4, or custom	15.4
	Pediatric custom lenses now available.							
BAUSCH & LOMB	Optima 38 1 Pack Visibility Tint	polymacon, 38.6%, cast-mold or RP III	14.0	8.4, 8.7	+4.00 to –9.00 in 0.25 steps	0.06 (–), 0.095 to 0.19 (+)	8.0 to 10.0	9.2
	Optima 38 Vial Visibility Tint	polymacon, 38.6%, cast-mold or RP III	14.0	8.4, 8.7, 9.0	+5.00 to –5.00 in 0.25 steps; –5.00 to –12.00 in 0.50 steps	0.06 (–), 0.095 to 0.19 (+)	8.0 to 10.0	9.2
	Optima 38 SP 2 Pack Visibility Tint	polymacon, 38.6%, cast-mold or RP III	14.0	8.4, 8.7, 9.0	+5.00 to –9.00 in 0.25 steps	0.06 (–), 0.095 to 0.19 (+)	8.0 to 10.0	9.2
	Plano T	polymacon, 38.6%, spin-cast	14.5		Pl	0.15		9.2
	SofLens® Series B3	polymacon, 38.6%, spin-cast	13.5		+6.00 to –20.00 in 0.50 steps above ±5.00	0.12 to 0.21	12.1 (–), 8.5 (+)	9.2
	SofLens® Series B4	polymacon, 38.6%, spin-cast	14.5		+6.00 to –9.00 in 0.50 steps above ±5.00	0.12 to 0.21	13.4 (–), 10.0 (+)	9.2
	SofLens® Series HO3	polymacon, 38.6%, spin-cast	13.5		–8.00 to –20.00 in 0.50 steps	0.035	9.0	9.2
	SofLens® Series HO4	polymacon, 38.6%, spin-cast	14.5		–8.00 to –20.00 in 0.50 steps	0.035	9.0	9.2
	Discontinued March 30, 1998. Will continue to sell while supplies last.							
	SofLens® Series U3	polymacon, 38.6%, spin-cast	13.5		+6.00 to –9.00 in 0.50 steps above ±5.00	0.07 (–3.00), 0.12 (+3.00)	12.4 (–), 7.8 (+)	9.2
	SofLens® Series U4	polymacon, 38.6%, spin-cast	14.5		+6.00 to –9.00 in 0.50 steps above ±5.00	0.07 (–3.00), 0.12 (+3.00)	13.6 (–), 7.8 (+)	9.2
	0.25, 0.50, 0.75 discontinued March 30, 1998. Will continue to sell while supplies last. All other powers still manufactured.							
BENZ RESEARCH & DEVELOPMENT CORP.	Benz Lens Blue Visibility Tint	hioxifilcon A, 59%, lathe-cut	14.5	median	+10.00 to –10.00	0.10 (–3.00) wet	11.0	21

DAILY WEAR SPHERICAL (CONTINUED)

MFR.	LENS	MATERIAL, % H_2O, PROCESS	DIAMETER (mm)	BASE CURVE (mm)	POWER (D)	CENTER THICKNESS (mm)	OPTIC ZONE (mm)	dK+ VALUE
BLANCHARD CONTACT LENS	Esstech SV	polymacon, 38%, lathe-cut	14.0	8.3, 8.7, 9.1	+6.00 to –6.00 in 0.25 steps*	0.08 (–) 0.15 (+)	N/A	8.4
	*High resolution optics free of spherical aberration. Masks up to +1.00 cylinder.							
CALIFORNIA OPTICS	C.O.Soft 55 DW™	methafilcon, 55%, lathe-cut	14.2	8.4	Pl to –6.00	variable	8.0	18.8
	C.O.Soft 55 DW™	methafilcon, 55%, lathe-cut	13.0, 13.5	8.4	Pl to ±30.00	variable	7.0, 9.5	18.8
	C.O.Soft 55 DW™	methafilcon, 55%, lathe-cut	15.0	8.9	Pl to –6.00	variable	8.0	18.8
	C.O.Soft 55 DW™	methafilcon, 55%, lathe-cut	15.0	8.6	Pl to –6.00	variable	8.0	18.8
	C.O.Soft 55 DW™	methafilcon, 55%, lathe-cut	14.0, 14.5, 15.0	8.3, 8.6, 8.9, 9.2	Pl to ±30.00	variable	8.0 to 9.5	18.8
CIBA VISION CORP.	CIBASOFT® Visitint® Light Blue Visibility Tint	tefilcon, 37.5%, lathe-cut	13.8	8.3, 8.6, 8.9	+6.00 to –6.00 in 0.25 steps; –6.50 to –10.00 in 0.50 steps	0.07 (–3.00), 0.14 (+3.00)	varies w/power (7.0 to 12.0)	8.9
			14.5	8.6, 8.9, 9.2	Pl to –6.00 in 0.25 steps; –6.50 to –10.00 in 0.50 steps			
	STD™ Visitint® Light Blue Visibility Tint	tefilcon, 37.5%, CIBACAST® mold	13.8	8.3, 8.6, 8.9	+6.00 to –6.00 in 0.25 steps	0.10 (–3.00), 0.17 (+3.00)	(7.0 to 12.8)	8.9
CONTACT LENS LABS, INC.	CLL-38 Clear, Visibility Tint	polymacon, 38%, lathe-cut, pitch-polished	14.0	8.3, 8.5, 8.7, 8.9	Pl to –15.00 in 0.25 steps	0.06	8.5	8.4
					Pl to +10.00			
CONTINENTAL SOFT LENS, INC.	Continental Spherical	ocufilcon B, 53%, lathe-cut	12.0 to 22.0	6.4 to 15.5	±40.00	varies	varies	16.5
COOPERVISION INC.	Cooper Clear™	tetrafilcon A, 43%, lathe-cut	14.0	8.3, 8.6	Pl to –6.50 in 0.25 steps; –6.50 to –10.00 in 0.50 steps	0.03 to 0.12	12.8	9.3
			14.4	8.7			13.2	
			14.4	8.7	Pl to +6.00 in 0.25 steps	0.08 to 0.28		
			14.0	8.3, 8.6				
	CooperThin®	polymacon, 38%, cast-mold	14.0	8.4	–0.25 to –5.00 in 0.25 steps; –5.50 to –10.00 in 0.50 steps	0.08	12.75 to 7.5	8.4
			14.5	8.6	–0.25 to –5.00 in 0.25 steps; –5.50 to –6.50 in 0.50 steps			
	Hydrasoft® Standard	methafilcon B, 55%, lathe-cut, pitch-polished	14.2	8.3, 8.6	+10.00 to –12.00 in 0.50 steps after ±8.00	0.10	8.5	18.8
			15.0	8.6, 8.9, 9.2	+10.00 to -20.00 in 0.50 steps after –10.00	0.12		

DAILY WEAR SPHERICAL (CONTINUED)

MFR.	LENS	MATERIAL, % H_2O, PROCESS	DIAMETER (mm)	BASE CURVE (mm)	POWER (D)	CENTER THICKNESS (mm)	OPTIC ZONE (mm)	dK+ VALUE
COOPERVISION INC.	Silver 2 Visibility Handling Tint	polymacon, 38%, cast-molded	14.0	8.4, 8.7, 9.0 Plus available only in 8.7	Pl to ±8.00			8.4
	Silver 7 Light Blue Handling Tint	polymacon, 38%, cast-molded	14.0	8.3, 8.6, 8.9 Plus available only in 8.6	Pl to ±8.00			8.4
	Vantage® Light Blue Handling Tint	tetrafilcon A, 43%, lathe-cut	14.0	8.3, 8.6, 8.9	Pl to –6.50 in 0.25 steps;	0.03 to 0.12	9.0 to 11.5	9.3
			14.4	8.7	–6.50 to –10.00 in 0.50 steps	0.08 to 0.28		
			14.0 14.7	8.3, 8.6 8.7	Pl to +6.00 in 0.25 steps			
EPCON LABS	Epcon Soft	polymacon, 38%, lathe-cut	14.0	8.4, 8.7, 9.0	–20.00 to +6.50	0.05 (–3.00)	varies w/power	8.4
IDEAL OPTICS, INC.	Ideal Soft	polymacon, 38.6%, lathe-cut	14.0	8.6, 8.9	–20.00 to +20.00	0.06	12.4 to 11.4	
				8.3	–20.00 to Pl			
KONTUR KONTACT LENS CO.	Kontur 55 Custom Sphere	methafilcon A, 55%, lathe-cut	12.0 to 16.0	7.00 to 9.80	+30.00 to –30.00			18.8
	Kontur 55 Sphere	methafilcon A, 55%, lathe-cut	15.0	8.3, 8.6, 8.9	+10.00 to –20.00	0.10 to 0.40	8.0	18.8
METRO OPTICS, INC.	Metro Lite Light Blue Visibility Tint	polymacon, 38%, lathe-cut	13.5	8.3, 8.6, 8.9	–20.00 to +20.00 in 0.50 steps above ±7.00	0.10	9.0	8.4
			14.0	Series M	Pl to –7.00	0.06		
	Metro Soft II	polymacon, 38%, lathe-cut	13.5	8.3, 8.6, 8.9	–20.00 to +20.00 in 0.50 steps above ±7.00	0.10 (–3.00)	9.0	8.4
	Metro Soft II Series M	polymacon, 38%, lathe-cut	14.0	Series M	Pl to –7.00 in 0.25 steps	0.06 (–3.00)	9.0	8.4
	Satureyes Available with Light Blue Visibility Tint or Clear	hioxifilcon A, 55%, lathe-cut	14.2	8.1, 8.4, 8.7	+10.00 to –10.00 in 0.50 steps above ±7.00	0.14 (–3.00)	9.0	20.0
OCU-EASE OPTICAL PRODUCTS INC.	Ocuflex 53 Handling tint available.	ocufilcon B, 53%, lathe-cut	14.0, 14.5, 15.0	8.2, 8.4, 8.6, 8.8, interchangeable	–20.00 to +12.00	0.13 (–); 0.18 (+)	8.0	18.1
	Ocuflex 53 Handling tint available. Other parameters available upon request.	ocufilcon B, 53%, lathe-cut	14.0, 14.5, 15.0	8.2, 8.4, 8.6, 8.8, interchangeable	12.25 to +20.00	varies	8.0	18.1
	Ocuflex 65 Spherical	ocufilcon E, 65%, lathe-cut	14.5, 15.0	8.45, 8.65, 8.85, interchangeable	–20.00 to +12.00		8.0	22.0 ± 2.0
OCULAR SCIENCES, INC.	EDGE® III Edge to Edge Visibility Tint	polymacon, 38%, cast-molded	14.0	8.3, 8.6, 8.9	–0.25 to –8.00 in 0.50 steps above –6.00	0.10 (–3.00)	8.0 to 12.5	8.4

DAILY WEAR SPHERICAL (CONTINUED)

MFR.	LENS	MATERIAL, % H_2O, PROCESS	DIAMETER (mm)	BASE CURVE (mm)	POWER (D)	CENTER THICKNESS (mm)	OPTIC ZONE (mm)	dK+ VALUE
OCULAR SCIENCES, INC.	EDGE® III Thin Edge to Edge Visibility Tint	polymacon, 38%, cast-molded	14.5	8.4, 8.7, 9.0	–0.25 to –8.00 in 0.50 steps above –6.00	0.07 (–3.00)	8.0 to 13.0	8.4
	Hydron Mini	polymacon, 38%, lathe-cut	13.0	8.1 to 8.9 in 0.20 steps	Pl to ±20.00 in 0.50 steps above ±10.00	0.10 (–3.00)	8.0 to 11.0	8.4
	Hydron Zero 6 Softblue (plus) Full Iris Visibility Tint	polymacon, 38%, lathed/molded	14.0	8.4, 8.7, 9.0	+0.25 to +10.00 in 0.50 steps above +5.00	variable	8.0	8.4
	Hydron Zero 6 Softblue Full Iris Visibility Tint	polymacon, 38%, lathed/molded	14.0	8.4, 8.7, 9.0	–0.25 to –10.00 in 0.50 steps above –6.00	0.06 (–3.00)	8.0 to 12.50	8.4
OPTECH, INC.	Fre–Flex® Bandage Lens	focofilcon A, 55%, lathe-cut	17.0	10.2	plano	0.14	N/A	15.5
	Free–Flex® Custom	focofilcon A, 55%, lathe-cut	10.0 to 17.5		–40.00 to +40.00	varies	varies	15.5
	Free-Flex® Custom Keratoconus	focofilcon A, 55%, lathe-cut	14.0	8.4	–40.00 to +40.00	0.30	6.10 to 9.45	15.5
	Free-Flex® Custom Piggyback	focofilcon A, 55%, lathe-cut	10.0 to 17.5	6.0, 11.0	any Pl groove diameter	varies	varies	15.5
	Free-Flex® Pediatric Diagnostic Set	focofilcon A, 55%, lathe-cut	7.4, 7.6, 7.8, 8.4	12.5, 13.0, 13.5, 14.0	+20.00	0.38	6.7	15.5
	Fre–Flex® Stock	focofilcon A, 55%, lathe-cut	14.0 15.0	8.6 9.2	–20.00 to +20.00	0.10 (–3.00), 0.13 (–3.00)	8.0 (–3.00)	15.5
PARAGON VISION SCIENCES, FLEXLENS™ PRODUCTS	Flexlens Custom Piggyback Also available in methafilcon A, 55%.	hefilcon A, 45%, lathe-cut	12.5 to 16.0 in 0.50 steps	6.00 to 10.80 in 0.30 steps	anterior cutout, 6.5 to 12.5mm	0.15	varies	11.3
	Flexlens Custom Sphere Also available in methafilcon A, 55%.	hefilcon A, 45%, lathe-cut	12.5 to 22.0 in 0.50 steps	6.20 to 11.00 in 0.30 steps	+50.00 to –50.00	0.10 (–3.00), 0.25 (+3.00)	varies	11.3
	Flexlens Harrison Keratoconus Also available in methafilcon A, 55%.	hefilcon A, 45%, lathe-cut	10.0 to 16.0 in 0.50 steps	6.00 to 9.90 in 0.30 steps	–20.00 to +30.00	varies	varies	11.3
	Flexlens Harrison Post Refractive Surgery Lens Also available in methafilcon A, 55%.	hefilcon A, 45%	10.0 to 16.0 in 0.50 steps	6.00 to 9.90 in 0.30 steps	–20.00 to +30.00 in 0.50 steps	0.28	varies	11.3

DAILY WEAR SPHERICAL (CONTINUED)

MFR.	LENS	MATERIAL, % H_2O, PROCESS	DIAMETER (mm)	BASE CURVE (mm)	POWER (D)	CENTER THICKNESS (mm)	OPTIC ZONE (mm)	dK+ VALUE
PARAGON VISION SCIENCES, FLEXLENS™ PRODUCTS	Flexlens Pediatric	hefilcon A, 45%, lathe-cut	10.0 to 16.0 in 0.50 steps	6.00 to 10.80 in 0.30 steps	Pl to +50.00	varies	varies	11.3
	Also available in methafilcon A, 55%.							
	Flexlens Tricurve Keratoconus	hefilcon A, 45%, lathe-cut	10.0 to 16.0 in 0.50 steps	6.00 to 9.90 in 0.30 steps	+30.00 to –20.00	varies	varies	11.3
	Also available in methafilcon A, 55%.							
PREMIER CONTACT LENS, CO., LLC	Softact II	polymacon, 38%, lathe-cut	14.0	8.4, 8.7, 9.0	–20.00 to +20.00 in 0.25 steps to ±12.00 and in 0.50 steps over ±12.00	0.06 to 0.32	varies	8.4
SODERBERG CONTACT LENS	Continental Spherical	ocufilcon B, 53%, lathe-cut	12.0 to 22.0	6.4 to 15.5	±40.00	varies	varies	16.5
	Flexlens Custom Sphere Visibility Tint	helfilcon B*, 45%, lathe-cut	12.5 to 22.0 in 0.50 steps	6.2 to11.0 in 0.30 steps	±50.00	varies	varies	11.3
	*Also available in methafilcon A, 55%.							
SUNSOFT	Revolution™ Light Blue Visibility Tint	methafilcon A, 55%, patented molding process	14.0	8.5	Pl to –10.00 in 0.25 steps	varies w/power; 0.10 (–3.00)	8.0	18.8
				8.7	+4.00 to –6.00 in 0.25 steps			
	Sunflex®	methafilcon A, 55%, lathe-cut	15.0	8.3, 8.6, 8.9	+10.00 to –20.00 in 0.50 steps above –10.00	0.10; 0.13 (–3.00)	8.0	18.8
	Sunflex® Prism Ballast	methafilcon A, 55%, lathe-cut	15.0	8.3, 8.9	+10.00 to –20.00 in 0.50 steps above –10.00	0.10; 0.13 (–3.00)	8.0	18.8
UNILENS CORP.	Sof-Form® II	polymacon, 38%, lathe-cut	14.0	8.3, 8.5, 8.7, 8.9	+9.75 to –10.00 in 0.25 steps	0.07 (–3.00)	8.0	8.4
	Sof-Form® II Custom	polymacon, 38%, lathe-cut	any	any	any			
	Sof-Form® 55 Spherical	methafilcon A, 55%, lathe-cut	14.0 15.0	8.3, 8.6, 8.9	+9.75 to –10.00 in 0.25 steps	0.06 (Pl)	8.0	18.8
	Sof-Form® 55 Custom	methafilcon A, 55%, lathe-cut	any	any	any			
UNITED CONTACT LENS, INC.	UCL 55%	ocufilcon C, 55%	14.0	8.3	sph: +20.00 to –20.00 in 0.50 steps after ±9.00	0.13 (–3.00)	8.0 to 8.5	18.8
			14.5, 15.0	8.3, 8.6, 8.9				
VALLEY CONTAX	Flexlens Custom Spheres	hefilcon A, 45%, available with handling tint; lathe-cut, prism ballast	12.5 to 16.0 in 0.50 steps	6.2 to 11.0 in 0.30 steps	–10.50 to –20.00 in 0.25 steps; –20.50 to –30.00 in 0.50 steps; +10.00 to +30.00 in 0.50 steps	NA	NA	NA

DAILY WEAR SPHERICAL (CONTINUED)

MFR.	LENS	MATERIAL, % H_2O, PROCESS	DIAMETER (mm)	BASE CURVE (mm)	POWER (D)	CENTER THICKNESS (mm)	OPTIC ZONE (mm)	dK+ VALUE
VALLEY CONTAX	Flexlens Custom Spheres	methafilcon A, 55%, available clear or with enhancer tint; lathe-cut, prism ballast	12.5 to 16.0 in 0.50 steps; 16.5 to 22.0 in 0.50 steps	6.2 to 11.0 in 0.30 steps; 9.0 to 10.0 in 0.50 steps	–30.00 (1.00); +30.00 (1.00); –10.00 to +10.00 in 0.25 steps	NA	NA	NA
	Flexlens Standard Spheres	hefilcon A, 45%, available with handling tint; lathe-cut methafilcon A, 55%, available clear or with enhancer tint; lathe-cut	14.5, 15.0	8.3 to 9.2 in 0.30 steps	–10.00 to +10.00 in 0.25 steps	NA	NA	NA
WESLEY-JESSEN	Aquaflex® Spheres	tetrafilcon A, 43%	13.2 (standard Vault minus)	0: 9.1 I: 8.8 II: 8.5 III: 8.2 IV: 7.9	Pl to –9.75 in 0.25 steps	0.14 (–3.00)	11.4	9.3
	Aquaflex® Spheres	tetrafilcon A, 43%	13.8 (super Vault Thin™ minus)	I 9.1 II: 8.8 III: 8.5 IV: 8.2	–0.25 to –20.00 in 0.25 steps	0.06 (–3.00)	12.0	9.3
	Aquaflex® Spheres	tetrafilcon A, 43%	13.8 (super Vault Thin™ low plus)	I: 9.1 II: 8.8 III: 8.5 IV: 8.2	+0.25 to +9.75 in 0.25 steps	0.21 (+3.00)	9.0	9.3
	ClearView™	polymacon, 38%, lathe-cut	13.8	8.4, 8.7	+4.00 to –10.00	0.08 (–3.00)	5.1	8.4
	CSI® Daily Wear Clear	crofilcon A, 38.6%, lathe-cut	13.8 14.8	8.0, 8.3, 8.6 8.6, 8.9, 9.35	+8.00 to –20.00 in 0.50 steps above –10.00 Pl to –20.00 in 0.50 steps above –10.00	0.06 (–3.00)	10.9 to 6.5	13.0
	CSI® Daily Wear Locator Tint Visibility Tint Edge to Edge	crofilcon A, 38.6%, lathe-cut	13.8	8.0, 8.3, 8.6	+8.00 to –6.00	0.06 (–3.00)	10.9 to 6.5	13.0
	DuraSoft 2® LiteTint Visibility Tint	phemfilcon A, 38%, lathe-cut	14.5 13.8	8.3, 8.6, 9.0 8.0, 8.3, 8.6 (median)	+20.00 to –20.00 in 0.25 steps to ±10.00, 0.50 steps over ±10.00	0.05 (–3.00)	8.0	9.03
	DuraSoft 2® D_2-T3 D_2-T4	phemfilcon A, 38%, lathe-cut	13.5 (D_2-T3) 14.5 (D_2-T4)	8.2 steep, 8.5 median 8.3 steep, 8.6 median, 9.0 flat	+20.00 to –20.00 in 0.25 steps to ±10.00, 0.50 steps over ±10.00	0.07 (–3.00)	8.0	9.03
	SOFT MATE B	bufilcon A, 45%, lathe-cut	14.3 14.8 Call for Parameters	8.7 9.0	+7.00 to –12.00 in 0.50 steps above +4.00 & –6.00	0.07 (–3.00)	7.5 to 8.0	12.0
WESTCON CONTACT LENS CO., INC.	Horizon™ 38 Custom	polymacon, 38%, lathe-cut	Call for Parameters			varies	varies	8.4
	Horizon™ 38 Sphere	polymacon, 38%, lathe-cut	14.0, 14.5	8.3, 8.6, 8.9,	+10.00 to –20.00	0.06 (–3.00)	varies	8.4

DAILY WEAR SPHERICAL (CONTINUED)

MFR.	LENS	MATERIAL, % H_2O, PROCESS	DIAMETER (mm)	BASE CURVE (mm)	POWER (D)	CENTER THICKNESS (mm)	OPTIC ZONE (mm)	dK+ VALUE
WESTCON CONTACT LENS CO., INC.	Horizon™ 55 Sphere	methafilcon A, 55%, lathe-cut	14.0, 14.5, 15.0	8.3, 8.6, 8.9	+10.00 to –20.00	varies	varies	18.8
	Horizon™ Custom	methafilcon A, 55%, lathe-cut	Call for Parameters			varies	varies	18.8
	Horizon™ Specialty Division I	methafilcon A, 55%, lathe-cut	14.0, 14.5, 15.0	8.0, 8.3, 8.6, 8.9, 9.2	+20.00 to –20.00	varies	varies	18.8
	Horizon™ Specialty Division II	methafilcon A, 55%, lathe-cut	15.5 to 18.0 in 0.50 steps	8.6 to 10.1 in 0.30 steps	+20.00 to –20.00	varies	varies	18.8
	Horizon™ Specialty Division III (Large Diameter)	methafilcon A, 55%, lathe-cut	Call for Specifications.		PI	varies	varies	18.8
	PRISM Sphere	methafilcon A, 55%, lathe-cut	14.5	8.6	+2.00 to –6.00 in 0.25 steps	varies	varies	18.8

TORIC

MFR.	LENS	MATERIAL, % H_2O, PROCESS	DIAMETER (mm)	BASE CURVE (mm)	SPHERE POWER (D)	CYLINDER POWER (D), SURFACE TYPE	AXIS	CENTER THICKNESS (mm)	OPTIC ZONE (mm)	dK+ VALUE
ACCUGEL LABS	Accugel Toric Division I Daily Wear	droxifilcon, 46.6%, lathe-cut, prism ballast	14.0	8.9	+3.00 to –6.00	–0.75 to –3.00, back surface	any 5° increments	all lenticular	8.0	18.0
	Accugel Toric Division 2 Daily Wear	droxifilcon, 46.6%, lathe-cut, prism ballast	14.0	8.0 to 9.2 in 0.1 steps	+10.00 to –20.00	–0.50 to –5.00, back surface	any	all lenticular	8.0	18.0
	Accugel Toric Division 3 Daily Wear	droxifilcon, 46.6%, lathe-cut, prism ballast	<14.0 >14.0	<8.0 >9.2	>+10.00 or >–20.00	> –5.00, back surface	8.0	all lenticular	8.0	18.0
	Toric Markings: all lenses dot at 6:00.									
ACCULENS, INC.	Accusoft Toric Division I Daily Wear	methafilcon A, 55%, lathe-cut, prism ballast	15.0	8.6, 8.9	+4.00 to –6.00	–0.75 to –2.00, back surface	any 1° steps	0.10 to 0.25	8.0	18.8
	Accusoft Toric Division II Daily Wear	methafilcon A, 55%, lathe-cut, prism ballast	15.0	8.3, 8.6, 8.9	+4.25 to +10.00, –6.25 to –10.00	–2.25 to –3.50, back surface	any 1° steps	0.10 to 0.45	8.0	18.8
	Accusoft Toric Division III Daily Wear	methafilcon A, 55%, lathe-cut prism ballast	15.0	8.3, 8.6, 8.9	–10.00 to –20.00	–3.75 to –5.00 back surface	any 1° steps	0.10 to 0.45	8.0	18.8
	Toric Markings: all lenses dot at 6:00.									

TORIC (CONTINUED)

MFR.	LENS	MATERIAL, % H_2O, PROCESS	DIAMETER (mm)	BASE CURVE (mm)	SPHERE POWER (D)	CYLINDER POWER (D), SURFACE TYPE	AXIS	CENTER THICKNESS (mm)	OPTIC ZONE (mm)	dK+ VALUE
ALDEN OPTICAL LABS, INC.	**Alden Classic Toric** Daily Wear	polymacon, 38%, lathe-cut, prism ballast	13.0, 13.5, 14.0	7.7, 7.9, 8.1, 8.3, 8.5, 8.7, 8.9	Pl to ±30.00	–0.50 to –5.00, front surface	any, 1° steps			8.4
	Clear and Enhancer tint. Available with visitint. Custom designs also available. Colors available: Aqua, Azure, Blue, Brown, Gray, Green, Jade, Yellow, Walnut. All colors available in 3 saturations: #1 (light), #2 (medium), #3 (dark).									
AMERICAN BIOCURVE, INC.	**Biocurve Toric Division 1** Daily Wear	methafilcon A, 55%, prism ballast, 1.5pd	14.5	8.8	–6.00 to +3.00 in 0.25 steps	–0.75 to –2.00 in 0.25 steps	180° ± 20°, 1° steps; 90° ± 20°, 1° steps	0.08 to 0.18	8.0	18.8
	Biocurve Toric Division 2 Daily Wear	methafilcon A, 55%, prism ballast, 1.5pd	14.0, 14.5	8.4, 8.6, 8.8, 9.0	–20.00 to +10.00 in 0.25 steps	–0.75 to –3.00 in 0.25 steps	any, 1° steps	0.08 to 0.25	8.0	18.8
	Biocurve Toric Division 3 Daily Wear	methafilcon A, 55%, prism ballast, 1.5pd	14.0, 14.5 15.0	8.2 to 9.0 in 0.20 steps 8.9	–20.00 to +10.00 in 0.25 steps	–0.75 to –7.00 in 0.25 steps	any, 1° steps	0.08 to 0.25	8.0	18.8
	Toric Markings: all lenses laser line at 6:00. Inquire about availability of handling tint.									
	Biocurve Toric Division 4 Daily Wear	methafilcon A, 55%, prism ballast, 1.5pd	13.5, 14.0, 14.5 15.0	8.0 to 9.0 in 0.20 steps 8.9	any	–0.50 to –10.00 in 0.25 steps	any, 1° steps	0.08 to 0.30	8.0	18.8
	Toric Markings: all lenses laser line at 6:00. Inquire about availability of handling tint.									
AQUA-SITE	**Aqua-Cyl** Daily Wear	ocufilcon B, 53%, lathe-cut, prism ballast, thin zone	14.5 or custom	8.6, 8.8, 9.0, or custom	-25.00 to +10.00 or custom	–6.00 or custom, back surface	any	varies w/ power	8.0	15.4
	Toric Markings: scribe at 6:00. Double Slab Toric and Pediatric Custom lenses available.									
BAUSCH & LOMB	**Optima™ Toric Core** Daily Wear	hefilcon B, 45%, prism ballast	14.0	8.3, 8.6	+2.00 to –6.00	–0.75, –1.25, –1.75, –2.25; front surface	90°/180° ±30° in 5° increments	0.10 to 0.28	8.0	13.0
	Optima™ Toric Select Daily Wear	hefilcon B, 45%, prism ballast	14.0	8.3, 8.6	+2.25 to +6.00, –6.25 to –9.00	–2.75, –3.25, –3.75, –4.25; front surface	125° to 145°, 35° to 55° in 5° increments	0.10 to 0.33	8.0	13.0
	If lens contains any of the following parameters			8.9	any one of the above parameters					
	Toric Marking: 3 laser marks at 5:00, 6:00, 7:00 (30° apart).									
	SofLens 66 Toric Daily Wear Visibility tint	alphafilcon A, 66%, castmold Lo-Torque	14.5	8.5	plano to –5.00 in 0.25 steps	–0.75 D –1.25 D –1.75 D	10° increments around the clock	0.195 mm @ –3.00D	8.0	32
	Toric Markings: 3 marks at 5:00, 6:00, 7:00.									
BIO-COMPATIBLES EYECARE, INC.	**Proclear Tailor Made Toric** Daily Wear	omafilcon A, 59%, lathe-cut, prism ballast	13.6 to 15.2 in 0.20 steps	8.0 to 9.3 in 0.10 steps	+10.00 to –10.00 in 0.25 steps	–0.75 to –5.00 in 0.25 steps; back surface	0° to 180°	varies	8.0	25
	Toric Markings: scribe at 3:00, 6:00, 9:00.									
CALIFORNIA OPTICS	**C.O.Soft 55 Toric™ Division I** Daily Wear	methafilcon A, 55%, lathe-cut, prism ballast	15.0	8.9	+3.00 to –6.00	–0.75 to –2.00 in 0.25 steps, back surface	any	varies	8.0	18.8

TORIC (CONTINUED)

MFR.	LENS	MATERIAL, % H_2O, PROCESS	DIAMETER (mm)	BASE CURVE (mm)	SPHERE POWER (D)	CYLINDER POWER (D), SURFACE TYPE	AXIS	CENTER THICKNESS (mm)	OPTIC ZONE (mm)	dK+ VALUE
CALIFORNIA OPTICS	**C.O.Soft 55 Toric™ Division II** Daily Wear	methafilcon A, 55%, lathe-cut, prism ballast	14.5, 15.0	8.6, 8.9	+10.00 to –10.00	–0.75 to –5.00 in 0.25 steps, back surface	any	varies	8.0	18.8
	C.O.Soft 55 Toric™ Division III Daily Wear Toric Markings: dot at 6:00.	methafilcon A, 55%, lathe-cut, prism ballast	15.0	9.2	+10.00 to –10.00	–0.75 to –5.00 in 0.25 steps, back surface	any	varies	8.0	18.8
	C.O.Soft 55 Toric™ Division III Custom Daily Wear	methafilcon A, 55%, lathe-cut, prism ballast	14.0, 14.5, 15.0	8.3, 8.6, 8.9, 9.2	+20.00 to –20.00	–0.75 to –10.00, back surface	any	varies	8.0	18.8
	C.O.Soft 55 Toric™ Custom FT Daily Wear	methafilcon A, 55%, lathe-cut, prism ballast or thin zone	14.0, 14.5, 15.0	8.6, 8.9, 9.2	+4.00 to –6.00	–0.75 to –2.50 front surface	any	varies	8.0	18.8
	C.O.Soft 55 Toric™ Custom BT Daily Wear Toric Markings: dot at 6:00.	methafilcon A, 55%, lathe-cut, thin zone	14.0, 14.5, 15.0	8.6, 8.9, 9.2	Pl to ±20.00	–0.75 to –5.00 in 0.25 steps	any	varies	8.0	18.8
CIBA VISION CORP.	**TORISOFT®** Daily Wear	tefilcon, 37.5%, lathe-cut, thin zones	14.5	8.6, 8.9, 9.2* *minus powers only	+4.00 to –6.00 in 0.25 steps; –6.50, –7.00	–1.00, –1.75; double front surface	8.6 & 8.9 BC: 0° to 180°; 10° steps. 9.2 BC: 180° ± 20°, 90° ± 20°; 10° steps	0.095 (–3.00), 0.175 (+3.00)	8.9	
				8.6, 8.9	Pl to –6.00 in 0.25 steps, –6.50,–7.00	–2.50	180° ± 90°, 90° ± 20°			
CONTINENTAL SOFT LENS, INC.	**CONTINENTAL Toric** Daily Wear Toric Markings: scribe at 6:00.	ocufilcon B, 53%, lathe-cut, prism ballast	13.0 to 15.0	7.0 to 10.0	±25.00	–0.50 to –11.00	all	varies	varies	16.5
COOPERVISION, INC.	**Alliance™ Toric** Blue Handling Tint Daily Wear	tetrafilcon A, 43%, fully lathe-cut	15.0	8.5, 8.8, 9.1	+20.00 to –20.00 in 0.25 steps	–0.50 to –10.00 in 0.25 steps	0° to 180°; 1° steps	0.06 (–), 0.25 (+)	8.0	9.3
	Cooper Toric™ Handling Tint Daily Wear	tetrafilcon A, 42.5%, lathe-cut front, cast-mold back	14.4	8.4, 8.7	+4.00 to –6.00 in 0.25 steps	–0.75, –1.25, –1.75, –2.25	full circle 0° to 180°, 10° steps	0.06 to 0.17	8.6	9.3
	Hydrasoft® Toric Div. I Standard Toric Daily Wear Flexible Wear	methafilcon B, 55%, lathe-cut, pitch polished, prism ballast	14.2 15.0	8.6 8.9	+3.00 to –6.00 in 0.25 steps	–0.75 to –2.00 in 0.25 steps, back surface	180° ± 20°, 90° ± 20°; 1° steps	0.07 to 0.40	8.0	18.8

TORIC (CONTINUED)

MFR.	LENS	MATERIAL, % H_2O, PROCESS	DIAMETER (mm)	BASE CURVE (mm)	SPHERE POWER (D)	CYLINDER POWER (D), SURFACE TYPE	AXIS	CENTER THICKNESS (mm)	OPTIC ZONE (mm)	dK+ VALUE
COOPER-VISION, INC.	**Hydrasoft® Toric Div. II Specialty Toric** Daily Wear Flexible Wear	methafilcon B, 55%, lathe-cut, pitch polished, prism ballast	15.0 14.2	8.6, 8.9 8.3, 8.6	+10.00 to −20.00 in 0.25 steps	−0.75 to −5.00 in 0.25 steps, back surface	any, 1° steps	0.07 to 0.40	8.0	18.8
	Hydrasoft® Toric Div. III Aphakic Daily Wear Flexible Wear	methafilcon B, 55%, lathe-cut, pitch polished, prism ballast	15.0	8.6, 8.9	+10.25 to +20.00 in 0.25 steps	−0.75 to −10.00, back surface	any, 1° steps	varies	8.0	18.8
	Hydrasoft® Toric Div. III Custom Toric Daily Wear Flexible Wear	methafilcon B, 55%, lathe-cut, pitch polished, prism ballast	15.0 14.2	8.3, 8.6, 8.9, 9.2 8.3, 8.6	+10.00 to −20.00 in 0.25 steps	−0.50 to −10.00 in 0.25 steps, back surface	any, 1° steps	0.07 to 0.40	8.0	18.8
	Preference® Toric™ Handling Tint Daily Wear	tetrafilcon A, 42.5%, lathe-cut front, cast-mold back, prism ballast	14.4	8.4, 8.7	+6.00 to −8.00 in 0.25 steps; −6.50 to −8.00 in −0.50 steps	−0.75, −1.25, −1.75, −2.25, back surface	full circle, 5° steps	0.06 to 0.17 varies with power	8.6	9.3
	Toric Markings: all lenses laser mark at 6:00.									
GREAT LAKES CONTACT LENS, INC.	**Flexlens Toric Lens Paragon Vision Sciences**	either hefilcon A, 45% or methafilcon, 55%, lathe prism ballast	14.0 to 15.0	8.0 to 9.2	Sphere +6.75 to −10.00	−0.50 to −10.00	any axis			
KONTUR KONTACT LENS CO.	**Kontur 55 Toric Div. I** Daily Wear	methafilcon A, lathe-cut, prism ballast	15.0	8.6, 8.9	+4.00 to −6.00	−0.75 to −2.00, back surface	any, 1° steps	0.10 to 0.25	8.0	18.8
	Kontur 55 Toric Div. II Daily Wear	methafilcon A, lathe-cut, prism ballast	15.0	8.3, 8.6, 8.9	+4.25 to +10.00, −6.25 to −10.00	−2.25 to −3.50, back surface	any, 1° steps	0.10 to 0.45	8.0	18.8
	Kontur 55 Toric Div. III Daily Wear	methafilcon A, lathe-cut, prism ballast	15.0	8.3, 8.6, 8.9	−10.00 to −20.00	−3.75 to −5.00, back surface	any, 1° steps	0.10 to 0.45	8.0	18.8
	Kontur 55 Toric Div. IV Custom Daily Wear	methafilcon A, lathe-cut, prism ballast	15.0	8.3, 8.6, 8.9	over +10.00 or −20.00	over −5.00, back surface	any, 1° steps	0.10 to 0.45	8.0	18.8
	Toric Markings: all lenses dot at 6:00.									
METRO OPTICS, INC.	**Metro Soft II Toric** Daily Wear	polymacon, 38%, lathe-cut, prism ballast	14.0	8.4, 8.7, 9.0	−10.00 to +10.00 in 0.25 steps	−0.75 to −6.00 in 0.25 steps	any, 5° steps	0.14	9.0	8.4
	Satureyes Toric Light Blue Visibility Tint also available Daily Wear	hioxifilcon A, 55%, lathe-cut, prism ballast	14.2	8.4, 8.7	−10.00 to +5.00 in 0.25 steps	−0.75 to −6.00 in 0.25 steps	any, 5° steps	0.14	9.0	20
	Toric Markings: Three vertical lines, one at 6:00 and one 10° to either side.									

TORIC (CONTINUED)

MFR.	LENS	MATERIAL, % H_2O, PROCESS	DIAMETER (mm)	BASE CURVE (mm)	SPHERE POWER (D)	CYLINDER POWER (D), SURFACE TYPE	AXIS	CENTER THICKNESS (mm)	OPTIC ZONE (mm)	dK+ VALUE
OCU-EASE OPTICAL PRODUCTS, INC.	**Ocuflex 53 Custom** Daily Wear	ocufilcon B, 53%, lathe-cut, prism ballast	14.5 15.0 (No interchanges)	8.6 8.8	+4.00 to −7.00	−0.50 to −3.00 in 0.25 steps, back surface	any	0.13 (−), 0.18 (+)	8.0	18.1
	Other parameters available on request. Handling tint available.									
	Ocuflex 53 Special Custom Daily Wear	ocufilcon B, 53%, lathe-cut, prism ballast	14.0 14.5, 15.0 (interchangeable)	8.4, 8.6, 8.8, 9.0	−20.00 to +20.00	−0.50 to −6.00 in 0.25 steps, back surface	any	0.13 (−), 0.18 (+)	8.0	18.1
	Handling tint available.									
	Ocuflex 65 Daily Wear	ocufilcon E, 65%, lathe-cut, prism ballast	14.0, 14.5, 15.0	8.45, 8.65, 8.85	+12.00 to −12.50 in 0.25 steps	up to −6.00 in 0.25 steps, back surface	any	0.13 (−), 0.18 (+)	8.0	22.0
	Toric Markings: all lenses black dot and scribe at 6:00.									
OCULAR SCIENCES, INC.	**HYDRON ULTRA T** Daily Wear	ocufilcon A, 43%, Spin-cast, front surface 0.75 pd BD	14.5	8.7 nominal	Pl to −6.00	−1.00, −1.50, −2.00; front surface	full circle, 10° steps	0.15 (−3.00)	8.0 (−3.00)	11.2
	Toric Markings: scribe at 5:30, 6:00, 6:30.									
OPTECH, INC.	**Fre-Flex® Custom Toric** Daily Wear	focofilcon A, 55%, lathe-cut, 2.0 pd BD	15.0	9.0	−20.00 to +20.00	−0.50 to −8.00, back surface	any	0.14 (−3.00)	8.0	15.5
	Fre-Flex® Special Design Toric Daily Wear	focofilcon A, 55%, lathe-cut, 2.0 pd BD	10.00 to 17.5	6.0 to 11.0	−30.00 to +30.00	−0.50 to −16.00, back surface	any	0.14 (−3.00)	8.0	15.5
	Toric Markings: all lenses scribe at 6:00.									
PARAGON VISION SCIENCES, FLEXLENS™ PRODUCTS	**Flexlens Toric** Daily Wear	hefilcon A, 45%, lathe-cut, prism ballast	14.0, 14.5, 15.0	8.0, 8.3, 8.6, 8.9, 9.2	+6.75 to −10.00	−0.50 to −10.00, back surface	any	0.15 (−3.00), 0.26 (+3.00)	7.5	11.3
	Also available in Methafilcon A, 55%.									
SODERBERG CONTACT LENS	**Continental Toric**	ocufilcon B, 53%, lathe-cut, prism ballast	13.0 to 15.0	7.0 to 10.0	±25.00	−0.50 to −11.00	any	varies	varies	16.5
	Toric Marking: Scribe at 6:00.									
	Flexlens Toric Visibility Tint	hefilcon B*, 45%, lathe-cut, prism ballast	14.0, 14.5, 15.0	8.0, 8.3, 8.6, 8.9, 9.2	+6.75 to −10.00 in 0.25 steps	−0.50 to −10.00 in 0.25 steps	any	varies	7.5	11.3
	Toric Marking: PVS laser marking. *Also available in methafilcon A, 55%.									
SPECIALTY ULTRAVI - SION, INC.	**Specialty T-FRP™** Daily Wear	ocufilcon A, 43%, molded, prism ballast	14.5	Aspheric (8.9 nominal)	+1.00 to −8.00 (−6.00 to −8.00 in 0.50D)	−1.00, 1.50, −2.00, front surface	10° around the clock	0.15	8.0	11.2
	Toric Markings: scribe at 6:00 and 15° on either side.									
SUNSOFT	**Eclipse®** Daily Wear Extended Wear Flexible Wear	methafilcon A, 55%, lathe-cut, prism ballast	14.5	8.7	+2.00 to −6.00 in 0.25 steps	−0.75 to −2.50 in 0.25 steps, back surface	180° ± 30°, 90° ± 30°; 5° steps	varies w/ power	8.8	18.8

TORIC (CONTINUED)

MFR.	LENS	MATERIAL, % H_2O, PROCESS	DIAMETER (mm)	BASE CURVE (mm)	SPHERE POWER (D)	CYLINDER POWER (D), SURFACE TYPE	AXIS	CENTER THICKNESS (mm)	OPTIC ZONE (mm)	dK+ VALUE
SUNSOFT	**Multiples®, Div. I** Visibility Tint Daily Wear Extended Wear Flexible Wear	methafilcon A, 55%, front molded/ back lathed, prism ballast	15.0	8.5, 8.9	+3.00 to −6.00 in 0.25 steps	−0.50 to −2.00 in 0.25 steps	full circle 5° steps	varies w/power	8.0	18.8
	Multiples®, Div. II Visibility Tint Daily Wear Extended Wear Flexible Wear	methafilcon A, 55%, front molded/ back lathed, prism ballast	15.0	8.5, 8.9	+6.00 to −8.00 in 0.25 steps	−0.50 to −6.00 in 0.25 steps	full circle 5° steps	varies w/power	8.0	18.8
	Sunsoft Toric 15.0® Div. I Daily Wear Extended Wear Flexible Wear	methafilcon A, 55%, lathe-cut, prism ballast	15.0	8.9	+3.00 to −6.00 in 0.25 steps	−0.75 to −2.00 in 0.25 steps, back surface	180° ± 20°, 90° ± 20°; 1° steps	varies w/ power	8.0	18.8
	Sunsoft Toric 15.0® Div. II Daily Wear Extended Wear Flexible Wear	methafilcon A, 55%, lathe-cut, prism ballast	15.0	8.3, 8.9	+10.00 to −20.00 in 0.25 steps	−0.75 to −7.00 in 0.25 steps, back surface	any	varies w/ power	8.0	18.8
	Toric Markings: all lenses target mark at 6:00.									
UNILENS CORP. USA	**Sof-Form® 55 Toric** Daily Wear	methafilcon A, 55%, lathe-cut, prism ballast	15.0	8.6, 8.9	+9.75 to −20.00	−0.25 to −5.00	1° steps	0.07 to 0.40	8.0 (−), 7.0 (+)	18.8
	Sof-Form® 55 Toric Custom	methafilcon A, 55%	any	any	any	any	any	any	any	18.8
	Toric Markings: All lenses laser scribe at 6:00.									
UNITED CONTACT LENS, INC.	**UCL Bifocal Toric** Daily Wear	ocufilcon C, 55%, prism ballast	14.5 to 15.0	8.3, 8.6, 8.9, 9.2	+20.00 to −20.00 in 0.25 steps	−1.00 to −3.00	any	0.08 to 0.30	1.7, 2.0, 2.3, 2.6, 2.9, 3.2	18.8
	UCL Custom Daily Wear	ocufilcon C, 55%, prism ballast	Any parameters not listed below					0.40	8.5	18.8
	UCL Multi Toric Daily Wear	ocufilcon C, 55%, prism ballast	14.7	8.3, 8.7, 9.0	+20.00 to −20.00 in 0.25 steps	−1.00 to −3.00	any	0.06 to 0.22	8.0 to 10.0	18.8
	UCL Toric Daily Wear	ocufilcon C, 55%, prism ballast	14.5 to 15.0	8.3, 8.6, 8.9, 9.2	+20.00 to −20.00	−0.75 to −7.00	any	0.12	8.0	18.8
	Toric Markings: all lenses scribe at 6:00.									

TORIC (CONTINUED)

MFR.	LENS	MATERIAL, % H_2O, PROCESS	DIAMETER (mm)	BASE CURVE (mm)	SPHERE POWER (D)	CYLINDER POWER (D), SURFACE TYPE	AXIS	CENTER THICKNESS (mm)	OPTIC ZONE (mm)	dK+ VALUE
VALLEY CONTAX	**Flexlens Custom Toric** Visibility Tint (methafilcon only) Daily Wear	hefilcon A, 45%, (available w/ handling tint), methafilcon A, 55%, (available clear or w/ enhancer tint), both numerically controlled lathe-cut, prism ballast	14.0, 14.5, 15.0	8.0, 8.3, 8.6, 8.9, 9.2	any	any	any	NA	NA	NA
	Flexlens Standard Toric Visibility Tint (methafilcon only) Daily Wear	hefilcon A, 45%, (available w/ handling tint), methafilcon A, 55%, (available clear or w/ enhancer tint), both numerically controlled lathe-cut, prism ballast	14.0, 14.5, 15.0	8.0, 8.3, 8.6, 8.9, 9.2	+6.75 to –10.00 in 0.25 steps	–0.50 to –10.00 in 0.25 steps	any	NA	NA	NA
WESLEY-JESSEN	**CSI® Toric** Edge to Edge Visibility Tint Daily Wear	crofilcon A, 38.6%, lathe-cut, back surface toric	14.0	8.3, 8.6	+4.00 to –8.00	–1.00, –1.75, –2.50; back surface	10° around the clock; 180° ± 20°, 90° ± 20°; 5° steps	0.10 (–3.00)	7.6	13.0
	Toric Markings: 3 laser marks (6:00 and 20° on either side).									
	D2® OptiFit® Toric Daily Wear Handling Tint	phemfilcon A, 38%, lathe-cut, thin zone	14.5	standard: median	+4.00 to –8.00	–0.75 to –2.75 in 0.50 steps, back surface	full circle 5° steps	0.07	8.0	9.03
				made-to-order: steep, median, flat	+10.00 to –20.00	–0.75 to –9.75 in 0.50 steps, back surface				
	Toric Markings: 3 laser marks (6:00 and 20° on either side).									
	D2® OptiFit® Toric for light eyes	phemfilcon A, 38%, lathe-cut, thin zone	14.5	made-to-order: steep, median, flat	+10.00 to –20.00	–0.75 to –9.75 in 0.50 steps, back surface	full circle 5° steps	0.07	8.0	9.03
	Colors: Aquamarine, Jade Green, Sky Blue, Violet-Blue									
	D2® OptiFit® Toric Colors	phemfilcon A, 38%, lathe-cut, thin zone	14.5	made-to-order: steep, median, flat	+4.00 to –8.00 in 0.25 steps; +4.50 to +10.00 in 0.50 steps; –8.50 to –20.00 in 0.50 steps	–0.75 to –9.75 in 0.50 steps, back surface	full circle 5° steps	0.07	8.0	9.03

TORIC (CONTINUED)

MFR.	LENS	MATERIAL, % H_2O, PROCESS	DIAMETER (mm)	BASE CURVE (mm)	SPHERE POWER (D) (mm)	CYLINDER POWER (D) SURFACE TYPE	AXIS	CENTER THICKNESS (mm)	OPTIC ZONE (mm)	dK+ VALUE
WESLEY-JESSEN	**D3® OptiFit® Toric** Flexible Wear	phemfilcon A, 55%, lathe-cut, thin zone	14.5	standard: median	+4.00 to –8.00	–0.75 to –2.25 in 0.50 steps, back surface	180° ± 30°, 90° ± 30°; 5° steps	0.07	8.0	16.1
				made-to-order: steep, median, flat	+4.00 to –8.00	–0.75 to –5.75 in 0.50 steps, back surface	full circle 5° steps			
	Toric Markings: bi-directional at 6:00, 20° apart.									
	D3® OptiFit® Toric Colors Flexible Wear	phemfilcon A, 55%, lathe-cut, thin zone	14.5	all made-to-order: steep, median, flat	+4.00 to –8.00	–0.75 to –5.75 in 0.50 steps, back surface	full circle 5° steps	0.07	5.0	16.1
	Colors: Aqua, Baby Blue, Sapphire Blue, Chestnut Brown, Mist Gray, Emerald Green, Jade Green, Hazel, Violet. **Complements Colors:** Blue, Blue-Violet, Brown, Gray, Green. Toric Markings: bi-directional at 6:00, 20° apart.									
	Hydrocurve 3 Extended Wear Flexible Wear	bufilcon A, 55%, lathe-cut, prism ballast	14.5	8.8	+4.00 to –8.00	–0.75, –1.25, –2.00; back surface	1° steps around the clock	0.06 (–3.00)	8.2	16
	Toric Markings: 3 laser marks (6:00 and 30° either side), axis number lasered on lens.									
WESTCON CONTACT LENS CO., INC.	**Horizon 55 Toric ™ (STD)** Daily Wear	methafilcon A, 55%, lathe-cut, prism ballast, 1.8 pd BD	14.5	8.6	+2.00 to –6.00 in 0.25 steps	–0.75 to –2.50 in 0.25 steps, back surface	180° ± 30°, 90° ± 30°; 1° steps	varies	varies	18.8
	Toric Markings: scribe mark at 6:00.									
	Horizon™ Toric Custom Daily Wear	methafilcon A, 55%, lathe-cut, prism ballast, 1.8 pd BD	Please contact Westcon Contact Lens Co. for any parameters not listed above.							
	Horizon™ Toric Division I Daily Wear	methafilcon A, 55%, lathe-cut, prism ballast, 1.8 pd BD	14.0, 14.5, 15.0	8.3, 8.6, 8.9	+4.00 to –8.00 in 0.25 steps	–0.75 to –2.50 in 0.25 steps, back surface	any, 1° steps	varies	varies	18.8
	Toric Markings: scribe at 6:00.									
	Horizon™ Toric Division II Daily Wear	methafilcon A, 55%, lathe-cut, prism ballast, 1.8 pd BD	14.0, 14.5, 15.0	8.3, 8.6, 8.9	+10.00 to –10.00 in 0.25 steps	–0.75 to –5.00 in 0.25 steps, back surface	any, 1° steps	varies	varies	18.8
	Toric Markings: scribe at 6:00.									
	Horizon™ Toric Division III Daily Wear	methafilcon A, 55%, lathe-cut, prism ballast, 1.8 pd BD	14.0, 14.5, 15.0	8.3, 8.6, 8.9, 9.2	+20.00 to –20.00 in 0.25 steps	–0.75 to –10.00 in 0.25 steps, back surface	any, 1° steps	varies	varies	18.8
	Toric Markings: scribe at 6:00.									
	Westhin Toric Division I	polymacon*, 38%, lathe-cut, double slab-off	14.2	8.6	+4.00 to –7.00	–0.75 to –2.00		varies	varies	8.4
	Division II			8.3, 8.6, 8.9	+9.75 to –12.00	–0.75 to –4.00				
	Division III Daily Wear			8.3, 8.6, 8.9	+20.00 to –20.00	–0.75 to –6.00, back surface				
	*Also available in methafilcon A, 55%, with dk+ value of 18.8. Toric Markings: mark at 3:00 and 9:00.									

BIFOCAL/MULTIFOCAL

MFR.	LENS	MATERIAL, % H_2O, PROCESS	DIAMETER (mm)	BASE CURVE (mm)	POWER (D)	ADDITIONS POWER (D), TYPE	CENTER THICKNESS (mm)	OPTIC ZONE (mm)	dK+ VALUE
ACUITY ONE, LLC	**Ultravue P** Daily Wear Visibility handling tint	Benz 45G, 49%, lathed-cut	14.5	8.3, 8.6, 8.9	Standard: +4.00 to –6.00 in 0.25 steps Custom: +20.00 to –20.00 in 0.25 steps	Standard +1.50 to +3.00 in 0.50 steps Custom: +1.00 to +4.00 in 0.50 steps	(–) 0.15 to 0.20 (+) 0.20 to +0.96	2.3, 2.6, 2.9	15×10^{-11}
	Ultravue C Daily Wear Visibility handling tint	Benz 45G, 49%, lathed-cut	14.5	8.3, 8.6, 8.9	Standard: +4.00 to –6.00 in 0.25 steps Custom: +20.00 to –20.00 in 0.25 steps	Varies up to 4.00 spherical central near aspherical annular intermediate and distance	(–) 0.15 to 0.20 (+) 0.20 to +0.96	1.7, 2.0, 2.3	15×10^{-11}
AERO CONTACT LENS, INC.	**LifeStyle 4-Vue™ Series 1** Daily Wear	polymacon, 38%, lathe-cut	14.5	8.8	+7.00 to –8.00 in 0.25 steps	zonal	0.17		16.0
	LifeStyle 4-Vue™ Series 2 Daily Wear	polymacon, 38%, lathe-cut	14.5	8.5	+7.00 to –8.00 in 0.25 steps	+1.75, zonal	0.17		16.0
	LifeStyle 4-Vue™ Hi-Add Daily Wear	polymacon, 38%, lathe-cut	14.5	8.5, 8.8	+7.00 to –8.00 in 0.25 steps	+2.50, zonal			16.0
	LifeStyle X-tra™ Daily Wear	polymacon, 38%, lathe-cut	14.5	8.5	+4.00 to –5.00	+1.00, +1.50, +2.00, +2.50			16.0
	SimulVue™ Daily Wear	hefilcon A, 45%, lathe-cut	14.5	8.4, 8.7, 9.0	–8.00 to +6.00 in 0.25 steps	+2.00, +2.50, +3.00; seg. sizes: 2.35, 2.55; concentric bifocal	0.14	9.0	11.6
	SoftSITE® Blue Visibility Tint Daily Wear	polymacon, 38%	14.5	8.4, 8.7	–8.00 to +6.00 in 0.25 steps	progressive +2.50 of ADD, or custom		N/A	N/A
	Unilens™ Daily Wear	hefilcon A, 45%, lathe-cut, aspheric	14.5	8.4, 8.7, 9.0	–8.00 to +6.00 in 0.25 steps	varies up to +1.75 through aspheric optics, near center	0.16	9.0	11.6
	Unilens™ 38 Blue Visibility Tint	polymacon, 38%	14.5	8.4, 8.7, 9.0	–8.00 to +6.00 in 0.25 steps	varies up to +1.75 through aspheric optics			16.0
BAUSCH & LOMB	**Occasions™ Multifocal** Visibility Tint Daily Wear	polymacon, 38.6%, shape-cast	14.0	8.6	+6.00 to –9.00 in 0.25 steps	+1.50, aspheric simultaneous	0.08 to 0.21	8.0 to 9.0	9.2
BLANCHARD CONTACT LENS	**Esstech PS Multifocal** Daily Wear	polymacon, 38%, lathe-cut	14.0	8.3, 8.7, 9.1	+6.00 to –6.00 in 0.25 steps	progressive adds +1.75 to +2.25, front aspheric near, intermediate & distance seen concurrently	0.14 (–) 0.15 (+)		8.4

BIFOCAL/MULTIFOCAL (CONTINUED)

MFR.	LENS	MATERIAL, % H_2O, PROCESS	DIAMETER (mm)	BASE CURVE (mm)	POWER (D)	ADDITIONS POWER (D), TYPE	CENTER THICKNESS (mm)	OPTIC ZONE (mm)	dK+ VALUE
BLANCHARD CONTACT LENS	**Esstech PSD Multifocal** Daily Wear	polymacon, 38%, lathe-cut	14.0	8.3, 8.7, 9.1	+6.00 to –6.00 in 0.25 steps	progressive adds up to +1.50, front aspheric near, intermediate & distance seen concurrently	0.14 (–) 0.15 (+)		8.4
	Quattro™ Aspheric Multifocal Blue Visitint	Hioxifilcon B, 48%, lathed	14.5	8.4, 8.8	+6.00 to –6.00 in 0.25 steps	progressive adds up to +2.25D, Front Aspheric near, intermediate and distance seen concurrently	0.08 (–) 0.12 (+)		15
CALIFORNIA OPTICS	**C.O.Soft 55 Custom Progressive Multifocal** Daily Wear	methafilcon A, 55%, lathe-cut	14.5, 15.0	8.3, 8.6, 8.9, 9.2	Pl to ±10.00	+1.00 to +3.50, center near progressive design	varies		18.8
	C.O.Soft 55 Toric Custom Progressive Multifocal Daily Wear Toric markings: dot at 6:00.	methafilcon A, 55%, lathe-cut, prism ballast, back surface	14.5, 15.0	8.3, 8.6, 8.9, 9.2	Pl to ±10.00, cyl: –0.75 to –5.00	+1.00 to +3.50, center near progressive design	varies		18.8
	C.O.Soft 55 Custom Bi-focal Daily Wear	methafilcon A, 55%, lathe-cut	14.5, 15.0	8.3, 8.6, 8.9, 9.2	Pl to ±10.00	+1.00 to +3.50, center add concentric design	varies	1.5, 2.0, 2.1, 3.0 for near	18.8
	C.O.Soft 55 Custom Bi-focal Toric Daily Wear Toric markings: dot at 6:00.	methafilcon A, 55%, lathe-cut, prism ballast, back surface	14.5, 15.0	8.3, 8.6, 8.9, 9.2	Pl to ±10.00 cyl: –0.75 to –5.00	+1.00 to +3.50, center near concentric design	varies	1.5, 2.0, 2.1, 3.0 for near	18.8
	C.O.Soft 55 Crescent Bi-focal Custom Daily Wear	methafilcon A, 55%, lathe-cut	14.5, 15.0	8.6, 8.9, 9.2	Pl to ±10.00	+1.00 to +4.00, one piece crescent design	varies		18.8
	C.O.Soft 55 Toric Crescent Bi-focal Custom Daily Wear Toric markings: dot at 6:00.	methafilcon A, 55%, lathe-cut, prism ballast, back surface	14.5, 15.0	8.6, 8.9, 9.2	Pl to ±10.00, cyl: –0.75 to –5.00	+1.00 to +4.00, one piece crescent design	varies		18.8
IDEAL OPTICS, INC.	**PolyVue®** Daily Wear	polymacon, 38%, lathe-cut	14.0	8.3, 8.6	+8.00 to –10.00	L: to +2.00 or H: to +3.25, front aspheric	N/A	N/A	N/A
LENS DYNAMICS, INC.	**Esstech** Daily Wear	polymacon, 38%, lathe-cut	14.5	8.3, 8.7, 9.1	+6.00 to –7.00	to +2.50	15.0		
THE LIFESTYLE COMPANY, INC.	**LifeStyle 4-Vue™** Daily Wear	polymacon, 38%, lathe-cut	14.5	8.5, 8.8	+7.00 to –8.00 in 0.25 steps	progressive to +1.50	0.17 (–3.00)	8.7 to 6.4	

BIFOCAL/MULTIFOCAL (CONTINUED)

MFR.	LENS	MATERIAL, % H_2O, PROCESS	DIAMETER (mm)	BASE CURVE (mm)	POWER (D)	ADDITIONS POWER (D), TYPE	CENTER THICKNESS (mm)	OPTIC ZONE (mm)	dK+ VALUE
THE LIFESTYLE COMPANY, INC.	**LifeStyle 4-Vue™ Hi-Add** Daily Wear	polymacon, 38%, lathe-cut	14.5	8.5, 8.8	+7.00 to –6.00 in 0.25 steps	progressive to +2.25			
	LifeStyle MV2, Monovision 2 Daily Wear Light Blue Handling Tint	polymacon, 38%, cast molded	14.5	8.5	Distance Lens –5.00 to +4.00 Near Lens –4.00 to +5.00	Concentric central area for intermediated range in both distance & near lenses.		Central intermediate area very small	
	Note: The distance lens is spherical with distance in periphery or lens with a very narrow concentric intermediate power in the center, and the Near lens is spherical with near in the periphery of lens with corrections intermediate power in the center.								
	LifeStyle X-tra™ Daily Wear	polymacon, 38%, lathe-cut	14.5	8.5	+4.00 to –5.00 in 0.25 steps	multifocal +1.00, +1.50, +2.00, +2.50	0.17 (–3.00)		
OCU-EASE OPTICAL PRODUCTS, INC.	**Ocuflex 53** Daily Wear Handling tint available	ocufilcon B, 53%, lathe-cut, aspheric	14.5	8.2, 8.4, 8.6,	+6.00 to –8.00 in 0.25 steps	L: +0.75 to +2.00 or H: +2.25 to +3.00 aspheric	0.13 (–) 0.23 (+)	center add 1.5mm or 1.9mm, 8.0 distance	18.1
	Ocuflex 53 Toric Multifocal Daily Wear Handling tint available	ocufilcon B, 53%, lathe-cut, aspheric	14.5	8.2, 8.4, 8.6	+4.00 to –7.00 in 0.25 steps Cyl: up to –3.00 in 0.25 steps, Axis: 90° ± 20°, 180 ± 20°	L: +0.75 to +2.00 or H: +2.25 to +3.00 aspheric	0.13 (–) 0.23 (+)	center add 1.9mm, 8.0 distance	18.1
OCULAR SCIENCES, INC.	**Hydron Echelon** Daily Wear	polymacon, 38%, lathed-molded	14.0	8.7	+4.00 to –6.00	+1.50, +2.00, +2.50; concentric, phase plate (4.55 & 4.21)	0.08 (–3.00)	8.7 to 6.4	8.4
PREFERRED OPTICS, INC.	**ADDvantage 38 High ADD Series** Daily Wear	polymacon, 38%, lathe-cut	14.0	8.4, 8.7	+10.00 to –6.00	progressive adds +1.50 to +2.50, aspheric near intermediate & distance seen concurrently	0.15 (–) 0.17 (+)	8.0	8.4
	ADDvantage 38 Low ADD Series Daily Wear	polymacon, 38%, lathe-cut	14.0	8.4, 8.7	+6.00 to –6.00	progressive adds to +1.50, aspheric near intermediate & distance seen concurrently	0.15 (–) 0.17 (+)	8.0	8.4
PREMIER CONTACT LENS CO.	**FULFOCUS** Daily Wear	polymacon, 38%, lathe-cut	14.2	8.4	+4.00 to –6.50 in 0.25 steps	+1.00 to +3.00, aspheric	0.06 to 0.32	varies w/ power	8.6
				8.7	+6.00 to –12.50 in 0.25 steps				8.4
				9.0	+4.00 to –6.50				
SODERBERG CONTACT LENS	**Lifestyle 4-Vue™**	polymacon, 38%, lathe-cut	14.5	8.5, 8.8	+7.00 to –8.00 in 0.25 steps	to +1.75 progressive	0.17	16.0	
	Lifestyle 4-Vue™ Hi-Add	polymacon, 38%, lathe-cut	14.5	8.5, 8.8	+7.00 to –8.00 in 0.25 steps	to +2.50 progressive		16.0	

BIFOCAL/MULTIFOCAL (CONTINUED)

MFR.	LENS	MATERIAL, % H_2O, PROCESS	DIAMETER (mm)	BASE CURVE (mm)	POWER (D)	ADDITIONS POWER (D), TYPE	CENTER THICKNESS (mm)	OPTIC ZONE (mm)	dK+ VALUE
SODERBERG CONTACT LENS	**Lifestyle MV2**	polymacon, 38%, lathe-cut	14.5	8.5	Distance +4.00 to –5.00 in 0.25 steps; near +5.00 to –4.00 in 0.25 steps	monovision	varies	varies	16.0
	SimulVue™	hefilcon A, 45%, lathe-cut	14.5	8.4, 8.7, 9.0	–8.00 to +6.00 in 0.25 steps	+2.00, +2.50, +3.00 concentric bifocal seg sizes 2.35, 2.55	0.14	9.0	11.6
	SoftSITE® Visibility Tint	polymacon, 38%, lathe-cut	14.5	8.4, 8.7	–8.00 to +6.00 in 0.25 steps	to +2.50 progressive	0.10	8.0	8.4
	Ultravue C	Benz 45 G, 48%, lathe-cut	14.5	8.3, 8.6, 8.9	±20.00 in 0.25 steps	+100 to +400 in 0.50 steps aspheric annular	varies	1.7, 2.0, 2.3	15 x 10^{-11}
	Ultravue P	Benz 45 G, 48%, lathe-cut	14.5	8.3, 8.6, 8.9	+4.00 to –6.00 in 0.25 steps	+1.50 to +3.00 in 0.50 steps sphere	varies	2.3, 2.6, 2.9	15 x 10^{-11}
	Unilens™	hefilcon A 45%, lathe-cut aspheric	14.5	8.4, 8.7, 9.0	–8.00 to +6.00 in 0.25 steps	to +1,75 aspheric progressive	0.16	9.0	11.3
	Unilens 38 Visibility Tint	polymacon, 38%, lathe-cut	14.5	8.4, 8.7, 9.0	–8.00 to +6.00 in 0.25 steps	to +1.75 front aspheric	0.10	8.0	8.4
SPECIALTY ULTRAVISION, INC.	**Specialty Progressive™** Blue Handling Tint Daily Wear	methafilcon A, 55%, fully molded	14.5	8.4 (–) 8.6 (+)	+4.00 to –5.00	+1.50, progressive aspheric (+3.00 effective add w/enhanced monovision fit)	0.18 (–3.00)	8.0	18.8
UNILENS CORP. USA	**SimulVue™ 38** Daily Wear Blue Visibility Tint	polymacon, 38%, lathe-cut	14.5	8.4, 8.7	–8.00 to +6.00 in 0.25D steps concentric bifocal, with near center add	+2.00, +2.50, +3.00, (+3.50 limited parameters) Seg. Size 2.35, 2.55	0.10	8.0	8.4
	SoftSITE® Daily Wear Blue Visibility Tint	polymacon, 38%, lathe-cut	14.5	8.4, 8.7	–8.00 to +8.00 in 0.25 steps	+1.75 to +2.50 of ADD, multiple front aspheres	0.10	8.0	8.4
	Custom parameters available. Planned replacement program available.								
	Unilens™ 38 Blue Visibility Tint	polymacon, 38%, lathe-cut	14.5	8.4, 8.7	+6.00 to –8.00 in 0.25 steps	up to +1.75, front surface aspheric	0.10	8.0	8.4
	Custom parameters available. Planned replacement program available.								
	Unilens E.M.A. Blue Visibility Tint	polymacon, 38%, lathe-cut	14.5	8.5, 8.8	–10.00 to +6.00D	Low add High add Front aspheric, near center	0.10	8.0	8.4
	6 month planned replacement.								

BIFOCAL/MULTIFOCAL (CONTINUED)

MFR.	LENS	MATERIAL, % H_2O, PROCESS	DIAMETER (mm)	BASE CURVE (mm)	POWER (D)	ADDITIONS POWER (D), TYPE	CENTER THICKNESS (mm)	OPTIC ZONE (mm)	dK+ VALUE
UNITED CONTACT LENS, INC.	**UCL Bifocal**	ocufilcon C, 55%	14.5, 15.0	8.3, 8.6, 8.9, 9.2	+20.00 to −20.00 in 0.25 steps	+1.00 to +3.50 in 0.25 steps	0.08, 0.30	1.7, 2.0, 2.3, 2.6, 2.9, 3.2	18.8
	UCL Multifocal	ocufilcon C, 55%	14.7	8.3, 8.7, 9.0	+20.00 to −20.00	up to +3.00	0.06 to 0.22	8.0 to 10.0	18.8
WESSLEY-JESSEN	**Hydrocurve II Bifocal** Custom Tint Available Daily Wear	bufilcon A, 45%, lathe-cut	14.8	9.0	+4.00 to −6.00	simultaneous dist. & near, aspheric +1.50 add w/ additional progressive power	0.05 (−3.00)	dist. 4	12.0
WESTCON CONTACT LENS CO., INC.	**Horizon™ 55 BI-CON**	methafilcon A, 55%, lathe-cut, double slab-off	14.0, 14.5, 15.0	8.3, 8.6, 8.9	+10.00 to −10.00 in 0.25 steps	+1.00 to +4.00 in 0.25 steps, concentric with near in center, simultaneous vision	0.14 to 0.37	8.3 distance; 2.0, 2.5, 3.0 & 3.5 near	18.8
	Horizon™ 55 BI-CON Toric	methafilcon A, 55%, lathe-cut, back surface toric, double slab-off	14.0, 14.5, 15.0	8.3, 8.6, 8.9	+10.00 to −10.00 in 0.25 steps, Cyl: −0.75 to −5.00 in 0.25 steps	+1.00 to +4.00 in 0.25 steps, concentric with near in center, simultaneous vision	0.14 to 0.37	8.3 distance; 2.0, 2.5, 3.0 & 3.5 near	18.8
	All cylinder axis range available in 1° steps. Custom lenses also available. Toric Markings: mark at 3:00 and 9:00.								
WORLD OPTICS INC.	**ABerCON™ D**	polymacon, 38.6%, computer-controlled lathe-cut	14	8.3, 8.7, 9.1	+10.00 to −10.00 in 0.25 steps	up to 1.50, masks astigmatism to 1.50, front aspheric, single vision w/up to 1.50D depth of focus	Averages: 0.16 (+), 0.13 (−)	10.0 to 14.0	8.4
	ABerCON™ N	polymacon, 38.6%, computer-controlled lathe-cut	14	8.3, 8.7, 9.1	+10.00 to −10.00 in 0.25 steps	up to +2.25, masks astigmatism to 1.50, front aspheric, center near, simultaneous mulitfocal	Averages: 0.17 (+), 0.15 (−)	9.5 to 12.0	8.4
	ABerCON™ N250	polymacon, 38.6%, computer-controlled lathe-cut	14	8.3, 8.7, 9.1	+10.00 to −10.00 in 0.25 steps	up to +2.75, masks astigmatism to 1.50, front aspheric, center near, simultaneous multifocal	Averages: 0.17 (+), 0.15 (−)	9.5 to 12.0	8.4

ENHANCER AND OPAQUE TINTS

MFR.	LENS	MATERIAL, % H_2O, PROCESS	DIAMETER (mm)	BASE CURVE (mm)	POWER (D)	CENTER THICKNESS (mm)	OPTIC ZONE (mm)	dK+ VALUE
ALDEN OPTICAL LABS, INC.	**Alden Classic Tinted** Daily Wear	polymacon, 38%, lathe-cut	13.0, 13.5, 14.0	7.7, 7.9, 8.1, 8.3, 8.5, 8.7, 8.9	Pl to ±30.00 Powers are the same as conventional contact lenses	0.12 (−3.00)	varies w/power	8.4
	Colors: Aqua, Azure, Blue, Brown, Gray, Green, Jade, Yellow, Walnut. All colors available in 3 saturations: #1 (light), #2 (medium), #3 (dark). Custom designs also available.							

ENHANCER AND OPAQUE TINTS (CONTINUED)

MFR.	LENS	MATERIAL, % H_2O, PROCESS	DIAMETER (mm)	BASE CURVE (mm)	POWER (D)	CENTER THICKNESS (mm)	OPTIC ZONE (mm)	dK+ VALUE
BAUSCH & LOMB	**Natural Tint-03** Flexible Wear	polymacon, 38.6 %	13.5		–1.00 to –5.00, –5.50, –6.00	0.035	12.4	9.2
	Transparent Colors: Aqua, Crystal Blue, Jade Green, Sable Brown (tint dia. 11mm solid).							
	Natural Tint-04 Flexible Wear	polymacon, 38.6%	14.5		–1.00 to –5.00, –5.50, –6.00; Pl (daily wear)	0.035	13.6	9.2
	Transparent Colors: Aqua, Crystal Blue, Jade Green, Sable Brown (tint dia. 11mm solid).							
	Optima 38 Natural Tint	polymacon, 38.6%, cast-mold or RP III	14.0	8.4, 8.7	Pl +5.00 to –5.00 in 0.25 steps, –5.50 to –9.00 in 0.50 steps	0.06 (–), 0.095 to 0.19 (+)	8.0 to 10.0	9.2
	Transparent Colors: Aqua, Crystal Blue, Jade Green (tint dia. 11mm solid).							
	SofLens® Series Natural Tint-B3 Daily Wear	polymacon, 38.6%, spin-cast	13.5		–0.25 to –5.00, –5.50, –6.00	0.12	12.1	9.2
	Colors: Aqua, Blue, Brown, Green (tint dia. 11mm solid).							
	SofLens® Series Natural Tint-U3 Daily Wear	polymacon, 38.6%, spin-cast	13.5		–1.00 to –5.00, –5.50, –6.00	0.07	12.4	9.2
	Colors: Aqua, Blue, Brown, Green (tint dia. 11mm solid).							
	SofLens® Series Natural Tint-U4 Daily Wear	polymacon, 38.6%, spin-cast	14.5		–1.00 to –5.00, –5.50, –6.00	0.07	13.6	9.2
	Colors: Aqua, Blue, Brown, Green (tint dia. 11mm solid).							
CIBA VISION CORP.	**CIBASOFT® SoftColors®** Daily Wear	tefilcon, 37.5%, lathe-cut	13.8	8.3, 8.6, 8.9	+6.00 to –6.00 in 0.25 steps,–6.50 to –10.00 in 0.50 steps	0.07 (–3.00) 0.14 (+3.00)	varies w/power (7.0 to 12.0)	8.9
			14.5	8.6, 8.9, 9.2	Pl to –6.00 in 0.25 steps, –6.50 to –10.00 in 0.50 steps			
	Colors: Amber, Aqua, Blue, Royal Blue, Green, Evergreen.							
	ILLUSIONS® Opaque Daily Wear	tefilcon, 37.5%, lathe-cut	13.8	8.3, 8.6, 8.9	+4.00 to –6.00 in 0.25 steps	0.10 (–3.00) 0.17 (+3.00)	varies w/power (7.0 to 12.8)	8.9
	Colors: Soft Amber, Deep Blue, Soft Blue, Deep Green, Soft Green, Grey.							
COOPERVISION INC.	**Natural Touch®**	polymacon, 38%, cast-mold	13.8	8.4, 8.7	+1.00 to –6.00	0.06 (–3.00)	5.1 (12.0 tint zone)	8.4
	Colors: Aqua Seas, Baby Blue, Hazel, Sophisticated Blue, Sultry Grey, Willow Green.							
	Vantage® Accents Daily Wear	tetrafilcon A, 43%, lathe-cut	14.0	8.3, 8.6	Pl to –6.50 in 0.25 steps	0.03 to 0.12	5.0 (clear pupil zone)	9.3
			14.4	8.7				
	Colors: Auburn, Misty Brown, Sky Blue, Spring Green, Turquoise, Violet Blue.							
	Vantage® Thin Accents Flexible Wear	tetrafilcon A, 43%, lathe-cut	14.0	8.4	Pl to –6.50 in 0.25 steps	0.03 to 0.082	12.8	9.3
			14.4	8.7			13.2	
	Colors: Auburn, Misty Brown, Sky Blue, Spring Green, Turquoise, Violet Blue.							
METRO OPTICS, INC.	**Metro Tint** Daily Wear	polymacon, 38%, lathe-cut	13.5	8.3, 8.6, 8.9	–20.00 to +20.00 in 0.50 steps above ±7.00	0.10	9.0	8.4
			14.0	Series M	Pl to –7.00	0.06		
	Colors: Aqua, Blue, Green.							

ENHANCER AND OPAQUE TINTS (CONTINUED)

MFR.	LENS	MATERIAL, % H_2O, PROCESS	DIAMETER (mm)	BASE CURVE (mm)	POWER (D)	CENTER THICKNESS (mm)	OPTIC ZONE (mm)	dK+ VALUE
OCULAR SCIENCES, INC.	**Hydron Versa-Scribe Softints** Daily Wear Flexible Wear Extended Wear	polymacon, 38%, cast-mold	14.0	8.6	Pl to – 6.00	0.04 (–3.00)	8.0	8.4
	Colors: Aqua, Blue, Green, Full iris tint.							
WESLEY-JESSEN	**DuraSoft® 2 Colors** Daily Wear	phemfilcon A, 38%, lathe-cut	14.5	8.3, 8.6	+4.00 to –6.00	0.07 (3.00)	5.0 (clear pupil zone)	9.03
	Colors: Blue, Gray, Green, Hazel.							
	DuraSoft® 2 Colors for Light Eyes Daily Wear	phemfilcon A, 38%, lathe-cut	14.5	8.3 steep 8.6 median 9.0 flat	Pl to –4.00 +4.00 to –8.00 Pl to –4.00 all in 0.25 steps	0.07 (–3.00)	5.0 (clear pupil zone)	9.03
	Colors: Aquamarine, Jade Green, Sky Blue, Violet Blue.							
	DuraSoft® 3 Colors Flexible Wear	phemfilcon A, 55%, lathe-cut	14.5	8.6 median 8.3 steep 9.00 flat	–8.00 to +6.00 Pl to –4.00	0.05 (–3.00)	5.0 (clear pupil zone)	16.1
	Colors: Aqua-Opaque, Baby Blue-Enhance, Baby Blue-Opaque, Chestnut Brown-Opaque, Emerald Green-Opaque, Hazel-Opaque, Jade Green-Opaque, Misty Gray-Opaque, Sapphire Blue-Opaque, Violet-Opaque. All colors available in three base curves, powers +20.00 to –20.00. Call customer service for more information regarding custom designs.							
	DuraSoft® 3 Complements Colors Flexible Wear	phemfilcon A, 55%, lathe-cut	14.5	8.6 median	–8.00 to +6.00	0.05 (–3.00)	5.0 (clear pupil zone)	16.1
	Colors: Complements Blue, Complements Brown, Complements Green, Complements Blue-Violet, Complements Shadow Gray. All colors available in three base curves; powers +20.00 to –20.00 (0.25D steps up to ±10.00D, –0.50D steps above ±10.00D). Call customer service for more information regarding custom designs.							
	WildEyes Daily Wear	phemfilcon A, 55%, lathe-cut	14.5	8.6	Pl to –4.00	0.05 (–3.00)	5.0 (clear pupil zone)	16.1
	Designs: Wildfire, White-Out, Starry Eyed, Pool Shark, Zoomin', Hypnotica, Cat-Eye, Red Hot.							

PROSTHETIC/THERAPEUTIC

MFR.	LENS	MATERIAL, % H_2O, PROCESS	DIAMETER (mm)	BASE CURVE (mm)	POWER (D)	CENTER THICKNESS (mm)	OPTIC ZONE (mm)	dK+ VALUE
ALDEN OPTICAL LABS, INC.	**Alden Classic Prosthetic** Daily Wear	polymacon, 38%, lathe-cut	13.0, 13.5, 14.0	7.7, 7.9, 8.1, 8.3, 8.5, 8.7, 8.9	Pl to ±30.00	0.12 (–3.00)	varies w/power	8.4
	Colors: Opaque Black pupil-Diameter size: 2.0 to 13.0 in 0.50 steps (available on clear or standard transparent tinted lens). Opaque Black annular-Outside diameter size: 2.0 to 13.0 in 0.50 steps; inside diameter size: 1.0 to 8.0 in 0.50 steps (available on clear or standard transparent tinted lens). Custom designs also available.							
CALIFORNIA OPTICS	**C.O.Soft 55 Custom Sphere** Daily Wear	methafilcon A, 55%, lathe-cut	13.0, 15.0, 16.0, 18.0, 20.0, 25.0	7.5, 8.3, 8.6, 8.9, 9.2, 9.6, 10.5	Pl to ±30.00	varies	7.0 to 9.5	18.8
CONTINENTAL SOFT LENS, INC.	**Continental 45 Sphere** Clear Tint Daily Wear	hefilcon A, 45%, custom-lathed	12.00 to 17.5	7.50 to 10.50	Pl to ±30.00	varies	varies	13.2
COOPERVISION INC.	**Permalens® Therapeutic**	perfilcon A, 71%, lathe-cut	13.5 14.2 15.0	7.7, 8.0, 8.3 8.6 9.0	Pl Pl Pl	0.24		34.0

PROSTHETIC/THERAPEUTIC (CONTINUED)

MFR.	LENS	MATERIAL, % H_2O, PROCESS	DIAMETER (mm)	BASE CURVE (mm)	POWER (D)	CENTER THICKNESS (mm)	OPTIC ZONE (mm)	dK+ VALUE
CUSTOM COLOR CONTACTS	**Custom Made Prosthetic Lenses**	hema	varies	8.3, 8.6, 8.9 or custom	±spheres	varies	varies	varies
GREAT LAKES CONTACT LENSES, INC.	**Flexlens Harrison Keratoconus, Paragon Vision Sciences**	hefilcon A, 45%, methafilcon A, 55%, Lathe	10.0 to 16.0	6.0 to 9.9	–20.00 to +10.00			
	Flexlens Piggy Back Lens, Paragon Vision Sciences	hefilcon A, 45%, methafilcon A, 55%, Lathe	12.0 to 16.0	6.0 to 10.8	Anterior cut out. Power is put in RGP Lens.			
SODERBERG CONTACT LENS	**Flexlens Harrison Keratoconus** Visibility Tint Daily Wear	hefilcon A, 45%*, lathe-cut *Also available in methafilcon A, 55%.	10.0 to 16.0 in 0.5mm steps	6.0 to 9.9 in 0.3mm steps	–20.00 to +10.00 in 0.50 steps; –20.50 to +30.00 in 0.50 steps; –10.50 to +30.00 in 0.50 steps	varies	varies	11.3
	Flexlens Harrison Post-Refractive Surgery Lens (PRS) Visibility Tint Daily Wear	hefilcon A, 45%*, lathe-cut *Also available in methafilcon A, 55%.	10.0 to 16.0 in 0.5mm steps	6.0 to 9.9 in 0.3mm steps	–20.00 to +10.00 in 0.50 steps; –20.50 to –30.00 in 0.50 steps; +10.50 to +30.00 in 0.50 steps	varies	varies	11.3
	Flexlens Piggyback (RGP lens not included) Visibility Tint Daily Wear	hefilcon A, 45%*, lathe-cut *Also available in methafilcon A, 55%.	12.5 to 16.0 in 0.5mm steps	6.0 to 10.8 in 0.3mm steps		varies	6.5 to 12.5 anterior cut out	
	Flexlens Tri-Curve Keratoconus Visibility Tint Daily Wear	hefilcon A, 45%*, lathe-cut *Also available in methafilcon A, 55%.	10.0 to 16.0 in 0.5mm steps	6.0 to 9.9 in 0.3mm steps	–20.00 to +10.00 in 0.50 steps; –20.50 to –30.00 in 0.50 steps; +10.50 to +30.00 in 0.50 steps	varies	varies	11.3
VALLEY CONTAX	**Flexlens Adult Aphakic Lens** Visibility Tint (methafilcon only) Daily Wear Custom also available	hefilcon A, 45%, available w/ handling tint methafilcon A, 55%, available clear or w/enhancer tint; numerically controlled lathe-cut	12.5 to 16.0 in 0.50 steps	6.0 to 10.8 in 0.30 steps	Pl to +10.00 in 0.25 steps; +10.50 to +30.00 in 0.50 steps; +30.50 to +50.00 in 1.00 steps			

PROSTHETIC/THERAPEUTIC (CONTINUED)

MFR.	LENS	MATERIAL, % H_2O, PROCESS	DIAMETER (mm)	BASE CURVE (mm)	POWER (D)	CENTER THICKNESS (mm)	OPTIC ZONE (mm)	dK+ VALUE
VALLEY CONTAX	**Flexlens Harrison Keratoconus Lens** Visibility Tint (methafilcon only) Daily Wear Custom also available	hefilcon A, 45%, available w/ handling tint methafilcon A, 55%, available clear or w/enhancer tint; numerically controlled lathe-cut	10.0 to 16.0 in 0.50 steps	6.0 to 9.9 in 0.30 steps	–20.00 to +10.00 in 0.50 steps; –20.50 to –30.00 in 0.50 steps; +10.50 to +30.00 in 0.50 steps			
	Flexlens Harrison Post Refractive Surgery Lens Visibility Tint (methafilcon only) Daily Wear Custom also available	hefilcon A, 45%, available w/ handling tint methafilcon A, 55%, available clear or w/enhancer tint; numerically controlled lathe-cut	10.0 to 16.0 in 0.50 steps	6.0 to 9.9 in 0.30 steps	–20.00 to +10.00 in 0.50 steps; –20.50 to –30.00 in 0.50 steps; +10.50 to +30.00 in 0.50 steps			
	Flexlens Pediatric Aphakic Lens Visibility Tint (methafilcon only) Daily Wear Custom also available	hefilcon A, 45%, available w/ handling tint methafilcon A, 55%, available clear or w/enhancer tint; numerically controlled lathe-cut	10.0 to 16.0 in 0.50 steps	6.0 to 10.8 in 0.30 steps	Pl to +10.00 in 0.25 steps; +10.50 to +30.00 in 0.50 steps; +30.50 to +50.00 in 1.00 steps			
	Flexlens Piggy Back Lens Visibility Tint (methafilcon only) Daily Wear Custom also available Anterior cutout 6.5mm to 12.5mm.	hefilcon A, 45%, available w/ handling tint methafilcon A, 55%, available clear or w/enhancer tint; numerically controlled lathe-cut	12.5 to 16.0 in 0.50 steps	6.0 to 10.8 in 0.30 steps				
	Flexlens Tricurve Keratoconus Lens Visibility Tint (methafilcon only) Daily Wear Custom also available	hefilcon A, 45%, available w/ handling tint methafilcon A, 55%, available clear or w/enhancer tint; numerically controlled lathe-cut	10.0 to 16.0 in 0.50 steps	6.0 to 9.9 in 0.30 steps	–20.00 to +10.00 in 0.50 steps; –20.50 to –30.00 in 0.50 steps; +10.50 to +30.00 in 0.50 steps			
WESLEY-JESSEN SPECIAL EYES FOUNDATION	**DuraSoft® 2** Opaque & Enhancer tints available. Profits support vision education.	phemfilcon A, 55%, lathe-cut	13.8, 14.5	8.3, 8.6, 9.0	Pl to ±20.00		clear or black pupil 3.7 or 5.0 (made-to-order available) iris dia. 12.5	9.01

PROSTHETIC/THERAPEUTIC (CONTINUED)

MFR.	LENS	MATERIAL, % H_2O, PROCESS	DIAMETER (mm)	BASE CURVE (mm)	POWER (D)	CENTER THICKNESS (mm)	OPTIC ZONE (mm)	dK+ VALUE
WESLEY-JESSEN SPECIAL EYES FOUNDATION	**DuraSoft® 3**	phemfilcon A, 55%, lathe-cut	13.8, 14.5	8.3, 8.6, 9.0 (made-to-order available)	Pl to ±20.00		clear or black pupil 3.7 or 5.0 (made-to-order available) iris dia. 12.5	16.1
	Opaque & Enhancer tints available. Profits to support vision education. **Colors:** DuraSoft® Colors for Light Eyes enhancement colors: Aquamarine, Sky Blue, Violet Blue, Jade Green. DuraSoft® Colors opaque colors: Aqua, Baby Blue, Sapphire Blue, Black, Chestnut Brown, Misty Gray, Emerald Green, Jade Green, Hazel, Violet. DuraSoft® 3 Complements: Blue, Blue Violet, Brown, Shadow Gray, Green.							
	Photo Image Process	Now available. (Formerly available from Narcissus Eye Research Foundation.) Contact Wesley-Jessen for more information.						

PLANNED REPLACEMENT LENSES

MFR.	LENS	MATERIAL, % H_2O, PROCESS	DIAMETER (mm)	BASE CURVE (mm)	POWER (D)	CENTER THICKNESS (mm)	OPTIC ZONE (mm)	dK+ VALUE
BAUSCH & LOMB	**Gold Medalist Toric** Visibility Tint	hefilcon C, 57%, lathe-cut	14.0	8.3, 8.6	+4.00 to –6.00 in 0.25 steps; Cyl: –0.75, –1.25, –1.75; Axis: 90° ±20°, 180° ±20° in 10° steps	0.010 to 0.028	8.0	17
	Optima FW Visibility Tint Flexible Wear	polymacon, 38.6%, cast-mold or RP III	14.0	8.4, 8.7, 9.0	+4.00 to –9.00 in 0.25 steps	0.026 to 0.035	8.0 to 10.0	9.2
BIO-COMPATIBLES EYECARE, INC.	**Proclear™** Daily Wear (6-month replacement)	omafilcon A, 59%, phosphoryl-choline, lathe-cut	14.2	8.2, 8.5, 8.8	+6.00 to –8.00 in 0.25 steps; –8.50 to –10.00 in 0.50 steps; +6.50 to +10.00 in 0.50 steps	0.07 (–3.00)	9.0	33 (Boundary Layer Method) 25 (Corrected Edge Method)
	Proclear™ Compatibles Daily Wear (1-month replacement)	omafilcon A, 62%, phosphoryl-choline, cast-mold	14.2	8.6	Pl to –6.00 in 0.25 steps; –6.50 to –10.00 in 0.50 steps; +0.50 to +4.00 in 0.25 steps; +4.50 to +6.00 in 0.50 steps	0.065 (–3.00)		34 (Boundary Layer Method) 27 (Corrected Edge Method)
CALIFORNIA OPTICS	**C.O.SOFT 55 Sphere™**	methafilcon, 55%, lathe-cut	14.5	8.7	+4.00 to –6.00 in 0.25 steps	0.10 to 0.25	8.0	18.8
	C.O.SOFT 55 Toric™ Division I	methafilcon, 55%, lathe-cut prism ballast	14.5	8.7	+4.00 to –6.00; Cyl: –0.75 to –3.25 in 0.50 steps; Axis: 0° - 180° in 5° steps	variable	8.0	18.8
	C.O.SOFT 55 Toric™ Division II	methafilcon, 55%, lathe-cut prism ballast	14.5	8.7	+10.00 to –10.00; Cyl: –0.75 to –5.00; Axis: 0° - 180° in 5° steps	variable	8.0	18.8
	C.O.SOFT 55 Toric™ Division III	methafilcon, 55%, lathe-cut, prism ballast	any	any	±20.00; Cyl: –0.75 to –10.00; Axis: 0° - 180°	variable	8.0	18.8
	Toric Markings: dot at 6:00.							

PLANNED REPLACEMENT LENSES (CONTINUED)

MFR.	LENS	MATERIAL, % H_2O, PROCESS	DIAMETER (mm)	BASE CURVE (mm)	POWER (D)	CENTER THICKNESS (mm)	OPTIC ZONE (mm)	dK+ VALUE
CIBA VISION CORP.	**Focus® SoftColors®** Monthly Daily Wear Extended Wear Flexible Wear **Colors:** Aqua, Evergreen, Royal Blue.	vifilcon A, 55%, CIBACAST® mold	14.0	8.6, 8.9	–8.00 to +6.00 in 0.25 steps	0.10 (–3.00) 0.16 (+3.00)	7.8	16.0
	Focus® Toric Monthly Daily Wear Extended Wear Flexible Wear Toric Markings: 3, 6, 9° (back surface).	vifilcon A, 55%, CIBACAST® mold	14.5	8.9, 9.2	sphere: –6.00 to +4.00 in 0.25 steps; Cyl: –1.00, –1.75; 0° to 180° in 10° steps; Axis: 10° around clock	0.15 (–3.00) 0.26 (+3.00)	8.0	16.0
	Focus® Visitint® Monthly Daily Wear Extended Wear Flexible Wear	vifilcon A, 55%, CIBACAST® mold	14.0	8.6, 8.9	–8.00 to +6.00 in 0.25 steps; –8.50 to –10.00 in 0.50 steps	0.10 (–3.00) 0.16 (+3.00)	7.8	16.0
COOPERVISION INC.	**Frequency™ 55** Blue Handling Tint Daily Wear	methafilcon A, 55%, mold	14.2	8.7, 9.0	+8.00 to –10.00, –0.25 to –8.00	0.08 (–3.00)		
	Preference® Planned Replacement Light Blue Handling Tint Edge to Edge Flexible Wear	tetrafilcon A, 43%, lathe-cut	14.4	8.4, 8.7	–0.25 to –6.50 in 0.25 steps; –6.50 to –10.00 in 0.50 steps	0.03 to 0.082	13.2	9.3
	Preference® Standard Light Blue Handling Tint Edge to Edge Daily Wear	tetrafilcon A, 43%, lathe-cut	14.0 14.4	8.3, 8.6 8.7	–0.25 to –6.50 in 0.25 steps; –6.50 to –10.00 in 0.50 steps; Pl to +6.00 in 0.25 steps	0.03 to 0.12 (–) 0.08 to 0.23 (+)	12.8 13.2	9.3
	Preference® Toric™ Handling Tint Daily Wear Toric Markings: Laser at 6:00.	tetrafilcon A, 42.5%, lathe-cut	14.4	8.4, 8.7	sphere: +6.00 to –8.00 in 0.25 steps (0.50 steps after –6.00); Cyl: –0.75, –1.25, –1.75, –2.25; Axis: full circle in 5° steps	0.06 to 0.17 varies w/power	8.6	9.3
METRO OPTICS, INC.	**Satureyes** Available with Light Blue Visibility Tint or Clear	hioxifilcon A, 55%, lathe-cut	14.2	8.1, 8.4, 8.7	+10.00 to –10.00 in 0.50 steps above ±7.00	0.14 (–3.00)	9.0	20.0
OCULAR SCIENCES, INC.	**EDGE® III ProActive** Edge to Edge Visibility Tint Daily Wear	polymacon, 38%, cast-molded	14.0	8.7 8.4, 8.7, 9.0	+0.25 to +5.00 –0.25 to –8.00 in 0.50 steps above –6.00	Variable 0.06 (–3.00)	8.0 to 12.5	8.4

PLANNED REPLACEMENT LENSES (CONTINUED)

MFR.	LENS	MATERIAL, % H_2O, PROCESS	DIAMETER (mm)	BASE CURVE (mm)	POWER (D)	CENTER THICKNESS (mm)	OPTIC ZONE (mm)	dK+ VALUE
OCULAR SCIENCES, INC.	**EDGE® III ProActive XT** Edge to Edge Visibility Tint Daily Wear	polymacon, 38%, cast-molded	14.0	8.7	+0.25 to +5.00	varies	8.0 to 12.5	8.4
				8.4, 8.7, 9.0	−0.25 to −8.00 in 0.50 steps above −6.00	0.06 (−3.00)		
	Hydron ProActive 55 Edge to Edge Visibility Tint Daily Wear Extended Wear Flexible Wear	ocufilcon D, 55%, cast-molded	14.2	8.7	−0.25 to −10.00 in 0.50 steps above −6.00	0.09 (−3.00)	10.1	19.7
SUNSOFT	**Multiples®** Sphere Visibility Tint Daily Wear Extended Wear Flexible Wear	methafilcon A, 55%, front molded/ back lathed	15.0	8.5, 8.9	+6.00 to −8.00 in 0.25 steps	varies w/power, 0.16 (−3.00)	8.0	18.8
	Multiples® Toric Div. I Visibility Tint Daily Wear Extended Wear Flexible Wear	methafilcon A, 55%, front molded/back lathed, prism ballast	15.0	8.5, 8.9	Sphere: +3.00 to −6.00 in 0.25 steps; Cyl: −0.50 to −2.00 in 0.25 steps	varies w/power	8.0	18.8
	Toric Markings: target mark at 6:00.							
	Multiples® Toric Div. II Visibility Tint Daily Wear Extended Wear Flexible Wear	methafilcon A, 55%, front molded/back lathed, prism ballast	15.0	8.5, 8.9	Sphere: +6.00 to −8.00 in 0.25 steps; Cyl: −0.50 to −6.00 in 0.25 steps	varies w/power	8.0	18.8
	Toric Markings: target mark at 6:00.							
VISTAKON	**SUREVUE®** Visibility Tint UV blocker (≥ 70% UV-A, ≥ 95% UV-B)	etafilcon A, 58%, stabilized soft mold	14.0	8.4, 8.8	−0.50 to −6.00 in 0.25 steps; −6.50 to −9.00 in 0.50 steps	0.105 (−3.00)	8.0	28.0
			14.4	9.1	+0.50 to +6.00 in 0.25 steps	0.20(+3.00)		
	For use as 2-week daily wear frequent replacement lens.							
	VISTAVUE™ Visibility Tint	genfilcon A, 48%, stabilized soft mold	14.0	8.6	−0.50 to−6.00 in 0.25 steps; −6.50 to −9.00 in 0.50 steps	0.07 (−3.00)	8.0	13.0
	For use as 2-week daily wear frequent replacement lens.							
WESLEY-JESSEN	**Gentle Touch** Daily Wear Flexible Wear Non-ionic Non-HEMA	netrafilcon A, 65%, lathe-cut w/spc	14.5	8.2, 8.5	+6.00 to −10.00 in 0.50 steps above +4.00 and −6.00	0.10	9.6	34.5

DISPOSABLE LENSES

MFR.	LENS	MATERIAL, % H_2O, PROCESS	DIAMETER (mm)	BASE CURVE (mm)	POWER (D)	CENTER THICKNESS (mm)	OPTIC ZONE (mm)	dK+ VALUE
BAUSCH & LOMB	**Optima FW** Visibility Tint	polymacon, 38.6%, cast-mold or RP III	14.0	8.4, 8.7, 9.0	+4.00 to −9.00 in 0.25 steps	0.026 to 0.035	8.0 to 10.0	9.2

DISPOSABLE LENSES (CONTINUED)

MFR.	LENS	MATERIAL, % H_2O, PROCESS	DIAMETER (mm)	BASE CURVE (mm)	POWER (D)	CENTER THICKNESS (mm)	OPTIC ZONE (mm)	dK+ VALUE
BAUSCH & LOMB	**SeeQuence®** Visibility Tint	polymacon, 38.6%, spin-cast	14.0		–0.50 to –9.00 in 0.25 steps	0.035 varies w/power 0.032 to 0.038	13.6	9.2
	SofLens 66™ Visibility Tint	alphafilcon A, 66%, cast-mold	14.2	F/M S/M	+0.50 to +6.00, –0.50 to –6.00 in 0.25 steps (–6.50 to –9.00 in 0.50 steps) plus powers available in F/M only	0.09 to 0.12	9.0	32.0
CIBA VISION CORP.	**Focus®** 1-2 wks. Visitint (formerly NewVues®)	vifilcon A, 55%, CIBACAST® mold	14.0	8.4, 8.8	+4.00 to –6.00 in 0.25 steps; –6.50 to –10.00 in 0.50 steps	0.06 (–3.00) 0.12 (+3.00)	7.2	16.0
	Focus® 1-2 wks. soft colors (formerly NewVues®) SoftColors®) **Colors:** Aqua, Evergreen, Royal Blue.	vifilcon A, 55%, CIBACAST® mold	14.0	8.4, 8.8	+4.00 to –6.00 in 0.25 steps	0.06 (–3.00) 0.12 (–13.00)	7.2	16.0
	Focus® Dailies™ Daily Wear	nelfilcon A, 69%, lightstream	8.6	13.8	–0.50 to –6.00 in 0.25 steps	0.10 (–3.00)	7.6 to 8.0	26.0
OCULAR SCIENCES, INC.	**Hydron Biomedics 38** Edge to Edge Visibility Tint Flexible Wear Extended Wear	polymacon, 38%, cast-molded	14.0	8.6	–0.25 to –10.00 in –0.50 steps above –6.00	0.04 (–3.00)	8.0	8.4
	Hydron Biomedics 55 Edge to Edge Visibility Tint Flexible Wear Extended Wear	ocufilcon D, 55%, cast-molded	14.2	8.6, 8.9(–) 8.8 (+)	–0.25 to –10.00 in 0.50 steps above –6.00 +0.25 to +5.00	0.07 (–3.00) variable	8.0	19.7
SPECIALTY ULTRAVISION, INC.	**Specialty Choice A.B.™** Blue Handling Tint Daily Wear	methafilcon A, 55%, fully molded	14.5	8.7	+4.00 to –8.00	0.09 (–3.00)	8.5	18.8
VISTAKON	**1-Day ACUVUE®** For use as daily wear, single-use, daily disposable lens UV blocker (≥ 70% UV-A, ≥ 95% UV-B)	etafilcon A, 58%, stabilized soft mold	14.2	8.5, 9.0	–0.50 to –6.00 in 0.25 steps; –6.50 to –9.00 in 0.50 steps +0.50 to +6.00 in 0.25 steps	0.07 (–3.00) 0.20 (+3.00)	8.0	28.0
	ACUVUE® Visibility Tint UV blocker (≥ 70% UV-A, ≥ 95% UV-B) For use as 1 - 7 days single-use, EW disposable lens or 2wks DW frequent replacement lens. "AV" mark on front surface for inside/outside indication. Also available without "AV" mark.	etafilcon A, 58%, stabilized soft mold	14.0 14.4	8.4, 8.8 8.8 only 9.3 9.1	–0.50 to –6.00 in 0.25 steps; –6.50 to –9.00 in 0.50 steps –9.50 to –11.00 in 0.50 steps –0.50 to –6.00 in 0.25 steps; –6.50 to –9.00 in 0.50 steps +0.50 to +6.00 in 0.25 steps; +6.50 to +8.00 in 0.50 steps	0.07 (–3.00) 0.17 (+3.00)	8.0	28.0

DISPOSABLE LENSES (CONTINUED)

MFR.	LENS	MATERIAL, % H_2O, PROCESS	DIAMETER (mm)	BASE CURVE (mm)	POWER (D)	CENTER THICKNESS (mm)	OPTIC ZONE (mm)	dK+ VALUE
WESLEY-JESSEN	**Fresh Look Colors**	phemfilcon A, 55%, wet molding	14.5	median	+6.00 to –8.00 in 0.25 steps	0.08	9.0 (5.0 clear pupil zone)	16.1
	Colors: Blue, Green, Hazel, Violet.							
	Fresh Look Color Blends	phemfilcon A, 55%, wet molding	14.5	median	pl to –4.00 in 0.25 steps	0.08	9.0 (5.0 clear pupil zone)	16.1
	Colors: Blue, Brown, Gray, Green.							
	Fresh Look Color Enhancers	phemfilcon A, 55%, wet molding	14.5	median	+6.00 to –8.00 in 0.25 steps	0.08	9.0 (5.0 clear pupil zone)	16.1
	Colors: Aqua, Blue, Green.							
	Fresh Look Lite Tint	phemfilcon A, 55%, wet molding	14.5	median	+6.00 to –8.00 in 0.25 steps	0.08	9.0	16.1
	Fresh Look Toric	phemfilcon A, 55%, back surface, prism ballast, wet molding	14.5	median	Sphere: Pl to –6.00 in 0.25 steps; Cyl: –0.75, –1.25, –1.75; Axis: 90° & 180° ± 20° in 10° increments	0.11 (–3.00)	8.0	16.1
	PRECISION UV™ Visibility Tint Edge to Edge Daily Wear Extended Wear Flexible Wear	surfilcon A, 74%, molded (90% effective in blocking UV radiation)	14.4	8.4 8.7	+8.00 to –10.00 in 0.50 steps above +5.00 and –6.00 +10.00 to –16.00	0.14 (–3.00) 0.26 (+3.00)	8.18 (–3.00) 8.01 (+3.00)	38.9
WORLD OPTICS INC.	**ActiFresh™ 400** with UV blocker up to 98% SoftBlue, handling tint Daily Wear	2.7% MMA/nVP Copolymer non-ionic, lidosilcon, 73%, spincast	14.3	8.4, 8.8	+6.00 to –8.00 in 0.25 steps; –8.50 to –10.00 in 0.50 steps; –10.00 to –15.00 in 0.50 steps (8.8)	0.12 mm (–3.00DS)	8.0	36

DISPOSABLE/PLANNED REPLACEMENT BIFOCAL/MULTIFOCAL

MFR.	LENS	MATERIAL, % H_2O, PROCESS	DIAMETER (mm)	BASE CURVE (mm)	POWER (D)	ADDITIONS POWER (D), TYPE	CENTER THICKNESS (mm)	OPTIC ZONE (mm)	dK+ VALUE
BLANCHARD CONTACT LENS	**Quattro™** Aspheric Multifocal Blue visibility tint	hioxifilcon B, 48%, lathe-cut	14.5	8.8, 8.4	+6.00 to –6.00 in 0.25D steps	Progressive adds up to +2.25D, front aspheric; near, intermediate and distance seen concur-rently	0.08 (–) 0.12 (+)		15

DISPOSABLE/PLANNED REPLACEMENT BIFOCAL/MULTIFOCAL (CONTINUED)

MFR.	LENS	MATERIAL, % H_2O, PROCESS	DIAMETER (mm)	BASE CURVE (mm)	POWER (D)	ADDITIONS POWER (D), TYPE	CENTER THICKNESS (mm)	OPTIC ZONE (mm)	dK+ VALUE
SODERBERG CONTACT LENS	**Lifestyle MV2** Multifocal monthly replacement	polymacon, 38%, lathe-cut	14.5	8.5	Distance +400 to –500 in 0.25 steps; near +500 to –400 in 0.25 steps	monovision	varies	varies	16.0
	Lifestyle Xtra Multifocal	polymacon, 38%, lathe-cut	14.5	8.5	+4.00 to –5.00 in 0.25 steps	+1.00, +1.50, +2.00, +2.50 multifocal	varies	varies	16.0
	Lifestyle Xtra Multifocal quarterly replacement	polymacon, 38%, lathe-cut	14.5	8.5	+4.00 to –5.00 in 0.25 steps	+1.00, +1.50, +2.00, +2.50 multifocal	varies	varies	16.0
	Softsite Seasons Multifocal visibility tint quarterly replacement	polymacon, 38%, lathe-cut	14.5	8.4, 8.7	±8.00 in 0.25 steps	up to +2.50 progressive	0.10	8.0	16.0
SUNSOFT	**Additions™** Blue Handling Tint Daily Wear Flexible Wear Extended Wear Planned replacement quarterly.	methafilcon A, 55%, molded front/back lathed	14.2	8.4, 8.7	+6.00 to –6.00 in 0.25 steps	Add A +0.75 to +1.25D, Add B +1.50 to +2.00D, Add C +2.25 to +2.50D. aspheric with stabilized near center	varies w/power	8.0	18.8
VISTAKON	**Acuvue® Bifocal** Visibility tint UV blocker (≥ 70% UV-A, ≥ 95% UV-B)	etafilcon A, 58%, stabilized soft mold	14.2	8.5	Distance: +4.00 to –6.00 in 0.25 steps	Near adds: +1.00 to +2.50 in 0.50 steps, Design: 5 zones concentric, center distance	0.075 (–3.00) 0.165 (+3.00)	8.0	28.0

2. COMPARISON AND CONVERSION TABLES

TABLE 2

RELATIVE MAGNIFICATION PRODUCED BY CONTACT AND SPECTACLE LENSES

The percentage increase (or decrease) in the size of the retinal image afforded by contact lenses in comparison with orthodox spectacles fitted at 12 mm from the cornea.

SPECTACLE REFRACTION	EQUIVALENT POWER OF CONTACT LENS SYSTEM	PERCENTAGE INCREASE AFFORDED BY CONTACT LENS	SPECTACLE REFRACTION	EQUIVALENT POWER OF CONTACT LENS SYSTEM	PERCENTAGE INCREASE AFFORDED BY CONTACT LENS	SPECTACLE REFRACTION	EQUIVALENT POWER OF CONTACT LENS SYSTEM	PERCENTAGE INCREASE AFFORDED BY CONTACT LENS
–20	–15.73	27.2	–8	–7.07	12.9	+6	+6.10	–4.7
–18	–14.41	24.8	–6	–5.42	10.5	+8	+8.29	–7.4
–16	–13.06	22.5	–4	–3.69	7.8	+10	+10.62	–10.3
–14	–11.65	20.1	–2	–1.88	5.4	+12	+13.07	–13.8
–12	–10.19	17.8	+2	+1.96	1.2	+14	+15.64	–17.3
–10	–8.66	15.3	+4	+3.99	–1.7			

Bennet AG. *Optics of Contact Lenses.* 4th ed. London: Hatton Press; 1966.

TABLE 3

INDEX OF REFRACTION OF LENS MATERIAL

	CROWN GLASS	1.6-INDEX CROWNLITE GLASS	HILITE GLASS	8-INDEX GLASS	CR–39 PLASTIC	HIRI PLASTIC	1.6-INDEX PLASTIC	POLY–CARBONATE THIN–LITE PLASTIC
INDEX OF REFRACTION The higher the number, the thinner the material	1.523	1.601	1.701	1.805	1.498	1.56	1.6	1.586
SPECIFIC GRAVITY The higher the number, the heavier the material	2.5	2.67	2.99	3.37	1.32	1.216	1.34	1.20
DISPERSION The higher the number, the less chromatic aberration (Abbe value)	59	42.24	31	25	58	38	37	31
PERSONALITY	temperable, coatable, ease in handling, vast availability	chemically temperable, ease in handling, limited availability	chemically temperable, fairly easy to handle, SV and multifocals; vacuum coatings cause lens to become highly sensitive to scratching	SV, difficult to temper, highly reflective so A/R coatings recommended, but have same problems as hilite; mfrs suggest having patient sign liability waiver when ground thin. Multifocal available in laminate.	strong, tintable, coatable, ease in handling, vast availability	SV and bifocal, tints well before SRC, edges well, must be SRC, extremely brittle	SV only, tints well before SRC, edges well, must be SRC	SV and multifocal, strongest lens material available, limited tintability, must be SPC, no fast fabrication, special edging equipment needed, a must for children and athletes

SV = single-vision lenses. A/R = antireflective. SRC = scratch-resistant coating.

TABLE 4

CYLINDER POWER IN OFF-AXIS MERIDIAN

DEGREES FROM CYLINDER AXIS

0	5	10	15	20	25	30	35	40	45	50	55	60	65	70	75	80	85	90
100	.99	.97	.93	.88	.82	.75	.67	.59	.50	.41	.33	.25	.18	.12	.07	.03	.01	.00

PERCENTAGE OF CYLINDER POWER IN OFF-AXIS MERIDIAN

To determine cylinder power in an off–axis meridian, place straightedge on diagram above so that it intersects center dot and upper-scale position for number of degrees that the meridian sought is off axis. Percentage of cylinder power in the meridian sought is indicated on lower scale at point of intersection with straightedge.

Example: 2.00 D cyl × 75° What is the power at 90° that is 15° off axis?
Reading on lower scale is 0.07; therefore, power in 90th meridian is 0.14 D.

TABLE 5

CORNEAL RADIUS EQUIVALENCE DIOPTERS/MILLIMETERS

DIOPTERS	mm	DIOPTERS	mm	DIOPTERS	mm	DIOPTERS	mm	DIOPTERS	mm	DIOPTERS	mm	DIOPTERS	mm	DIOPTERS	mm
20.00	16.875	36.00	9.375	39.00	8.653	42.00	8.035	45.00	7.500	48.00	7.031	51.00	6.617	54.00	6.250
22.00	15.340	36.12	9.343	39.12	8.627	42.12	8.012	45.12	7.480	48.12	7.013	51.12	6.602	54.12	6.236
24.00	14.062	36.25	9.310	39.25	8.598	42.25	7.988	45.25	7.458	48.25	6.994	51.25	6.585	54.25	6.221
26.00	12.980	36.37	9.279	39.37	8.572	42.37	7.965	45.37	7.438	48.37	6.977	51.37	6.569	54.37	6.207
27.00	12.500	36.50	9.246	39.50	8.544	42.50	7.941	45.50	7.417	48.50	6.958	51.50	6.553	54.50	6.192
28.00	12.053	36.62	9.216	39.62	8.518	42.62	7.918	45.62	7.398	48.62	6.941	51.62	6.538	54.62	6.179
29.00	11.638	36.75	9.183	39.75	8.490	42.75	7.894	45.75	7.377	48.75	6.923	51.75	6.521	54.75	6.164
29.50	11.441	36.87	9.153	39.87	8.465	42.87	7.872	45.87	7.357	48.87	6.906	51.87	6.506	54.87	6.150
30.00	11.250	37.00	9.121	40.00	8.437	43.00	7.848	46.00	7.336	49.00	6.887	52.00	6.490	55.00	6.136
30.50	11.065	37.12	9.092	40.12	8.412	43.12	7.826	46.12	7.317	49.12	6.870	52.12	6.475	55.12	6.123
31.00	10.887	37.25	9.060	40.25	8.385	43.25	7.803	46.25	7.297	49.25	6.852	52.25	6.459	55.25	6.108
31.50	10.714	37.37	9.031	40.37	8.360	43.37	7.781	46.37	7.278	49.37	6.836	52.37	6.444	55.37	6.095
32.00	10.547	37.50	9.000	40.50	8.333	43.50	7.758	46.50	7.258	49.50	6.818	52.50	6.428	55.50	6.081
32.50	10.385	37.62	8.971	40.62	8.308	43.62	7.737	46.62	7.239	49.62	6.801	52.62	6.413	55.62	6.068
33.00	10.227	37.75	8.940	40.75	8.282	43.75	7.714	46.75	7.219	49.75	6.783	52.75	6.398	55.75	6.054
33.50	10.075	37.87	8.912	40.87	8.257	43.87	7.693	46.87	7.200	49.87	6.767	52.87	6.383	55.87	6.041
34.00	9.926	38.00	8.881	41.00	8.231	44.00	7.670	47.00	7.180	50.00	6.750	53.00	6.367	56.00	6.027
34.25	9.854	38.12	8.853	41.12	8.207	44.12	7.649	47.12	7.162	50.12	6.733	53.12	6.353	56.50	5.973
34.50	9.783	38.25	8.823	41.25	8.181	44.25	7.627	47.25	7.142	50.25	6.716	53.25	6.338	57.00	5.921
34.75	9.712	38.37	8.795	41.37	8.158	44.37	7.606	47.37	7.124	50.37	6.700	53.37	6.323	57.50	5.869
35.00	9.643	38.50	8.766	41.50	8.132	44.50	7.584	47.50	7.105	50.50	6.683	53.50	6.308	58.00	5.819
35.25	9.574	38.62	8.738	41.62	8.109	44.62	7.563	47.62	7.087	50.62	6.667	53.62	6.294	58.50	5.769
35.50	9.507	38.75	8.708	41.75	8.083	44.75	7.541	47.75	7.068	50.75	6.650	53.75	6.279	59.00	5.720
35.75	9.440	38.87	8.682	41.87	8.060	44.87	7.521	47.87	7.050	50.87	6.634	53.87	6.265	60.00	5.625

TABLE 6

VERTEX DISTANCE CONVERSION SCALE (mm)

SPECTACLE LENS	PLUS LENSES								MINUS LENSES							
POWER	8	9	10	11	12	13	14	15	8	9	10	11	12	13	14	15
4.00	4.12	4.12	4.12	4.12	4.25	4.25	4.25	4.25	3.87	3.87	3.87	3.87	3.87	3.75	3.75	3.75
4.50	4.62	4.75	4.75	4.75	4.75	4.75	4.75	4.87	4.37	4.37	4.25	4.25	4.25	4.25	4.25	4.25
5.00	5.25	5.25	5.25	5.25	5.25	5.37	5.37	5.37	4.75	4.75	4.75	4.75	4.75	4.75	4.62	4.62
5.50	5.75	5.75	5.75	5.87	5.87	5.87	6.00	6.00	5.25	5.25	5.25	5.12	5.12	5.12	5.12	5.12
6.00	6.25	6.37	6.37	6.37	6.50	6.50	6.50	6.62	5.75	5.62	5.62	5.62	5.62	5.50	5.50	5.50
6.50	6.87	6.87	7.00	7.00	7.00	7.12	7.12	7.25	6.12	6.12	6.12	6.00	6.00	6.00	6.00	5.87
7.00	7.37	7.50	7.50	7.62	7.62	7.75	7.75	7.75	6.62	6.62	6.50	6.50	6.50	6.37	6.37	6.37
7.50	8.00	8.00	8.12	8.12	8.25	8.25	8.37	8.50	7.12	7.00	7.00	6.87	6.87	6.87	6.75	6.75
8.00	8.50	8.62	8.75	8.75	8.87	8.87	9.00	9.12	7.50	7.50	7.37	7.37	7.25	7.25	7.25	7.25
8.50	9.12	9.25	9.25	9.37	9.50	9.50	9.62	9.75	8.00	7.87	7.87	7.75	7.75	7.62	7.62	7.50
9.00	9.75	9.75	9.87	10.00	10.12	10.25	10.37	10.37	8.37	8.37	8.25	8.25	8.12	8.00	8.00	8.00
9.50	10.25	10.37	10.50	10.62	10.75	10.87	11.00	11.12	8.87	8.75	8.62	8.62	8.50	8.50	8.37	8.37
10.00	10.87	11.00	11.12	11.25	11.37	11.50	11.62	11.75	9.25	9.12	9.12	9.00	8.87	8.87	8.75	8.75
10.50	11.50	11.62	11.75	11.87	12.00	12.12	12.25	12.50	9.62	9.62	9.50	9.37	9.37	9.25	9.12	9.12
11.00	12.00	12.25	12.37	12.50	12.75	12.87	13.00	13.12	10.12	10.00	9.87	9.75	9.75	9.62	9.50	9.50
11.50	12.62	12.87	13.00	13.12	13.37	13.50	13.75	13.87	10.50	10.37	10.37	10.25	10.12	10.00	9.87	9.87
12.00	13.25	13.50	13.62	13.87	14.00	14.25	14.50	14.62	11.00	10.87	10.75	10.62	10.50	10.37	10.25	10.12
12.50	13.87	14.12	14.25	14.50	14.75	15.00	15.25	15.37	11.37	11.25	11.12	11.00	10.87	10.75	10.62	10.50
13.00	14.50	14.75	15.00	15.25	15.50	15.62	16.00	16.12	11.75	11.62	11.50	11.37	11.25	11.12	11.00	10.87
13.50	15.12	15.37	15.62	15.87	16.12	16.37	16.62	16.87	12.25	12.00	11.87	11.75	11.62	11.50	11.37	11.25
14.00	15.75	16.00	16.25	16.50	16.75	17.12	17.50	17.75	12.62	12.50	12.25	12.12	12.00	11.87	11.75	11.50
14.50	16.50	16.75	17.00	17.25	17.50	17.87	18.25	18.50	13.00	12.75	12.62	12.50	12.37	12.25	12.00	11.87
15.00	17.00	17.37	17.75	18.00	18.25	18.62	19.00	19.37	13.37	13.25	13.00	12.87	12.75	12.50	12.37	12.25
15.50	17.75	18.00	18.25	18.75	19.00	19.37	19.75	20.25	13.75	13.62	13.50	13.25	13.00	12.87	12.75	12.62
16.00	18.25	18.75	19.00	19.37	19.75	20.25	20.50	21.00	14.25	14.00	13.75	13.62	13.50	13.25	13.00	12.87
16.50	19.00	19.37	19.75	20.25	20.50	21.00	21.50	21.87	14.50	14.37	14.12	14.00	13.75	13.62	13.50	13.25
17.00	19.75	20.25	20.50	21.00	21.50	22.00	22.25	22.87	15.00	14.75	14.50	14.25	14.12	14.00	13.75	13.50
17.50	20.50	20.75	21.25	21.75	22.25	22.75	23.25	23.75	15.37	15.12	14.87	14.75	14.50	14.25	14.00	13.87
18.00	21.00	21.50	22.00	22.50	23.00	23.50	24.00	24.62	15.75	15.50	15.25	15.00	14.75	14.62	14.37	14.12
18.50	21.75	22.25	22.75	23.25	23.75	24.50	25.00	25.62	16.12	15.87	15.62	15.37	15.12	14.87	14.75	14.50
19.00	22.50	23.00	23.50	24.00	24.75	25.25	26.00	26.50	16.50	16.25	16.00	15.75	15.50	15.25	15.00	14.75

TABLE 7

MJK SPHEROCYLINDRICAL VERTEX CHART

VERTEX DISTANCE = 13.00 mm					CYLINDER INCREMENT = 0.25 DIOPTER						SPHERE INCREMENT = 0.125 DIOPTER		
SR	**SRV**	**–0.25**	**–0.50**	**–0.75**	**–1.00**	**–1.25**	**–1.50**	**–1.75**	**–2.00**	**–2.25**	**–2.50**	**–2.75**	**–3.00**
–3.00	–2.87	–0.25	–0.50	–0.75	–1.00	–1.25	–1.25	–1.50	–1.75	–2.00	–2.25	–2.50	–2.75
–3.25	–3.12	–0.25	–0.50	–0.75	–1.00	–1.25	–1.25	–1.50	–1.75	–2.00	–2.25	–2.50	–2.75
–3.50	–3.37	–0.25	–0.50	–0.75	–1.00	–1.25	–1.25	–1.50	–1.75	–2.00	–2.25	–2.50	–2.75
–3.75	–3.62	–0.25	–0.50	–0.75	–1.00	–1.00	–1.25	–1.50	–1.75	–2.00	–2.25	–2.50	–2.75
–4.00	–3.75	–0.25	–0.50	–0.75	–1.00	–1.00	–1.25	–1.50	–1.75	–2.00	–2.25	–2.50	–2.50
–4.25	–4.00	–0.25	–0.50	–0.75	–1.00	–1.00	–1.25	–1.50	–1.75	–2.00	–2.25	–2.50	–2.50
–4.50	–4.25	–0.25	–0.50	–0.75	–1.00	–1.00	–1.25	–1.50	–1.75	–2.00	–2.25	–2.25	–2.50
–4.75	–4.50	–0.25	–0.50	–0.75	–1.00	–1.00	–1.25	–1.50	–1.75	–2.00	–2.25	–2.25	–2.50
–5.00	–4.75	–0.25	–0.50	–0.75	–0.75	–1.00	–1.25	–1.50	–1.75	–2.00	–2.25	–2.25	–2.50
–5.25	–4.87	–0.25	–0.50	–0.75	–0.75	–1.00	–1.25	–1.50	–1.75	–2.00	–2.25	–2.25	–2.50
–5.50	–5.12	–0.25	–0.50	–0.75	–0.75	–1.00	–1.25	–1.50	–1.75	–2.00	–2.00	–2.25	–2.50
–5.75	–5.37	–0.25	–0.50	–0.75	–0.75	–1.00	–1.25	–1.50	–1.75	–2.00	–2.00	–2.25	–2.50
–6.00	–5.62	–0.25	–0.50	–0.75	–0.75	–1.00	–1.25	–1.50	–1.75	–2.00	–2.00	–2.25	–2.50
–6.25	–5.75	–0.25	–0.50	–0.75	–0.75	–1.00	–1.25	–1.50	–1.75	–1.75	–2.00	–2.25	–2.50
–6.50	–6.00	–0.25	–0.50	–0.75	–0.75	–1.00	–1.25	–1.50	–1.75	–1.75	–2.00	–2.25	–2.50
–6.75	–6.25	–0.25	–0.50	–0.75	–0.75	–1.00	–1.25	–1.50	–1.75	–1.75	–2.00	–2.25	–2.50
–7.00	–6.37	–0.25	–0.50	–0.50	–0.75	–1.00	–1.25	–1.50	–1.75	–1.75	–2.00	–2.25	–2.50
–7.25	–6.62	–0.25	–0.50	–0.50	–0.75	–1.00	–1.25	–1.50	–1.75	–1.75	–2.00	–2.25	–2.50
–7.50	–6.87	–0.25	–0.50	–0.50	–0.75	–1.00	–1.25	–1.50	–1.50	–1.75	–2.00	–2.25	–2.50
–7.75	–7.00	–0.25	–0.50	–0.50	–0.75	–1.00	–1.25	–1.50	–1.50	–1.75	–2.00	–2.25	–2.50
–8.00	–7.25	–0.25	–0.50	–0.50	–0.75	–1.00	–1.25	–1.50	–1.50	–1.75	–2.00	–2.25	–2.50
–8.25	–7.50	–0.25	–0.50	–0.50	–0.75	–1.00	–1.25	–1.50	–1.50	–1.75	–2.00	–2.25	–2.25
–8.50	–7.62	–0.25	–0.50	–0.50	–0.75	–1.00	–1.25	–1.50	–1.50	–1.75	–2.00	–2.25	–2.25
–8.75	–7.87	–0.25	–0.50	–0.50	–0.75	–1.00	–1.25	–1.50	–1.50	–1.75	–2.00	–2.25	–2.25
–9.00	–8.00	–0.25	–0.50	–0.50	–0.75	–1.00	–1.25	–1.25	–1.50	–1.75	–2.00	–2.25	–2.25
–9.25	–8.25	–0.25	–0.50	–0.50	–0.75	–1.00	–1.25	–1.25	–1.50	–1.75	–2.00	–2.00	–2.25
–9.50	–8.50	–0.25	–0.50	–0.50	–0.75	–1.00	–1.25	–1.25	–1.50	–1.75	–2.00	–2.00	–2.25
–9.75	–8.62	–0.25	–0.50	–0.50	–0.75	–1.00	–1.25	–1.25	–1.50	–1.75	–2.00	–2.00	–2.25
–10.00	–8.87	–0.25	–0.50	–0.50	–0.75	–1.00	–1.25	–1.25	–1.50	–1.75	–2.00	–2.00	–2.25
–10.25	–9.00	–0.25	–0.50	–0.50	–0.75	–1.00	–1.25	–1.25	–1.50	–1.75	–2.00	–2.00	–2.25
–10.50	–9.25	–0.25	–0.50	–0.50	–0.75	–1.00	–1.25	–1.25	–1.50	–1.75	–2.00	–2.00	–2.25
–10.75	–9.37	–0.25	–0.50	–0.50	–0.75	–1.00	–1.25	–1.25	–1.50	–1.75	–2.25	–2.00	–2.25
+4.00	+4.25	–0.25	–0.50	–0.75	–1.00	–1.25	–1.75	–2.00	–2.25	–2.50	–2.75	–3 00	–3.25
+4.25	+4.50	–0.25	–0.50	–0.75	–1.00	–1.50	–1.75	–2.00	–2.25	–2.50	–2.75	–3.00	–3.25
+4.50	+4.75	–0.25	–0.50	–0.75	–1.00	–1.50	–1.75	–2.00	–2.25	–2.50	–2.75	–3.00	–3.25
+4.75	+5.12	–0.25	–0.50	–0.75	–1.00	–1.50	–1.75	–2.00	–2.25	–2.50	–2.75	–3.00	–3.25
+5.00	+5.37	–0.25	–0.50	–0.75	–1.00	–1.50	–1.75	–2.00	–2.25	–2.50	–2.75	–3.00	–3.25
+5.25	+5.62	–0.25	–0.50	–0.75	–1.00	–1.50	–1.75	–2.00	–2.25	–2.50	–2.75	–3.00	–3.25
+5.50	+5.87	–0.25	–0.50	–0.75	–1.00	–1.50	–1.75	–2.00	–2.25	–2.50	–2.75	–3.00	–3.25
+5.75	+6.25	–0.25	–0.50	–0.75	–1.00	–1.50	–1.75	–2.00	–2.25	–2.50	–2.75	–3.00	–3.25
+6.00	+6.50	–0.25	–0.50	–0.75	–1.00	–1.50	–1.75	–2.00	–2.25	–2.50	–2.75	–3.00	–3.50
+6.25	+6.75	–0.25	–0.50	–1.00	–1.00	–1.50	–1.75	–2.00	–2.25	–2.50	–2.75	–3.25	–3.50
+6.50	+7.12	–0.25	–0.50	–1.00	–1.00	–1.50	–1.75	–2.00	–2.25	–2.50	–3.00	–3.25	–3.50
+6.75	+7.37	–0.25	–0.50	–1.00	–1.00	–1.50	–1.75	–2.00	–2.25	–2.50	–3.00	–3.25	–3.50
+7.00	+7.75	–0.25	–0.50	–1.00	–1.00	–1.50	–1.75	–2.00	–2.25	–2.75	–3.00	–3.25	–3.50
+7.25	+8 00	–0.25	–0.50	–1.00	–1.00	–1.50	–1.75	–2.00	–2.25	–2.75	–3.00	–3.25	–3.50
+7.50	+8.25	–0.25	–0.50	–1.00	–1.00	–1.50	–1.75	–2.00	–2.50	–2.75	–3.00	–3.25	–3.50
+7.75	+8.62	–0.25	–0.50	–1.00	–1.00	–1.50	–1.75	–2.00	–2.50	–2.75	–3.00	–3 25	–3.50
+8.00	+8.87	–0.25	–0.50	–1.00	–1.00	–1.50	–1.75	–2.25	–2.50	–2.75	–3.00	–3.25	–3.50
+8.25	+9.25	–0.25	–0.50	–1.00	–1.00	–1.50	–1.75	–2.25	–2.50	–2.75	–3.00	–3.25	–3.50
+8.50	+9 25	–0.25	–0.75	–1.00	–1.25	–1.50	–1.75	–2.25	–2.50	–2.75	–3.00	–3.25	–3.75
+8.75	+9.87	–0.25	–0.75	–1.00	–1.25	–1.50	–1.75	–2.25	–2.50	–2.75	–3.00	–3.25	–3.75
+9.00	+10.25	–0.25	–0.75	–1.00	–1.25	–1.50	–2.00	–2.25	–2.50	–2.75	–3.00	–3.50	–3.75
+9.25	+10.50	–0.25	–0.75	–1.00	–1.25	–1.50	–2.00	–2.25	–2.50	–2.75	–3.00	–3.50	–3.75
+9.50	+10.87	–0.25	–0.75	–1.00	–1.25	–1.50	–2.00	–2.25	–2.50	–2.75	–3.25	–3.50	–3.75
+9.75	+11.12	–0.25	–0.75	–1.00	–1.25	–1.50	–2.00	–2.25	–2.50	–2.75	–3.25	–3.50	–3.75
+10.00	+11.50	–0.25	–0.75	–1.00	–1.25	–1.50	–2.00	–2.25	–2.50	–3.00	–3.25	–3.50	–3.75
+10.25	+11.87	–0.25	–0.75	–1.00	–1.25	–1.75	–2.00	–2.25	–2.50	–3.00	–3.25	–3.50	–3.75
+10 50	+12.12	–0.25	–0.75	–1.00	–1.25	–1.75	–2.00	–2.25	–2.50	–3.00	–3 25	–3.50	–3.75
+10.75	+12.50	–0.25	–0.75	–1.00	–1.25	–1.75	–2.00	–2.25	–2.50	–3.00	–3.25	–3.50	–4.00
+11.00	+12.87	–0.25	–0.75	–1.00	–1.25	–1.75	–2.00	–2.25	–2.75	–3.00	–3.25	–3.50	–4.00
+11.25	+13.12	–0.25	–0.75	–1.00	–1.25	–1.75	–2.00	–2.25	–2.75	–3.00	–3.25	–3.50	–4.00
+11.50	+13.50	–0.25	–0.75	–1.00	–1.25	–1.75	–2.00	–2.25	–2.75	–3.00	–3.25	–3.75	–4.00
+11.75	+13.87	–0.25	–0.75	–1.00	–1.25	–1.75	–2.00	–2.25	–2.75	–3.00	–3.25	–3.75	–4.00

Example: Spectacle refraction (SR) at 13 mm = –5.75 – 2.50 × 180.
Matching up –5.75 on the left, gives effective spherical power (SRV) of –5.37.
Following underlined values to the right and reading in the –2.50 cylinder column gives a cylinder value of –2.00.

Corneal plane refraction = –5.37 – 2.00 × 180.

Legend: In this chart of spherocylindrical corneal plane refractions, the spherical value is calculated and rounded off to the nearest 0.12 diopter, while the cylinder value is rounded off to the nearest 0.25 diopter.

SECTION 5

VISION STANDARDS AND LOW VISION

1. VISION STANDARDS

TABLE 1

VISION STANDARDS FOR PILOTS

	WITHOUT RX[1]	REQUIRING RX[1] CORRECTED TO	NEAR VISION WITH/ WITHOUT RX	PHORIAS[2]	FIELDS	COLOR	PATHOLOGY
1st class	20/20	20/100 to 20/20	20/40 (J_3)	6 D eso/exo 1 Δ hyper	Normal	Normal	4
2nd class	20/20	20/100 to 20/20	20/40 (J_3)	6 D eso/exo 1 Δ hyper	Normal	3	5
3rd class	20/50	To 20/30	20/60 (J_6)	. . .	. . .	3	5

1. Each eye.
2. If exceeded, further evaluation required to determine bifoveal fixation and adequate vergence phoria relationship.
3. Able to distinguish aviation signal red, aviation signal green, and white.
4. No acute or chronic pathologic condition of either eye of adnexa that might interfere with its proper function, might progress to that degree, or be aggravated by flying.
5. No serious pathology.

Note: By amendment regulations (12/21/76) correction may be by spectacles or contact lenses.

TABLE 2

VISION STANDARDS FOR ADMISSION TO SERVICE ACADEMIES

US Coast Guard Academy	Minimum uncorrected 20/200 each eye; correctable to 20/20 each eye; refractive error not more than ±5.50 D any meridian; astigmatism not over 3.00 D; anisometropia not exceeding 3.50 D; full visual fields; normal color vision; no chronic, disfiguring, disabling, ocular pathology.
US Merchant Marine Academy	Minimum uncorrected 20/100 each eye; correctable to 20/20 each eye; refractive error as for Coast Guard Academy; color vision normal by Farnsworth lantern test or pseudoisochromatic; plates; certain pathologies may disqualify.
US Naval Academy	Uncorrected vision 20/20 each eye; limited waivers if correctable to 20/20 each eye and to refraction standards, Coast Guard Academy; color vision normal–no waivers; no chronic, disfiguring, disabling ocular pathology.
US Military Academy	Distance vision correctable to 20/20 each eye; refractive error as for Coast Guard Academy; able to distinguish vivid red and green; ET less than 15 prism diopters; XT less than 10 prism diopters; hypertropia less than 2 prism diopters; certain pathologies may disqualify.
US Air Force Academy	Pilot: Uncorrected vision 20/20 or better each eye, far and near; refractive error hyperopia no greater than +1.75 D and nearsightedness less than plano in any one meridian; the astigmatic error must not exceed 0.75 D. Navigator: Uncorrected vision 20/70 or better correctable with ordinary glasses to 20/20 each eye; near acuity 20/20 or better each eye, uncorrected; hyperopia not greater than +3.00 D and myopia not greater than –1.50 D any meridian; astigmatism not to exceed 2.00 D. Commission: Distance acuity correctable 20/40 one eye and 20/70 other, or 20/30 one eye and 20/100 other; near acuity correctable to 20/20 (J_1) one eye and 20/30 (J_2) in other; refractive error of equivalent sphere not more than ±8.00 D; no chronic, disfiguring, disabling ocular pathology.

Based on information as of 17 May, 1983, Medical Examination Review Board, Department of Defense.

TABLE 3

VISION STANDARDS FOR COMMERCIAL DRIVERS

	VISUAL ACUITY	VISUAL FIELD				
	BINOC	MONOC	BINOC	COLOR	OTHER	RETEST
Alabama	20/70	No	No	No	No	No
Alaska	20/40	No	No	No	No	Periodic
Arizona	20/40	No	No	No	No	Periodic
Arkansas	20/50	NS	NS	NS	NS	NS
California	20/40	70, 70	NS	R,G,A	NS	Periodic
Colorado	20/40	Yes	Yes	Yes	ST	Periodic
Connecticut	20/40	Yes	Yes	Yes	ST	No
Delaware	20/40	No	No	No	No	Periodic
Florida	20/70	No	No	No	No	Periodic
Georgia	20/60	140, 140	140	No	No	Periodic
Hawaii	20/40	70, 70	140	R,G,A	ST, EC	Periodic
Idaho	20/40	NS	NS	NS	NS	Periodic
Illinois	20/40	70, 70	140	NS	NS	Periodic
Indiana	20/50	No	No	No	NS	Periodic
Iowa	20/70	No	No	No	NS	Periodic
Kansas	20/40	NS	NS	NS	NS	Periodic
Kentucky	20/45, PV	No	No	No	No	No
Louisiana	20/40	No	No	No	No	Periodic
Maine	20/40	NS	NS	NS	NS	No
Maryland	20/40	140, 140	140	No	No	Periodic
Massachusetts	20/40	90, 90	120	Yes	No	Periodic
Michigan	20/40	70, 70	140	NS	NS	Periodic
Minnesota	20/40	NS	NS	NS	NS	Periodic
Mississippi	20/40	90, 90	180	No	ST	No
Missouri	20/40	55, 55	No	No	No	Periodic
Montana	20/40	75, 75	No	Yes	ST	Periodic
Nebraska	20/40	70, 70	140	Yes	No	Periodic
Nevada	20/40	No	No	No	No	Periodic
New Hampshire	20/40	NS	NS	NS	NS	Periodic
New Jersey	20/40	70, 70	No	R,G,A	No	NS
New Mexico	20/40	NS	NS	NS	NS	Periodic
New York	20/40	NS	NS	NS	NS	Periodic
North Carolina	20/50	No	70	Yes	No	Periodic
North Dakota	20/40	70, 70	140	No	No	Periodic
Ohio	20/40	70, 70	No	No	No	Periodic
Oklahoma	20/40	No	No	No	No	No
Oregon	20/40	No	110	No	No	No
Pennsylvania	20/40	No	140	No	No	No
Rhode Island	20/40	60, 60	120	Yes	No	Periodic
South Carolina	PV	NS	NS	NS	NS	Periodic
South Dakota	20/40	No	No	No	No	Periodic
Tennessee	20/40	No	No	No	No	No
Texas	20/50	No	No	No	No	Periodic
Utah	20/40	NS	NS	Yes	ST	Periodic
Vermont	20/40	NS	NS	NS	NS	No
Virginia	20/40	100, 100	100	No	NS	Periodic
Washington	20/40	No	140	R,G,A	No	Periodic
West Virginia	20/40	No	No	No	No	No
Wisconsin	20/40	70, 70	140	No	No	Periodic
Wyoming	20/40	No	No	No	No	Periodic

Key: Visual acuity is expressed in Snellen notation; visual field is given in degrees along the horizontal meridian; color abbreviations: R = red, G = green, A = amber; abbreviations for other conditions: EC = eye coordination; ST = stereopsis (absence of); NS = standard not specified; No = no standard; PV = default to private vehicle standard.

Source: US Dept of Transportation. *Visual Disorders and Commercial Drivers*. Washington, DC: Federal Highway Administration, Office of Motor Carriers; Nov 1991. US Dept of Transportation publication FHWA-MC-92-003, HCS-10/1-92(200)E.

2. LOW-VISION AIDS

Under federal regulation, a patient is considered legally blind when the best vision attained in the better eye is 20/200 or less, or when, whatever the acuity achieved, the field of vision of the better eye is 20° or less. While most states have adopted these standards, individual variations may exist at the local level.

Patients whose vision is reduced or inadequate for their visual tasks — those whose best corrected vision ranges from 20/50 downward toward the 20/200 level — can frequently be aided by the same techniques and devices used for the legally blind and visually rehabilitated. These modalities include rehabilitation training programs and optical and nonoptical aids. They often can help restore independence and mobility, allowing the patient to remain productive.

For those patients considered partially sighted rather than partially blind, increased vision is obtained by magnification or approximation. For distance, this may be accomplished by telescopic devices. Although difficult to use while moving about, these instruments may be quite effective for distinguishing a street sign or the number of a house or bus. They are also useful aids in the theater or classroom and at sporting events.

Telescopic devices can be obtained in magnifications of 2.2, 2.5, 3.0, 3.5, 4.0, 6.0, 8.0, and 10× from suppliers such as Vision, Keeler, Nikon, Selsi, Walters, and Zeiss. Some are fixed focus; others may be refocused for viewing closer material. Telescopes fitted with reading cap lenses permit reading at greater distances than high-plus aids. A familiar example of this system is the surgical loupe.

Because the field diminishes as the power increases, the magnification of telescopic devices should be kept to the minimum needed to secure desired acuity. Differences in design and construction of these devices may cause slight variations in the fields produced at a given magnification. A representative sample may be drawn from the devices produced by Designs for Vision:

MAGNIFICATION	FIELD AT 20 FEET
2.2 standard	12°
2.2 wide Angle	17°
3.0 standard	8°
3.0 wide angle	12°
4.0 standard	6°

Near vision can be augmented by higher adds, high-plus "Micro" lenses (American Optical, Lucerne Optical), binocular loupes, and handheld or stand magnifiers. The higher plus values permit approximation to increase the angle subtended with little or no demand on accommodation. The add to obtain J_5 can be estimated by the inverse of the best distance vision obtained. For example, if best distance vision is 20/200, the add is 200/20, or 10 D.

Greater detail can be obtained through increased add power or supplementary magnifiers. If the patient will not read at extremely close range, lower adds may be used in combination with magnifiers. Required magnification at desired working distance can also be provided by a telemicroscope system modified with a reading cap or objective lens, as in a surgical loupe.

When binocular function is present, prism base-in may be required in the near prescription (about 1 prism diopter per diopter of add). Plastic-lens, half-eye spectacles of 6, 8, or 10 D with incorporated prism are available from American Optical and Lucerne Optical. Handheld magnifiers ranging from 23 to 83 are available from Bausch & Lomb, Coburn, Coil, Eschenbach, McLeod, and Selsi. Once again, the higher powers have reduced fields of view. Patients with physical infirmities can use stand magnifiers that rest on the material and remain in focus as they are moved across the page.

Nonoptical aids include reading masks, large-print publications, heavily ruled stationery, check-writing guides, large playing cards, and easy-to-thread needles. Also available are fixed-power opaque projection magnifiers (Nesbit Co) and closed-circuit television devices with variable magnification.

Television permits a greater range of magnification and can, when polarity is reversed, provide a white-on-black image instead of the usual black-on-white. This effect, for many, is an additional aid. Products are available from Telesensory Systems and Visualtek. Advances in electronics have also made possible talking clocks, calculators, computers, and word processors whose "voices" open the way to gainful employment for the visually impaired.

A *Catalogue of Optical Aids* is available from the New York Association for the Blind, 111 East 59th Street, New York, NY 10022. Available from the American Foundation for the Blind, 15 West 16th Street, New York, NY 10011, are Aid for the 80's, *Products for People with Visual Handicaps*, and a *Catalogue of Publications,* all of which can further help the visually impaired. The Talking Books Program can be joined by applying to the National Library Science for the Blind and Physically Handicapped, Library of Congress, Washington, DC 20542.

For those with clouded vision, absorptive lenses provide glare protection and can help improve acuity. Neutral gray lenses with 5% to 15% transmission are specifically recommended for achromatopes, who may also require the protection of wide side shield frames. Albinotic patients are aided by brown tints with 75% transmission indoors and 25% outdoors. Retinitis pigmentosa patients generally require daytime outdoor protection with the darker sunglass tints. Many are aided in night vision by the Kalichrome lenses (Bausch & Lomb) and the Hazemaster line (American Optical).

SECTION 6

EVALUATION OF PERMANENT VISUAL IMPAIRMENT

The purpose of this section is to provide criteria and a method for evaluating permanent impairments of the visual system and relating them to permanent impairment of the whole person. The visual system consists of the eyes, ocular adnexa, and visual pathways.

Visual impairment occurs in the presence of a deviation from normal in one or more of the functions of the eye, which include (1) corrected visual acuity for near and far objects; (2) visual field perception; and (3) ocular motility with diplopia. Evaluation of visual impairment is based on evaluation of the three functions. Although not all of the functions are equally important, vision is imperfect without coordination of all three. Other ocular functions and disturbances are considered to the extent that they affect one or more of the three functions. Impairment percents representing the functions are *combined* (Combined Values Chart, p.75).

If an ocular or adnexal disturbance or deformity interferes with visual function and is not reflected in diminished visual acuity, decreased visual fields, or ocular motility with diplopia, the significance of the disturbance or deformity should be evaluated by the examining physician. In that situation, the physician may *combine* an additional 5% to 10% impairment with the impaired visual function of the involved eye. Abnormalities that might result in such impairments include media opacities, corneal or lens opacities, and abnormalities resulting in such symptoms as epiphora, photophobia, or metamorphopsia.

Permanent deformities of the orbit, such as scars or cosmetic defects that do not alter ocular function, also may be considered to be factors causing whole-person impairments as high as 10%. If facial disfigurement due to scarring above the upper lip is evaluated by means of *the Guides to the Evaluation of Permanent Impariment* on the ear, nose, throat, and related structures, then any overlapping impairment percentage due to ocular scarring should be subtracted from the greater value.

Equipment

The following equipment is necessary to test the functions of the visual system.

1. *Visual Acuity Test Charts*: For distance vision tests, the Snellen test chart with nonserif block letters or numbers, the illiterate E chart, or Landolt's broken-ring chart are acceptable. For near vision, charts with print similar to that of the Snellen chart, with Revised Jaeger Standard print, or with American point-type notation for use at 35 cm (14 in) are acceptable. The 10 equally difficult block letters (D, K, R, H, V, C, N, Z, S, and O) of Louise L. Sloan are recommended for testing distance vision. Each letter subtends a visual angle of 5 minutes and a stroke width of 1 minute.
2. *Visual Field Testing:* The standard for testing visual fields is the traditional stimulus III-4e of the Goldmann perimeter. Other acceptable perimeters and stimuli are listed in **Table 1.** The tangent screen may be used for diplopia testing.
3. *Refraction Equipment:* The necessary equipment consists of a phoropter or a combination of hand-held lenses and a retinoscope.

TABLE 1

STIMULI EQUIVALENT TO THE GOLDMANN KINETIC STIMULUS

	Phakic	Aphakic
Goldmann (kinetic)	III-4E	IV-4e
ARC perimeter (kinetic)	3 mm white at radius 330 mm	6 mm white at radius 330 mm
Allergan-Humphrey (static, size 3)	10 dB	6 dB
Octopus (static, size 3)	7 dB	3 dB

Preparation for Medical Evaluation

Before using the information in this section, the reader should become familiar with Chapters 1 and 2 and the Glossary of *the Guides to the Evaluation of Permanent Impairment*, which discuss the purpose of the Guides and the situations in which they are useful and also provide basic definitions. Chapters 1 and 2 discuss the methods for examining patients and preparing reports. A medical evaluation report should include information such as the following.

A. *Medical Evaluation*
- History of medical condition
- Results of most recent clinical evaluation
- Assessment of current clinical status and statement of further medical plans
- Diagnosis

B. *Analysis of Findings*
- Impact of medical condition on life activities
- Explanation for concluding that the condition is stable and unlikely to change during the next year
- Explanation for concluding that the individual is or is not likely to suffer further impairment by engaging in ordinary activities
- Explanation for concluding that accommodations or restrictions are or are not warranted

C. Comparison of Analysis with Impairment Criteria

- Description of clinical findings and how these findings relate to specific criteria
- Explanation of each impairment estimate
- Summary of all impairment estimates
- Overall estimate of whole-person impairment

CENTRAL VISUAL ACUITY

Test chart illumination of at least 5 foot-candles is recommended to attain a distinct contrast of 0.85 or greater and a comfortable luminance of approximately 85 ± 5 candelas per square meter. The chart or reflecting surface should not be dirty or discolored. The far test distance simulates infinity at 6 m (20 ft) or at no less than 4 m (13 ft 1 in). The near test distance should be fixed at 35 cm (14 in) in keeping with the Revised Jaeger Standard. Adequate and comfortable illumination must be diffused onto the test card at a level about three times greater than that of usual room illumination. **Table 2** shows standards for distance and near visual acuity.

There are no universally accepted standards for contrast and glare sensitivity testing and glare disability testing. Thus, the results of such testing are not incorporated in visual tests of central visual acuity. However, such testing, if it is done with generally accepted methods, may be the basis for an additional impairment of visual function of the involved eye as high as 10%.

Central vision should be measured and recorded for distance and for near objects, without correction and with best corrected conventional spectacle refraction. If a patient is well adapted to contact lenses and wishes to wear them, best corrected vision with contact lenses is acceptable as the basis for estimating impairment. In certain ocular conditions, particularly in the presence of corneal abnormalities, contact lens-corrected vision may be better than that which can be obtained with spectacle correction. If the patient does not already wear contact lenses, it is not necessary to fit a contact lens to determine best corrected visual acuity.

Visual acuity for distance should be recorded in the Snellen notation, using a fraction in which the numerator is the test distance in feet or meters and the denominator is the distance at which the smallest letter discriminated by the patient would subtend 5 minutes of arc and at which an eye with 20/20 vision would see that letter. The fraction notation is one of convenience that does not indicate percentage of visual acuity. A similar Snellen notation using centimeters or inches, or a comparable Revised Jaeger Standard or American point type notation, may be used in designating near visual acuity.

The values shown in **Table 2** for distance and near visual acuity and loss were used to develop **Table 3**. **Table 3** combines both types of loss to derive an overall estimate of loss of central vision in an eye. Using **Table 3**, the examiner identifies the Snellen rating for near vision along the top row and the Snellen rating for distance along the first column. Reading down from the former and across from the latter, the examiner locates two impairment values for loss of central vision where the column and row cross. It can be seen that each impairment percentage for loss of central vision is the mean of the impairment percentages for the losses of distance acuity and near visual acuity. **Tables 2** and **3** were developed in 1955 by the Council on Industrial Health of the American Medical Association.

TABLE 2

VISUAL ACUITY NOTATIONS WITH CORRESPONDING PERCENTAGES OF LOSS OF CENTRAL VISION

FOR DISTANCE

ENGLISH	SNELLEN NOTATIONS METRIC 6	SNELLEN NOTATIONS METRIC 4	% LOSS
20/15	6/5	4/3	0
20/20	6/6	4/4	0
20/25	6/7.5	4/5	5
20/30	6/10	4/6	10
20/40	6/12	4/8	15
20/50	6/15	4/10	25
20/60	6/20	4/12	35
20/70	6/22	4/14	40
20/80	6/24	4/16	45
20/100	6/30	4/20	50
20/125	6/38	4/25	60
20/150	6/50	4/30	70
20/200	6/60	4/40	80
20/300	6/90	4/60	85
20/400	6/120	4/80	90
20/800	6/240	4/160	95

FOR NEAR

NEAR SNELLEN INCHES	NEAR SNELLEN CENTIMETERS	REVISED JAEGER STANDARD	AMERICAN POINT-TYPE	% LOSS
14/14	35/35	1	3	0
14/18	35/45	2	4	0
14/21	35/53	3	5	5
14/24	35/60	4	6	7
14/28	35/70	5	7	10
14/35	35/88	6	8	50
14/40	35/100	7	9	55
14/45	35/113	8	10	60
14/60	35/150	9	11	80
14/70	35/175	10	12	85
14/80	35/200	11	13	87
14/88	35/220	12	14	90
14/112	35/280	13	21	95
14/140	35/350	14	23	98

Monocular aphakia or monocular pseudophakia is considered to be an additional central vision impairment. If either is present, the remaining central vision is decreased by 50%, as shown by **Table 3.** With monocular pseudophakia, despite a normal Snellen acuity, there is more light scattering and a greater likelihood of glare, diminished contrast sensitivity, and spherical aberration than with a normal phakic eye. Also, capsular opacification, lens decentralization with visualization of the lens edge or positioning hole, or pupillary abnormalities may occur, and there is total loss of accomodation. For these reasons an initial 50% impairment in the central visual acuity of the pseudophakic eye is allowed, to which 50% of the observed impairment for loss of central vision is added.

Determining the Loss of Central Vision in One Eye
First, measure and record the best central visual acuity for distance and the best acuity for near vision, with and without conventional corrective spectacles or contact lenses.

Then consult **Table 3** to derive the overall loss, combining the values for best corrected near and distance acuities. Allow, if indicated, for the additional loss of central vision that results from monocular aphakia or pseudophakia.

Example: A 55-year-old man's Snellen rating for distance vision of the left eye was 20/30, and the rating for near vision of the same eye was 14/24. The man's native lens was present. **Table 3** indicates that the loss of central vision of the eye was 9%.

VISUAL FIELDS

While central visual acuity represents the ability to discern fine details, visual field acuity represents visual ability over a wider breadth of view while the subject is looking straight ahead. There are two elements to the visual field evaluation. One is the peripheral-most location at which a standard object

TABLE 3

LOSS IN % OF CENTRAL VISION* IN A SINGLE EYE.

SNELLEN RATING FOR DISTANCE IN FEET	APPROXIMATE SNELLEN RATING FOR NEAR IN INCHES													
	14/14	14/18	14/21	14/24	14/28	14/35	14/40	14/45	14/60	14/70	14/80	14/88	14/112	14/140
20/15	0	0	3	4	5	25	27	30	40	43	44	45	48	49
	50	50	52	52	53	63	64	65	70	72	72	73	74	75
20/20	0	0	3	4	5	25	27	30	40	43	44	46	48	49
	50	50	52	52	53	63	64	65	70	72	72	73	74	75
20/25	3	3	5	6	8	28	30	33	43	45	46	48	50	52
	52	52	53	53	54	64	65	67	72	73	73	74	75	76
20/30	5	5	8	9	10	30	32	35	45	48	49	50	53	54
	53	53	54	54	55	65	66	68	73	74	74	75	76	77
20/40	8	8	10	11	13	33	35	38	48	50	51	53	55	57
	54	54	55	56	57	67	68	69	74	75	76	77	78	79
20/50	13	13	15	16	18	38	40	43	53	55	56	58	60	62
	57	57	58	58	59	69	70	72	77	78	78	79	80	81
20/60	16	16	18	20	22	41	44	46	56	59	60	61	64	65
	58	58	59	60	61	70	72	73	78	79	80	81	82	83
20/70	18	18	21	22	23	43	46	48	58	61	62	63	66	67
	59	59	61	61	62	72	73	74	79	81	81	82	83	84
20/80	20	20	23	24	25	45	47	50	60	63	64	65	68	69
	60	60	62	62	63	73	74	75	80	82	82	83	84	85
20/100	25	25	28	29	30	50	52	55	65	68	69	70	73	74
	63	63	64	64	65	75	76	78	83	84	84	85	87	87
20/125	30	30	33	34	35	55	57	60	70	73	74	75	78	79
	65	65	67	67	68	78	79	80	85	87	87	88	89	90
20/150	34	34	37	38	39	59	61	64	74	77	78	79	82	83
	67	67	68	69	70	80	81	82	87	88	89	90	91	92
20/200	40	40	43	44	45	65	67	70	80	83	84	85	88	89
	70	70	72	72	73	83	84	85	90	91	92	93	94	95
20/300	43	43	45	46	48	68	70	73	83	85	86	88	90	92
	72	72	73	73	74	84	85	87	91	93	93	94	95	96
20/400	45	45	48	49	50	70	72	75	85	88	89	90	93	94
	73	73	74	74	75	85	86	88	93	94	94	95	97	97
20/800	48	48	50	51	53	73	75	78	88	90	91	93	95	97
	74	74	75	76	77	87	88	89	94	95	96	97	98	99

*Upper number shows % loss of central vision without allowance for monocular aphakia or monocular pseudophakia; lower number shows % loss of central vision with allowance for monocular aphakia or monocular pseudophakia.

can be detected. The other is the quality of visual functioning at every point within the field of view.

For the purpose of evaluating impairment in a standard fashion, a patient's visual field is evaluated as the ability to see a standard stimulus, either in terms of the peripheral-most extent along eight meridians at which the stimulus is seen (method 1) or in terms of the proportion of a predefined region in which the standard stimulus is or is not visible (method 2).

With either method, tests that have been performed for medical diagnosis may be used for calculation of impairment or to determine that a certain level of impairment has been exceeded. Sometimes, however, the available test results are not adequate for this purpose, so a specific examination must be done to allow determination of impairment. **Figure 1** shows a type of chart that is used to measure visual fields.

The traditional standard stimulus is the III-4e kinetic stimulus of the Goldmann perimeter. The IV-4e stimulus should be used in aphakic patients without a lens implant or contact lens. The equivalent stimuli with other instruments are given in **Table 1**.

Determining Loss of Monocular Visual Fields

In method 1 of measuring the visual field, the peripheral-most extent over which the static stimulus is seen is noted in each of eight principal meridians. The normal extent of these meridians is given in **Table 4**; the total extent summed over eight meridians

TABLE 4

NORMAL VISUAL FIELDS FOR EIGHT PRINCIPAL MERIDIANS.

DIRECTION OF VISION	DEGREES OF FIELD
Temporally	85
Down temporally	85
Direct down	65
Down nasally	50
Nasally	60
Up nasally	55
Direct up	45
Up temporally	55
Total	500

Figure 1. Example of Perimetric Charts Used to Plot Extent or Outline of Visual Field Along Eight Principal Meridians Separated by 45° Intervals.

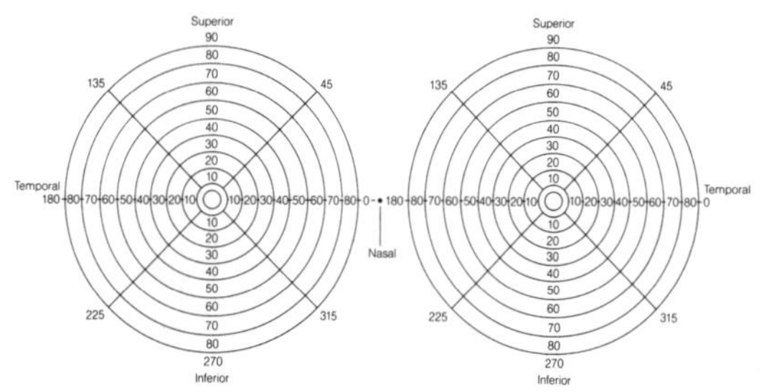

is 500. To calculate the percentage of retained vision, one adds the extent of the visual field along each of the eight meridians, considering the maximum normal values for the meridians given in **Table 4**, then divides by 5 to determine the percentage of visual field perception that remains. One must subtract the percentage of visual field remaining from 100% to obtain the percentage of visual field lost. **Table 5** tabulates the losses of monocular visual fields calculated by this method.

If the boundary of the visual field coincides with a principal meridian, as in hemianopia or nasal step, the value used for that meridian is the midpoint. Thus, in a hemianopic patient in whom the vertical meridian is split by the III-4e isopter from the point of fixation (0°) up to 40°, that meridian is given a value of 20°. In the case of a nasal step extending from 30° to 60° with the standard stimulus, a value of 45° is used for the nasal meridian.

If a meridian passes through a scotoma, the width of the scotoma is subtracted from the maximum number of degrees for that meridian. The visual field loss in each eye is increased by 5% for an inferior quadrant loss and by 10% for an inferior hemianopic loss, because major loss of a visual field below has more of a functional consequence than an equivalent field loss above. The increase of 5% or 10% is *added* to the percentage representing the visual field loss.

In method 2, an Esterman grid is used (**Figs. 2A** and **2B**). The extent over which the standard stimulus is seen or not seen in an ordinary monocular field test is transferred onto the Esterman 100 unit monocular grid. A simple count of the number of dots seen within the field among the 100 dots that are in the grid gives the percentage of retained vision. A count of the number of dots *not* seen gives the percentage lost. The Esterman grid is available from the American Academy of Ophthalmology, 655 Beech St., P.O. Box 7424, San Francisco, CA 94120-7424.

When it is available, a binocular field test performed with both eyes open and the chin in the middle of the instrument is preferred if method 2 is to be used, except for patients with one eye or those with a strabismic deviation of one eye (heterotropia). The binocular field result is determined by using the Esterman 120-unit binocular grid, and the dot count is multiplied by 5/6 to obtain the percentage of retained or lost field.

Some automated machines can perform a test of one or two eyes with a method corresponding to method 2, presenting the standard stimulus at the 100 or 120 prescribed locations and recording the result.

If a medical test of visual fields is already available, it may or may not be valid for determining visual impairment. Kinetic visual field tests should not be used if the standard stimulus was not among those plotted. An exception may occur if a stimulus stronger than the standard was plotted and the field is quite restricted. The loss is gauged by calculating the percentage of loss with the stronger stimulus; then it is certain that the percentage loss with the standard stimulus would be greater.

Another way of using a previously determined diagnostic field occurs if it covers only part of the maximum visual field, for example, only the central 30°. Methods 1 and 2 will yield the desired percentage calculation only if the patient can visualize the standard stimulus within the tested region. Thus, if the 10-decibel (dB) stimulus of the Allergan-Humphrey instrument is seen only inside 15° along all eight meridians but is not seen outside 15°, in considering the 20° or 30° field one may calculate that the retained vision is 24% (15° x 8/5). However, if the 10-dB stimulus is seen out to the edge of the 30° field along each meridian and for an unknown extent beyond, one cannot calculate the percentage of retained vision or visual loss. In such an instance, one can document the loss only if the visual field examination covers a larger field.

If an automated central field examination is normal, it is acceptable as documentation that the entire field is normal, if the ocular history and examination do not suggest lesions that would affect the outer extent of the field.

Figure 2A.–Esterman 120-unit *Binocular* Scoring Grid* for Use with Both Eyes Open.

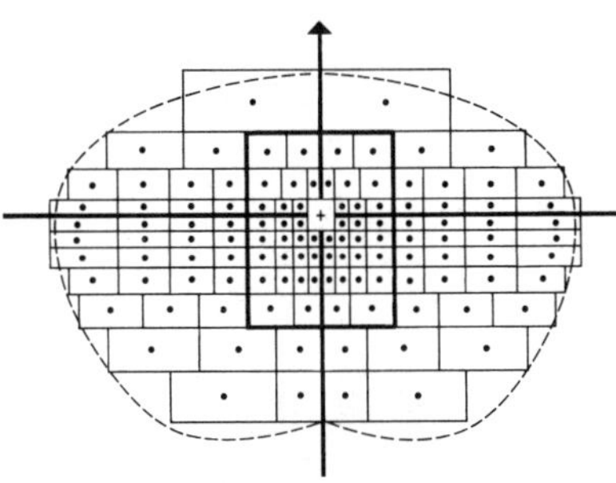

Figure 2B.–Esterman 100-unit *Monocular* Scoring Grid* for Arc or Bowl Perimeter or Similar Automated Instrument Providing Full Monocular Field Analysis.

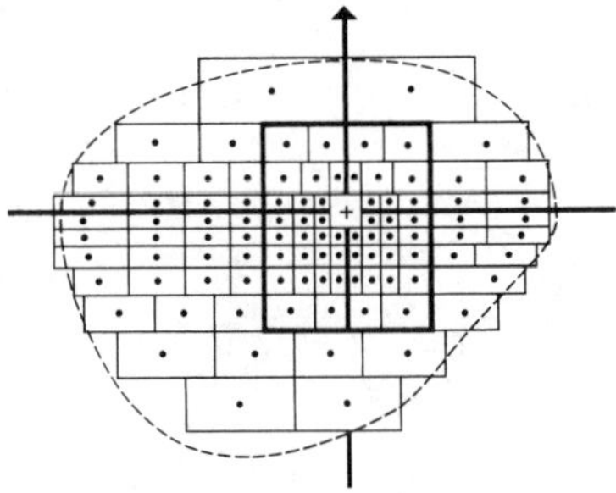

Examples of determining visual field impairments follow.

Example 1: Determine the visual field impairment and percentage of retained visual field in Field 1, right eye (below) using method 1.

Direction of vision	Degrees of field	Comments
Temporally	77	
Down temporally	84	
Direct down	55	65° maximum from table,minus 10° of scotoma between 15° and 25°
Down nasally	50	Not 55°, because maximum from table is 50°
Nasally	37	Midway between 22° and 52°
Up nasally	15	
Direct up	10	
Up temporally	33	40° peripheral extent, minus 7° excluded by isopter between 10° and 17°
Total	361	361 divided by 5 = 72

Thus, the retained visual field is 72%, and the impairment is 28%.

Field 1

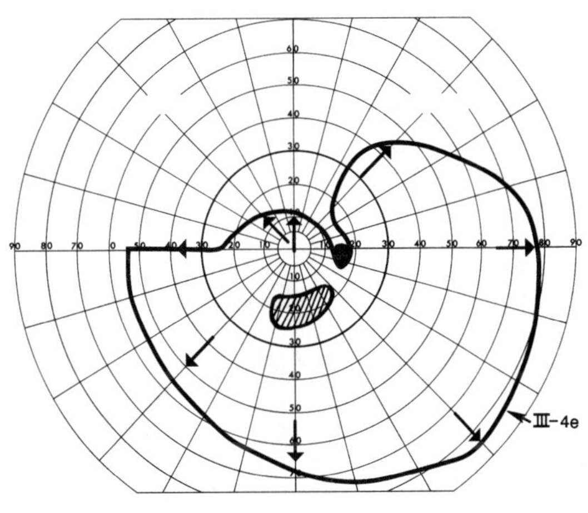

*Grids may be obtained from the American Academy of Ophthalmology, 655 Beech St., San Francisco, CA 94120

Example 2: Determine the percentage of field loss in *Field 2*, left eye (below) using method 2.

Solution: Twenty-seven of the dots are excluded by the standard isopter. This is considered to be a 27% visual field loss, with 73% of the visual field retained.

Example 3: Calculate the visual field using method 1 and the diagnostic results shown in Field 3, right eye (below).

A line is drawn around the location where visibility is better than 10 dB, the standard stimulus for the Humphrey Visual Field Analyzer. Although the field may extend slightly beyond the 30° edge of the tested region, it is obvious that the field is quite restricted. The eight meridians are summed as follows.

Direction of vision	Degree of field	Comments
Temporally	30	
Down temporally	5	
Direct down	3	Midpoint between 6 and 0°
Down nasally	0	
Nasally	8	Midpoint between 15 and 0°
Up nasally	15	
Direct up	17.5	
Up temporally	20	
Total	98.5	98.5 divided by 5 = 19.7, or about 20%

Thus, the patient retains 20% of the visual field and has an 80% loss.

Field 2

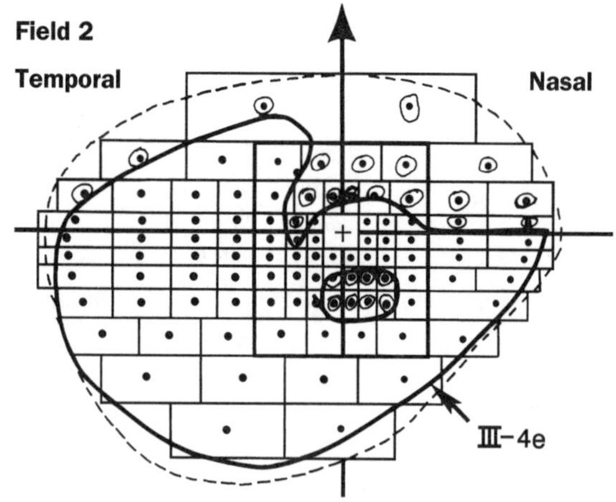

Field 3

Nasal

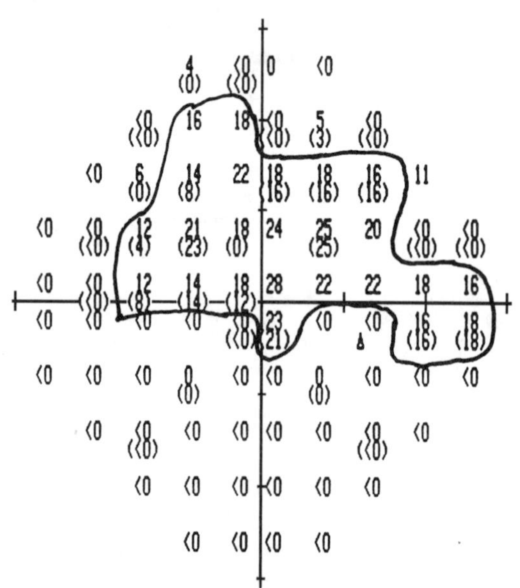

Temporal

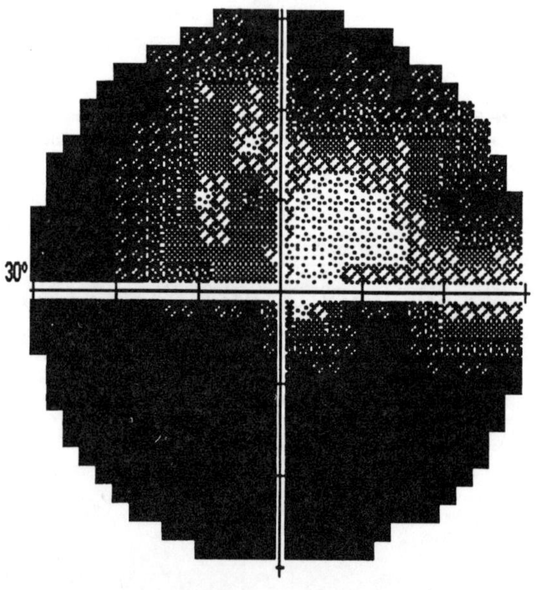

TABLE 5

LOSS OF MONOCULAR VISUAL FIELD

TOTAL DEGREES		% OF
LOST	RETAINED	LOSS
0	500*	0
5	495	1
10	490	2
15	485	3
20	480	4
25	475	5
30	470	6
35	465	7
40	460	8
45	455	9
50	450	10
55	445	11
60	440	12
65	435	13
70	430	14
75	425	15
80	420	16
85	415	17
90	410	18
95	405	19
100	400	20
105	395	21
110	390	22
115	385	23
120	380	24
125	375	25
130	370	26
135	365	27
140	360	28
145	355	29
150	350	30
155	345	31
160	340	32
165	335	33
170	330	34
175	325	35
180	320	36
185	315	37
190	310	38
195	305	39
200	300	40
205	295	41
210	290	42
215	285	43
220	280	44
225	275	45
230	270	46
235	265	47
240	260	48
245	255	49
250	250	50
255	245	51
260	240	52
265	235	53
270	230	54
275	225	55
280	220	56
285	215	57
290	210	58
295	205	59
300	200	60
305	195	61
310	190	62
315	185	63
320	180	64
325	175	65
330	170	66
335	165	67
340	160	68
345	155	69
350	150	70
355	145	71
360	140	72
365	135	73
370	130	74
375	125	75
380	120	76
385	115	77
390	110	78
395	105	79
400	100	80
405	95	81
410	90	82
415	85	83
420	80	84
425	75	85
430	70	86
435	65	87
440	60	88
445	55	89
450	50	90
455	45	91
460	40	92
465	35	93
470	30	94
475	25	95
480	20	96
485	15	97
490	10	98
495	5	99
500	0	100

*Or more.

ABNORMAL OCULAR MOTILITY AND BINOCULAR DIPLOPIA

Unless a patient has diplopia within 30° of the center of fixation, the diplopia rarely causes significant visual impairment. An exception is diplopia on looking downward. The extent of diplopia in the various directions of gaze is determined on an arc perimeter at 33 cm or with a bowl perimeter. A tangent screen also is acceptable for evaluating the central 30°. Examination is made in each of the eight major meridians by using a small test light or the projected light of approximately Goldmann III-4e without adding colored lenses or correcting prisms.

To determine the impairment of ocular motility, the patient is seated with both eyes open and the chin resting in the chin rest and centered so that the eyes are equidistant from the sides of the central fixation target.

The presence of diplopia is then plotted along the eight meridians of a suitable visual field chart (**Fig. 1**). The impairment percentage for loss of ocular motility due to diplopia in the meridian of maximum impairment, according to **Fig. 3**, is *combined* with any other visual impairment (Combined Values Chart, p. 75).

Example 1: Diplopia within the central 20° is estimated to be a 100% impairment of ocular motility (**Fig. 3**). This is equivalent to the total loss of vision of one eye, which is estimated to be a 25% impairment of the visual system and a 24% whole-person impairment (**Table 6**).

Figure 3. Percentage Loss of Ocular Motility of One Eye in Diplopia Fields.

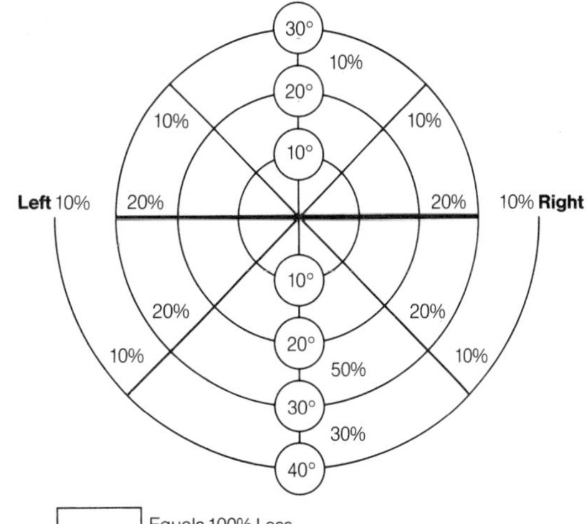

Example 2: Diplopia on looking horizontally off center from 20° to 30° is equivalent to 20% loss of ocular motility. Diplopia of the same eye when looking diagonally from 30° to 40° is equivalent to 10% loss of ocular motility. The impairments from diplopia are added, and the total loss of ocular motility is 30%.

STEPS IN DETERMINING IMPAIRMENT OF THE VISUAL SYSTEM AND OF THE WHOLE PERSON

Step 1: Determine and record the percentage loss of central vision for each eye separately, combining the losses of near and distance vision.

Step 2: Determine and record the percentage loss of visual field for each eye separately (monocular) or for both eyes together (binocular).

Step 3: Determine and record the percentage loss of ocular motility.

Procedure with Monocular Visual Fields Test

If the percentage loss of visual field is calculated for each eye separately (monocular), *combine* (Combined Values Chart, p. 75) the percentage loss of central vision with the percentage loss of visual field in each eye and record the values.

Example 1:

Right Eye

Loss of central vision
(both near and distance) 56%

Loss of visual field 32%

56% *combined* with 32%
(Combined Values) 70%

Thus, the estimated impairment of the right eye is 70%.

Left Eye

Loss of central vision
(both near and distance) 46%

Loss of visual field 32%

46% *combined* with 32%
(Combined Values) 63%

Estimated impairment of the left eye is 63%.

Again using the Combined Values, *combine* the percentage for impairment of ocular motility with the combined value for central vision and visual field in the eye manifesting the greater impairment, the right eye in example 1. Disregard the loss of ocular motility in the other eye.

TABLE 6

IMPAIRMENT OF THE VISUAL SYSTEM AS IT RELATES TO IMPAIRMENT OF THE WHOLE PERSON

% IMPAIRMENT OF		% IMPAIRMENT OF		% IMPAIRMENT OF		% IMPAIRMENT OF		% IMPAIRMENT OF		% IMPAIRMENT OF	
VISUAL SYSTEM	WHOLE PERSON	VISUAL SYSTEM	WHOLE PERSON	VISUAL SYSTEM	WHOLE PERSON	VISUAL SYSTEM	WHOLE PERSON	VISUAL SYSTEM	WHOLE PERSON	VISUAL SYSTEM	WHOLE PERSON
0	0	15	14	30	28	45	42	60	57	75	71
1	1	16	15	31	29	46	43	61	58	76	72
2	2	17	16	32	30	47	44	62	59	77	73
3	3	18	17	33	31	48	45	63	59	78	74
4	4	19	18	34	32	49	46	64	60	79	75
5	5	20	19	35	33	50	47	65	61	80	76
6	6	21	20	36	34	51	48	66	62	81	76
7	7	22	21	37	35	52	49	67	63	82	77
8	8	23	22	38	36	53	50	68	64	83	78
9	8	24	23	39	37	54	51	69	65	84	79
10	9	25	24	40	38	55	52	70	66	85	80
11	10	26	25	41	39	56	53	71	67	86	81
12	11	27	25	42	40	57	54	72	68	87	82
13	12	28	26	43	41	58	55	73	69	88	83
14	13	29	27	44	42	59	56	74	70	89	84
										90-100	85

	% IMPAIRMENT VISUAL SYSTEM	% IMPAIRMENT WHOLE PERSON
Total loss of vision one eye	25	24
Total loss of vision both eyes	100	85

Example 2:
In the patient described above, the eye with the greater motility loss has a 25% motility impairment.

Right Eye
Impairment of central vision and visual field . . .70%
Loss of ocular motility 25%
70% *combined* with 25%
(Combined Values Chart) 78%

The examiner may *combine* as much as a 10% impairment for an ocular abnormality or dysfunction that he or she believes is not adequately reflected in the visual acuity, visual fields, or diplopia testing (Combined Values Chart). In the above example, an impairment of 78% combined with a 10% impairment would result in a visual impairment of the right eye of 80%.

Step 4: After determining the level of impairment of each eye, use **Table 7** to determine visual system impairment. In the above example, considering impairments of 80% and 63%, impairment of the visual system is seen from **Table 7** to be 67%.

Step 5: Consult **Table 6** to ascertain the impairment of the whole person that is contributed by impairment of the visual system. A 67% impairment of the patient's visual system, as shown in the example above, is equivalent to a 63% impairment of the whole person (**Table 6**).

Procedure with Binocular Esterman Field Test
If the percentage loss of visual fields is determined for both eyes together by means of the Esterman binocular grid, consult **Table 7** to ascertain the impairment of the visual system due to loss of central vision.

Example 3:

Right Eye
Loss of central vision for both near and
distance is 56%

Left Eye
Loss of central vision for both near and
distance is 46%
From **Table 7** it is seen that impairment due to
the loss of central vision of both eyes is . .49%

Using the Combined Values Chart, *combine* the impairment due to loss of central vision with the impairment due to binocular visual field loss.

Binocular visual field testing is not recommended when loss of ocular motility is present.

With the patient in example 3:
Impairment due to loss of central vision of
both eyes is 49%
Impairment due to binocular visual field loss
is determined to be 20%
Combine the central vision and visual field losses
(Combined Values Chart); the impairment
of the visual system is 59%

Consult **Table 6** to ascertain the impairment of the whole person that is contributed by the visual system. In example 3, the 59% visual system impairment is equivalent to a 56% whole-person impairment (**Table 6**).

OTHER CONDITIONS

Up to an additional 10% impairment may be *combined* with the whole-person impairment related to the visual system for such conditions as permanent deformities of the orbit, scars, and other cosmetic deformities that do not otherwise alter ocular function. *Combine* the estimates by means of the Combined Values Chart.

Example:
Impairment due to loss of central vision
of both eyes 49%
Impairment due to binocular visual field loss . . .20%
Impairment of visual system
(Combined Values Chart) 59%
Impairment of whole person related to visual
system (**Table 6**) 56%
10% impairment for orbital scar and
deformity 10%
Whole-person impairment
(Combined Values Chart) 60%

REFERENCES
1. Sloan LL. New test charts for the measurement of visual acuity. *Am J Ophthalmol.* 1959;48:808-813.
2. Report of Working Group 39, Committee on Vision, National Academy of Sciences. Recommended standard procedures for the clinical measurement and specification of visual acuity. *Adv Ophthalmol.* 1980;41:103-143.
3. Esterman B. Grid for scoring visual field, II perimeter. *Arch Ophthalmol.* 1968;79:400-406.
4. Keeney AH, Duerson HL Jr. Collated near-vision test card. *Am J Ophthalmol.* 1958;46:592-594.
5. Keeney AH. *Ocular Examination: Basis and Technique.* 2nd ed. St Louis, Mo: CV Mosby Co; 1976.
6. Newell FW. *Ophthalmology: Principles and Concepts.* 7th ed. St Louis, Mo: CV Mosby Co; 1992.
7. Esterman B. Functional scoring of the binocular visual field. *Ophthalmology.* 1982;89:1226-1234.
8. Esterman B, Blance E, Wallach M, Bonelli A. Computerized scoring of the functional field: preliminary report. Doc *Ophthalmol Proc Ser.* 1985;42:333-339.
9. Anderson DR. *Perimetry: With and Without Automation.* 2nd ed. St Louis, Mo: CV Mosby Co; 1987.
10. American Academy of Ophthalmology. Contrast sensitivity and glare testing in the evaluation of anterior segment disease. *Ophthalmology.* 1990;97:1233-1237.
11. Frisen L. *Clinical Tests of Vision.* New York, NY: Raven Press; 1990.

TABLE 7

VISUAL SYSTEM

The values in this table are based on the following formula:

$$\frac{3 \times \text{impairment value of better eye} + \text{impairment value of worse eye}}{4} = \text{impairment of visual system}$$

The guides to the table are percentage impairment values for each eye. The percentage for the worse eye is read at the side of the table. The percentage for the better eye is read at the bottom of the table. At the intersection of the column for the worse eye and the column for the better eye is the impairment of visual system value.

For example, when there is 60% impairment of one eye and 30% impairment of the other eye, read down the side of the table until you come to the larger value (60%). Then follow across the row until it is intersected by the column headed by 30% at the bottom of the page. At the intersection of these two columns is printed the number 38. This number (38) represents the percentage impairment of the visual system when there is 60% impairment of one eye and 30% impairment of the other eye.

If bilateral aphakia is present and corrected central vision has been used in evaluation, impairment of the visual system is weighted by an additional 25% decrease in the value of the remaining corrected vision. For example, a 38% impairment (62% remaining) would be increased to 38% + (25%) (62%) = 54%.

% Impairment Worse Eye \ % Impairment Better Eye	0	1	2	3	4	5	6	7	8	9	10	11	12	13	14	15	16	17	18	19	20	21	22	23	24
0	0																								
1	0	1																							
2	1	1	2																						
3	1	2	2	3																					
4	1	2	3	3	4																				
5	1	2	3	4	4	5																			
6	2	2	3	4	5	5	6																		
7	2	3	3	4	5	6	6	7																	
8	2	3	4	4	5	6	7	7	8																
9	2	3	4	5	5	6	7	8	8	9															
10	3	3	4	5	6	6	7	8	9	9	10														
11	3	4	4	5	6	7	7	8	9	10	10	11													
12	3	4	5	5	6	7	8	8	9	10	11	11	12												
13	3	4	5	6	6	7	8	9	9	10	11	12	12	13											
14	4	4	5	6	7	7	8	9	10	10	11	12	13	13	14										
15	4	5	5	6	7	8	8	9	10	11	11	12	13	14	14	15									
16	4	5	6	6	7	8	9	9	10	11	12	12	13	14	15	15	16								
17	4	5	6	7	7	8	9	10	10	11	12	13	13	14	15	16	16	17							
18	5	5	6	7	8	8	9	10	11	11	12	13	14	14	15	16	17	17	18						
19	5	6	6	7	8	9	9	10	11	12	12	13	14	15	15	16	17	18	18	19					
20	5	6	7	7	8	9	10	10	11	12	13	13	14	15	16	16	17	18	19	19	20				
21	5	6	7	8	8	9	10	11	11	12	13	14	14	15	16	17	17	18	19	20	20	21			
22	6	6	7	8	9	9	10	11	12	12	13	14	15	15	16	17	18	18	19	20	21	21	22		
23	6	7	7	8	9	10	10	11	12	13	13	14	15	16	16	17	18	19	19	20	21	22	22	23	
24	6	7	8	8	9	10	11	11	12	13	14	14	15	16	17	17	18	19	20	20	21	22	23	23	24
25	6	7	8	9	9	10	11	12	12	13	14	15	15	16	17	18	18	19	20	21	21	22	23	24	24
26	7	7	8	9	10	10	11	12	13	13	14	15	16	16	17	18	19	19	20	21	22	22	23	24	25
27	7	8	8	9	10	11	11	12	13	14	14	15	16	17	17	18	19	20	20	21	22	23	23	24	25
28	7	8	9	9	10	11	12	12	13	14	15	15	16	17	18	18	19	20	21	21	22	23	24	24	25
29	7	8	9	10	10	11	12	13	13	14	15	16	16	17	18	19	19	20	21	22	22	23	24	25	25
30	8	8	9	10	11	11	12	13	14	14	15	16	17	17	18	19	20	20	21	22	23	23	24	25	26
31	8	9	9	10	11	12	12	13	14	15	15	16	17	18	18	19	20	21	21	22	23	24	24	25	26
32	8	9	10	10	11	12	13	13	14	15	16	16	17	18	19	19	20	21	22	22	23	24	25	25	26
33	8	9	10	11	11	12	13	14	14	15	16	17	17	18	19	20	20	21	22	23	23	24	25	26	26
34	9	9	10	11	12	12	13	14	15	15	16	17	18	18	19	20	21	21	22	23	24	24	25	26	27
35	9	10	10	11	12	13	13	14	15	16	16	17	18	19	19	20	21	22	22	23	24	25	25	26	27
36	9	10	11	11	12	13	14	14	15	16	17	17	18	19	20	20	21	22	23	23	24	25	26	26	27
37	9	10	11	12	12	13	14	15	15	16	17	18	18	19	20	21	21	22	23	24	24	25	26	27	27
38	10	10	11	12	13	13	14	15	16	16	17	18	19	19	20	21	22	22	23	24	25	25	26	27	28
39	10	11	11	12	13	14	14	15	16	17	17	18	19	20	20	21	22	23	23	24	25	26	26	27	28
40	10	11	12	12	13	14	15	15	16	17	18	18	19	20	21	21	22	23	24	24	25	26	27	27	28
41	10	11	12	13	13	14	15	16	16	17	18	19	19	20	21	22	22	23	24	25	25	26	27	28	28
42	11	11	12	13	14	14	15	16	17	17	18	19	20	20	21	22	23	23	24	25	26	26	27	28	29
43	11	12	12	13	14	15	15	16	17	18	18	19	20	21	21	22	23	24	24	25	26	27	27	28	29
44	11	12	13	13	14	15	16	16	17	18	19	19	20	21	22	22	23	24	25	25	26	27	28	28	29
45	11	12	13	14	14	15	16	17	17	18	19	20	20	21	22	23	23	24	25	26	26	27	28	29	29
46	12	12	13	14	15	15	16	17	18	18	19	20	21	21	22	23	24	24	25	26	27	27	28	29	30
47	12	13	13	14	15	16	16	17	18	19	19	20	21	22	22	23	24	25	25	26	27	28	28	29	30
48	12	13	14	14	15	16	17	17	18	19	20	20	21	22	23	23	24	25	26	26	27	28	29	29	30
49	12	13	14	15	15	16	17	18	18	19	20	21	21	22	23	24	24	25	26	27	27	28	29	30	30

% Impairment Worse Eye \ % Impairment Better Eye	25	26	27	28	29	30	31	32	33	34	35	36	37	38	39	40	41	42	43	44	45	46	47	48	49
25	25																								
26	25	26																							
27	26	26	27																						
28	26	27	27	28																					
29	26	27	28	28	29																				
30	26	27	28	29	29	30																			
31	27	27	28	29	30	30	31																		
32	27	28	28	29	30	31	31	32																	
33	27	28	29	29	30	31	32	32	33																
34	27	28	29	30	30	31	32	33	33	34															
35	28	28	29	30	31	31	32	33	34	34	35														
36	28	29	29	30	31	32	32	33	34	35	35	36													
37	28	29	30	30	31	32	33	33	34	35	36	36	37												
38	28	29	30	31	31	32	33	34	34	35	36	37	37	38											
39	29	29	30	31	32	32	33	34	35	35	36	37	38	38	39										
40	29	30	30	31	32	33	33	34	35	36	36	37	38	39	39	40									
41	29	30	31	31	32	33	34	34	35	36	37	37	38	39	40	40	41								
42	29	30	31	32	32	33	34	35	35	36	37	38	38	39	40	41	41	42							
43	30	30	31	32	33	33	34	35	36	36	37	38	39	39	40	41	42	42	43						
44	30	31	31	32	33	34	34	35	36	37	37	38	39	40	40	41	42	43	43	44					
45	30	31	32	32	33	34	35	35	36	37	38	38	39	40	41	41	42	43	44	44	45				
46	30	31	32	33	33	34	35	36	36	37	38	39	39	40	41	42	42	43	44	45	45	46			
47	31	31	32	33	34	34	35	36	37	37	38	39	40	40	41	42	43	43	44	45	46	46	47		
48	31	32	32	33	34	35	35	36	37	38	38	39	40	41	41	42	43	44	44	45	46	47	47	48	
49	31	32	33	33	34	35	36	36	37	38	39	39	40	41	42	42	43	44	45	45	46	47	48	48	49

% Impairment Better Eye (columns) / % Impairment Worse Eye (rows)

% Impairment Worse Eye	0	1	2	3	4	5	6	7	8	9	10	11	12	13	14	15	16	17	18	19	20	21	22	23	24	25	26	27	28	29	30	31	32	33	34	35	36	37	38	39	40	41	42	43	44	45	46	47	48	49	
50	13	13	14	15	16	16	17	18	19	19	20	21	22	22	23	24	25	25	26	27	28	28	29	30	31	31	32	33	34	34	35	36	37	37	38	39	40	40	41	42	43	43	44	45	46	46	47	48	49	49	50
51	13	14	14	15	16	17	17	18	19	20	20	21	22	23	23	24	25	26	26	27	28	29	29	30	31	32	32	33	34	35	35	36	37	38	38	39	40	41	41	42	43	44	44	45	46	47	47	48	49	50	51
52	13	14	15	15	16	17	18	18	19	20	21	21	22	23	24	24	25	26	27	27	28	29	30	30	31	32	33	33	34	35	36	36	37	38	39	39	40	41	42	42	43	44	45	45	46	47	48	48	49	50	52
53	13	14	15	16	16	17	18	19	19	20	21	22	22	23	24	25	25	26	27	28	28	29	30	31	31	32	33	34	34	35	36	37	37	38	39	40	40	41	42	43	43	44	45	46	46	47	48	49	49	50	53
54	14	14	15	16	17	17	18	19	20	20	21	22	23	23	24	25	26	26	27	28	29	29	30	31	32	32	33	34	35	35	36	37	38	38	39	40	41	41	42	43	44	44	45	46	47	47	48	49	50	50	54
55	14	15	15	16	17	18	18	19	20	21	21	22	23	24	24	25	26	27	27	28	29	30	30	31	32	33	33	34	35	36	36	37	38	39	39	40	41	42	42	43	44	45	45	46	47	48	48	49	50	51	55
56	14	15	16	16	17	18	19	19	20	21	22	22	23	24	25	25	26	27	28	28	29	30	31	31	32	33	34	34	35	36	37	37	38	39	40	40	41	42	43	43	44	45	46	46	47	48	49	49	50	51	56
57	14	15	16	17	17	18	19	20	20	21	22	23	23	24	25	26	26	27	28	29	29	30	31	32	32	33	34	35	35	36	37	38	38	39	40	41	41	42	43	44	44	45	46	47	47	48	49	50	50	51	57
58	15	15	16	17	18	18	19	20	21	21	22	23	24	24	25	26	27	27	28	29	30	30	31	32	33	33	34	35	36	36	37	38	39	39	40	41	42	42	43	44	45	45	46	47	48	48	49	50	51	51	58
59	15	16	16	17	18	19	19	20	21	22	22	23	24	25	25	26	27	28	28	29	30	31	31	32	33	34	34	35	36	37	37	38	39	40	40	41	42	43	43	44	45	46	46	47	48	49	49	50	51	52	59
60	15	16	17	17	18	19	20	20	21	22	23	23	24	25	26	26	27	28	29	29	30	31	32	32	33	34	35	35	36	37	38	38	39	40	41	41	42	43	44	44	45	46	47	47	48	49	50	50	51	52	60
61	15	16	17	18	18	19	20	21	21	22	23	24	24	25	26	27	27	28	29	30	30	31	32	33	33	34	35	36	36	37	38	39	39	40	41	42	42	43	44	45	45	46	47	48	48	49	50	51	51	52	61
62	16	16	17	18	19	19	20	21	22	22	23	24	25	25	26	27	28	28	29	30	31	31	32	33	34	34	35	36	37	37	38	39	40	40	41	42	43	43	44	45	46	46	47	48	49	49	50	51	52	52	62
63	16	17	17	18	19	20	20	21	22	23	23	24	25	26	26	27	28	29	29	30	31	32	32	33	34	35	35	36	37	38	38	39	40	41	41	42	43	44	44	45	46	47	47	48	49	50	50	51	52	53	63
64	16	17	18	18	19	20	21	21	22	23	24	24	25	26	27	27	28	29	30	30	31	32	33	33	34	35	36	36	37	38	39	39	40	41	42	42	43	44	45	45	46	47	48	48	49	50	51	51	52	53	64
65	16	17	18	19	19	20	21	22	22	23	24	25	25	26	27	28	28	29	30	31	31	32	33	34	34	35	36	37	37	38	39	40	40	41	42	43	43	44	45	46	46	47	48	49	49	50	51	52	52	53	65
66	17	17	18	19	20	20	21	22	23	23	24	25	26	26	27	28	29	29	30	31	32	32	33	34	35	35	36	37	38	38	39	40	41	41	42	43	44	44	45	46	47	47	48	49	50	50	51	52	53	53	66
67	17	18	18	19	20	21	21	22	23	24	24	25	26	27	27	28	29	30	30	31	32	33	33	34	35	36	36	37	38	39	39	40	41	42	42	43	44	45	45	46	47	48	48	49	50	51	51	52	53	54	67
68	17	18	19	19	20	21	22	22	23	24	25	25	26	27	28	28	29	30	31	31	32	33	34	34	35	36	37	37	38	39	40	40	41	42	43	43	44	45	46	46	47	48	49	49	50	51	52	52	53	54	68
69	17	18	19	20	20	21	22	23	23	24	25	26	26	27	28	29	29	30	31	32	32	33	34	35	35	36	37	38	38	39	40	41	41	42	43	44	44	45	46	47	47	48	49	50	50	51	52	53	53	54	69
70	18	18	19	20	21	21	22	23	24	24	25	26	27	27	28	29	30	30	31	32	33	33	34	35	36	36	37	38	39	39	40	41	42	42	43	44	45	45	46	47	48	48	49	50	51	51	52	53	54	54	70
71	18	19	19	20	21	22	22	23	24	25	25	26	27	28	28	29	30	31	31	32	33	34	34	35	36	37	37	38	39	40	40	41	42	43	43	44	45	46	46	47	48	49	49	50	51	52	52	53	54	55	71
72	18	19	20	20	21	22	23	23	24	25	26	26	27	28	29	29	30	31	32	32	33	34	35	35	36	37	38	38	39	40	41	41	42	43	44	44	45	46	47	47	48	49	50	50	51	52	53	53	54	55	72
73	18	19	20	21	21	22	23	24	24	25	26	27	27	28	29	30	30	31	32	33	33	34	35	36	36	37	38	39	39	40	41	42	42	43	44	45	45	46	47	48	48	49	50	51	51	52	53	54	54	55	73
74	19	19	20	21	22	22	23	24	25	25	26	27	28	28	29	30	31	31	32	33	34	34	35	36	37	37	38	39	40	40	41	42	43	43	44	45	46	46	47	48	49	49	50	51	52	52	53	54	55	55	74
75	19	20	20	21	22	23	23	24	25	26	26	27	28	29	29	30	31	32	32	33	34	35	35	36	37	38	38	39	40	41	41	42	43	44	44	45	46	47	47	48	49	50	50	51	52	53	53	54	55	56	75
76	19	20	21	21	22	23	24	24	25	26	27	27	28	29	30	30	31	32	33	33	34	35	36	36	37	38	39	39	40	41	42	42	43	44	45	45	46	47	48	48	49	50	51	51	52	53	54	54	55	56	76
77	19	20	21	22	22	23	24	25	25	26	27	28	28	29	30	31	31	32	33	34	34	35	36	37	37	38	39	40	40	41	42	43	43	44	45	46	46	47	48	49	49	50	51	52	52	53	54	55	55	56	77
78	20	20	21	22	23	23	24	25	26	26	27	28	29	29	30	31	32	32	33	34	35	35	36	37	38	38	39	40	41	41	42	43	44	44	45	46	47	47	48	49	50	50	51	52	53	53	54	55	56	56	78
79	20	21	21	22	23	24	24	25	26	27	27	28	29	30	30	31	32	33	33	34	35	36	36	37	38	39	39	40	41	42	42	43	44	45	45	46	47	48	48	49	50	51	51	52	53	54	54	55	56	57	79
80	20	21	22	22	23	24	25	25	26	27	28	28	29	30	31	31	32	33	34	34	35	36	37	37	38	39	40	40	41	42	43	43	44	45	46	46	47	48	49	49	50	51	52	52	53	54	55	55	56	57	80
81	20	21	22	23	23	24	25	26	26	27	28	29	29	30	31	32	32	33	34	35	35	36	37	38	38	39	40	41	41	42	43	44	44	45	46	47	47	48	49	50	50	51	52	53	53	54	55	56	56	57	81
82	21	21	22	23	24	24	25	26	27	27	28	29	30	30	31	32	33	33	34	35	36	36	37	38	39	39	40	41	42	42	43	44	45	45	46	47	48	48	49	50	51	51	52	53	54	54	55	56	57	57	82
83	21	22	22	23	24	25	25	26	27	28	28	29	30	31	31	32	33	34	34	35	36	37	37	38	39	40	40	41	42	43	43	44	45	46	46	47	48	49	49	50	51	52	52	53	54	55	55	56	57	58	83
84	21	22	23	23	24	25	26	26	27	28	29	29	30	31	32	32	33	34	35	35	36	37	38	38	39	40	41	41	42	43	44	44	45	46	47	47	48	49	50	50	51	52	53	53	54	55	56	56	57	58	84
85	21	22	23	24	24	25	26	27	27	28	29	30	30	31	32	33	33	34	35	36	36	37	38	39	39	40	41	42	42	43	44	45	45	46	47	48	48	49	50	51	51	52	53	54	54	55	56	57	57	58	85
86	22	22	23	24	25	25	26	27	28	28	29	30	31	31	32	33	34	34	35	36	37	37	38	39	40	40	41	42	43	43	44	45	46	46	47	48	49	49	50	51	52	52	53	54	55	55	56	57	58	58	86
87	22	23	23	24	25	26	26	27	28	29	29	30	31	32	32	33	34	35	35	36	37	38	38	39	40	41	41	42	43	44	44	45	46	47	47	48	49	50	50	51	52	53	53	54	55	56	56	57	58	59	87
88	22	23	24	24	25	26	27	27	28	29	30	30	31	32	33	33	34	35	36	36	37	38	39	39	40	41	42	42	43	44	45	45	46	47	48	48	49	50	51	51	52	53	54	54	55	56	57	57	58	59	88
89	22	23	24	25	25	26	27	28	28	29	30	31	31	32	33	34	34	35	36	37	37	38	39	40	40	41	42	43	43	44	45	46	46	47	48	49	49	50	51	52	52	53	54	55	55	56	57	58	58	59	89
90	23	23	24	25	26	26	27	28	29	29	30	31	32	32	33	34	35	35	36	37	38	38	39	40	41	41	42	43	44	44	45	46	47	47	48	49	50	50	51	52	53	53	54	55	56	56	57	58	59	59	90
91	23	24	24	25	26	27	27	28	29	30	30	31	32	33	33	34	35	36	36	37	38	39	39	40	41	42	42	43	44	45	45	46	47	48	48	49	50	51	51	52	53	54	54	55	56	57	57	58	59	60	91
92	23	24	25	25	26	27	28	28	29	30	31	31	32	33	34	34	35	36	37	37	38	39	40	40	41	42	43	43	44	45	46	46	47	48	49	49	50	51	52	52	53	54	55	55	56	57	58	58	59	60	92
93	23	24	25	26	26	27	28	29	29	30	31	32	32	33	34	35	35	36	37	38	38	39	40	41	41	42	43	44	44	45	46	47	47	48	49	50	50	51	52	53	53	54	55	56	56	57	58	59	59	60	93
94	24	24	25	26	27	27	28	29	30	30	31	32	33	33	34	35	36	36	37	38	39	39	40	41	42	42	43	44	45	45	46	47	48	48	49	50	51	51	52	53	54	54	55	56	57	57	58	59	60	60	94
95	24	25	25	26	27	28	28	29	30	31	31	32	33	34	34	35	36	37	37	38	39	40	40	41	42	43	43	44	45	46	46	47	48	49	49	50	51	52	52	53	54	55	55	56	57	58	58	59	60	61	95
96	24	25	26	26	27	28	29	29	30	31	32	32	33	34	35	35	36	37	38	38	39	40	41	41	42	43	44	44	45	46	47	47	48	49	50	50	51	52	53	53	54	55	56	56	57	58	59	59	60	61	96
97	24	25	26	27	27	28	29	30	30	31	32	33	33	34	35	36	36	37	38	39	39	40	41	42	42	43	44	45	45	46	47	48	48	49	50	51	51	52	53	54	54	55	56	57	57	58	59	60	60	61	97
98	25	25	26	27	28	28	29	30	31	31	32	33	34	34	35	36	37	37	38	39	40	40	41	42	43	43	44	45	46	46	47	48	49	49	50	51	52	52	53	54	55	55	56	57	58	58	59	60	61	61	98
99	25	26	26	27	28	29	29	30	31	32	32	33	34	35	35	36	37	38	38	39	40	41	41	42	43	44	44	45	46	47	47	48	49	50	50	51	52	53	53	54	55	56	56	57	58	59	59	60	61	62	99
100	25	26	27	27	28	29	30	30	31	32	33	33	34	35	36	36	37	38	39	39	40	41	42	42	43	44	45	45	46	47	48	48	49	50	51	51	52	53	54	54	55	56	57	57	58	59	60	60	61	62	100
% Impairment Better Eye	0	1	2	3	4	5	6	7	8	9	10	11	12	13	14	15	16	17	18	19	20	21	22	23	24	25	26	27	28	29	30	31	32	33	34	35	36	37	38	39	40	41	42	43	44	45	46	47	48	49	

% Impairment Worse Eye (rows) / % Impairment Better Eye (columns)

% Impairment Worse Eye	50	51	52	53	54	55	56	57	58	59	60	61	62	63	64	65	66	67	68	69	70	71	72	73	74
50	50																								
51	50	51																							
52	51	51	52																						
53	51	52	52	53																					
54	51	52	53	53	54																				
55	51	52	53	54	54	55																			
56	52	52	53	54	55	55	56																		
57	52	53	53	54	55	56	56	57																	
58	52	53	54	54	55	56	57	57	58																
59	52	53	54	55	55	56	57	58	58	59															
60	53	53	54	55	56	56	57	58	59	59	60														
61	53	54	54	55	56	57	57	58	59	60	60	61													
62	53	54	55	55	56	57	58	58	59	60	61	61	62												
63	53	54	55	56	56	57	58	59	59	60	61	62	62	63											
64	54	54	55	56	57	57	58	59	60	60	61	62	63	63	64										
65	54	55	55	56	57	58	58	59	60	61	61	62	63	64	64	65									
66	54	55	56	56	57	58	59	59	60	61	62	62	63	64	65	65	66								
67	54	55	56	57	57	58	59	60	60	61	62	63	63	64	65	66	66	67							
68	55	55	56	57	58	58	59	60	61	61	62	63	64	64	65	66	67	67	68						
69	55	56	56	57	58	59	59	60	61	62	62	63	64	65	65	66	67	68	68	69					
70	55	56	57	57	58	59	60	60	61	62	63	63	64	65	66	66	67	68	69	69	70				
71	55	56	57	58	58	59	60	61	61	62	63	64	64	65	66	67	67	68	69	70	70	71			
72	56	56	57	58	59	59	60	61	62	62	63	64	65	65	66	67	68	68	69	70	71	71	72		
73	56	57	57	58	59	60	60	61	62	63	63	64	65	66	66	67	68	69	69	70	71	72	72	73	
74	56	57	58	58	59	60	61	61	62	63	64	64	65	66	67	67	68	69	70	70	71	72	73	73	74
75	56	57	58	59	59	60	61	62	62	63	64	65	65	66	67	68	68	69	70	71	71	72	73	74	74
76	57	57	58	59	60	60	61	62	63	63	64	65	66	66	67	68	69	69	70	71	72	72	73	74	75
77	57	58	58	59	60	61	61	62	63	64	64	65	66	67	67	68	69	70	70	71	72	73	73	74	75
78	57	58	59	59	60	61	62	62	63	64	65	65	66	67	68	68	69	70	71	71	72	73	74	74	75
79	57	58	59	60	60	61	62	63	63	64	65	66	66	67	68	69	69	70	71	72	72	73	74	75	75
80	58	58	59	60	61	61	62	63	64	64	65	66	67	67	68	69	70	70	71	72	73	73	74	75	76
81	58	59	59	60	61	62	62	63	64	65	65	66	67	68	68	69	70	71	71	72	73	74	74	75	76
82	58	59	60	60	61	62	63	63	64	65	66	66	67	68	69	69	70	71	72	72	73	74	75	75	76
83	58	59	60	61	61	62	63	64	64	65	66	67	67	68	69	70	70	71	72	73	73	74	75	76	76
84	59	59	60	61	62	62	63	64	65	65	66	67	68	68	69	70	71	71	72	73	74	74	75	76	77
85	59	60	60	61	62	63	63	64	65	66	66	67	68	69	69	70	71	72	72	73	74	75	75	76	77
86	59	60	61	61	62	63	64	64	65	66	67	67	68	69	70	70	71	72	73	73	74	75	76	76	77
87	59	60	61	62	62	63	64	65	65	66	67	68	68	69	70	71	71	72	73	74	74	75	76	77	77
88	60	60	61	62	63	63	64	65	66	66	67	68	69	69	70	71	72	72	73	74	75	75	76	77	78
89	60	61	61	62	63	64	64	65	66	67	67	68	69	70	70	71	72	73	73	74	75	76	76	77	78
90	60	61	62	62	63	64	65	65	66	67	68	68	69	70	71	71	72	73	74	74	75	76	77	77	78
91	60	61	62	63	63	64	65	66	66	67	68	69	69	70	71	72	72	73	74	75	75	76	77	78	78
92	61	61	62	63	64	64	65	66	67	67	68	69	70	70	71	72	73	73	74	75	76	76	77	78	79
93	61	62	62	63	64	65	65	66	67	68	68	69	70	71	71	72	73	74	74	75	76	77	77	78	79
94	61	62	63	63	64	65	66	66	67	68	69	69	70	71	72	72	73	74	75	75	76	77	78	78	79
95	61	62	63	64	64	65	66	67	67	68	69	70	70	71	72	73	73	74	75	76	76	77	78	79	79
96	62	62	63	64	65	65	66	67	68	68	69	70	71	71	72	73	74	74	75	76	77	77	78	79	80
97	62	63	63	64	65	66	66	67	68	69	69	70	71	72	72	73	74	75	75	76	77	78	78	79	80
98	62	63	64	64	65	66	67	67	68	69	70	70	71	72	73	73	74	75	76	76	77	78	79	79	80
99	62	63	64	65	65	66	67	68	68	69	70	71	71	72	73	74	74	75	76	77	77	78	79	80	80
100	63	63	64	65	66	66	67	68	69	69	70	71	72	72	73	74	75	75	76	77	78	78	79	80	81

% Impairment Worse Eye	75	76	77	78	79	80	81	82	83	84	85	86	87	88	89	90	91	92	93	94	95	96	97	9[illegible]	99	100
75	75																									
76	75	76																								
77	76	76	77																							
78	76	77	77	78																						
79	76	77	78	78	79																					
80	76	77	78	79	79	80																				
81	77	77	78	79	80	80	81																			
82	77	78	78	79	80	81	81	82																		
83	77	78	79	79	80	81	82	82	83																	
84	77	78	79	80	80	81	82	83	83	84																
85	78	78	79	80	81	81	82	83	84	84	85															
86	78	79	79	80	81	82	82	83	84	85	85	86														
87	78	79	80	80	81	82	83	83	84	85	86	86	87													
88	78	79	80	81	81	82	83	84	84	85	86	87	87	88												
89	79	79	80	81	82	82	83	84	85	85	86	87	88	88	89											
90	79	80	80	81	82	83	83	84	85	86	86	87	88	89	89	90										
91	79	80	81	81	82	83	84	84	85	86	87	87	88	89	90	90	91									
92	79	80	81	82	82	83	84	85	85	86	87	88	88	89	90	91	91	92								
93	80	80	81	82	83	83	84	85	86	86	87	88	89	89	90	91	92	92	93							
94	80	81	81	82	83	84	84	85	86	87	87	88	89	90	90	91	92	93	93	94						
95	80	81	82	82	83	84	85	85	86	87	88	88	89	90	91	91	92	93	94	94	95					
96	80	81	82	83	83	84	85	86	86	87	88	89	89	90	91	92	92	93	94	95	95	96				
97	81	81	82	83	84	84	85	86	87	87	88	89	90	90	91	92	93	93	94	95	96	96	97			
98	81	82	82	83	84	85	85	86	87	88	88	89	90	91	91	92	93	94	94	95	96	97	97	[illegible]		
99	81	82	83	83	84	85	86	86	87	88	89	89	90	91	92	92	93	94	95	95	96	97	98	[illegible]	99	
100	81	82	83	84	84	85	86	87	87	88	89	90	90	91	92	93	93	94	95	96	96	97	98	[illegible]	99	100

% Impairment Better Eye

TABLE 8

COMBINED VALUES CHART

The values are derived from the formula A + B (1 – A) = combined value of A and B, where A and B are the decimal equivalents of the impairment ratings. In the chart all values are expressed as percents. To combine any two impairment values, locate the larger of the values on the side of the chart and read along that row until you come to the column indicated by the smaller value at the bottom of the chart. At the intersection of the row and the column is the combined value.

For example, to combine 35% and 20% read down the side of the chart until you come to the larger value, 35%. Then read across the 35% row until you come to the column indicated by 20% at the bottom of the chart. At the intersection of the row and column is the number 48. Therefore, 35% combined with 20% is 48%. Due to the construction of this chart, the larger impairment value must be identified at the side of the chart.

If three or more impairment values are to be combined, select any two and find their combined values as above. Then use that value and the third value to locate the combined value of all. This process can be repeated indefinitely, the final value in each instance being the combination of all the previous values. In each step of this process the larger impairment value must be identified at the side of the chart.

	1	2	3	4	5	6	7	8	9	10	11	12	13	14	15	16	17	18	19	20	21	22	23	24	25	26	27	28	29	30	31	32	33	34	35	36	37	38	39	40	41	42	43	44	45	46	47	48	49	50
1	2																																																	
2	3	4																																																
3	4	5	6																																															
4	5	6	7	8																																														
5	6	7	8	9	10																																													
6	7	8	9	10	11	12																																												
7	8	9	10	11	12	13	14																																											
8	9	10	11	12	13	14	14	15																																										
9	10	11	12	13	14	14	15	16	17																																									
10	11	12	13	14	15	15	16	17	18	19																																								
11	12	13	14	15	15	16	17	18	19	20	21																																							
12	13	14	15	16	16	17	18	19	20	21	22	23																																						
13	14	15	16	16	17	18	19	20	21	22	23	23	24																																					
14	15	16	17	17	18	19	20	21	22	23	23	24	25	26																																				
15	16	17	18	18	19	20	21	22	23	24	24	25	26	27	28																																			
16	17	18	19	19	20	21	22	23	24	24	25	26	27	28	29	29																																		
17	18	19	19	20	21	22	23	24	24	25	26	27	28	29	29	30	31																																	
18	19	20	20	21	22	23	24	25	25	26	27	28	29	29	30	31	32	33																																
19	20	21	21	22	23	24	25	25	26	27	28	29	30	30	31	32	33	34	34																															
20	21	22	22	23	24	25	26	26	27	28	29	30	30	31	32	33	34	34	35	36																														
21	22	23	23	24	25	26	27	27	28	29	30	30	31	32	33	34	34	35	36	37	38																													
22	23	24	24	25	26	27	27	28	29	30	31	31	32	33	34	34	35	36	37	38	38	39																												
23	24	25	25	26	27	28	28	29	30	31	31	32	33	34	35	35	36	37	38	38	39	40	41																											
24	25	26	26	27	28	29	29	30	31	32	32	33	34	35	35	36	37	38	38	39	40	41	41	42																										
25	26	27	27	28	29	30	30	31	32	33	33	34	35	36	36	37	38	39	39	40	41	42	42	43	44																									
26	27	27	28	29	30	30	31	32	33	33	34	35	36	36	37	38	39	39	40	41	42	42	43	44	45	45																								
27	28	28	29	30	31	31	32	33	34	34	35	36	36	37	38	39	39	40	41	42	42	43	44	45	45	46	47																							
28	29	29	30	31	32	32	33	34	34	35	36	37	37	38	39	40	40	41	42	42	43	44	45	45	46	47	47	48																						
29	30	30	31	32	33	33	34	35	35	36	37	38	38	39	40	40	41	42	42	43	44	45	45	46	47	47	48	49	50																					
30	31	31	32	33	34	34	35	36	36	37	38	38	39	40	41	41	42	43	43	44	45	45	46	47	48	48	49	50	50	51																				
31	32	32	33	34	34	35	36	37	37	38	39	39	40	41	41	42	43	43	44	45	45	46	47	48	48	49	50	50	51	52	52																			
32	33	33	34	35	35	36	37	37	38	39	39	40	41	42	42	43	44	44	45	46	46	47	48	48	49	50	50	51	52	52	53	54																		
33	34	34	35	36	36	37	38	38	39	40	40	41	42	42	43	44	44	45	46	46	47	48	48	49	50	50	51	52	52	53	54	54	55																	
34	35	35	36	37	37	38	39	39	40	41	41	42	43	43	44	45	45	46	47	47	48	49	49	50	51	51	52	52	53	54	54	55	56	56																
35	36	36	37	38	38	39	40	40	41	42	42	43	43	44	45	45	46	47	47	48	49	49	50	51	51	52	53	53	54	55	55	56	56	57	58															
36	37	37	38	39	39	40	40	41	42	42	43	44	44	45	46	46	47	48	48	49	49	50	51	51	52	53	53	54	55	55	56	56	57	58	58	59														
37	38	38	39	40	40	41	41	42	43	43	44	45	45	46	46	47	48	48	49	50	50	51	51	52	53	53	54	55	55	56	57	57	58	58	59	60	60													
38	39	39	40	40	41	42	42	43	44	44	45	45	46	47	47	48	49	49	50	50	51	52	52	53	54	54	55	55	56	57	57	58	58	59	60	60	61	62												
39	40	40	41	41	42	43	43	44	44	45	46	46	47	48	48	49	49	50	51	51	52	52	53	54	54	55	55	56	57	57	58	59	59	60	60	61	62	62	63											
40	41	41	42	42	43	44	44	45	45	46	47	47	48	48	49	50	50	51	51	52	53	53	54	54	55	56	56	57	57	58	59	59	60	60	61	62	62	63	63	64										
41	42	42	43	43	44	45	45	46	46	47	47	48	49	49	50	50	51	52	52	53	53	54	55	55	56	56	57	58	58	59	59	60	60	61	62	62	63	63	64	65	65									
42	43	43	44	44	45	45	46	47	47	48	48	49	50	50	51	51	52	52	53	54	54	55	55	56	57	57	58	58	59	59	60	61	61	62	62	63	63	64	65	65	66	66								
43	44	44	45	45	46	46	47	48	48	49	49	50	50	51	52	52	53	53	54	54	55	56	56	57	57	58	58	59	60	60	61	61	62	62	63	64	64	65	65	66	66	67	68							
44	45	45	46	46	47	47	48	48	49	50	50	51	51	52	52	53	54	54	55	55	56	56	57	57	58	59	59	60	60	61	61	62	62	63	64	64	65	65	66	66	67	68	68	69						
45	46	46	47	47	48	48	49	49	50	51	51	52	52	53	53	54	54	55	55	56	57	57	58	58	59	59	60	60	61	62	62	63	63	64	64	65	65	66	66	67	68	68	69	69	70					
46	47	47	48	48	49	49	50	50	51	51	52	52	53	54	54	55	55	56	56	57	57	58	58	59	60	60	61	61	62	62	63	63	64	64	65	65	66	67	67	68	68	69	69	70	70	71				
47	48	48	49	49	50	50	51	51	52	52	53	53	54	54	55	55	56	57	57	58	58	59	59	60	60	61	61	62	62	63	63	64	64	65	66	66	67	67	68	68	69	69	70	70	71	71	72			
48	49	49	50	50	51	51	52	52	53	53	54	54	55	55	56	56	57	57	58	58	59	59	60	60	61	62	62	63	63	64	64	65	65	66	66	67	67	68	68	69	69	70	70	71	71	72	72	73		
49	50	50	51	51	52	52	53	53	54	54	55	55	56	56	57	57	58	58	59	59	60	60	61	61	62	62	63	63	64	64	65	65	66	66	67	67	68	68	69	69	70	70	71	71	72	72	73	73	74	
50	51	51	52	52	53	53	54	54	55	55	56	56	57	57	58	58	59	59	60	60	61	61	62	62	63	63	64	64	65	65	66	66	67	67	68	68	69	69	70	70	71	71	72	72	73	73	74	74	75	75

COMBINED VALUES CHART (CONTINUED)

	1	2	3	4	5	6	7	8	9	10	11	12	13	14	15	16	17	18	19	20	21	22	23	24	25
51	51	52	52	53	53	54	54	55	55	56	56	57	57	58	58	59	59	60	60	61	61	62	62	63	63
52	52	53	53	54	54	55	55	56	56	57	57	58	58	59	59	60	60	61	61	62	62	63	63	64	64
53	53	54	54	55	55	56	56	57	57	58	58	59	59	60	60	61	61	61	62	62	63	63	64	64	65
54	54	55	55	56	56	57	57	58	58	59	59	59	60	60	61	61	62	62	63	63	64	64	65	65	66
55	55	56	56	57	57	58	58	59	59	60	60	60	61	61	62	62	63	63	64	64	64	65	65	66	66
56	56	57	57	58	58	59	59	60	60	60	61	61	62	62	63	63	63	64	64	65	65	66	66	67	67
57	57	58	58	59	59	60	60	60	61	61	62	62	63	63	63	64	64	65	65	66	66	66	67	67	68
58	58	59	59	60	60	61	61	61	62	62	63	63	63	64	64	65	65	66	66	66	67	67	68	68	68
59	59	60	60	61	61	61	62	62	63	63	64	64	64	65	65	66	66	66	67	67	68	68	68	69	69
60	60	61	61	62	62	62	63	63	64	64	64	65	65	66	66	66	67	67	68	68	68	69	69	70	70
61	61	62	62	63	63	63	64	64	65	65	65	66	66	66	67	67	68	68	68	69	69	70	70	70	71
62	62	63	63	64	64	64	65	65	65	66	66	67	67	67	68	68	68	69	69	70	70	70	71	71	72
63	63	64	64	64	65	65	66	66	66	67	67	67	68	68	69	69	69	70	70	70	71	71	72	72	72
64	64	65	65	65	66	66	67	67	67	68	68	68	69	69	69	70	70	70	71	71	72	72	72	73	73
65	65	66	66	66	67	67	67	68	68	69	69	69	70	70	70	71	71	71	72	72	72	73	73	73	74
66	66	67	67	67	68	68	68	69	69	69	70	70	70	71	71	71	72	72	72	73	73	73	74	74	75
67	67	68	68	68	69	69	69	70	70	70	71	71	71	72	72	72	73	73	73	74	74	74	75	75	75
68	68	69	69	69	70	70	70	71	71	71	72	72	72	72	73	73	73	74	74	74	75	75	75	76	76
69	69	70	70	70	71	71	71	71	72	72	72	73	73	73	74	74	74	75	75	75	76	76	76	76	77
70	70	71	71	71	72	72	72	72	73	73	73	74	74	74	75	75	75	75	76	76	76	77	77	77	78
71	71	72	72	72	72	73	73	73	74	74	74	74	75	75	75	76	76	76	77	77	77	77	78	78	78
72	72	73	73	73	73	74	74	74	75	75	75	75	76	76	76	76	77	77	77	78	78	78	78	79	79
73	73	74	74	74	74	75	75	75	75	76	76	76	77	77	77	77	78	78	78	78	79	79	79	79	80
74	74	75	75	75	75	76	76	76	76	77	77	77	77	78	78	78	78	79	79	79	79	80	80	80	81
75	75	76	76	76	76	77	77	77	77	78	78	78	78	79	79	79	79	80	80	80	80	81	81	81	81
76	76	76	77	77	77	77	78	78	78	78	79	79	79	79	80	80	80	80	81	81	81	81	82	82	82
77	77	77	78	78	78	78	79	79	79	79	80	80	80	80	80	81	81	81	81	82	82	82	82	83	83
78	78	78	79	79	79	79	80	80	80	80	80	81	81	81	81	82	82	82	82	82	83	83	83	83	84
79	79	79	80	80	80	80	80	81	81	81	81	82	82	82	82	82	83	83	83	83	83	84	84	84	84
80	80	80	81	81	81	81	81	82	82	82	82	82	83	83	83	83	83	84	84	84	84	84	85	85	85
81	81	81	82	82	82	82	82	83	83	83	83	83	83	84	84	84	84	84	85	85	85	85	85	86	86
82	82	82	83	83	83	83	83	83	84	84	84	84	84	85	85	85	85	85	85	86	86	86	86	86	87
83	83	83	84	84	84	84	84	84	85	85	85	85	85	85	86	86	86	86	86	86	87	87	87	87	87
84	84	84	84	85	85	85	85	85	85	86	86	86	86	86	86	87	87	87	87	87	87	88	88	88	88
85	85	85	85	86	86	86	86	86	86	87	87	87	87	87	87	87	88	88	88	88	88	88	88	89	89
86	86	86	86	87	87	87	87	87	87	87	88	88	88	88	88	88	88	89	89	89	89	89	89	89	90
87	87	87	87	88	88	88	88	88	88	88	88	89	89	89	89	89	89	89	89	90	90	90	90	90	90
88	88	88	88	88	89	89	89	89	89	89	89	89	90	90	90	90	90	90	90	90	91	91	91	91	91
89	89	89	89	89	90	90	90	90	90	90	90	90	90	91	91	91	91	91	91	91	91	91	92	92	92
90	90	90	90	90	91	91	91	91	91	91	91	91	91	91	92	92	92	92	92	92	92	92	92	92	93
91	91	91	91	91	91	92	92	92	92	92	92	92	92	92	92	92	93	93	93	93	93	93	93	93	93
92	92	92	92	92	92	92	93	93	93	93	93	93	93	93	93	93	93	93	94	94	94	94	94	94	94
93	93	93	93	93	93	93	93	94	94	94	94	94	94	94	94	94	94	94	94	94	94	94	95	95	95
94	94	94	94	94	94	94	94	94	95	95	95	95	95	95	95	95	95	95	95	95	95	95	95	95	96
95	95	95	95	95	95	95	95	95	95	96	96	96	96	96	96	96	96	96	96	96	96	96	96	96	96
96	96	96	96	96	96	96	96	96	96	96	96	96	97	97	97	97	97	97	97	97	97	97	97	97	97
97	97	97	97	97	97	97	97	97	97	97	97	97	97	97	97	97	98	98	98	98	98	98	98	98	98
98	98	98	98	98	98	98	98	98	98	98	98	98	98	98	98	98	98	98	98	98	98	98	98	98	99
99	99	99	99	99	99	99	99	99	99	99	99	99	99	99	99	99	99	99	99	99	99	99	99	99	99

	26	27	28	29	30	31	32	33	34	35	36	37	38	39	40	41	42	43	44	45	46	47	48	49	50
51	64	64	65	65	66	66	67	67	68	68	69	69	70	70	71	71	72	72	73	73	74	74	75	75	76
52	64	65	65	66	66	67	67	68	68	69	69	70	70	71	71	72	72	73	73	74	74	75	75	76	76
53	65	66	66	67	67	68	68	69	69	69	70	70	71	71	72	72	73	73	74	74	75	75	76	76	77
54	66	66	67	67	68	68	69	69	70	70	71	71	71	72	72	73	73	74	74	75	75	76	76	77	77
55	67	67	68	68	69	69	69	70	70	71	71	72	72	73	73	73	74	74	75	75	76	76	77	77	78
56	67	68	68	69	69	70	70	71	71	71	72	72	73	73	74	74	74	75	75	76	76	77	77	78	78
57	68	69	69	69	70	70	71	71	72	72	72	73	73	74	74	75	75	75	76	76	77	77	78	78	79
58	69	69	70	70	71	71	71	72	72	73	73	74	74	74	75	75	76	76	76	77	77	78	78	79	79
59	70	70	70	71	71	72	72	73	73	73	74	74	75	75	75	76	76	77	77	77	78	78	79	79	80
60	70	71	71	72	72	72	73	73	74	74	74	75	75	76	76	76	77	77	78	78	78	79	79	80	80
61	71	72	72	72	73	73	73	74	74	75	75	75	76	76	77	77	77	78	78	79	79	79	80	80	81
62	72	72	73	73	73	74	74	75	75	75	76	76	76	77	77	78	78	78	79	79	79	80	80	81	81
63	73	73	73	74	74	74	75	75	76	76	76	77	77	77	78	78	79	79	79	80	80	80	81	81	82
64	73	74	74	74	75	75	76	76	76	77	77	77	78	78	78	79	79	79	80	80	81	81	81	82	82
65	74	74	75	75	76	76	76	77	77	77	78	78	78	79	79	79	80	80	80	81	81	81	82	82	83
66	75	75	76	76	76	77	77	77	78	78	78	79	79	79	80	80	80	81	81	81	82	82	82	83	83
67	76	76	76	77	77	77	78	78	78	79	79	79	80	80	80	81	81	81	82	82	82	83	83	83	84
68	76	77	77	77	78	78	78	79	79	79	80	80	80	80	81	81	81	82	82	82	83	83	83	84	84
69	77	77	78	78	78	79	79	79	80	80	80	80	81	81	81	82	82	82	83	83	83	84	84	84	85
70	78	78	78	79	79	79	80	80	80	81	81	81	81	82	82	82	83	83	83	84	84	84	84	85	85
71	79	79	79	79	80	80	80	81	81	81	81	82	82	82	83	83	83	83	84	84	84	85	85	85	86
72	79	80	80	80	80	81	81	81	82	82	82	82	83	83	83	83	84	84	84	85	85	85	85	86	86
73	80	80	81	81	81	81	82	82	82	82	83	83	83	84	84	84	84	85	85	85	85	86	86	86	87
74	81	81	81	82	82	82	82	83	83	83	83	84	84	84	84	85	85	85	85	86	86	86	86	87	87
75	82	82	82	82	83	83	83	83	84	84	84	84	85	85	85	85	86	86	86	86	87	87	87	87	88
76	82	82	83	83	83	83	84	84	84	84	85	85	85	85	86	86	86	86	87	87	87	87	88	88	88
77	83	83	83	84	84	84	84	85	85	85	85	86	86	86	86	86	87	87	87	87	88	88	88	88	89
78	84	84	84	84	85	85	85	85	85	86	86	86	86	87	87	87	87	87	88	88	88	88	89	89	89
79	84	85	85	85	85	86	86	86	86	86	87	87	87	87	87	88	88	88	88	88	89	89	89	89	90
80	85	85	86	86	86	86	86	87	87	87	87	87	88	88	88	88	88	89	89	89	89	89	90	90	90
81	86	86	86	87	87	87	87	87	87	88	88	88	88	88	89	89	89	89	89	90	90	90	90	90	91
82	87	87	87	87	87	88	88	88	88	88	88	89	89	89	89	89	90	90	90	90	90	90	91	91	91
83	87	88	88	88	88	88	88	89	89	89	89	89	89	90	90	90	90	90	90	91	91	91	91	91	92
84	88	88	88	89	89	89	89	89	89	90	90	90	90	90	90	91	91	91	91	91	91	92	92	92	92
85	89	89	89	89	90	90	90	90	90	90	90	91	91	91	91	91	91	91	92	92	92	92	92	92	93
86	90	90	90	90	90	90	90	91	91	91	91	91	91	91	92	92	92	92	92	92	92	93	93	93	93
87	90	91	91	91	91	91	91	91	91	92	92	92	92	92	92	92	92	93	93	93	93	93	93	93	94
88	91	91	91	91	92	92	92	92	92	92	92	92	93	93	93	93	93	93	93	93	94	94	94	94	94
89	92	92	92	92	92	92	93	93	93	93	93	93	93	93	93	94	94	94	94	94	94	94	94	94	95
90	93	93	93	93	93	93	93	93	93	94	94	94	94	94	94	94	94	94	94	95	95	95	95	95	95
91	93	93	94	94	94	94	94	94	94	94	94	94	94	95	95	95	95	95	95	95	95	95	95	95	96
92	94	94	94	94	94	94	95	95	95	95	95	95	95	95	95	95	95	95	96	96	96	96	96	96	96
93	95	95	95	95	95	95	95	95	95	95	96	96	96	96	96	96	96	96	96	96	96	96	96	96	97
94	96	96	96	96	96	96	96	96	96	96	96	96	96	96	96	96	97	97	97	97	97	97	97	97	97
95	96	96	96	96	96	97	97	97	97	97	97	97	97	97	97	97	97	97	97	97	97	97	97	97	98
96	97	97	97	97	97	97	97	97	97	97	97	97	98	98	98	98	98	98	98	98	98	98	98	98	98
97	98	98	98	98	98	98	98	98	98	98	98	98	98	98	98	98	98	98	98	98	98	98	98	98	99
98	99	99	99	99	99	99	99	99	99	99	99	99	99	99	99	99	99	99	99	99	99	99	99	99	99
99	99	99	99	99	99	99	99	99	99	99	99	99	99	99	99	99	99	99	99	99	99	99	99	99	100

COMBINED VALUES CHART (CONTINUED)

	51	52	53	54	55	56	57	58	59	60	61	62	63	64	65	66	67	68	69	70	71	72	73	74	75	76	77	78	79	80	81	82	83	84	85	86	87	88	89	90	91	92	93	94	95	96	97	98	99
51	76																																																
52	76	77																																															
53	77	77	78																																														
54	77	78	78	79																																													
55	78	78	79	79	80																																												
56	78	79	79	80	80	81																																											
57	79	79	80	80	81	81	82																																										
58	79	80	80	81	81	82	82	82																																									
59	80	80	81	81	82	82	82	83	83																																								
60	80	81	81	82	82	82	83	83	84	84																																							
61	81	81	82	82	82	83	83	84	84	84	85																																						
62	81	82	82	83	83	83	84	84	84	85	85	86																																					
63	82	82	83	83	83	84	84	84	85	85	86	86	86																																				
64	82	83	83	83	84	84	85	85	85	86	86	86	87	87																																			
65	83	83	84	84	84	85	85	85	86	86	86	87	87	87	88																																		
66	83	84	84	84	85	85	85	86	86	86	87	87	87	88	88	88																																	
67	84	84	84	85	85	85	86	86	86	87	87	87	88	88	88	88	89																																
68	84	85	85	85	86	86	86	87	87	87	88	88	88	88	89	89	89	90																															
69	85	85	85	86	86	86	87	87	87	88	88	88	89	89	89	89	90	90	90																														
70	85	86	86	86	87	87	87	87	88	88	88	89	89	89	90	90	90	90	91	91																													
71	86	86	86	87	87	87	88	88	88	88	89	89	89	90	90	90	90	91	91	91	92																												
72	86	87	87	87	87	88	88	88	89	89	89	89	90	90	90	93	91	91	91	92	92	92																											
73	87	87	87	88	88	88	88	89	89	89	89	90	90	90	91	91	91	91	92	92	92	92	93																										
74	87	88	88	88	88	89	89	89	89	90	90	90	90	91	91	91	91	92	92	92	92	93	93	93																									
75	88	88	88	89	89	89	89	90	90	90	90	91	91	91	91	92	92	92	92	93	93	93	93	94	94																								
76	88	88	89	89	89	89	90	90	90	90	91	91	91	91	92	92	92	92	93	93	93	93	94	94	94	94																							
77	89	89	89	89	90	90	90	90	91	91	91	91	91	92	92	92	92	93	93	93	93	94	94	94	94	94	95																						
78	89	89	90	90	90	90	91	91	91	91	91	92	92	92	92	93	93	93	93	93	94	94	94	94	95	95	95	95																					
79	90	90	90	90	91	91	91	91	91	92	92	92	92	92	93	93	93	93	93	94	94	94	94	95	95	95	95	95	96																				
80	90	90	91	91	91	91	91	92	92	92	92	92	93	93	93	93	93	94	94	94	94	94	95	95	95	95	95	96	96	96																			
81	91	91	91	91	91	92	92	92	92	92	93	93	93	93	93	94	94	94	94	94	94	95	95	95	95	95	96	96	96	96	96																		
82	91	91	92	92	92	92	92	92	93	93	93	93	93	94	94	94	94	94	94	95	95	95	95	95	96	96	96	96	96	96	97	97																	
83	92	92	92	92	92	93	93	93	93	93	93	94	94	94	94	94	94	95	95	95	95	95	95	96	96	96	96	96	96	97	97	97	97																
84	92	92	92	93	93	93	93	93	93	94	94	94	94	94	94	95	95	95	95	95	95	96	96	96	96	96	96	96	97	97	97	97	97	97															
85	93	93	93	93	93	93	94	94	94	94	94	94	94	95	95	95	95	95	95	96	96	96	96	96	96	96	97	97	97	97	97	97	97	98	98														
86	93	93	93	94	94	94	94	94	94	94	95	95	95	95	95	95	95	96	96	96	96	96	96	96	97	97	97	97	97	97	97	97	98	98	98	98													
87	94	94	94	94	94	94	94	95	95	95	95	95	95	95	95	96	96	96	96	96	96	96	96	97	97	97	97	97	97	97	98	98	98	98	98	98	98												
88	94	94	94	94	95	95	95	95	95	95	95	95	95	96	96	96	96	96	96	96	97	97	97	97	97	97	97	97	97	98	98	98	98	98	98	98	98	99											
89	95	95	95	95	95	95	95	95	95	96	96	96	96	96	96	96	96	96	97	97	97	97	97	97	97	97	97	98	98	98	98	98	98	98	98	98	99	99	99										
90	95	95	95	95	96	96	96	96	96	96	96	96	96	96	97	97	97	97	97	97	97	97	97	97	98	98	98	98	98	98	98	98	98	98	99	99	99	99	99	99									
91	96	96	96	96	96	96	96	96	96	96	96	97	97	97	97	97	97	97	97	97	97	97	98	98	98	98	98	98	98	98	98	98	98	99	99	99	99	99	99	99	99								
92	96	96	96	96	96	96	97	97	97	97	97	97	97	97	97	97	97	97	98	98	98	98	98	98	98	98	98	98	98	98	98	99	99	99	99	99	99	99	99	99	99	99							
93	97	97	97	97	97	97	97	97	97	97	97	97	97	97	98	98	98	98	98	98	98	98	98	98	98	98	98	98	99	99	99	99	99	99	99	99	99	99	99	99	99	99	100						
94	97	97	97	97	97	97	97	97	98	98	98	98	98	98	98	98	98	98	98	98	98	98	98	98	99	99	99	99	99	99	99	99	99	99	99	99	99	99	99	99	99	100	100	100					
95	98	98	98	98	98	98	98	98	98	98	98	98	98	98	98	98	98	98	98	99	99	99	99	99	99	99	99	99	99	99	99	99	99	99	99	99	99	99	99	100	100	100	100	100	100				
96	98	98	98	98	98	98	98	98	98	98	98	98	99	99	99	99	99	99	99	99	99	99	99	99	99	99	99	99	99	99	99	99	99	99	99	99	99	100	100	100	100	100	100	100	100	100			
97	99	99	99	99	99	99	99	99	99	99	99	99	99	99	99	99	99	99	99	99	99	99	99	99	99	99	99	99	99	99	99	99	99	100	100	100	100	100	100	100	100	100	100	100	100	100	100		
98	99	99	99	99	99	99	99	99	99	99	99	99	99	99	99	99	99	99	99	99	99	99	99	99	100	100	100	100	100	100	100	100	100	100	100	100	100	100	100	100	100	100	100	100	100	100	100	100	
99	100	100	100	100	100	100	100	100	100	100	100	100	100	100	100	100	100	100	100	100	100	100	100	100	100	100	100	100	100	100	100	100	100	100	100	100	100	100	100	100	100	100	100	100	100	100	100	100	100

SECTION 7

PRODUCT IDENTIFICATION GUIDE

To aid in quick identification, manufacturers participating in this section have furnished full-color photographs of selected ophthalmic products. Capsules and tablets are shown in actual size. Tubes, bottles, boxes, and other types of packaging appear in reduced size to fit available space.

For more information on any of the products in this section, please turn to the Pharmaceutical and Equipment Product Information Section, or check directly with the manufacturer. The page number of each product's text entry appears above its photograph.

While every effort has been made to guarantee faithful reproduction of the products in this section, changes in size, color, and design are always a possibility. Be sure to confirm a product's identity with the manufacturer or your pharmacist.

MANUFACTURERS INDEX

PRODUCT INDEX

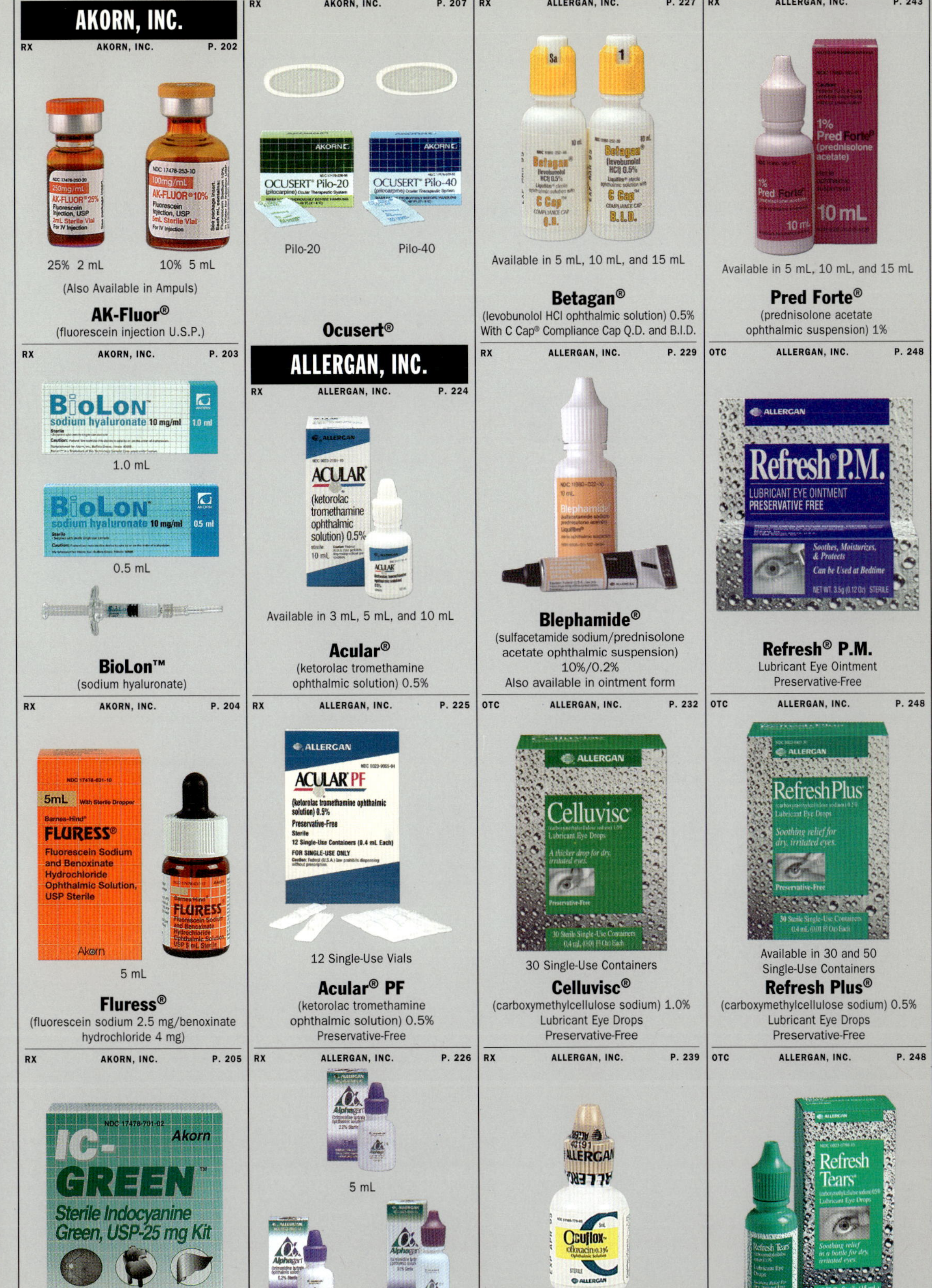

AKORN, INC.

RX AKORN, INC. P. 202

25% 2 mL — 10% 5 mL

(Also Available in Ampuls)

AK-Fluor®
(fluorescein injection U.S.P.)

RX AKORN, INC. P. 207

Pilo-20 — Pilo-40

Ocusert®

RX ALLERGAN, INC. P. 227

Available in 5 mL, 10 mL, and 15 mL

Betagan®
(levobunolol HCl ophthalmic solution) 0.5%
With C Cap® Compliance Cap Q.D. and B.I.D.

RX ALLERGAN, INC. P. 243

Available in 5 mL, 10 mL, and 15 mL

Pred Forte®
(prednisolone acetate ophthalmic suspension) 1%

RX AKORN, INC. P. 203

1.0 mL

0.5 mL

BioLon™
(sodium hyaluronate)

ALLERGAN, INC.

RX ALLERGAN, INC. P. 224

Available in 3 mL, 5 mL, and 10 mL

Acular®
(ketorolac tromethamine ophthalmic solution) 0.5%

RX ALLERGAN, INC. P. 229

Blephamide®
(sulfacetamide sodium/prednisolone acetate ophthalmic suspension) 10%/0.2%
Also available in ointment form

OTC ALLERGAN, INC. P. 248

Refresh® P.M.
Lubricant Eye Ointment
Preservative-Free

RX AKORN, INC. P. 204

5 mL

Fluress®
(fluorescein sodium 2.5 mg/benoxinate hydrochloride 4 mg)

RX ALLERGAN, INC. P. 225

12 Single-Use Vials

Acular® PF
(ketorolac tromethamine ophthalmic solution) 0.5%
Preservative-Free

OTC ALLERGAN, INC. P. 232

30 Single-Use Containers

Celluvisc®
(carboxymethylcellulose sodium) 1.0%
Lubricant Eye Drops
Preservative-Free

OTC ALLERGAN, INC. P. 248

Available in 30 and 50 Single-Use Containers

Refresh Plus®
(carboxymethylcellulose sodium) 0.5%
Lubricant Eye Drops
Preservative-Free

RX AKORN, INC. P. 205

6 - 25 mg vials and 10 mL ampules
Aqueous Solvent

IC-Green™

RX ALLERGAN, INC. P. 226

5 mL

10 mL — 15 mL

Alphagan®
(brimonidine tartrate ophthalmic solution) 0.2%

RX ALLERGAN, INC. P. 239

Available in 5 mL and 10 mL

Ocuflox®
(ofloxacin ophthalmic solution) 0.3%

OTC ALLERGAN, INC. P. 248

Available in 3 mL, 15 mL and 30 mL

Refresh Tears®
(carboxymethycellulose sodium) 0.5%
Lubricant Eye Drops

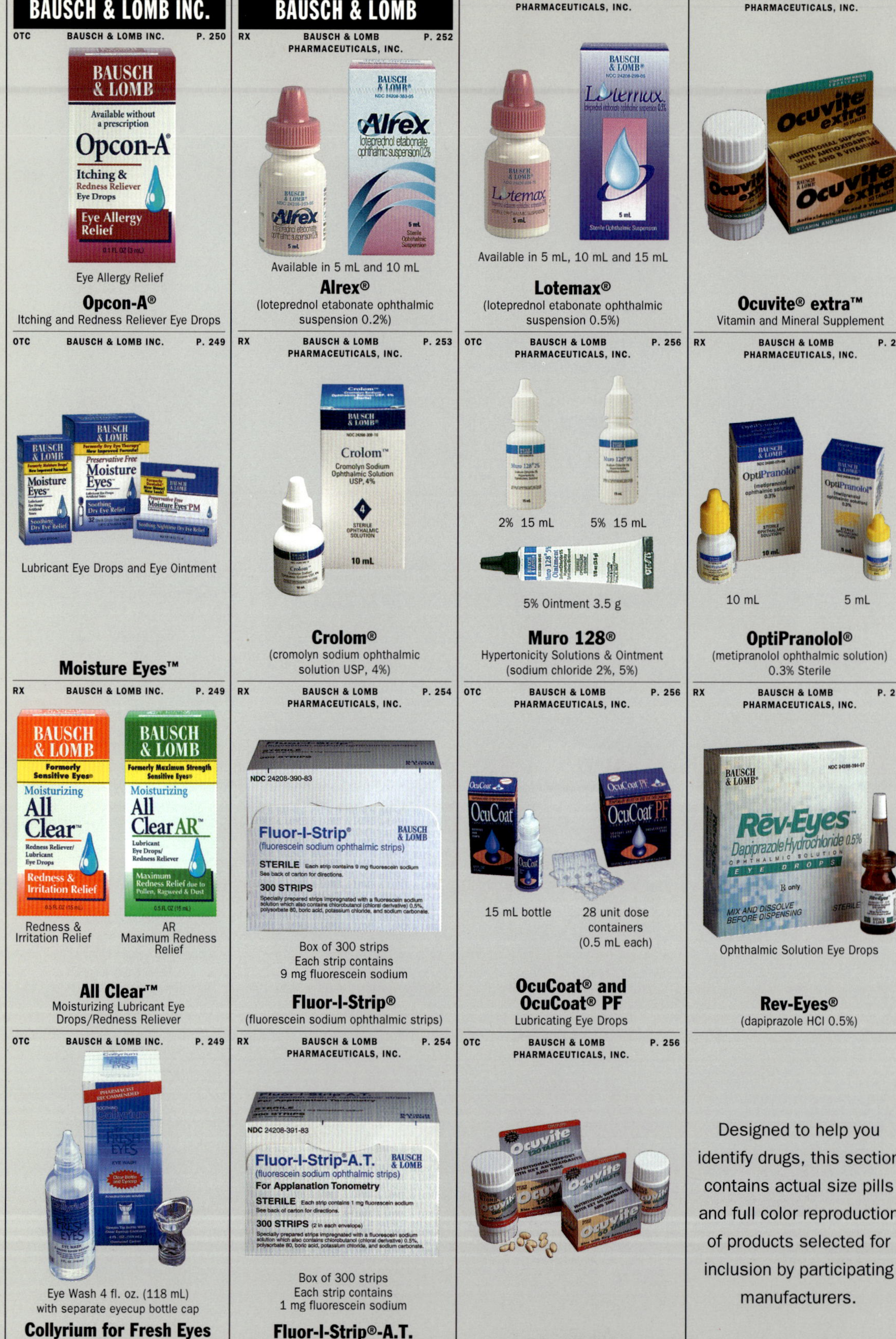
BAUSCH & LOMB INC.
BAUSCH & LOMB
OTC BAUSCH & LOMB INC. P. 250
BAUSCH & LOMB
Available without a prescription
Opcon-A
Itching & Redness Reliever Eye Drops
Eye Allergy Relief
Eye Allergy Relief
Opcon-A®
Itching and Redness Reliever Eye Drops
RX BAUSCH & LOMB PHARMACEUTICALS, INC. P. 252
BAUSCH & LOMB
Alrex
loteprednol etabonate ophthalmic suspension 0.2%
5 mL
Available in 5 mL and 10 mL
Alrex®
(loteprednol etabonate ophthalmic suspension 0.2%)
RX BAUSCH & LOMB PHARMACEUTICALS, INC. P. 254
BAUSCH & LOMB
Lotemax
5 mL
Sterile Ophthalmic Suspension
Available in 5 mL, 10 mL and 15 mL
Lotemax®
(loteprednol etabonate ophthalmic suspension 0.5%)
OTC BAUSCH & LOMB PHARMACEUTICALS, INC. P. 257
Ocuvite extra
Ocuvite® extra™
Vitamin and Mineral Supplement
OTC BAUSCH & LOMB INC. P. 249
BAUSCH & LOMB
Moisture Eyes
Preservative Free Moisture Eyes
Moisture Eyes PM
Lubricant Eye Drops and Eye Ointment
Moisture Eyes™
RX BAUSCH & LOMB PHARMACEUTICALS, INC. P. 253
BAUSCH & LOMB
Crolom™
Cromolyn Sodium Ophthalmic Solution USP, 4%
STERILE OPHTHALMIC SOLUTION
10 mL
Crolom®
(cromolyn sodium ophthalmic solution USP, 4%)
OTC BAUSCH & LOMB PHARMACEUTICALS, INC. P. 256
2% 15 mL
5% 15 mL
5% Ointment 3.5 g
Muro 128®
Hypertonicity Solutions & Ointment
(sodium chloride 2%, 5%)
RX BAUSCH & LOMB PHARMACEUTICALS, INC. P. 257
BAUSCH & LOMB
OptiPranolol
10 mL
5 mL
OptiPranolol®
(metipranolol ophthalmic solution)
0.3% Sterile
RX BAUSCH & LOMB INC. P. 249
BAUSCH & LOMB
Formerly Sensitive Eyes®
Moisturizing All Clear™
Redness & Irritation Relief
BAUSCH & LOMB
Formerly Maximum Strength Sensitive Eyes®
Moisturizing All Clear AR™
Maximum Redness Relief due to Pollen, Ragweed & Dust
Redness & Irritation Relief
AR Maximum Redness Relief
All Clear™
Moisturizing Lubricant Eye Drops/Redness Reliever
RX BAUSCH & LOMB PHARMACEUTICALS, INC. P. 254
NDC 24208-390-83
Fluor-I-Strip®
(fluorescein sodium ophthalmic strips)
BAUSCH & LOMB
STERILE
300 STRIPS
Box of 300 strips
Each strip contains
9 mg fluorescein sodium
Fluor-I-Strip®
(fluorescein sodium ophthalmic strips)
OTC BAUSCH & LOMB PHARMACEUTICALS, INC. P. 256
OcuCoat
OcuCoat PF
15 mL bottle
28 unit dose containers
(0.5 mL each)
OcuCoat® and
OcuCoat® PF
Lubricating Eye Drops
RX BAUSCH & LOMB PHARMACEUTICALS, INC. P. 258
BAUSCH & LOMB
Rēv-Eyes
Dapiprazole Hydrochloride 0.5%
OPHTHALMIC SOLUTION
EYE DROPS
MIX AND DISSOLVE BEFORE DISPENSING
STERILE
Ophthalmic Solution Eye Drops
Rev-Eyes®
(dapiprazole HCl 0.5%)
OTC BAUSCH & LOMB INC. P. 249
Collyrium
Fresh Eyes
Eye Wash 4 fl. oz. (118 mL)
with separate eyecup bottle cap
Collyrium for Fresh Eyes
Eye Wash
(a neutral borate solution)
RX BAUSCH & LOMB PHARMACEUTICALS, INC. P. 254
NDC 24208-391-83
Fluor-I-Strip-A.T.
BAUSCH & LOMB
(fluorescein sodium ophthalmic strips)
For Applanation Tonometry
STERILE
300 STRIPS
Box of 300 strips
Each strip contains
1 mg fluorescein sodium
Fluor-I-Strip®-A.T.
For Applanation Tonometry
(fluorescein sodium ophthalmic strips)
OTC BAUSCH & LOMB PHARMACEUTICALS, INC. P. 256
Ocuvite
Ocuvite®
Vitamin and Mineral Supplement
Designed to help you identify drugs, this section contains actual size pills and full color reproduction of products selected for inclusion by participating manufacturers.

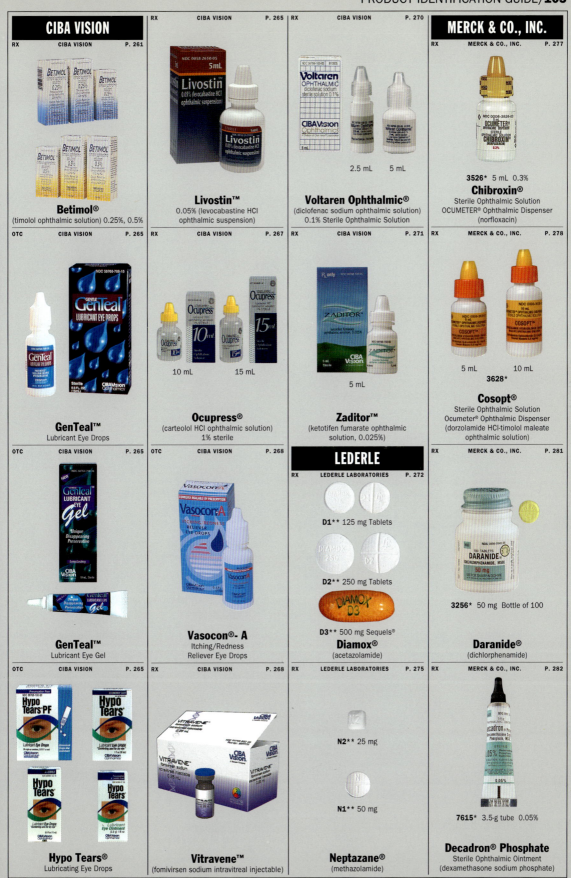

**Ledermark Identification Code

*Manufacturer's identification code

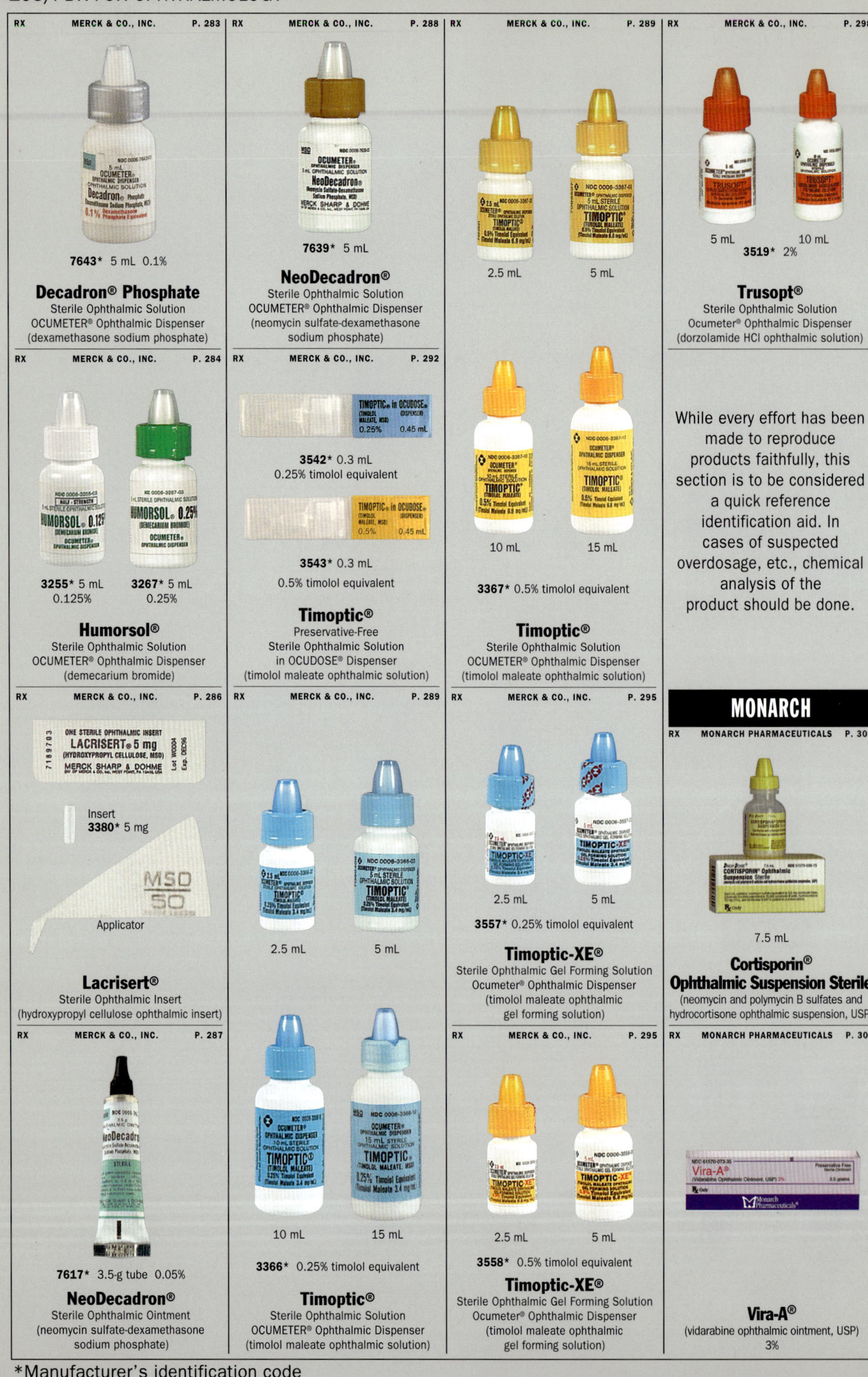

RX MERCK & CO., INC. P. 283

7643* 5 mL 0.1%

Decadron® Phosphate
Sterile Ophthalmic Solution
OCUMETER® Ophthalmic Dispenser
(dexamethasone sodium phosphate)

RX MERCK & CO., INC. P. 284

3255* 5 mL 0.125%
3267* 5 mL 0.25%

Humorsol®
Sterile Ophthalmic Solution
OCUMETER® Ophthalmic Dispenser
(demecarium bromide)

RX MERCK & CO., INC. P. 286

Insert
3380* 5 mg

Applicator

Lacrisert®
Sterile Ophthalmic Insert
(hydroxypropyl cellulose ophthalmic insert)

RX MERCK & CO., INC. P. 287

7617* 3.5-g tube 0.05%

NeoDecadron®
Sterile Ophthalmic Ointment
(neomycin sulfate-dexamethasone sodium phosphate)

RX MERCK & CO., INC. P. 288

7639* 5 mL

NeoDecadron®
Sterile Ophthalmic Solution
OCUMETER® Ophthalmic Dispenser
(neomycin sulfate-dexamethasone sodium phosphate)

RX MERCK & CO., INC. P. 292

3542* 0.3 mL
0.25% timolol equivalent

3543* 0.3 mL
0.5% timolol equivalent

Timoptic®
Preservative-Free
Sterile Ophthalmic Solution
in OCUDOSE® Dispenser
(timolol maleate ophthalmic solution)

RX MERCK & CO., INC. P. 289

2.5 mL 5 mL

10 mL 15 mL

3366* 0.25% timolol equivalent

Timoptic®
Sterile Ophthalmic Solution
OCUMETER® Ophthalmic Dispenser
(timolol maleate ophthalmic solution)

RX MERCK & CO., INC. P. 289

2.5 mL 5 mL

10 mL 15 mL

3367* 0.5% timolol equivalent

Timoptic®
Sterile Ophthalmic Solution
OCUMETER® Ophthalmic Dispenser
(timolol maleate ophthalmic solution)

RX MERCK & CO., INC. P. 295

2.5 mL 5 mL

3557* 0.25% timolol equivalent

Timoptic-XE®
Sterile Ophthalmic Gel Forming Solution
Ocumeter® Ophthalmic Dispenser
(timolol maleate ophthalmic gel forming solution)

RX MERCK & CO., INC. P. 295

2.5 mL 5 mL

3558* 0.5% timolol equivalent

Timoptic-XE®
Sterile Ophthalmic Gel Forming Solution
Ocumeter® Ophthalmic Dispenser
(timolol maleate ophthalmic gel forming solution)

RX MERCK & CO., INC. P. 298

5 mL 10 mL
3519* 2%

Trusopt®
Sterile Ophthalmic Solution
Ocumeter® Ophthalmic Dispenser
(dorzolamide HCl ophthalmic solution)

While every effort has been made to reproduce products faithfully, this section is to be considered a quick reference identification aid. In cases of suspected overdosage, etc., chemical analysis of the product should be done.

MONARCH

RX MONARCH PHARMACEUTICALS P. 302

7.5 mL

Cortisporin® Ophthalmic Suspension Sterile
(neomycin and polymycin B sulfates and hydrocortisone ophthalmic suspension, USP)

RX MONARCH PHARMACEUTICALS P. 306

Vira-A®
(vidarabine ophthalmic ointment, USP)
3%

*Manufacturer's identification code

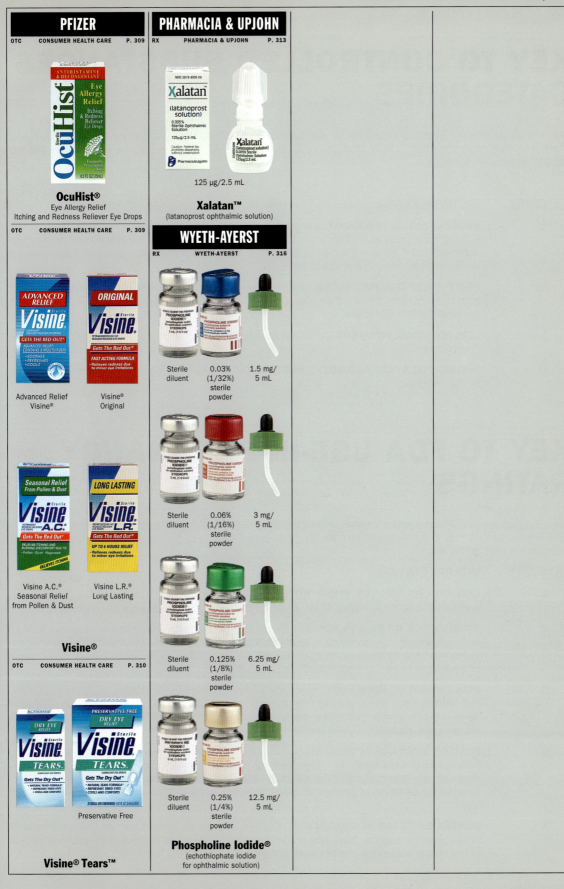

PFIZER

OTC CONSUMER HEALTH CARE P. 309

OcuHist®
Eye Allergy Relief
Itching and Redness Reliever Eye Drops

OTC CONSUMER HEALTH CARE P. 309

Advanced Relief Visine®

Visine® Original

Visine A.C.® Seasonal Relief from Pollen & Dust

Visine L.R.® Long Lasting

Visine®

OTC CONSUMER HEALTH CARE P. 310

Preservative Free

Visine® Tears™

PHARMACIA & UPJOHN

RX PHARMACIA & UPJOHN P. 313

125 µg/2.5 mL

Xalatan™
(latanoprost ophthalmic solution)

WYETH-AYERST

RX WYETH-AYERST P. 316

Sterile diluent | 0.03% (1/32%) sterile powder | 1.5 mg/ 5 mL

Sterile diluent | 0.06% (1/16%) sterile powder | 3 mg/ 5 mL

Sterile diluent | 0.125% (1/8%) sterile powder | 6.25 mg/ 5 mL

Sterile diluent | 0.25% (1/4%) sterile powder | 12.5 mg/ 5 mL

Phospholine Iodide®
(echothiophate iodide for ophthalmic solution)

KEY TO CONTROLLED SUBSTANCES CATEGORIES

Products listed with the symbols shown below are subject to the Controlled Substances Act of 1970. These drugs are categorized according to their potential for abuse. The greater the potential, the more severe the limitations on their prescription.

CATEGORY	INTERPRETATION
CII	**HIGH POTENTIAL FOR ABUSE.** Use may lead to severe physical or psychological dependence. Prescriptions must be written in ink, or typewritten and signed by the practitioner. Verbal prescriptions must be confirmed in writing within 72 hours, and may be given only in a genuine emergency. No renewals are permitted.
CIII	**SOME POTENTIAL FOR ABUSE.** Use may lead to low-to-moderate physical dependence or high psychological dependence. Prescriptions may be oral or written. Up to 5 renewals are permitted within 6 months.
CIV	**LOW POTENTIAL FOR ABUSE.** Use may lead to limited physical or psychological dependence. Prescriptions may be oral or written. Up to 5 renewals are permitted within 6 months.
CV	**SUBJECT TO STATE AND LOCAL REGULATION.** Abuse potential is low; a prescription may not be required.

KEY TO FDA USE-IN-PREGNANCY RATINGS

The U.S. Food and Drug Administration's use-in-pregnancy rating system weighs the degree to which available information has ruled out risk to the fetus against the drug's potential benefit to the patient. The ratings, and their interpretation, are as follows:

CATEGORY	INTERPRETATION
A	**CONTROLLED STUDIES SHOW NO RISK.** Adequate, well-controlled studies in pregnant women have failed to demonstrate a risk to the fetus in any trimester of pregnancy.
B	**NO EVIDENCE OF RISK IN HUMANS.** Adequate, well-controlled studies in pregnant women have not shown increased risk of fetal abnormalities despite adverse findings in animals, or, in the absence of adequate human studies, animal studies show no fetal risk. The chance of fetal harm is remote, but remains a possibility.
C	**RISK CANNOT BE RULED OUT.** Adequate, well-controlled human studies are lacking, and animal studies have shown a risk to the fetus or are lacking as well. There is a chance of fetal harm if the drug is administered during pregnancy; but the potential benefits may outweigh the potential risk.
D	**POSITIVE EVIDENCE OF RISK.** Studies in humans, or investigational or post-marketing data, have demonstrated fetal risk. Nevertheless, potential benefits from the use of the drug may outweigh the potential risk. For example, the drug may be acceptable if needed in a life-threatening situation or serious disease for which safer drugs cannot be used or are ineffective.
X	**CONTRAINDICATED IN PREGNANCY.** Studies in animals or humans, or investigational or post-marketing reports, have demonstrated positive evidence of fetal abnormalities or risk which clearly outweighs any possible benefit to the patient.

SECTION 8

PRODUCT INFORMATION ON PHARMACEUTICALS AND EQUIPMENT

This book is made possible through the courtesy of the manufacturers whose products appear in this and the following section. The information concerning each pharmaceutical product has been prepared by the manufacturer, and edited and approved by the manufacturer's medical department, medical director, or medical counsel.

For those products that have official package circulars, the descriptions in *Physicians' Desk Reference For Ophthalmology* must be in full compliance with Food and Drug Administration regulations pertaining to the labeling of prescription drugs. For more information, please turn to the Foreword. In presenting the following material, the publisher is not necessarily advocating the use of any product listed.

Akorn, Inc.
2500 MILLBROOK DRIVE
BUFFALO GROVE, IL 60089

NDC 17478 PRODUCT

-287- **AKBETA™** ℞
Levobunolol HCl 0.5%, sterile ophthalmic solution.
5mL: -10
10mL: -11
15mL: -12

-275-10 **AK-CIDE®** ℞
Sulfacetamide Sodium 100mg, Prednisolone Acetate 5mg, sterile ophthalmic suspension.
5mL

-276-35 **AK-CIDE® OINTMENT** ℞
Sulfacetamide Sodium 10%, Prednisolone Acetate 0.5%, sterile ophthalmic ointment.
3.5gm

-216-12 **AK-CON™** ℞
Naphazoline HCl 0.1%, sterile ophthalmic solution.
15mL

-279-10 **AK-DEX®** ℞
Dexamethasone Sodium Phosphate 0.1%, sterile ophthalmic solution.
5mL

-200- **AK-DILATE™ 2.5%** ℞
Phenylephrine HCl, sterile ophthalmic solution.
2mL: -20
15mL: -12

-205 **AK-DILATE™ 10%** ℞
Phenylephrine HCl, sterile ophthalmic solution.
5mL: -10

-254-10 **AK-FLUOR® 10% GLASS AMPUL** ℞
Fluorescein injection, USP, sterile aqueous ophthalmic solution.
5mL

-251-20 **AK-FLUOR® 25% GLASS AMPUL** ℞
Fluorescein injection, USP, sterile aqueous ophthalmic solution.
2mL

-253-10 **AK-FLUOR® 10% SINGLE DOSE VIAL** ℞
Fluorescein injection, USP, sterile aqueous ophthalmic solution.
5mL

-250-20 **AK-FLUOR® 25% SINGLE DOSE VIAL** ℞
Fluorescein injection, USP, sterile aqueous ophthalmic solution.
2mL

-623-12 **SODIUM CHLORIDE OPHTHALMIC SOLUTION USP, 5%**
Sodium Chloride 5%, sterile hypertonic ophthalmic solution.
15mL

-622-35 **SODIUM CHLORIDE OPHTHALMIC OINTMENT USP, 5%**
Sodium Chloride 5%, sterile ophthalmic ointment. (Preservative-Free)
3.5gm

-220-12 **AK-NEFRIN™**
Phenylephrine HCl 0.12%, sterile ophthalmic solution.
15mL

-805-60 **AKORN ANTIOXIDANTS**
Vitamin and mineral supplement.
60/btl.

-100- **AK-PENTOLATE™ 1%** ℞
Cyclopentolate HCl, sterile ophthalmic solution.
2mL: -20
15mL: -12

-097- **AK-PENTOLATE™ 2%** ℞
Cyclopentolate HCl, sterile ophthalmic solution.
2mL: -20
5mL: -10

-238-35 **AK-POLY-BAC™ OINTMENT** ℞
Polymyxin B Sulfate, Bacitracin Zinc, sterile ophthalmic ointment. (Preservative-Free)
3.5gm

-218-10 **AK-PRED™ 0.125%** ℞
Prednisolone Sodium Phosphate 0.125%, sterile ophthalmic solution.
5mL

-219- **AK-PRED™ 1%** ℞
Prednisolone Sodium Phosphate 1%, sterile ophthalmic solution.
5mL: -10
15mL: -12

-269- **AK-RINSE™** ℞
Irrigating solution.
4fl.oz.: -18

-790-11 **AK-SPORE®** ℞
Polymyxin B, Neomycin, Gramicidin, sterile ophthalmic solution.
10mL

-235-35 **AK-SPORE® OINTMENT** ℞
Polymyxin B, Neomycin, Bacitracin, sterile ophthalmic ointment. (Preservative-Free)
3.5gm

-232-35 **AK-SPORE® HC OINTMENT** ℞
Polymyxin B, Bacitracin, Neomycin, Hydrocortisone, sterile ophthalmic ointment. (Preservative-Free)
3.5gm

-237-11 **AK-SPORE® HC OTIC SOLUTION** ℞
Polymyxin B, Neomycin, Hydrocortisone, sterile otic solution.
10mL

-236-11 **AK-SPORE® HC OTIC SUSPENSION** ℞
Polymyxin B, Neomycin, Hydrocortisone, sterile otic suspension.
10mL

-221-12 **AK-SULF®** ℞
Sulfacetamide Sodium 10%, sterile ophthalmic solution.
15mL

-227-35 **AK-SULF® OINTMENT** ℞
Sulfacetamide Sodium 10%, sterile ophthalmic ointment.
3.5gm

-263-12 **AK-TAINE®** ℞
Proparacaine HCl 0.5%, sterile ophthalmic solution.
15mL

-290-10 **AKTOB™** ℞
Tobramycin 0.3%, sterile ophthalmic solution.
5mL

-233-35 **AK-TRACIN™ OINTMENT** ℞
Bacitracin, sterile ophthalmic ointment. (Preservative-Free)
3.5gm

Continued on next page

Product listing-Akorn—Cont.

-239-10 **AK-TROL®** ℞
Dexamethasone 0.1%, Neomycin Sulfate, Polymyxin B Sulfate, sterile ophthalmic suspension.
5mL

-240-35 **AK-TROL® OINTMENT** ℞
Dexamethasone 0.1%, Neomycin Sulfate, Polymyxin B Sulfate, sterile ophthalmic ointment.
3.5gm

-920- **AKORN BALANCED SALT SOLUTION** ℞
Sterile surgical solution. (Preservative-Free)
18mL: -19
500mL: -90

-060-12 **AKWA TEARS®**
Polyvinyl Alcohol, ocular lubricant solution.
15mL

-062-35 **AKWA TEARS® OINTMENT**
White Petrolatum, Mineral Oil, Lanolin Derivatives, sterile ophthalmic ointment. (Preservative-Free)
3.5gm

-214- **ATROPINE CARE™ 1%** ℞
Atropine Sulfate 1%, sterile ophthalmic solution.
2mL: -20
5mL: -10
15mL: -12

-930-90 **B-SALT FORTE™** ℞
Balanced Salt Solution Enriched with Bicarbonate, Dextrose and Glutathione. Sterile Surgical Solution (Preservative-Free)
515mL

BioLon™ ℞
1% Sodium Hyaluronate
10 mg/ml
1mL 0890-22
0.5mL 0891-22

-291-11 **Cromolyn Sodium** ℞
Ophthalmic Solution USP, 4%
10mL

0070-35 **Erythromycin** ℞
Sterile Ophthalmic Ointment
3.5gm

-610-12 **EyeSine™**
Tetrahydrozoline HCl 0.05%, sterile ophthalmic solution.
15mL

-311-10 **FLUORACAINE®** ℞
Fluorescein Sodium 0.25%, Proparacaine HCl 0.5%, sterile ophthalmic solution.
5mL

-400-01 **Fluorets™**
Fluorescein Sodium 1mg, individually wrapped, sterile ophthalmic strips.
100/box

0631-10 **FLURESS®** ℞
Fluorescein Sodium 0.25%, Benoxinate HCl 0.4% USP, sterile ophthalmic solution.
5mL

0077-0631-93 **FUL-GLO®**
Fluorescein Sodium USP 0.6mg, individually wrapped, sterile ophthalmic strips.
300/box

-283- **GENTAK®** ℞
Gentamicin Sulfate, sterile ophthalmic solution.
5mL: -10
15mL: -12

-284-35 **GENTAK® OINTMENT** ℞
Gentamicin Sulfate, sterile ophthalmic ointment.
3.5gm

-070-12 **GONAK™**
Hydroxypropyl Methylcellulose 2.5%, sterile ophthalmic solution.
15mL

0011-8361-01 **IC GREEN™ BASIC ICG OPHTHALMIC ANGIOGRAPHY KIT** ℞
25mg Indocyanine Green USP-Sterile with diluent

0806-60 **I-Sense Vitamins**
NDC: 17478-0806-60
60 Capsules per bottle

-820-06 **LID WIPES-SPF™ Sterile, Preservative-Free.** Hypo-allergenic, isotonic eyelid cleansing pad, for sensitive eyes.
30/box

228-05 **OCUSERT Pilo-20**
(pilocarpine) Ocular Therapeutic System
8 Sterile Systems/box

229-05 **OCUSERT Pilo-40**
(pilocarpine) Ocular Therapeutic System
8 Sterile Systems/box

-810-100 **Palmitate-A**
15,000 IU Vitamin A.
100/btl.

0077-0929-99 **ROSE BENGAL OPHTHALMIC STRIPS**
1.3mg Rose Bengal, individually wrapped, sterile ophthalmic strips
100/box

57217-9521-1 **Rosets™**
1.3mg Rose Bengal, individually wrapped, sterile ophthalmic strips.
100/box

-401-01 **Sno strips™**
Sterile, individually wrapped, tear flow test strips.
100/box

-061-12 **TEARS RENEWED®**
Dextran 70, Hydroxypropyl Methylcellulose 2906, sterile ophthalmic solution.
15mL

-063-35 **TEARS RENEWED® OINTMENT (Preservative and Lanolin Free)**
White petrolatum and light mineral oil, sterile ophthalmic ointment.
3.5gm

-230-35 **TERAK™ OINTMENT** ℞
Oxytetracycline HCl, Polymyxin B Sulfate, sterile ophthalmic ointment.
3.5gm

-0289- **Timolol Maleate** ℞
Sterile Ophthalmic Solution 0.25%
5mL: -10
10mL: -11
15mL: -12

-0288- **Timolol Maleate** ℞
Sterile Ophthalmic Solution 0.5%
5mL: -10
10mL: -11
15mL: -12

-703-11 **TRIMETHOPRIM SULFATE AND POLYMYXIN B SULFATE Sterile Opthalmic Solution** ℞
10mL

-101-12 **TROPICACYL® 0.5%** ℞
Tropicamide, sterile ophthalmic solution.
15mL

-102- **TROPICACYL® 1%** ℞
Tropicamide, sterile ophthalmic solution.
2mL: -20
15mL: -12

AK–FLUOR® ℞

Fluorescein Injection, USP
10% & 25% Sterile Solution

Description: AK-FLUOR® (Fluorescein Injection, USP) is a sterile solution in Water for Injection, of Fluorescein prepared with the aid of Sodium Hydroxide. Hydrochloric Acid and/or Sodium Hydroxide may be used to adjust pH (8.0–9.8). AK-FLUOR® is used intravenously as a diagnostic aid. The active ingredient exists as a sodium salt of fluorescein and is represented by the chemical structure:

NaO ... O ... COONa

Established Name: Fluorescein Sodium
Chemical Name: Spiro[isobenzofuran-1(3H),-9′[9H]xanthene]-3-one, 3′6′-dihydroxy, disodium salt
Clinical Pharmacology: The yellowish-green fluorescence of the product demarcates the vascular area under observation, distinguishing it from adjacent areas.
Indications and Usage: Indicated in diagnostic fluorescein angiography or angioscopy of the fundus and of the iris vasculature.
Contraindications: Contraindicated in those persons who have shown hypersensitivity to any component of this preparation.
Warnings: Care must be taken to avoid extravasation during injection as the high pH of fluorescein solution can result in severe local tissue damage. The following complications resulting from extravasation of fluorescein have been noted to occur: sloughing of the skin, superficial phlebitis, subcutaneous granuloma, and toxic neuritis along the median curve in the antecubital area. Complications resulting from extravasation can cause severe pain in the arm for up to several hours. When significant extravasation occurs, the injection should be discontinued and conservative measures to treat damaged tissues and to relieve pain should be implemented.
Precautions: Caution is to be exercised in patients with a history of allergy or bronchial asthma. An emergency tray including such items as 0.1% epinephrine for intravenous or intramuscular use; an antihistamine, soluble steroid, and aminophylline for intravenous use; oxygen should always be available in the event of possible reaction to fluorescein injection.[1]

Pediatric Use: Safety and effectiveness in children have not been established.

Carcinogenesis, Mutagenesis, Impairment of Fertility: There have been no long-term studies done using fluorescein in animals to evaluate carcinogenic potential.

Use in Pregnancy: Avoid angiography on patients who are pregnant, especially those in first trimester. There have been no reports of fetal complications for fluorescein injection during pregnancy.

Nursing Mothers: Caution should be exercised when AK-FLUOR® (Fluorescein Injection, USP) is administered to a nursing woman.

Patient Warning: Skin will attain a temporary yellowish discoloration. Urine attains a bright yellow color. Discoloration of the skin fades in 6 to 12 hours; urine fluorescence in 24 to 36 hours.

Adverse Reactions: Nausea and headache, gastrointestinal distress, syncope, vomiting, hypotension, and other symptoms and signs of hypersensitivity have occurred. Cardiac arrest, basilar artery ischemia, severe shock, convulsions, and thrombophlebitis at the injection site and rare cases of death have been reported.

Extravasation of the solution at the injection site causes intense pain at the site and a dull aching pain in the injected arm. (SEE WARNINGS.) Generalized hives and itching, bronchospasm and anaphylaxis have been reported. A strong taste may develop after injection.

The most common reaction is nausea.

Dosage and Administration: Inject the contents of the ampul or vial rapidly into the antecubital vein, *after taking precautions to avoid extravasation.* A syringe, filled with fluorescein, is attached to transparent tubing and a 25 gauge scalp vein needle for injection. Insert the needle and draw the patient's blood to the hub of the syringe so that a *small* air bubble separates the patient's blood in the tubing from the fluorescein. With the room lights on, slowly inject the blood back into the vein while watching the skin over the needle tip. If the needle has extravasated, the patient's blood will be seen to bulge the skin and the injection should be stopped before any fluorescein is injected. When assured that extravasation has not occurred, the room light may be turned off and the fluorescein injection completed. Luminescence appears in the retina and choroidal vessels in 9 to 14 seconds and can be observed by standard viewing equipment. If potential allergy is suspected, an intradermal skin test may be performed prior to intravenous administration, i.e., 0.05 mL injected intradermally to be evaluated 30 to 60 minutes following injection. For pediatric patients, the dose is calculated on the basis of 35 mg for each ten pounds of body weight.

Parenteral drug products should be inspected visually for particulate matter and discoloration, whenever solution and container permit.

How Supplied: AK-FLUOR®, 10% (Fluorescein Injection, USP—Sterile) 100 mg/mL

NDC 17478-253-10 12 × 5 mL Single Dose Vials

NDC 17478-254-10 25 × 5 mL Ampuls

AK-FLUOR®, 25% (Fluorescein Injection, USP—Sterile) 250 mg/mL

NDC 17478-250-20 12 × 2 mL Single Dose Vials

NDC 17478-251-20 12 × 2 mL Ampuls

Storage: Store at 15°–25°C (59°–77°F); protect from freezing.

Reference:

1. Schatz, Burton, Yannuzzi, Rabb. Interpretation of Fundus Fluorescein Angiography, p. 38, C.V. Mosby Co., St. Louis, Mo., 1978.

Rx only

AKORN
Buffalo Grove, IL 60089
Shown in Product Identification Guide, page 103

BIOLON™ ℞
sodium hyaluronate

Product Information

Description: BioLon™ is a sterile, nonpyrogenic, ***optically clear,*** viscoelastic preparation of highly purified, high molecular weight sodium hyaluronate. BioLon™ contains 10 mg/ml of sodium hyaluronate dissolved in a physiological sodium chloride phosphate buffer ***(pH 6.8 – 7.6).*** This high molecular weight polymer is made up of repeating disaccharide units of N-acetyl-glucosamine and sodium glucuronate linked by β-1,3 and β-1,4 glycosidic bonds.

Sodium hyaluronate is a physiological material that is widely distributed in the connective tissues of both animals and man. Chemically identical in all species, hyaluronate can be found in the vitreous and aqueous humor of the eye, the synovial fluid, the skin and the umbilical cord.

BioLon™ has the following properties:

- High molecular weight (mass average molecular weight approximately 3 million daltons)
- High viscosity

Each milliliter of BioLon™ contains: sodium hyaluronate, 10 mg; sodium chloride, 8.5 mg; disodium hydrogen phosphate dodecahydrate 0.56 mg; sodium dihydrogen phosphate dihydrate 0.045 mg; water for injection q.s. BioLon™ has an osmolality of 260–380 mOsm/kg and a viscosity of approximately 100,000 cps at a shear rate of 0.1 sec^{-1} (25°C). [See graphic below]

Indications: BioLon™ is indicated for use as a surgical aid to protect corneal endothelium during cataract extraction (extra-capsular) procedures, intraocular lens (IOL) implantation and anterior segment surgery. When introduced in the anterior segment of the eye during these surgical procedures, BioLon™ serves to maintain a deep anterior chamber.

In addition, BioLon™ helps to push back the vitreous face and prevent formation of a post-operative flat chamber.

Contraindications: When used as recommended there are no known contraindications to the use of BioLon™.

Warnings: Mixing of quaternary ammonium salts such as benzalkonium chloride with sodium hyaluronate results in the formation of a precipitate. ***The eye should not be irrigated with any solution containing benzylalkonium chloride if BioLon™ is to be used during surgery.***

Precautions:

- ***The BioLon™ syringe should be used only with the single-use cannula provided in the package.***
- Cannulas are intended for single patient use only. If reuse becomes necessary on the same patient during the surgical procedures, rinse the cannula thoroughly with sterile distilled water to remove all traces of residual material.
- Verify that the cannula is properly locked to the Luer Lock Adaptor. Do not overtighten the Luer Lock Adaptor; this can lead to loosening of the Leur Lock Adaptor from the barrel.
- Use only if the solution is clear.
- Care should be taken to avoid trapping air bubbles behind BioLon™.
- Instilling excessive amounts of BioLon™ into the anterior segment of the eye may cause increased intraocular pressure.
- Pre-existing glaucoma or compromised outflow and operative procedures and sequelae thereto, including enzymatic zonulysis, absence of an iridectomy, trauma to filtration structures, and by blood and lenticular remnants in the anterior chamber may increase post-operative intraocular pressure. Therefore,
  - → Do not overfill the eye chamber with BioLon™.
  - → Remove all remaining BioLon™ by irrigation and/or aspiration at the close of surgery.

Continued on next page

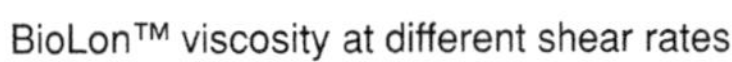

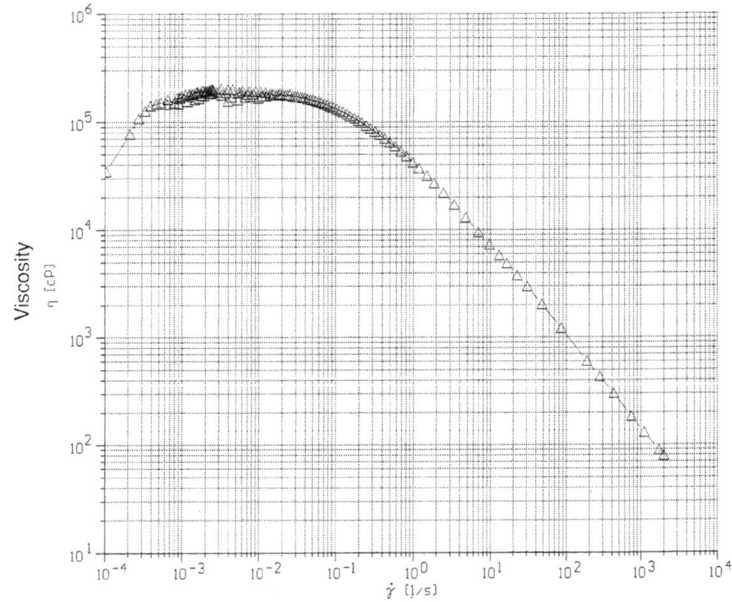

BioLon—Cont.

→ Carefully monitor the intraocular pressure, especially during the immediate post-operative period. If a significant rise is observed, treat appropriately.

- On rare occasions, viscoelastic products containing sodium hyaluronate have been observed to become slightly opaque or to form a slight precipitate upon instillation into the eye. The clinical significance, if any, of this phenomenon is not known. The physician should, however, be aware of this possibility, and, should it be observed, the cloudy or precipitated material should be removed by irrigation and/or aspiration.
- BioLon™ is a highly purified substance extracted from bacterial cells. However, physicians should be aware of immunological, allergic and other potential risks of the type that can occur from the injection of any biological substance since the presence of minute quantities of impurities (e.g., proteins) cannot be totally excluded.

Adverse Reactions: In clinical trials, 298 patients were treated with BioLon™ and 224 patients were treated with sodium hyaluronate, an approved comparative device on the U.S. market for more than five years. The incidences of adverse experiences that were reported in >1% of the patients are shown in Table I.

[See table below]

Adverse events which occurred in <1% and in at least 2 patients include: ocular hemorrhage, corneoscleral leak, suture related adverse events, vitreous in anterior chamber, hyphema and hematic Tyndall, synechiae, capsule rupture, and cyclytic membrane.

Dosage/Applications: Cataract Surgery and Intraocular Lens Implantation

Refrigerated BioLon™ should be allowed to attain room temperature (approximately 20 – 30 minutes) prior to use. The usual dose required is 0.2 to 0.5 ml of BioLon™. BioLon™ should be slowly and carefully introduced into the anterior segment of the eye using the provided cannula.

Injection of BioLon™ can be performed either before or after delivery of the lens. BioLon™ may also be used to cost surgical instruments and the intraocular lenses prior to insertion.

Additional BioLon™ can be injected during surgery to replace any BioLon™ lost during surgical manipulation (see Precautions section).

How Supplied: BioLon™ is supplied in sterile, disposable 2.25 ml syringes containing either 0.5 ml or 1.0 ml of 1% sodium hyaluronate in phosphate-buffered salt solution. Each product package contains a blister-packed syringe, a sterile, single-use ophthalmic cannula (anterior chamber irrigator) and a package insert.

Storage Instructions: Store in a cold dark place (2° – 8°C; 36° – 48°F). May be kept at 25°C (77°F) for up to one month. Protect from freezing. Bring to room temperature prior to use.

Caution: Federal law restricts this device to sale by or on the order of a physician.

Manufactured by: Bio-Technology General, (Israel) Ltd., Kiryat Weizmann, Rehovot 76326, Israel

Manufactured for: Akorn, Inc., Buffalo Grove, Illinois 60089

BIOLON™
sodium hyaluronate
Syringe Operating Instructions

1. Twenty to thirty minutes before use, remove the product box from the refrigerator, remove the blister pack from the box and allow the syringe to reach room temperature.
2. Peel off the blister Tyvek backing.

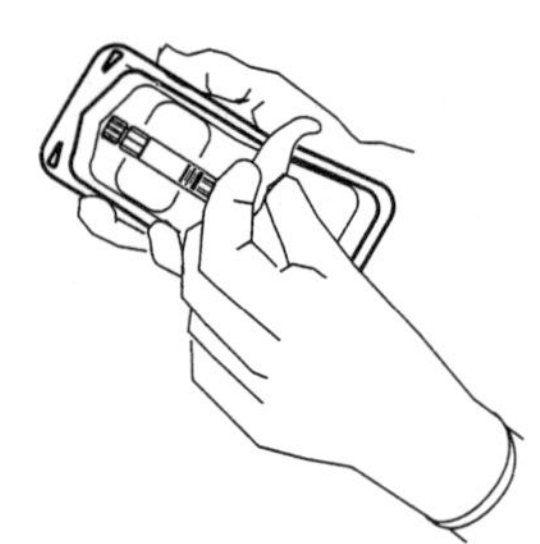

3. While holding the blister open side down, bend the blister and allow the syringe to fall gently onto the sterile surface. (Alternatively, hold the blister open side up and bend back the blister until the barrel's luer end is exposed. Gripping the luer end of the barrel, remove the syringe from the blister. **Do not remove the syringe from the plunger end).**

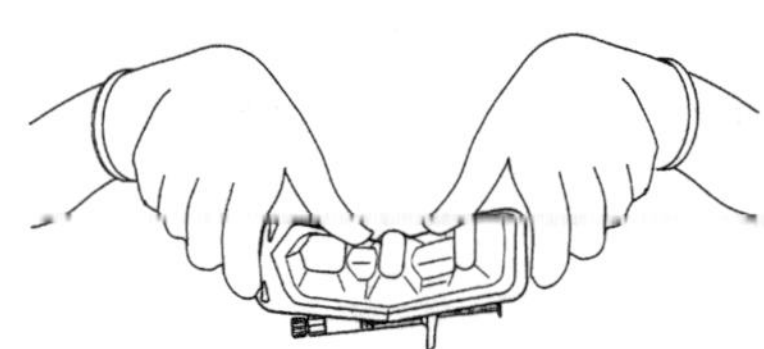

4. Remove the tip cap from the syringe and attach the cannula. **Attention:** Do not apply pressure to the plunger rod while the cannula is being affixed.

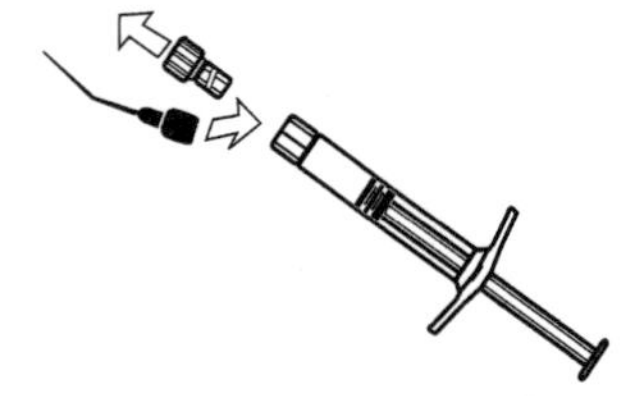

5. Apply gentle pressure to the plunger in order to expel air from the cannula and verify that the syringe is operating properly.

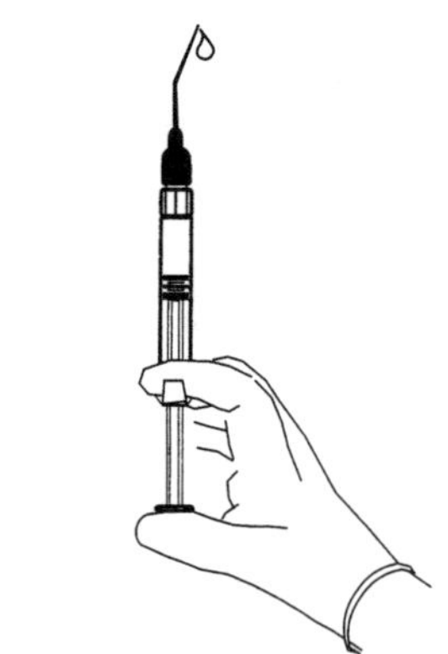

6. The syringe is ready for use.

1812-5020
9/98

Shown in Product Identification Guide, page 103

Table I*

	BIOLON		CONTROL	
	n=298	(%)	n=224	(%)
Increased Intraocular Pressure Requiring Treatment⁺	22	(7.4)	17	(7.6)
Superficial & Conjunctival Punctate Keratitis	12	(4.0)	5	(2.2)
Cystoid Macular Edema	8	(2.7)	2	(0.9)
Posterior Capsule Opacity	8	(2.7)	10	(4.5)
Seidel Phenomenon	4	(1.3)	4	(1.8)
Conjunctivitis	3	(1.0)	3	(1.3)
Corneal Edema	3	(1.0)	0	(0)
Corneal Erosion	3	(1.0)	0	(0)
Sphincter Damage	3	(1.0)	1	(0.4)
Uveitis	3	(1.0)	3	(1.3)

***There is no statistically significant difference in the number of adverse events between the two treatment groups.**
⁺Mean IOP BioLon™=36.7 mm Hg (30 mm Hg – 52 mm Hg)
⁺Mean IOP Control =33.6 mm Hg (28 mm Hg – 48 MM Hg)

FLURESS® ℞

Fluorescein Sodium and Benoxinate Hydrochloride Ophthalmic Solution, USP
Sterile

Description: Fluress® (Fluorescein Sodium and Benoxinate Hydrochloride Ophthalmic Solution, USP) is a sterile ophthalmic solution combining a disclosing agent with an anesthetic agent.

Fluorescein sodium is a disclosing agent with molecular formula $C_{20}H_{10}N_2O_5$, molecular weight 376.28, and chemical structure:

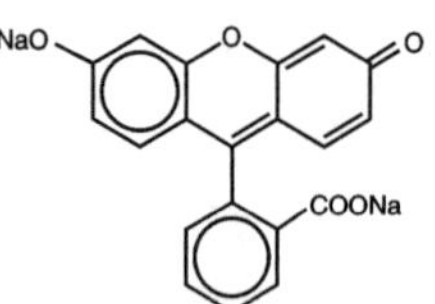

Chemical Name:
Spiro[isobenzofuran-1(3*H*), 9′-[9*H*]xanthene]-3-one, 3′6′dihydroxy, Disodium salt

Benoxinate Hydrochloride is an anesthetic agent with molecular formula $C_{17}H_{28}N_2O_3$-•HCl, molecular weight 344.88, and chemical structure:

[See chemical structure at top of next page]

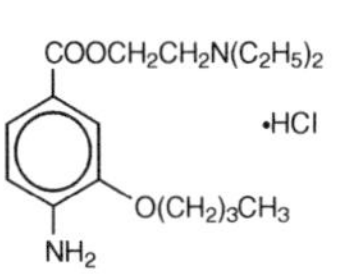

Chemical Name:
Benzoic acid, 4-amino-3-butoxyl-,2-(diethylamino) ethyl ester, monohydrochloride

Each mL contains:
Active: Benoxinate Hydrochloride 4 mg (0.4%), Fluorescein Sodium 2.5 mg (0.25%).
Preservative: Chlorobutanol 10 mg (1%).
Inactive: Povidone, Boric Acid, Sodium Hydroxide and/or Hydrochloric Acid (to adjust pH), Purified Water USP.

Clinical Pharmacology: Fluress® is the combination of a disclosing agent with a rapidly acting anesthetic agent of short duration.

Indications and Usage: For procedures requiring a disclosing agent in combination with an anesthetic agent such as tonometry, gonioscopy, removal of corneal foreign bodies and other short corneal or conjunctival procedures.

Contraindications: Known hypersensitivity to any component of this product.

Warnings: NOT FOR INJECTION—FOR TOPICAL OPHTHALMIC USE ONLY.
Prolonged use of a topical ocular anesthetic is not recommended. It may produce permanent corneal opacification with accompanying visual loss.

Precautions: Fluress® (Fluorescein Sodium and Benoxinate Hydrochloride Ophthalmic Solution, USP) should be used cautiously and sparingly in patients with known allergies, cardiac disease, or hyperthyroidism. The long-term toxicity is unknown; prolonged use may possibly delay wound healing. Although exceedingly rare with ophthalmic application of local anesthetics, systemic toxicity (manifested by central nervous system stimulation followed by depression) may occur.
Protection of the eye from irritating chemicals, foreign bodies and rubbing during the period of anesthesia is very important. Tonometers soaked in sterilizing or detergent solutions should be thoroughly rinsed with sterile distilled water prior to use. Patients should be advised to avoid touching the eye until the anesthesia has worn off.

Pregnancy:
Pregnancy Category C. Animal reproduction studies have not been conducted with Fluress®. It is also not known whether Fluress® can cause fetal harm when administered to a pregnant woman or can affect reproduction capacity. Fluress® should be given to a pregnant woman only if clearly needed.

Nursing Mothers:
Caution should be exercised when Fluress® is administered to a nursing woman.

Pediatric Use:
Safety and effectiveness in pediatric patients have not been established.

Adverse Reactions: Occasional temporary stinging, burning and conjunctival redness have been reported after use of ocular anesthetics, as well as a rare severe, immediate-type, apparently hyperallergic corneal reaction with acute, intense and diffuse epithelial keratitis, a gray, ground glass appearance, sloughing or large areas of necrotic epithelium, corneal filaments and sometimes iritis with descemetitis.
Allergic contact dermatitis with drying and fissuring of the fingertips has been reported.

Dosage and Administration: Removal of foreign bodies and sutures, and for tonometry: 1 to 2 drops (in single instillations) in each eye before operating.
Deep ophthalmic anesthesia: 2 drops in each eye at 90 second intervals for 3 instillations.
NOTE: The use of an eye patch is recommended.

How Supplied: 5 mL contained in a glass bottle with a separate sterile dropper applicator.

Storage:
Refrigerate at 2°–8°C (36°–46°F). User may store at room temperature for up to one month. Protect from light. Keep tightly closed.
CAUTION: Federal (USA) law prohibits dispensing without prescription.
U.S. PATENT NO. 3306820
CANADIAN PATENT NO. 835940
FLURESS® is a registered trademark of, and licensed by, Allergen Elite, Inc.
AKORN INC., Decatur, IL 62522

Shown in Product Identification Guide, page 103

IC-GREEN™ ℞
Sterile Indocyanine Green

Description: IC-GREEN™ is a sterile, water soluble, tricarbocyanine dye with a peak spectral absorption at 800–810 nm in blood plasma or blood. IC-GREEN™ contains not more than 5.0% sodium iodide. IC-GREEN™ is to be administered intravenously.
The Aqueous Solvent provided, (pH of 5.5 to 6.5) is a prepared Sterile Water for Injection used to dissolve IC-GREEN™.

Clinical Pharmacology: Following intravenous injection, IC-GREEN™ is rapidly bound to plasma protein, of which albumin is the principle carrier (95%). IC-GREEN™ undergoes no significant extrahepatic or enterohepatic circulation; simultaneous arterial and venous blood estimations have shown negligible renal, peripheral, lung or cerebro-spinal uptake of the dye. IC-GREEN™ is taken up from the plasma almost exclusively by the hepatic parenchymal cells and is secreted entirely into the bile. After biliary obstruction, the dye appears in the hepatic lymph, independently of the bile, suggesting that the biliary mucosa is sufficiently intact to prevent diffusion of the dye, though allowing diffusion of bilirubin. These characteristics make IC-GREEN™ a helpful index of hepatic function.

$C_{43}H_{47}N_2NaO_6S_2$ Molecular Weight 774.96

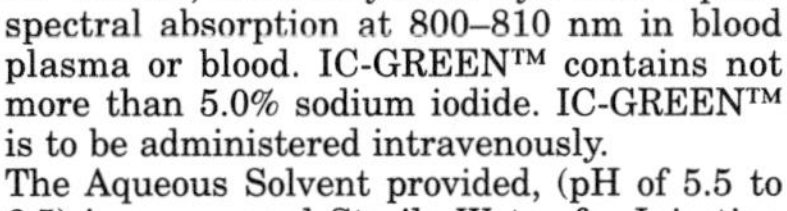

Indications: For determining cardiac output, hepatic function and liver blood flow, and for ophthalmic angiography.

Contraindications: IC-GREEN™ contains sodium iodide and should be used with caution in patients who have a history of allergy to iodides.

Warnings: Two anaphylactic deaths have been reported following IC-GREEN™ administration during cardiac catheterization. One of these was in a patient with a history of sensitivity to penicillin and sulfa drugs.
The Aqueous Solvent provided for this proiduct, pH 5.5 to 6.5, which is especially prepared Sterile Water for Injection, should be used to dissolve IC-GREEN™ because there have been reports of incompatibility with some commercially available Water for Injection.

Precautions: General: IC-GREEN™ Powder and Solution: IC-GREEN™ is unstable in aqueous solution and must be used within 10 hours. However, the dye is stable in plasma and whole blood so that samples obtained in discontinuous sampling techniques may be read hours later. Sterile techniques should be used in handling the dye solution as well as in the performance of the dilution curves.
IC-GREEN™ (sterile indocyanine green) powder may cling to the vial or lump together because it is freeze-dried in the vials. *This is not due to the presence of water*—the moisture content is carefully controlled.
Heparin preparations containing sodium bisulfate reduce the absorption peak of IC-GREEN™ in blood and, therefore, should not be used as an anticoagulant for the collection of samples for analysis.
The plasma fractional disappearance rate at the recommended 0.5 mg/kg dose has been reported to be significantly greater in women than in men, although there was no significant difference in the calculated value for clearance.
Radioactive iodine uptake studies should not be performed for at least a week following the use of IC-GREEN™.
Pregnancy Category C: Animal Reproduction studies have not been conducted with IC-GREEN™. It is also not known whether IC-GREEN™ can cause fetal harm when administered to a pregnant woman or can affect reproduction capacity. IC-GREEN™ should be given to a pregnant woman only if clearly indicated.

Nursing Mothers: It is not known whether this drug is excreted in human milk. Because many drugs are excreted in human milk, caution should be exercised when IC-GREEN™ is administered to a nursing woman.

Adverse Reactions: Anaphylactic or urticarial reactions have been reported in patients with or without history of allergy to iodides. If such reactions occur, treatment with the appropriate agents, e.g., epinephrine, antihistamines, and corticosteroids should be administered.

Drug Abuse and Dependence: IC-GREEN™ is not a controlled substance listed in any of the Drug Enforcement Administration schedules. Its use is not known to lead to dependence or abuse.

Overdosage: There are no data available describing the signs, symptoms, or laboratory findings accompanying overdosage. The LD_{50} after I.V. administration ranges between 60 and 80 mg/kg in mice, 50 and 70 mg/kg in rats and 50 and 80 mg/kg in rabbits.

Dosage And Administration: *INDICATOR-DILUTION STUDIES:* IC-GREEN™ permits recording of the indicator-dilution curves for both diagnostic and research purpose independently of fluctuations in oxygen saturation. In the performance of dye dilution curves, a known amount of dye is usually injected as a single bolus as rapidly as possible via a cardiac catheter into selected sites in the vascular system. A recording instrument (oximeter or densitometer) is attached to a needle or catheter for sampling of the dye-blood mixture from a systemic arterial sampling site.
Under sterile conditions, the IC-GREEN™ powder should be dissolved with the Aqueous Solvent provided for this product, and the solution used within 10 hours after it is prepared. If a precipitate is present, discard the solution. The amount of solvent to be used can be calculated from the dosage form which follows. It is recommended that the syringe used for injection of the dye be rinsed with this diluent. Isotonic saline should be used to flush the residual dye from the cardiac catheter into the circulation so as to avoid hemolysis. With the exception of the rinsing of the dye injection syringe, saline is used in all other parts of the catheterization procedure.
This matter of rinsing the dye syringe with distilled water may not be critical, since it is known that an amount of sodium chloride sufficient to make an isotonic solution may be added to dye *that has first been dissolved in distilled water.* This procedure has been used for constant-rate injection techniques without precipitation of the dye.

Continued on next page

IC-Green—Cont.

The usual doses of IC-GREEN™ which have been used for dilution curves are as follows:

Adults	5.0 mg
Children -	2.5 mg
Infants -	1.25 mg

These doses of the dye are usually injected in a ml volume. An average of five dilution curves are required in the performance of a diagnostic cardiac catheterization. The total dose of dye injected should be kept below 2 mg/kg.

Calibrating Dye Curves: To quantitate the dilution curves, standard dilutions of IC-GREEN™ in whole blood are made as follows. It is strongly recommended that the same dye that was used for the injections be used in the preparation of these standard dilutions. The most concentrated dye solution is made by accurately diluting 1 ml of the 5 mg/ml dye with 7 ml of distilled water. This concentration is then successively halved by diluting 4 ml of the previous concentration with 4 ml of distilled water. (If a 2.5 mg/ml concentration was used for the dilution curves, 1 ml of the 2.5 mg/ml dye is added to 3 ml of distilled water to make the most concentrated "standard" solution. This concentration is then successively halved by diluting 2 ml of the previous concentration with 2 ml of distilled water.) Then 0.2 ml portions (accurately measured from a calibrated syringe) of these dye solutions are added to 5 ml aliquots of the subject's blood, giving final concentrations of the dye in blood beginning with 24.0 mg/liter, approximately (actual concentration depends on the exact volume of dye added). This concentration is, of course, successively halved in the succeeding aliquots of the subject's blood. These aliquots of blood containing known amounts of dye, as well as a blank sample of which 0.2 ml of saline containing no dye has been added, are then passed through the detecting instrument and a calibration curve is constructed from the deflections recorded.

HEPATIC FUNCTION STUDIES: Due to its absorption spectrum, changing concentrations of IC-GREEN™ (sterile indocyanine green) in the blood can be monitored by ear densitometry or by obtaining blood specimens at timed intervals. The technique for both methods is as follows.

The patient should be studied in a fasting, basal state. The patient should be weighed and the dosage calculated on the basis of 0.5 mg/kg of body weight.

Under sterile conditions, the IC-GREEN™ powder should be dissolved with the Aqueous Solvent provided. Exactly 5 ml of aqueous solvent should be added to the 25 mg vial or exactly 10 ml of aqueous solvent should be added to the 50 mg vial, giving 5 mg of dye per ml of solution.

Inject the correct amount of dye into the lumen of an arm vein as rapidly as possible, without allowing the dye to escape outside the vein. (*If the photometric method is used, prior to injecting IC-GREEN™, withdraw 6 ml of venous blood from the patient's arm for serum blank and standard curve construction, and through the same needle, inject the correct amount of dye.*)

Ear Densitometry: Ear oximetry has also been used and makes it possible to monitor the appearance and disappearance of IC-GREEN™ without the necessity of withdrawal and spectrophotometric analysis of blood samples for calibration. An ear densitometer which has a compensatory photo-electric cell to correct for changes in blood volume and hematocrit, and a detection photocell which registers levels has been described. This device permits simultaneous measurement of cardiac output, blood volume and hepatic clearance of IC-GREEN™* and was found to provide a reliable index of plasma removal kinetice after single injections or continuous intrusions of IC-GREEN™. This technique was employed in newborn infants, healthy adults and in children and adults with liver disease. The normal subject has a removal rate of 18–24% per minute. Due to the absence of extrahepatic removal, IC-GREEN™ was found to be ideally suited for serial study of severe chronic liver disease and to provide a stable measurement of hepatic blood flow. In larger doses, IC-GREEN™ has proven to be particularly valuable in detecting drug-induced alterations of hepatic function and in the detection of mild liver injury.

---

*Dichromatic earpiece densitometer supplied by The Waters Company, Rochester, Minnesota.

Using the ear densitometer, a dosage of 0.5 mg/kg in normal subjects gives the following clearance pattern.

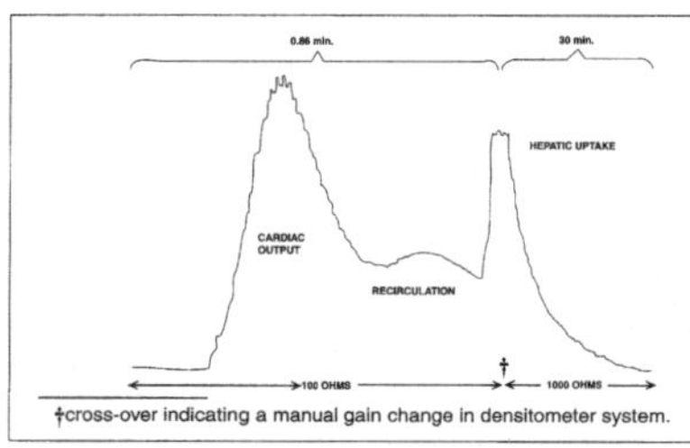

†cross-over indicating a manual gain change in densitometer system.

Photometric Method-

Determination Using Percentage Retention of Dye:

A typical curve obtained by plotting dye concentration versus optical density is shown below. Percent retention can be read from this plot.

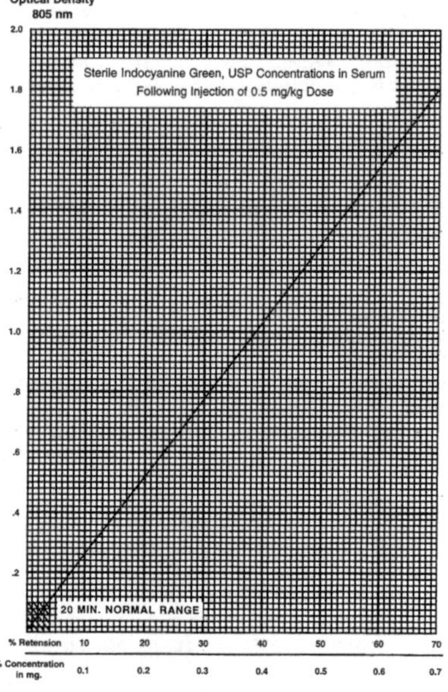

If more accurate results are desired, a curve using the patient's blood and the vial of IC-GREEN™ being used in the determination can be constructed as follows:

1. Take 6 ml of non-dye-containing venous blood from the patient's arm. Place in a test tube and allow the blood to clot. The serum is separated by centrifugation.
2. Pipette 1 ml of the serum into a microcuvette.
3. Add 1 lambda (λ) of the 5 mg/ml aqueous IC-GREEN™ (sterile indocyanine green) solution to the serum, giving a dilution of 5 mg/liter, the standard for 50% retention. (The addition of 2 lambda (λ) of the 5 mg/ml IC-GREEN™ solution would give 100% retention; however, this concentration cannot be read on the spectrophotometer.)
4. The optical density of this solution is read at 805 nm, using normal serum as the blank.
5. Using graph paper similar to that used in the illustration, plot the 50% figure obtained in Step 4, and draw a line connecting this point with the zero coordinates.

Percentage Retention: A single 20-minute sample (withdrawn from a vein in the opposite arm to that injected) is allowed to clot, centrifuged and its optical density is determined at 805 nm using the patient's normal serum as the blank. Dye concentration is read from the curve above. A single 20-minute sample of serum in healthy subjects should contain no more than 4% of the initial concentration of the dye. The use of percentage retention is less accurate than percentage disappearance rate, but provides reproducible results. Hemolysis does not interfere with a reading.

Determination Using Disappearance Rate of Dye: To calculate the percentage disappearance rate, obtain samples at 5, 10, 15 and 20 minutes after injecting the dye. Prepare the sample as in the previous section and measure the optical densities at 805 nm, using the patient's normal serum as the blank. The IC-GREEN™ concentration in each timed specimen can be determined by using the concentration curve illustrated. Plot values on semilogarithmic paper.

Specimens containing IC-GREEN™ should be read at the same temperature since its optical density is influenced by temperature variations.

Normal Values: Percentage disappearance rate in healthy subjects is 18–24% per minute. Normal biological half-time is 2.5–3.0 minutes.

OPHTHALMIC ANGIOGRAPHY STUDIES: The excitation and emission spectra (Figure 1) and the absorption spectra (Figure 2) of IC-GREEN™ make it useful in ophthalmic angiography. The peak absorption and emission of IC-GREEN™ lie in a region (800–850 nm) where transmission of energy by the pigment epithelium is more efficient than in the region of visible light energy. IC-GREEN™ also has the property of being nearly 98% bound to blood protein, and therefore, excessive dye extravasation does not take place in the highly fenestrated choroidal vasculature It is, therefore, useful in both absorption and fluorescence infrared angiography of the choroidal vasculature when using appropriate filters and film in a fundus camera.

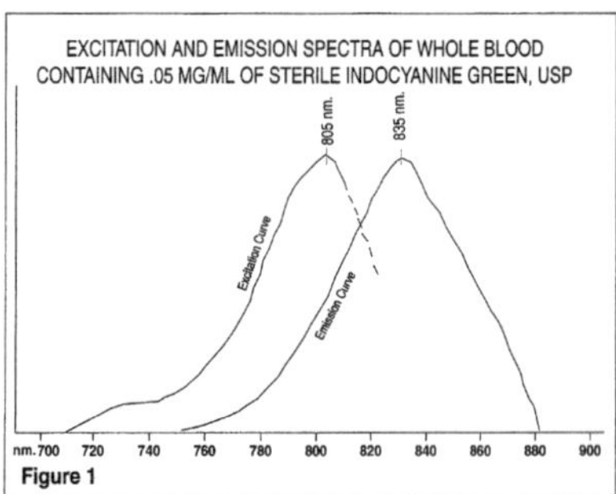

Figure 1

Dosages up to 40 mg IC-GREEN™ dye in 2 ml of aqueous solvent have been found to give optimal angiograms, depending on the imaging equipment and technique used. The antecubital vein injected IC-GREEN™ dye bolus should immediately be followed by a 5 ml bolus of normal saline.

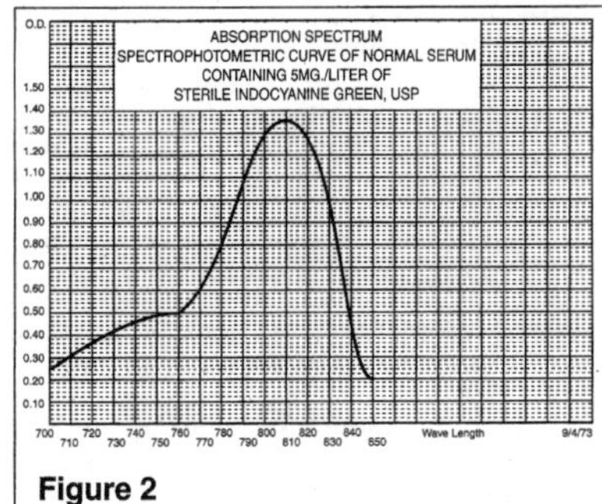

Figure 2

Clinically, angiograms of uniformly good quality can be assured only after taking care to optimize the contributions of all possible factors such as, patient cooperation and dye injection. The foregoing injection regimen is designed to provide delivery of a spatially limited dye bolus of optimal concentration to the choroidal vasculature following intravenous injection.

HOW SUPPLIED

AVAILABILITY

IC-GREEN™, Six each 25 mg vials and 10 ml ampules Aqueous solvent, NDC 17478-701-2.

Manufactured for:
Akorn, Inc
Buffalo Grove, IL 60089
Shown in Product Identification Guide, page 103

OCUSERT® Pilo-20 ℞
[*ok "u-sĕrt*]
(pilocarpine)
Ocular Therapeutic System
20 µg/hr. for one week
and
OCUSERT® Pilo-40 ℞
(pilocarpine)
Ocular Therapeutic System
40 µg/hr. for one week

Description: OCUSERT® pilocarpine system is an elliptically shaped unit designed for continuous release of pilocarpine following placement in the cul-de-sac of the eye. Clinical evaluation in appropriate patients has demonstrated therapeutic efficacy of the system in the eye for one week. Two strengths are available, Pilo-20 and Pilo-40.

OCUSERT® systems contain a core reservoir consisting of pilocarpine and alginic acid. Pilocarpine is designated chemically as 2(3H)-Furanone,3-ethyldihydro-4[(1-methyl-1H-imidazol-5-yl) methyl]-, (3S-cis)- and has the following structural formula:

The core is surrounded by a hydrophobic ethylene/vinyl acetate (EVA) copolymer membrane which controls the diffusion of pilocarpine from the OCUSERT® system into the eye. The Pilo-40 membrane contains di(2-ethylhexyl) phthalate, which increases the rate of diffusion of pilocarpine across the EVA membrane. Of the total content of pilocarpine in the Pilo-20 or Pilo-40 system (5 mg or 11 mg, respectively), a portion serves as the thermodynamic diffusional energy source to release the drug and remains in the unit at the end of the week's use. The alginic acid component of the core is not released from the system. The readily visible white margin around the system contains titanium dioxide. The Pilo-20 system is 5.7 × 13.4 mm on its axes and 0.3 mm thick; the Pilo-40 system is 5.5 × 13 mm on its axes and 0.5 mm thick.

Release Rate Concept: With the OCUSERT® system form of therapy, the particular strength is described by the rated release, the mean release rate of drug from the system over seven days, in micrograms per hour. To cover the range of drug therapy needed to control the increased intraocular pressure associated with the glaucomas, two rated releases of pilocarpine from the OCUSERT® system are available, 20 and 40 micrograms per hour, for one week.

During the first few hours of the seven day time course, the release rate is higher than that prevailing over the remainder of the one-week period. The system releases drug at three times the rated value in the first hours and drops to the rated value in approximately six hours. A total of 0.3 mg to 0.7 mg pilocarpine (Pilo-20 or Pilo-40, respectively) is released during this initial six-hour period (one drop of 2% pilocarpine ophthalmic solution contains 1 mg pilocarpine). During the remainder of the seven day period the release rate is within ± 20% of the rated value.

Clinical Pharmacology: Pilocarpine is released from the OCUSERT® system as soon as it is placed in contact with the conjunctival surfaces. Pilocarpine is a direct acting parasympathomimetic drug which produces pupillary constriction, stimulates the ciliary muscle, and increases aqueous humor outflow facility. Because of its action on ciliary muscle, pilocarpine induces transient myopia, generally more pronounced in younger patients. In association with the increase in outflow facility, there is a decrease in intraocular pressure.

Preclinical Results: The levels of ^{14}C-pilocarpine in the ocular tissues of rabbits following OCUSERT® system and eyedrop administration have been determined. The OCUSERT® system produces constant low pilocarpine levels in the ciliary body and iris. Following ^{14}C-pilocarpine eyedrop treatment, the initial levels of pilocarpine in the cornea, aqueous humor, ciliary body and iris are 3 to 5 times higher than the corresponding levels with the OCUSERT® system, declining over the next six hours to approximately the tissue concentrations maintained by the OCUSERT® system. In contrast, in the conjunctiva, lens, and vitreous the ^{14}C-pilocarpine concentrations remain consistently high from eyedrops and do not return to the constant low levels maintained by the OCUSERT® system. Pilocarpine does not accumulate in ocular tissues during OCUSERT® system use. These studies in rabbits have not been done in humans.

Clinical Results: The ocular hypotensive effect of both the Pilo-20 and Pilo-40 systems is fully developed within 1½ to 2 hours after placement in the cul-de-sac. A satisfactory ocular hypotensive response is maintained around-the-clock. Intraocular pressure reduction for an entire week is achieved with the OCUSERT® system from either 3.4 mg or 6.7 mg pilocarpine (20 or 40 µg/hour times 24 hours/day times 7 days, respectively), as compared with 28 mg administered as a 2% ophthalmic solution four times a day.

During the first several hours after insertion of an OCUSERT® pilocarpine system into the conjunctival cul-de-sac, induced myopia may occur. In contrast to the fluctuating and high levels of induced myopia typical of pilocarpine administration by eyedrop, the amount of induced myopia with OCUSERT® systems decreases after the first several hours to a low baseline level, approximately 0.5 diopters or less, which persists for the therapeutic life of the OCUSERT® system. Pilocarpine-induced miosis approximately parallels the induced myopia.

Of the 302 patients who used the OCUSERT® system in clinical studies for more than two weeks, 229 (75%) preferred it to previously used pilocarpine eyedrops. This percentage increased with further wearing experience.

Indications and Usage: OCUSERT® pilocarpine system is indicated for control of elevated intraocular pressure in pilocarpine responsive patients. Clinical studies have demonstrated OCUSERT® system efficacy in certain glaucomatous patients.

The patient should be instructed on the use of the OCUSERT® system and should read the package insert instructions for use. The patient should demonstrate to the ophthalmologist his ability to place, adjust and remove the units.

Concurrent Therapy: OCUSERT® systems have been used concomitantly with various ophthalmic medications. The release rate of pilocarpine from the OCUSERT® system is not influenced by carbonic anhydrase inhibitors, epinephrine or timolol ophthalmic solutions, fluorescein, or anesthetic, antibiotic, or anti-inflammatory steroid ophthalmic solutions. Systemic reactions consistent with an increased rate of absorption from the eye of an autonomic drug, such as epinephrine, have been observed. The occurrence of mild bulbar conjunctival edema, which is frequently present with epinephrine ophthalmic solutions, is not influenced by the OCUSERT® pilocarpine system.

Contraindications: OCUSERT® pilocarpine system is contraindicated where pupillary constriction is undesirable, such as for glaucomas associated with acute inflammatory disease of the anterior segment of the eye, and glaucomas occurring or persisting after extracapsular cataract extraction where posterior synechiae may occur.

Warnings: Patients with acute infectious conjunctivitis or keratitis should be given special consideration and evaluation prior to the use of the OCUSERT® pilocarpine system.

Damaged or deformed systems should not be placed or retained in the eye. Systems believed to be associated with an unexpected increase in drug action should be removed and replaced with a new system.

Precautions:

General

OCUSERT® pilocarpine system safety in retinal detachment patients and in patients with filtration blebs has not been established. The conjunctival erythema and edema associated with epinephrine ophthalmic solutions are not substantially altered by concomitant OCUSERT® pilocarpine system therapy. The use of pilocarpine drops should be considered when intense miosis is desired in certain ocular conditions.

Drug Interactions

Although ophthalmic solutions have been used effectively in conjunction with the OCUSERT® system, systemic reactions consistent with an increased rate of absorption from the eye of an autonomic drug, such as epinephrine, have been observed. In rare instances, reactions of this type can be severe.

Carcinogenesis, Mutagenesis, Impairment of Fertility

No long-term carcinogenicity and reproduction studies in animals have been conducted with the OCUSERT® system.

Pregnancy Category C

Although the use of the OCUSERT® pilocarpine system has not been reported to have adverse effect on pregnancy, the safety of its use in pregnant women has not been absolutely established. While systemic absorption of pilocarpine from the OCUSERT® system is highly unlikely, pregnant women should use it only if clearly needed.

Continued on next page

Ocusert Pilo—Cont.

Nursing Mothers
It is not known whether pilocarpine is excreted in human milk. Because many drugs are excreted in human milk, caution should be exercised when the OCUSERT® system is used by a nursing woman.

Pediatric Use
Safety and effectiveness in children have not been established.

Adverse Reactions: Ciliary spasm is encountered with pilocarpine usage but is not a contraindication to continued therapy unless the induced myopia is debilitating to the patient. Irritation from pilocarpine has been infrequently encountered and may require cessation of therapy depending on the judgement of the physician. True allergic reactions are uncommon but require discontinuation of therapy should they occur. Corneal abrasion and visual impairment have been reported with use of the OCUSERT® System.

Although withdrawal of the peripheral iris from the anterior chamber angle by miosis may reduce the tendency for narrow angle closure, miotics can occasionally precipitate angle closure by increasing the resistance to aqueous flow from posterior to anterior chamber. Miotic agents may also cause retinal detachment; thus, care should be exercised with all miotic therapy especially in young myopic patients.

Some patients may notice signs of conjunctival irritation, including mild erythema with or without a slight increase in mucous secretion when they first use OCUSERT® pilocarpine systems. These symptoms tend to lessen or disappear after the first week of therapy. In rare instances a sudden increase in pilocarpine effects has been reported during system use.

Dosage and Administration: *Initiation of Therapy:* A patient whose intraocular pressure has been controlled by 1% or 2% pilocarpine eyedrop solution has a higher probability of pressure control with the Pilo-20 system than a patient who has used a higher strength pilocarpine solution and might require Pilo-40 therapy. However, there is no direct correlation between the OCUSERT® system (Pilo-20 or Pilo-40) and the strength of pilocarpine eyedrop solutions required to achieve a given level of pressure lowering. The OCUSERT® system reduces the amount of drug necessary to achieve adequate medical control; therefore, therapy may be started with the OCUSERT® Pilo-20 system irrespective of the strength of pilocarpine solution the patient previously required. Because of the patient's age, family history, and disease status or progression, however, the ophthalmologist may elect to begin therapy with the Pilo-40. The patient should then return during the first week of therapy for evaluation of his intraocular pressure, and as often thereafter as the ophthalmologist deems necessary.

If the pressure is satisfactorily reduced with the OCUSERT® Pilo-20 system the patient should continue its use, replacing each unit every 7 days. If the physician desires intraocular pressure reduction greater than that achieved by the Pilo-20 system, the patient should be transferred to the Pilo-40 system. If necessary, an epinephrine ophthalmic solution or a carbonic anhydrase inhibitor may be used concurrently with OCUSERT® system.

After a satisfactory therapeutic regimen has been established with the OCUSERT® pilocarpine system, the frequency of follow-up should be determined by the ophthalmologist according to the status of the patient's disease process.

Placement and Removal of the OCUSERT® System: The OCUSERT® system is readily placed in the eye by the patient, according to patient instructions provided in the package. The instructions also describe procedures for removal of the system. It is strongly recommended that the patient's ability to manage the placement and removal of the system be reviewed at the first patient visit after initiation of therapy.

Since the pilocarpine-induced myopia from the OCUSERT® systems may occur during the first several hours of therapy (average of 1.4 diopters in a group of young subjects), the patient should be advised to place the system into the conjunctival cul-de-sac at bedtime. By morning the induced myopia is at a stable level (about 0.5 diopters or less in young subjects).

Sanitary Handling: Patients should be instructed to wash their hands thoroughly with soap and water before touching or manipulating the OCUSERT® system. In the event a displaced unit contacts unclean surfaces, rinsing with cool tap water before replacing is advisable. Obviously bacteriologically contaminated units should be discarded and replaced with a fresh unit.

OCUSERT® System Retention in the Eye: During the initial adaptation period, the OCUSERT® unit may slip out of the conjunctival cul-de-sac onto the cheek. The patient is usually aware of such movement and can replace the unit without difficulty.

In those patients in whom retention of the OCUSERT® unit is a problem, superior cul-de-sac placement is often more desirable. The OCUSERT® unit can be manipulated from the lower to the upper conjunctival cul-de-sac by a gentle digital massage through the lid, a technique readily learned by the patient. If possible the unit should be moved before sleep to the upper conjunctival cul-de-sac for best retention. Should the unit slip out of the conjunctival cul-de-sac during sleep, its ocular hypotensive effect following loss continues for a period of time comparable to that following instillation of eyedrops. The patient should be instructed to check for the presence of the OCUSERT® unit before retiring at night and upon arising.

How Supplied: OCUSERT® Pilo-20 or Pilo-40 systems are available in packages containing eight individual sterile systems.

Storage and Handling: Store under refrigeration (36°–46°F).

Rx only

MANUFACTURED FOR:
AKORN, Inc., Buffalo Grove, IL 60089
BY:
ALZA Corporation, Palo Alto, California 94304
Edition Date: September 1998
7140641-7

Shown in Product Identification Guide, page 103

Alcon Laboratories, Inc.

and its affiliates
CORPORATE HEADQUARTERS:
6201 SOUTH FREEWAY
FORT WORTH, TX 76134

Address Inquiries to:

Pharmaceuticals/Consumer Products	800-451-3937
(Therapeutic Drugs/Lens Care)	
Surgical	800-862-5266
(Instrumentation/Surgical Meds)	
Systems	800-289-1991
(Medical Management Information Systems)	

ALOMIDE® 0.1% ℞
(lodoxamide tromethamine ophthalmic solution)

Description: ALOMIDE® is a sterile ophthalmic solution containing the mast cell stabilizer lodoxamide tromethamine for topical administration to the eyes. Lodoxamide tromethamine is a white, crystalline, water-soluble powder with a molecular weight of 553.91.

Chemical Name: N,N[1]-(2-chloro-5-cyano-m-phenylene)dioxamic acid tromethamine salt
Empirical Formula: $C_{19}H_{28}O_{12}N_5Cl$

Each mL of ALOMIDE® Ophthalmic Solution contains: Active: 1.78 mg lodoxamide tromethamine equivalent to 1 mg lodoxamide. **Preservative:** benzalkonium chloride 0.007%. **Inactive:** mannitol, hydroxypropyl methylcellulose 2910, sodium citrate, citric acid, edetate disodium, tyloxapol, hydrochloric acid and/or sodium hydroxide (adjust pH), and purified water.

Clinical Pharmacology: Lodoxamide tromethamine is a mast cell stabilizer that inhibits the *in vivo* Type 1 immediate hypersensitivity reaction. Lodoxamide therapy inhibits the increases in cutaneous vascular permeability that are associated with reagin or IgE and antigen-mediated reactions.

In vitro studies have demonstrated the ability of lodoxamide to stabilize rodent mast cells and prevent antigen-stimulated release of histamine. In addition, lodoxamide prevents the release of other mast cell inflammatory mediators (i.e., SRS-A, slow-reacting substances of anaphylaxis, also known as the peptidoleukotrienes) and inhibits eosinophil chemotaxis. Although lodoxamide's precise mechanism of action is unknown, the drug has been reported to prevent calcium influx into mast cells upon antigen stimulation.

Lodoxamide has no intrinsic vasoconstrictor, antihistaminic, cyclooxygenase inhibition, or other anti-inflammatory activity.

The disposition of ^{14}C-lodoxamide was studied in six healthy adult volunteers receiving a 3 mg (50 µCi) oral dose of lodoxamide. Urinary excretion was the major route of elimination. The elimination half-life of ^{14}C-lodoxamide was 8.5 hours in urine. In a study conducted in twelve healthy adult volunteers, topical administration of ALOMIDE® 0.1% (lodoxamide tromethamine ophthalmic solution), one drop in each eye four times per day for ten days, did not result in any measurable lodoxamide plasma levels at a detection limit of 2.5 ng/mL.

Indications and Usage: ALOMIDE® Ophthalmic Solution 0.1% is indicated in the treatment of the ocular disorders referred to by the terms vernal keratoconjunctivitis, vernal conjunctivitis, and vernal keratitis.

Contraindications: Hypersensitivity to any component of this product.

Warnings: Not for injection. As with all ophthalmic preparations containing benzalkonium chloride, patients should be instructed not to wear soft contact lenses during treatment with ALOMIDE® Ophthalmic Solution. Do not touch the dropper tip to any surface, as this may contaminate the solution.

Precautions: General: Patients may experience a transient burning or stinging upon instillation of ALOMIDE® Ophthalmic Solution. Should these symptoms persist, the patient should be advised to contact the prescribing physician.

Carcinogenesis, Mutagenesis, Impairment of Fertility: A long-term study with lodoxamide tromethamine in rats (two-year oral administration) showed no neoplastic or tumorigenic effects at doses 100 mg/kg/day (more than 5000 times the proposed human clinical dose). No evidence of mutagenicity or genetic damage was seen in the Ames *Salmonella* Assay, Chromosomal Aberration in CHO Cells Assay, or

Mouse Forward Lymphoma Assay. In the BALB/c-3T3 Cells Transformation Assay, some increase in the number of transformed foci was seen at high concentrations (greater than 4000 µg/mL). No evidence of impairment of reproductive function was shown in laboratory animal studies.

Pregnancy: Pregnancy Category B. Reproduction studies with lodoxamide tromethamine administered orally to rats and rabbits in doses of 100 mg/kg/day (more than 5000 times the proposed human clinical dose) produced no evidence of developmental toxicity. There are, however, no adequate and well-controlled studies in pregnant women. Because animal reproduction studies are not always predictive of human response, ALOMIDE® 0.1% (lodoxamide tromethamine ophthalmic solution) should be used during pregnancy only if clearly needed.

Nursing Mothers: It is not known whether lodoxamide tromethamine is excreted in human milk. Because many drugs are excreted in human milk, caution should be exercised when ALOMIDE® Ophthalmic Solution 0.1% is administered to nursing women.

Pediatric Use: Safety and effectiveness in pediatric patients below the age of 2 have not been established.

Adverse Reactions: During clinical studies of ALOMIDE® Ophthalmic Solution 0.1%, the most frequently reported ocular adverse experiences were transient burning, stinging, or discomfort upon instillation, which occurred in approximately 15% of the subjects. Other ocular events occurring in 1 to 5% of the subjects included ocular itching/pruritus, blurred vision, dry eye, tearing/discharge, hyperemia, crystalline deposits, and foreign body sensation. Events that occurred in less than 1% of the subjects included corneal erosion/ulcer, scales on lid/lash, eye pain, ocular edema/swelling, ocular warming sensation, ocular fatigue, chemosis, corneal abrasion, anterior chamber cells, keratopathy/keratitis, blepharitis, allergy, sticky sensation, and epitheliopathy.

Nonocular events reported were headache (1.5%) and (at less than 1%) heat sensation, dizziness, somnolence, nausea, stomach discomfort, sneezing, dry nose, and rash.

Overdosage: There have been no reports of ALOMIDE® 0.1% (lodoxamide tromethamine ophthalmic solution) overdose following topical ocular application. Accidental overdose of an oral preparation of 120 to 180 mg of lodoxamide resulted in a temporary sensation of warmth, profuse sweating, diarrhea, lightheadedness, and a feeling of stomach distension; no permanent adverse effects were observed. Side effects reported following systemic oral administration of 0.1 mg to 10.0 mg of lodoxamide include a feeling of warmth or flushing, headache, dizziness, fatigue, sweating, nausea, loose stools, and urinary frequency/urgency. The physician may consider emesis in the event of accidental ingestion.

Dosage and Administration: The dose for adults and children greater than two years of age is one to two drops in each affected eye four times daily for up to 3 months.

How Supplied: ALOMIDE® Ophthalmic Solution 0.1% is supplied in plastic ophthalmic DROP-TAINER® dispenser as follows:

10 mL: **NDC** 0065-0345-10

Storage: Store at 15°C–27°C (59°F–80°F).

Rx Only

AZOPT™ ℞

(brinzolamide ophthalmic suspension) 1%

Description: AZOPT™ (brinzolamide ophthalmic suspension) 1% contains a carbonic anhydrase inhibitor formulated for multidose topical ophthalmic use. Brinzolamide is described chemically as: (R)-(+)-4-Ethylamino-2-(3-methoxypropyl)-3,4-dihydro-2H-thieno [3,2-e]-1,2-thiazine-6-sulfonamide-1,1-doxide. Its empirical formula is $C_{12}H_{21}N_3O_5S_3$. Brinzolamide has a molecular weight of 383.5 and a melting point of about 131°C. It is a white powder, which is insoluble in water, very soluble in methanol and soluble in ethanol.

AZOPT 1% is supplied as a sterile, aqueous suspension of brinzolamide which has been formulated to be readily suspended and slow settling, following shaking. It has a pH of approximately 7.5 and an osmolality of 300 mOsm/kg. Each mL of AZOPT 1% contains 10 mg brinzolamide. Inactive ingredients are mannitol, carbomer 974P, tyloxapol, edetate disodium, sodium chloride, hydrochloric acid and/or sodium hydroxide (to adjust pH), and purified water. Benzalkonium chloride 0.01% is added as a preservative.

Clinical Pharmacology: Carbonic anhydrase (CA) is an enzyme found in many tissues of the body including the eye. It catalyzes the reversible reaction involving the hydration of carbon dioxide and the dehydration of carbonic acid. In humans, carbonic anhydrase exists as a number of isoenzymes, the most active being carbonic anhydrase II (CA-II), found primarily in red blood cells (RBCs), but also in other tissues. Inhibition of carbonic anhydrase in the ciliary processes of the eye decreases aqueous humor secretion, presumably by slowing the formation of bicarbonate ions with subsequent reduction in sodium and fluid transport.

The result is a reduction in intraocular pressure (IOP).

AZOPT 1% contains brinzolamide, an inhibitor of carbonic anhydrase II (CA-II). Following topical ocular administration, brinzolamide inhibits aqueous humor formation and reduces elevated intraocular pressure. Elevated intraocular pressure is a major risk factor in the pathogenesis of optic nerve damage and glaucomatous visual field loss.

Following topical ocular administration, brinzolamide is absorbed into the systemic circulation. Due to its affinity for CA-II, brinzolamide distributes extensively into the RBCs and exhibits a long half-life in whole blood (approximately 111 days). In humans, the metabolite N-desethyl brinzolamide is formed, which also binds to CA and accumulates in RBCs. This metabolite binds mainly to CA-I in the presence of brinzolamide. In plasma, both parent brinzolamide and N-desethyl brinzolamide concentrations are low and generally below assay quantitation limits (<10 ng/mL). Binding to plasma proteins is approximately 60%. Brinzolamide is eliminated predominantly in the urine as unchanged drug. N-Desethyl brinzolamide is also found in the urine along with lower concentrations of the N-desmethoxypropyl and O-desmethyl metabolites.

An oral pharmacokinetic study was conducted in which healthy volunteers received 1 mg capsules of brinzolamide twice per day for up to 32 weeks. This regimen approximates the amount of drug delivered by topical ocular administration of AZOPT (brinzolamide ophthalmic suspension) 1% dosed to both eyes three times per day and simulates systemic drug and metabolite concentrations similar to those achieved with long-term topical dosing. RBC CA activity was measured to assess the degree to systemic CA inhibition. Brinzolamide saturation of RBC CA-II was achieved within 4 weeks (RBC concentrations of approximately 20 µM). N-Desethyl brinzolamide accumulated in RBCs to steady-state within 20–28 weeks reaching concentrations ranging from 6–30 µM. The inhibition of CA-II activity at steady-state was approximately 70–75%, which is below the degree of inhibition expected to have a pharmacological effect on renal function or respiration in healthy subjects.

In two, three-month clinical studies, AZOPT (brinzolamide ophthalmic suspension) 1% dosed three times per day (TID) in patients with elevated intraocular pressure (IOP), produced significant reductions in IOPs (4–5 mmHg). These IOP reductions are equivalent to the reductions observed with TRUSOPT* (dorzolamide hydrochloride ophthalmic solution) 2% dosed TID in the same studies.

In two clinical studies in patients with elevated intraocular pressure, AZOPT 1% was associated with less stinging and burning upon instillation than TRUSOPT* 2%.

Indications and Usage: AZOPT™ Ophthalmic Suspension 1% is indicated in the treatment of elevated intraocular pressure in patients with ocular hypertension or open-angle glaucoma.

Contraindications: AZOPT™ is contraindicated in patients who are hypersensitive to any component of this product.

Warnings: AZOPT™ is a sulfonamide and although administered topically it is absorbed systemically. Therefore, the same types of adverse reactions that are attributable to sulfonamides may occur with topical administration of AZOPT. Fatalities have occurred, although rarely, due to severe reactions to sulfonamides including Stevens-Johnson syndrome, toxic epidermal necrolysis, fulminant hepatic necrosis, agranulocytosis, aplastic anemia, and other blood dyscrasias. Sensitization may recur when a sulfonamide is re-administered irrespective of the route of administration. If signs of serious reactions or hypersensitivity occur, discontinue the use of this preparation.

Precautions

General:

Carbonic anhydrase activity has been observed in both the cytoplasm and around the plasma membranes of the corneal endothelium. The effect of continued administration of AZOPT on the corneal endothelium has not been fully evaluated. The management of patients with acute angle-closure glaucoma requires therapeutic interventions in addition to ocular hypotensive agents. AZOPT has not been studied in patients with acute angle-closure glaucoma.

AZOPT has not been studied in patients with severe renal impairment (CrCl <30 mL/min). Because AZOPT and its metabolite are excreted predominantly by the kidney, AZOPT is not recommended in such patients.

AZOPT has not been studied in patients with hepatic impairment and should be used with caution in such patients.

There is a potential for an additive effect on the known systemic effects of carbonic anhydrase inhibition in patients receiving an oral carbonic anhydrase inhibitor and AZOPT. The concomitant administration of AZOPT and oral carbonic anhydrase inhibitors is not recommended.

Information For Patients:

AZOPT™ is a sulfonamide and although administered topically, it is absorbed systemically; therefore, the same type of adverse reactions attributable to sulfonamides may occur with topical administration. Patients should be advised that if serious or unusual ocular or systemic reactions or signs of hypersensitivity occur, they should discontinue the use of the product and consult their physician (see **Warnings**).

Vision may be temporarily blurred following dosing with AZOPT. Care should be exercised in operating machinery or driving a motor vehicle.

Patients should be instructed to avoid allowing the tip of the dispensing container to contact the eye or surrounding structures or other surfaces, since the product can become contaminated by common bacteria known to cause oc-

Continued on next page

Azopt—Cont.

ular infections. Serious damage to the eye and subsequent loss of vision may result from using contaminated solutions.

Patients should also be advised that if they have ocular surgery or develop an intercurrent ocular condition (e.g., trauma or infection), they should immediately seek their physician's advice concerning the continued use of the present multidose container.

If more than one topical ophthalmic drug is being used, the drugs should be administered at least ten minutes apart. The preservative in AZOPT™ Ophthalmic Suspension, benzalkonium chloride, may be absorbed by soft contact lenses. Contact lenses should be removed during instillation of AZOPT, but may be reinserted 15 minutes after instillation.

Drug Interactions:

AZOPT™ Ophthalmic Suspension 1% contains a carbonic anhydrase inhibitor. Acid-base and electrolyte alterations were not reported in the clinical trials with brinzolamide. However, in patients treated with oral carbonic anhydrase inhibitors, rare instances of drug interactions have occurred with high-dose salicylate therapy. Therefore, the potential for such drug interaction should be considered in patients receiving AZOPT.

Carcinogenesis, Mutagenesis, Impairment of Fertility:

Carcinogenicity data on brinzolamide are not available. The following tests for mutagenic potential were negative: (1) *in vivo* mouse micronucleus assay; (2) *in vivo* sister chromatid exchange assay; and (3) Ames *E. coli* test. The *in vitro* mouse lymphoma forward mutation assay was negative in the absence of activation, but positive in the presence of microsomal activation.

In reproduction studies of brinzolamide in rats, there were no adverse effects on the fertility or reproductive capacity of males or females at doses up to 18 mg/kg/day (375 times the recommended human ophthalmic dose).

Pregnancy:

Teratogenic Effects: Pregnancy Category C. Developmental toxicity studies with brinzolamide in rabbits at oral doses of 1, 3, and 6 mg/kg/day (20, 62, and 125 times the recommended human ophthalmic dose) produced maternal toxicity at 6 mg/kg/day and a significant increase in the number of fetal variations, such as accessory skull bones, which was only slightly higher than the historic value at 1 and 6 mg/kg. In rats, statistically decreased body weights of fetuses from dams receiving oral doses of 18 mg/kg/day (375 times the recommended human ophthalmic dose) during gestation were proportional to the reduced maternal weight gain, with no statistically significant effects on organ or tissue development. Increases in unossified sternebrae, reduced ossification of the skull, and unossified hyoid that occurred at 6 and 18 mg/kg were not statistically significant. No treatment-related malformations were seen. Following oral administration of ^{14}C-brinzolamide to pregnant rats, radioactivity was found to cross the placenta and was present in the fetal tissues and blood.

There are no adequate and well-controlled studies in pregnant women. AZOPT should be used during pregnancy only if the potential benefit justifies the potential risk to the fetus.

Nursing Mothers:

In a study of brinzolamide in lactating rats, decreases in body weight gain in offspring at an oral dose of 15 mg/kg/day (312 times the recommended human ophthalmic dose) were seen during lactation. No other effects were observed. However, following oral administration of ^{14}C-brinzolamide to lactating rats, radioactivity was found in milk at concentrations below those in the blood and plasma.

It is not known whether this drug is excreted in human milk. Because many drugs are excreted in human milk and because of the potential for serious adverse reactions in nursing infants from AZOPT, a decision should be made whether to discontinue nursing or to discontinue the drug, taking into account the importance of the drug to the mother.

Pediatric Use:

Safety and effectiveness in pediatric patients have not been established.

Adverse Reactions:

In clinical studies of AZOPT (brinzolamide ophthalmic suspension) 1%, the most frequently reported adverse events associated with AZOPT 1% were blurred vision and bitter, sour or unusual taste. These events occurred in approximately 5–10% of patients. Blepharitis, dermatitis, dry eye, foreign body sensation, headache, hyperemia, ocular discharge, ocular discomfort, ocular keratitis, ocular pain, ocular pruritus and rhinitis were reported at an incidence of 1–5%.

The following adverse reactions were reported at an incidence below 1%: allergic reactions, alopecia, chest pain, conjunctivitis, diarrhea, diplopia, dizziness, dry mouth, dyspnea, dyspepsia, eye fatigue, hypertonia, keratoconjunctivitis, keratopathy, kidney pain, lid margin crusting or sticky sensation, nausea, pharyngitis, tearing and urticaria.

Overdosage: Although no human data are available, electrolyte imbalance, development of an acidotic state, and possible nervous system effects may occur following oral administration of an overdose. Serum electrolyte levels (particularly potassium) and blood pH levels should be monitored.

Dosage and Administration: Shake well before use. The recommended dose is 1 drop of AZOPT Ophthalmic Suspension in the affected eye(s) three times daily.

AZOPT may be used concomitantly with other topical ophthalmic drug products to lower intraocular pressure.

If more than one topical ophthalmic drug is being used, the drugs should be administered at least ten minutes apart.

How Supplied: AZOPT™ Ophthalmic Suspension 1% is supplied in plastic DROP-TAINER® dispensers with a controlled dispensing-tip as follows:

NDC 0065-0275-24	2.5 mL
NDC 0065-0275-05	5 mL
NDC 0065-0275-10	10 mL
NDC 0065-0275-15	15 mL

Storage: Store AZOPT Ophthalmic Suspension 1% at 4–30°C (39–86°F).

Rx Only

U.S. Patent Numbers: 5,240,923; 5,378,703; 5,461,081; patents pending.

*TRUSOPT is a registered trademark of Merck & Co., Inc.

BETOPTIC® S ℞

(betaxolol HCl)
0.25% as base
Sterile Ophthalmic Suspension

Description: BETOPTIC S Ophthalmic Suspension 0.25% contains betaxolol hydrochloride, a cardioselective beta-adrenergic receptor blocking agent, in a sterile resin suspension formulation. Betaxolol hydrochloride is a white, crystalline powder, with a molecular weight of 343.89.

Chemical Name:

(±)-1-[p-[2-(cyclopropylmethoxy)ethyl]phenoxy]-3-(isopropylamino)-2-propanol hydrochloride.

Each mL of BETOPTIC S Ophthalmic Suspension contains: Active: betaxolol HCl 2.8 mg equivalent to 2.5 mg of betaxolol base. Preservative: benzalkonium chloride 0.01%. Inactive: Mannitol, Poly(Styrene-Divinyl Benzene) sulfonic acid, Carbomer 934P, edetate disodium, hydrochloric acid or sodium hydroxide (to adjust pH) and purified water.

Clinical Pharmacology: Betaxolol HCl, a cardioselective (beta-1-adrenergic) receptor blocking agent, does not have significant membrane-stabilizing (local anesthetic) activity and is devoid of intrinsic sympathomimetic action. Orally administered beta-adrenergic blocking agents reduce cardiac output in healthy subjects and patients with heart disease. In patients with severe impairment of myocardial function, beta-adrenergic receptor antagonists may inhibit the sympathetic stimulatory effect necessary to maintain adequate cardiac function.

When instilled in the eye, BETOPTIC S Ophthalmic Suspension 0.25% has the action of reducing elevated intraocular pressure, whether or not accompanied by glaucoma. Ophthalmic betaxolol has minimal effect on pulmonary and cardiovascular parameters.

Elevated IOP presents a major risk factor in glaucomatous field loss. The higher the level of IOP, the greater the likelihood of optic nerve damage and visual field loss. Betaxolol has the action of reducing elevated as well as normal intraocular pressure and the mechanism of ocular hypotensive action appears to be a reduction of aqueous production as demonstrated by tonography and aqueous fluorophotometry. The onset of action with betaxolol can generally be noted within 30 minutes and the maximal effect can usually be detected 2 hours after topical administration. A single dose provides a 12-hour reduction in intraocular pressure.

In controlled, double-masked studies, the magnitude and duration of the ocular hypotensive effect of BETOPTIC S Ophthalmic Suspension 0.25% and BETOPTIC Ophthalmic Solution 0.5% were clinically equivalent. BETOPTIC S Suspension was significantly more comfortable than BETOPTIC Solution.

Ophthalmic betaxolol solution at 1% (one drop in each eye) was compared to placebo in a crossover study challenging nine patients with reactive airway disease. Betaxolol HCl had no significant effect on pulmonary function as measured by FEV_1, Forced Vital Capacity (FVC), FEV_1/FVC and was not significantly different from placebo. The action of isoproterenol, a beta stimulant, administered at the end of the study was not inhibited by ophthalmic betaxolol.

No evidence of cardiovascular beta adrenergic-blockade during exercise was observed with betaxolol in a double-masked, crossover study in 24 normal subjects comparing ophthalmic betaxolol and placebo for effects on blood pressure and heart rate.

Indications and Usage: BETOPTIC S Ophthalmic Suspension 0.25% has been shown to be effective in lowering intraocular pressure and may be used in patients with chronic open-angle glaucoma and ocular hypertension. It may be used alone or in combination with other intraocular pressure lowering medications.

Contraindications: Hypersensitivity to any component of this product. BETOPTIC S Ophthalmic Suspension 0.25% is contraindicated in patients with sinus bradycardia, greater than a first degree atrioventricular block, cardiogenic shock, or patients with overt cardiac failure.

Warning: Topically applied beta-adrenergic blocking agents may be absorbed systemically. The same adverse reactions found with systemic administration of beta-adrenergic blocking agents may occur with topical administra-

tion. For example, severe respiratory reactions and cardiac reactions, including death due to bronchospasm in patients with asthma, and rarely death in association with cardiac failure, have been reported with topical application of beta-adrenergic blocking agents.
BETOPTIC S Ophthalmic Suspension 0.25% has been shown to have a minor effect on heart rate and blood pressure in clinical studies. Caution should be used in treating patients with a history of cardiac failure or heart block. Treatment with BETOPTIC S Ophthalmic Suspension 0.25% should be discontinued at the first signs of cardiac failure.

Precautions:

General: Diabetes Mellitus. Beta-adrenergic blocking agents should be administered with caution in patients subject to spontaneous hypoglycemia or to diabetic patients (especially those with labile diabetes) who are receiving insulin or oral hypoglycemic agents. Beta-adrenergic receptor blocking agents may mask the signs and symptoms of acute hypoglycemia.

Thyrotoxicosis. Beta-adrenergic blocking agents may mask certain clinical signs (e.g., tachycardia) of hyperthyroidism. Patients suspected of developing thyrotoxicosis should be managed carefully to avoid abrupt withdrawal of beta-adrenergic blocking agents, which might precipitate a thyroid storm.

Muscle Weakness. Beta-adrenergic blockade has been reported to potentiate muscle weakness consistent with certain myasthenic symptoms (e.g., diplopia, ptosis and generalized weakness).

Major Surgery. Consideration should be given to the gradual withdrawal of beta-adrenergic blocking agents prior to general anesthesia because of the reduced ability of the heart to respond to beta-adrenergically mediated sympathetic reflex stimuli.

Pulmonary. Caution should be exercised in the treatment of glaucoma patients with excessive restriction of pulmonary function. There have been reports of asthmatic attacks and pulmonary distress during betaxolol treatment. Although rechallenges of some such patients with ophthalmic betaxolol has not adversely affected pulmonary function test results, the possibility of adverse pulmonary effects in patients sensitive to beta blockers cannot be ruled out.

Information for Patients: Do not touch dropper tip to any surface, as this may contaminate the contents. Do not use with contact lenses in eyes.

Drug Interactions: Patients who are receiving a beta-adrenergic blocking agent orally and BETOPTIC S Ophthalmic Suspension 0.25% should be observed for a potential additive effect either on the intraocular pressure or on the known systemic effects of beta blockade.
Close observation of the patient is recommended when a beta blocker is administered to patients receiving catecholamine-depleting drugs such as reserpine, because of possible additive effects and the production of hypotension and/or bradycardia.
Betaxolol is an adrenergic blocking agent; therefore, caution should be exercised in patients using concomitant adrenergic psychotropic drugs.

Risk from anaphylactic reaction: While taking beta-blockers, patients with a history of atopy or a history of severe anaphylactic reaction to a variety of allergens may be more reactive to repeated accidental, diagnostic, or therapeutic challenge with such allergens. Such patients may be unresponsive to the usual doses of epinephrine used to treat anaphylactic reactions.

Ocular: In patients with angle-closure glaucoma, the immediate treatment objective is to reopen the angle by constriction of the pupil with a miotic agent. Betaxolol has little or no effect on the pupil. When BETOPTIC S Ophthalmic Suspension 0.25% is used to reduce elevated intraocular pressure in angle-closure glaucoma, it should be used with a miotic and not alone.

Carcinogenesis, Mutagenesis, Impairment of Fertility: Lifetime studies with betaxolol HCl have been completed in mice at oral doses of 6, 20 or 60 mg/kg/day and in rats at 3, 12 or 48 mg/kg/day; betaxolol HCl demonstrated no carcinogenic effect. Higher dose levels were not tested.
In a variety of *in vitro* and *in vivo* bacterial and mammalian cell assays, betaxolol HCl was nonmutagenic.

Pregnancy: Pregnancy Category C. Reproduction, teratology, and peri- and postnatal studies have been conducted with orally administered betaxolol HCl in rats and rabbits. There was evidence of drug related postimplantation loss in rabbits and rats at dose levels above 12 mg/kg and 128 mg/kg, respectively. Betaxolol HCl was not shown to be teratogenic, however, and there were no other adverse effects on reproduction at subtoxic dose levels. There are no adequate and well-controlled studies in pregnant women. BETOPTIC S should be used during pregnancy only if the potential benefit justifies the potential risk to the fetus.

Nursing Mothers: It is not known whether betaxolol HCl is excreted in human milk. Because many drugs are excreted in human milk, caution should be exercised when BETOPTIC S Ophthalmic Suspension 0.25% is administered to nursing women.

Pediatric Use: Safety and effectiveness in pediatric patients have not been established.

Adverse Reactions:

Ocular: In clinical trials, the most frequent event associated with the use of BETOPTIC S Ophthalmic Suspension 0.25% has been transient ocular discomfort. The following other conditions have been reported in small numbers of patients: blurred vision, corneal punctate keratitis, foreign body sensation, photophobia, tearing, itching, dryness of eyes, erythema, inflammation, discharge, ocular pain, decreased visual acuity and crusty lashes. Additional medical events reported with other formulations of betaxolol include allergic reactions, decreased corneal sensitivity, corneal punctate staining which may appear in dendritic formations, edema and anisocoria.

Systemic: Systemic reactions following administration of BETOPTIC S Ophthalmic Suspension 0.25% or BETOPTIC Ophthalmic Solution 0.5% have been rarely reported. These include:

Cardiovascular: Bradycardia, heart block and congestive failure.

Pulmonary: Pulmonary distress characterized by dyspnea, bronchospasm, thickened bronchial secretions, asthma and respiratory failure.

Central Nervous System: Insomnia, dizziness, vertigo, headaches, depression, lethargy, and increase in signs and symptoms of myasthenia gravis.

Other: Hives, toxic epidermal necrolysis, hair loss, and glossitis. Perversions of taste and smell have been reported.

Overdosage: No information is available on overdosage of humans. The oral LD50 of the drug ranged from 350–920 mg/kg in mice and 860–1050 mg/kg in rats. The symptoms which might be expected with an overdose of a systemically administered beta-1-adrenergic receptor blocking agent are bradycardia, hypotension and acute cardiac failure.
A topical overdose of BETOPTIC S Ophthalmic Suspension 0.25% may be flushed from the eye(s) with warm tap water.

Dosage and Administration: The recommended dose is one to two drops of BETOPTIC S Ophthalmic Suspension 0.25% in the affected eye(s) twice daily. In some patients, the intraocular pressure lowering responses to BETOPTIC S may require a few weeks to stabilize. As with any new medication, careful monitoring of patients is advised.
If the intraocular pressure of the patient is not adequately controlled on this regimen, concomitant therapy with pilocarpine and other miotics, and/or epinephrine and/or carbonic anhydrase inhibitors can be instituted.

How Supplied: BETOPTIC S Ophthalmic Suspension 0.25% is supplied as follows: 2.5, 5, 10 and 15 mL in plastic ophthalmic DROP-TAINER® dispensers.

2.5 mL: **NDC** 0065-0246-20
5 mL: **NDC** 0065-0246-05
10 mL: **NDC** 0065-0246-10
15 mL: **NDC** 0065-0246-15

Storage: Store upright at room temperature. Shake well before using.

Rx Only

U.S. Patents Nos. 4,252,984; 4,311,708; 4,342,783; 4,911,920.

BION® TEARS OTC

Lubricant Eye Drops

Description: BION® TEARS are specially designed to be physiologically compatible with the surface of the eye and to treat dry eye symptoms by replacing needed tear components. BION® TEARS advanced formula contains:
The unique DUASORB® polymeric system which combines with natural tears to soothe sensitive dry spots.
A special lubricating vehicle designed to match the electrolyte balance of sodium, potassium, calcium, magnesium, zinc and bicarbonate found in natural tears.
No preservatives or decongestants that may cause irritation or limit use. BION® TEARS may be used as often as necessary to provide relief.
BION® TEARS special formula requires special packaging. Airtight foil pouches are used to maintain the delicate balance of ingredients until the product is ready for use in the eye. **To ensure optimal effectiveness once the pouch is opened, the containers inside the pouch must be used within four days (96 hours).**

PLEASE READ THESE WARNINGS PRIOR TO USING BION® TEARS LUBRICANT EYE DROPS AND KEEP THIS INSERT FOR FUTURE REFERENCE.

Warnings: If you experience eye pain, changes in vision, continued redness or irritation of the eye, or if the condition worsens or persists for more than 72 hours, discontinue use and consult a doctor.
If solution changes color or becomes cloudy, do not use.
To avoid contamination, do not touch tip of container to any surface. Do not reuse. Once opened, discard. Keep this and all drugs out of the reach of children. In case of accidental ingestion, seek professional assistance or contact a Poison Control Center immediately.

How Supplied: BION® TEARS Lubricant Eye Drops are supplied in boxes of 28 0.015 fl. oz. single-use containers.

Product Code 0065-0419-28

BSS® ℞

Sterile Irrigating Solution
(balanced salt solution)

Description: BSS® Sterile Irrigating Solution is a sterile physiological balanced salt solution.

How Supplied:
15 mL Sterile DROP-TAINER® Bottle—NDC 0065079515

Continued on next page

BSS—Cont.

30 mL Sterile DROP-TAINER Bottle—NDC 0065079530
250 mL Glass Bottle—NDC 0065079525
500 mL Glass Bottle—NDC 0065079550
Storage: Store at 46° to 80° F (8° to 27° C).

BSS PLUS® ℞

Sterile Intraocular Irrigating Solution (Balanced Salt Solution Enriched with Bicarbonate, Dextrose and Glutathione)
U.S. Patent Nos. 4,443,432 and 4,550,022

Description: BSS PLUS® is a sterile intraocular irrigating solution for use during all intraocular surgical procedures, even those requiring a relatively long intraocular perfusion time (e.g., pars plana vitrectomy, phacoemulsification, extracapsular cataract extraction/lens aspiration, anterior segment reconstruction, etc.). The solution does not contain a preservative and should be prepared just prior to use in surgery.
How Supplied: BSS PLUS is supplied in two packages for reconstitution prior to use: a 500 mL bottle containing 480 mL (Part I) and a 20 mL vial (Part II)—NDC 0065080050. See package insert for information concerning reconstitution of the solution.
Storage: Store Part I and Part II at 46° to 80°F (8° to 27°C). Discard prepared solution after six hours.

CILOXAN® ℞

(Ciprofloxacin HCl)
0.3% as base
Sterile Ophthalmic Solution and Ointment

Description: CILOXAN® (Ciprofloxacin HCl) Ophthalmic Solution and Ointment are synthetic, sterile, multiple dose, antimicrobial for topical ophthalmic use. Ciprofloxacin is a fluoroquinolone antibacterial active against a broad spectrum of gram-positive and gram-negative ocular pathogens. It is available as the monohydrochloride monohydrate salt of 1-cyclopropyl-6-fluoro-1,4-dihydro-4-oxo-7-(1-piperazinyl)-3-quinoline-carboxylic acid. It is a faint to light yellow crystalline powder with a molecular weight of 385.8. Its empirical formula is $C_{17}H_{18}FN_3O_3 \bullet HCl \bullet H_2O$.
Ciprofloxacin differs from other quinolones in that it has a fluorine atom at the 6-position, a piperazine moiety at the 7-position, and a cyclopropyl ring at the 1-position.
Each mL of CILOXAN Ophthalmic Solution contains: **Active:** Ciprofloxacin HCl 3.5 mg equivalent to 3 mg base. **Preservative:** Benzalkonium Chloride 0.006%. **Inactive:** Sodium Acetate, Acetic Acid, Mannitol 4.6%, Edetate Disodium 0.05%, Hydrochloric Acid and/or Sodium Hydroxide (to adjust pH) and Purified Water. The pH is approximately 4.5 and the osmolality is approximately 300 mOsm.
Each gram of CILOXAN Ophthalmic Ointment contains: **Active:** Ciprofloxacin HCl 3.33 mg equivalent to 3 mg base. **Inactives:** Mineral Oil, White Petrolatum.
Clinical Pharmacology:
Systemic Absorption: A systemic absorption study was performed in which CILOXAN Ophthalmic Solution was administerd in each eye every two hours while awake for two days followed by every four hours while awake for an additional 5 days. The maximum reported plasma concentration of ciprofloxacin was less than 5 ng/mL. The mean concentration was usually less than 2.5 ng/mL. Ointment mean concentration levels have not been determined but are expected to be similar.
Microbiology: Ciprofloxacin has in vitro activity against a wide range of gram-negative and gram-positive organisms. The bactericidal action of ciprofloxacin results from interference with the enzyme DNA gyrase which is needed for the synthesis of bacterial DNA.
Ciprofloxacin has been shown to be active against most strains of the following organisms both in vitro and in clinical infections. (See INDICATIONS AND USAGE section).

Gram-Positive: *Staphylococcus aureus* (including methicillin-susceptible and methicillin-resistant strains)
Staphylococcus epidermidis
Streptococcus pneumoniae
Streptococcus (Viridans Group)

Gram-Negative:
Haemophilus influenzae
Pseudomonas aeruginosa
Serratia marcescens
Ciprofloxacin has been shown to be active in vitro against most strains of the following organisms, however, the clinical significance of these data is unknown:

Gram-Positive:
Bacillus species
Corynobacterium species
Enterococcus faecalis (Many strains are only moderately susceptible)
Staphylococcus haemolyticus
Staphylococcus hominis
Staphylococcus saprophyticus
Streptococcus pyogenes

Gram-Negative:
Acinetobacter caloacetius subsp anitratus
Aeromonas caviae
Aeromonas hydrophilia
Brucella melitensis
Campylobacter coli
Campylobacter jejuni
Citrobacter diversus
Citrobacter freundii
Edwardsiella tarda
Enterobacter aerogenes
Enterobacter cloacae
Eschricia coli
Haemophilius ducreyl
Haemophilius parainfluenzae
Klebsiella pneumoniae
Klebsiella oxytoca
Legionella pneumophilia
Moraxella (Branhamella) catarrhalis
Morganella morganii
Neisseria gonorrhea
Neisseria meningitidis
Pasteurella multocida
Proteus mirabilis
Proteus vulgaris
Providencia rettgeri
Providencia stuartii
Salmonella enteritidis
Salmonella typhi
Shigella sonneli
Shigella flexneri
Vibrio cholerae
Vibrio parahaemolyticus
Vibrio vulnificus
Yersinia enterocolitica
Other Organisms: Chlamydia trachomatis (only moderately susceptible) and Mycobacterium tuberculosis (only moderately susceptible).
Most strains of Pseudomonas cepacia and Burkholderia cepacia and some strains of Pseudomonas maltophilia and Stenotrophomonas maltophilia are resistant to ciprofloxacin as are most anaerobic bacteria, including Bacteroides fragilis and Clostridium difficile.
The minimal bactericidal concentration (MBC) generally does not exceed the minimal inhibitory concentration (MIC) by more than a factor of 2. Resistance to ciprofloxacin in vitro usually develops slowly (multiple-step mutation). Ciprofloxacin does not cross-react with other antimicrobial agents such as beta-lactams or aminoglycosides; therefore, organisms resistant to these drugs may be susceptible to ciprofloxacin. Organisms resistant to ciprofloxacin may be susceptible to beta-lactams or aminoglycosides.
Clinical Studies: Following therapy with CILOXAN® Ophthalmic Solution, 76% of the patients with corneal ulcers and positive bacterial cultures were clinically cured and complete re-epithelialization occurred in about 92% of the ulcers.
In 3 and 7 day multicenter trials, 52% of the patients with conjunctivitis and positive conjunctival cultures were clinically cured and 70–80% had all causative pathogens eradicated by the end of treatment. Following therapy with CILOXAN Ointment 75% of the patients with signs and symptoms of bacterial conjunctivitis and positive conjunctival cultures were clinically cured and approximately 80% had presumed pathogenes eradicated by the end of treatment (day 7).
Indications and Usage: CILOXAN Ophthalmic Solution and CILOXAN Ophthalmic Ointment are indicated for the treatment of infections caused by susceptible strains of the designated microorganisms in the conditions listed below:
Conjunctivitis — Solution and Ointment:
Haemophilus influenzae
Staphylococcus aureus
Staphylococcus epidermidis
Streptococcus pneumoniae
Streptococcus (Viridans Group)
Corneal Ulcers — Solution only:
Pseudomonas aeruginosa
Serratia marcescens*
Staphylococcus aureus
Staphylococcus epidermidis
Streptococcus pneumoniae
Streptococcus (Viridans Group)*
*Efficacy for these organisms was studied in fewer than 10 infections.
Contraindications: A history of hypersensitivity to ciprofloxacin or any other component of the medication is a contraindication to its use. A history of hypersensitivity to other quinolones may also contraindicate the use of ciprofloxacin.
Warnings: NOT FOR INJECTION INTO THE EYE.
Serious and occasionally fatal hypersensitivity (anaphylactic) reactions, some following the first dose, have been reported in patients receiving systemic quinolone therapy. Some reactions were accompanied by cardiovascular collapse, loss of consciousness, tingling, pharyngeal or facial edema, dyspnea, urticaria, and itching. Only a few patients had a history of hypersensitivity reactions. Serious anaphylactic reactions require immediate emergency treatment with epinephrine and other resuscitation measures, including oxygen, intravenous fluids, intravenous antihistamines, corticosteroids, pressor amines and airway management, as clinically indicated.
Precautions:
General: As with other antibacterial preparations, prolonged use of ciprofloxacin may result in overgrowth of nonsusceptible organisms, including fungi. If superinfection occurs, appropriate therapy should be initiated. Whenever clinical judgment dictates, the patient should be examined with the aid of magnification, such as slit lamp biomicroscopy and, where appropriate, fluorescein staining.
Ciprofloxacin should be discontinued at the first appearance of a skin rash or any other sign of hypersensitivity reaction. Ophthalmic ointments may retard corneal healing and cause visual blurring. Patients should be advised not to wear contact lenses if they have signs and symptoms of bacterial conjunctivitis.
In clinical studies of patients with bacterial corneal ulcer, a white crystalline precipitate located in the superficial portion of the corneal defect was observed in 35 (16.6%) of 210 patients. The onset of the precipitate was within

24 hours to 7 days after starting therapy. In one patient, the precipitate was immediately irrigated out upon its appearance. In 17 patients, resolution of the precipitate was seen in 1 to 8 days (seven within the first 24–72 hours), in five patients, resolution was noted in 10–13 days. In nine patients, exact resolution days were unavailable; however, at follow-up examinations, 18–44 days after onset of the event, complete resolution of the precipitate was noted. In three patients, outcome information was unavailable. The precipitate did not preclude continued use of ciprofloxacin, nor did it adversely affect the clinical course of the ulcer or visual outcome. (SEE ADVERSE REACTIONS).

Information for patients: Do not touch tip of any surface, as this may contaminate the product.

Drug Interactions: Specific drug interaction studies have not been conducted with ophthalmic ciprofloxacin. However, the systemic administration of some quinolones has been shown to elevate plasma concentrations of theophylline, interfere with the metabolism of caffeine, enhance the effects of the oral anticoagulant, warfarin, and its derivatives and has been associated with transient elevations in serum creatinine in patients receiving cyclosporine concomitantly.

Carcinogenesis, Mutagenesis, Impairment of Fertility: Eight in vitro mutagenicity tests have been conducted with ciprofloxacin and the test results are listed below:

Salmonella/Microsome Test (Negative)
E. coli DNA Repair Assay (Negative)
Mouse Lymphoma Cell Forward Mutation Assay (Positive)
Chinese Hamster V79 Cell HGPRT Test (Negative)
Syrian Hamster Embryo Cell Transformation Assay (Negative)
Saccharomyces cerevisiae Point Mutation Assay (Negative)
Saccharomyces cerevisiae Mitotic Crossover and Gene Conversion Assay (Negative)
Rat Hepatocyte DNA Repair Assay (Positive)

Thus, two of the eight tests were positive, but the results of the following three in vivo test systems gave negative results:

Rat Hepatocyte DNA Repair Assay
Micronucleus Test (Mice)
Dominant Lethal Test (Mice)

Long term carcinogenicity studies in mice and rats have been completed. After daily oral dosing for up to two years, there is no evidence that ciprofloxacin had any carcinogenic or tumorigenic effects in these species.

Pregnancy—Pregnancy Category C: Reproduction studies have been performed in rats and mice at doses up to six times the usual daily human oral dose and have revealed no evidence of impaired fertility or harm to the fetus due to ciprofloxacin. In rabbits, as with most antimicrobial agents, ciprofloxacin (30 and 100 mg/kg orally) produced gastrointestinal disturbances resulting in maternal weight loss and an increased incidence of abortion. No teratogenicity was observed at either dose. After intravenous administration, at doses up to 20 mg/kg, no maternal toxicity was produced and no embryotoxicity or teratogenicity was observed. There are no adequate and well controlled studies in pregnant women. CILOXAN® should be used during pregnancy only if the potential benefit justifies the potential risk to the fetus.

Nursing Mothers: It is not known whether topically applied ciprofloxacin is excreted in human milk; however, it is known that orally administered ciprofloxacin is excreted in the milk of lactating rats and oral ciprofloxacin has been reported in human breast milk after a single 500 mg dose. Caution should be exercised when CILOXAN is administered to a nursing mother.

Pediatric Use: Safety and effectiveness in pediatric patients below the age of 1 year (solution) and 2 years (ointment) have not been established.

Although ciprofloxacin and other quinolones cause arthropathy in immature Beagle dogs after oral administration, topical ocular administration of ciprofloxacin to immature animals did not cause any arthropathy and there is no evidence that the ophthalmic dosage form has any effect on the weight bearing joints.

Adverse Reactions: The most frequently reported drug related adverse reaction was local burning or discomfort. In corneal ulcer studies with frequent administration of the drug, white crystalline precipitates were seen in approximately 17% (solution) and 13% (ointment) of patients (SEE PRECAUTIONS). Other reactions occurring in less than 10% of patients included lid margin crusting, crystals/scales, foreign body sensation, itching, conjunctival hyperemia and a bad taste following instillation. Additional events occurring in less than 1% of patients included corneal staining, keratopathy/keratitis, allergic reactions, lid edema, tearing, photophobia, corneal infiltrates, nausea and decreased vision, blurred vision, dry eye, epitheliopathy, eye pain, irritation and dermatitis.

Overdosage: A topical overdose of CILOXAN Opthmalmic Solution may be flushed from the (eye(s) with warm tap water.

Dosage and Administration:

Bacterial Conjunctivitis: Solution: The recommended dosage regimen for the treatment of bacterial conjunctivitis is one or two drops of CILOXAN Ophthalmic Solution instilled into the conjunctival sac(s) every two hours while awake for two days and one or two drops every four hours while awake for the next five days. Ointment: Apply a ½″ ribbon into the conjunctival sac three times a day on the first two days, then apply a ½″ ribbon two times a day for the next five days.

Corneal Ulcers: The recommended dosage regimen for the treatment of corneal ulcers is two drops of the Solution into the affected eye every 15 minutes for the first six hours and then two drops into the affected eye every 30 minutes for the remainder of the first day. On the second day, instill two drops in the affected eye hourly. On the third through the fourteenth day, place two drops in the affected eye every four hours. Treatment may be continued after 14 days if corneal re-epithelialization has not occurred.

How Supplied: As a sterile ophthalmic solution in 2.5 mL (NDC 0065-0656-25) and 5 mL (NDC 0065-0656-05) in plastic DROP-TAINER® dispensers. Sterile ophthalmic ointment in 3.5 g ophthalmic tube (NDC 0065-0654-35).

Storage: Solution: Store at 2° to 30°C (36° to 86°F). Protect from light.

Ointment: Store at 36°F to 77°F (2°C to 25°C)

Animal Pharmacology: Ciprofloxacin and related drugs have been shown to cause arthropathy in immature animals of most species tested following oral administration. However, a one-month topical ocular study using immature Beagle dogs did not demonstrate any articular lesions.

Rx Only

U.S. Patent No. 4,670,444

⅛% ECONOPRED® ℞
1% ECONOPRED® PLUS ℞
(prednisolone acetate)
Ophthalmic Suspension

EMADINE™ ℞
(emedastine difumarate ophthalmic solution) 0.05%

Description: EMADINE™ (emedastine difumarate ophthalmic solution) 0.05% is a sterile ophthalmic solution containing emedastine, a relatively selective, H_1-receptor antagonist for topical administration to the eyes. Emedastine difumarate is a white, crystalline, water-soluble fine powder with a molecular weight of 534.57.

Chemical Name:
1H-Benzimidazole, 1-(2-ethoxyethyl)-2-(hexahydro-4-methyl-1H-1,4-diazepin-1-yl), (E)-2-butenedioate (1:2)

Each mL of EMADINE contains: Active: 0.884 mg emedastine difumarate equivalent to 0.5 mg emedastine. **Preservative:** benzalkonium chloride 0.01%. **Inactives:** Tromethamine; sodium chloride; hydroxypropyl methylcellulose; hydrochloric acid/sodium hydroxide (adjust pH); and purified water. It has a pH of approximately 7.4 and an osmolality of approximately 300 mOsm/kg. DM-00

Clinical Pharmacology: Emedastine is a relatively selective, histamine H_1 antagonist. *In vitro* examinations of emedastine's affinity for histamine receptors (H_1: Ki=1.3 nM, H_2: Ki=49,067 nM, and H_3: Ki=12,430 nM) demonstrate relative selectivity for the H_1 histamine receptor. *In vivo* studies have shown concentration-dependent inhibition of histamine-stimulated vascular permeability in the conjunctiva following topical ocular administration. Emedastine appears to be devoid of effects on adrenergic, dopaminergic and serotonin receptors.

Following topical administration in man, emedastine was shown to have low systemic exposure. In a study involving 10 normal volunteers dosed bilaterally twice daily for 15 days with emedastine ophthalmic solution 0.05%, plasma concentrations of the parent compound were generally below the quantitation limit of the assay (<0.3 ng/mL). Samples in which emedastine was quantifiable ranged from 0.30 to 0.49 ng/mL. The elimination half-life of oral emedastine in plasma is 3–4 hours. Approximately 44% of the oral dose is recovered in the urine over 24 hours with only 3.6% of the dose excreted as parent drug. Two primary metabolites, 5- and 6-hydroxyemedastine, are excreted in the urine as both free and conjugated forms. The 5′-oxoanalogs of 5- and 6-hydroxyemedastine and the N-oxide are also formed as minor metabolites.

In an environmental study, patients with allergic conjunctivitis were treated with EMADINE for six weeks. The results demonstrated that EMADINE provides relief of the signs and symptoms of allergic conjunctivitis.

In conjunctival antigen challenge studies, in which subjects were challenged with antigen both initially and up to four hours after dosing, EMADINE was demonstrated to be significantly more effective than placebo in preventing ocular itching associated with allergic conjunctivitis.

Indications and Usage: EMADINE (emedastine difumarate ophthalmic solution) 0.05% is indicated for the temporary relief of the signs and symptoms of allergic conjunctivitis.

Contraindications: EMADINE is contraindicated in persons with a known hypersensitivity to emedastine difumarate or any of its components.

Warnings: EMADINE is for topical use only and not for injection or oral use.

Precautions: Information for Patients: To prevent contaminating the dropper tip and solution, care should be taken not to touch the eyelids or surrounding areas with the dropper

Continued on next page

Emadine—Cont.

tip of the bottle. Keep the bottle tightly closed when not in use. Do not use if the solution has become discolored.

Patients should be advised not to wear a contact lens if their eye is red. EMADINE should not be used to treat contact lens related irritation. The preservative in EMADINE, benzalkonium chloride, may be absorbed by soft contact lenses. Patients who wear soft contact lenses and **whose eyes are not red,** should be instructed to wait at least ten minutes after instilling EMADINE before they insert their contact lenses.

Carcinogenesis, Mutagenesis, Impairment of Fertility: Emedastine difumarate demonstrated no carcinogenicity effects in lifetime studies in mice and rats at dietary doses more than 80,000 times and more than 26,000 times the maximum recommended ocular human use level of 0.002 mg/kg/day for a 50 kg adult, respectively. Higher dose levels were not tested. Emedastine difumarate was determined to be nonmutagenic in an *in vitro* bacterial reverse mutation (Ames) test, an *in vitro* modification of the Ames test, an *in vitro* mammalian chromosome aberration test, an *in vitro* mammalian forward mutation test, an *in vitro* mammalian DNA repair synthesis test, an *in vivo* mammalian sister chromatid exchange test and an *in vivo* mouse micronucleus test. There was no evidence of impaired fertility or reproductive capacity in rats at 15,000 times the maximum recommended ocular human use level.

Pregnancy: Pregnancy Category B. Teratology and peri- and post-natal studies have been conducted with emedastine difumarate in rats and rabbits. At 15,000 times the maximum recommended ocular human use level, emedastine difumarate was shown not to be teratogenic in rats and rabbits and no effects on peri/post-natal development were observed in rats. However, at 70,000 times the maximum recommended ocular human use level, emedastine difumarate was shown to increase the incidence of external, visceral and skeletal anomalies in rats. There are, however, no adequate and well controlled studies in pregnant women. Because animal studies are not always predictive of human response, this drug should be used during pregnancy only if clearly needed.

Nursing Mothers: Emedastine has been identified in breast milk in rats following oral administration. It is not known whether topical ocular administration could result in sufficient systemic absorption to produce detectable quantities in breast milk. Nevertheless, caution should be exercised when EMADINE™ (emedastine difumarate ophthalmic solution) 0.05% is administered to a nursing mother.

Pediatric Use: Safety and effectiveness in pediatric patients below the age of 3 years have not been established.

Adverse Reactions: In controlled clinical studies of EMADINE lasting for 42 days, the most frequent adverse reaction was headache 11%. The following adverse experiences were reported in less than 5% of patients: Abnormal dreams, asthenia, bad taste, blurred vision, burning or stinging, corneal infiltrates, corneal staining, dermatitis, discomfort, dry eye, foreign body sensation, hyperemia, keratitis, pruritus, rhinitis, sinusitis and tearing. Some of these events were similar to the underlying disease being studied.

Overdosage: Somnolence and malaise have been reported following daily oral administration. Oral ingestion of the contents of a 15 mL DROP-TAINER® dispenser would be equivalent to 7.5 mg. In case of overdosage, treatment is symptomatic and supportive.

Dosage and Administration: The recommended dose is one drop in the affected eye up to four times daily.

How Supplied: EMADINE (emedastine difumarate ophthalmic solution) 0.05% is supplied as follows: 5mL in opaque, plastic DROP-TAINER® dispenser.

5 mL: NDC 0065-0325-05

Storage

Store at 4°–30°C (39°–86°F)

Rx Only

U.S. Patents Nos. 4,430,343 and 5,441,958.

FLAREX® ℞

(fluorometholone acetate ophthalmic suspension)
Sterile

FLUORESCITE® INJECTION ℞

(fluorescein injection)

Description: FLUORESCITE® Injection is a sterile aqueous solution in two strengths for use intravenously as a diagnostic aid.

Chemical name:
Spiro[isobenzofuran-1(3*H*),9′-[9*H*] xanthene]-3-one, 3′6′ dihydroxy, disodium salt.

The solution contains Fluorescein Sodium (equivalent to Fluorescein 10% or 25%), Sodium Hydroxide and/or Hydrochloric Acid (to adjust pH), and Water for Injection.

Clinical Pharmacology: The yellowish-green fluorescence of the drug demarcates the vascular area under observation, distinguishing it from adjacent areas.

Indications and Usage: Indicated in diagnostic fluorescein angiography or angioscopy of the fundus and of the iris vasculature.

Contraindications: Contraindicated in those persons who have shown hypersensitivity to any component of this preparation.

Warning:

NOT FOR INTRATHECAL USE

FOR OPHTHALMIC USE ONLY. Care must be taken to avoid extravasation during injection as the high pH of fluorescein solution can result in severe local tissue damage. The following complications resulting from extravasation of fluorescein have been noted to occur: sloughing of the skin, superficial phlebitis, subcutaneous granuloma, and toxic neuritis along the median curve in the antecubital area. Complications resulting from extravasation can cause severe pain in the arm for up to several hours. When significant extravasation occurs, the injection should be discontinued and conservative measures to treat damaged tissue and to relieve pain should be implemented. Do not mix or dilute with other solutions or drugs in syringe. Flush intravenous cannulas before and after drugs are injected to avoid physical incompatibility reactions. Rare cases of death due to anaphylaxis have been reported (See PRECAUTIONS).

Precautions: General: Caution is to be exercised in patients with a history of allergy or bronchial asthma. An emergency tray including such items as 0.1% epinephrine for intravenous or intramuscular use; an antihistamine, soluble steroid, and aminophyllene for IV use; and oxygen should always be available in the event of possible reaction to fluorescein injection.[1]

Information for Patients: Skin will attain a temporary yellowish discoloration. Urine attains a bright yellow color. Discoloration of the skin fades in 6 to 12 hours; urine fluorescein in 24 to 36 hours.

Carcinogenesis, Mutagenesis, Impairment of Fertility: There have been no long-term studies done using fluorescein in animals to evaluate carcinogenic potential.

Use in Pregnancy: Avoid angiography on patients who are pregnant, especially those in first trimester. There have been no reports of fetal complications from fluorescein injection during pregnancy.

Nursing Mothers: Fluorescein has been demonstrated to be execreted in human milk. Caution should be exercised when fluorescein is administered to a nursing woman.

Adverse Reactions: Nausea and headache, gastrointestinal distress, syncope, vomiting, hypotension, and other symptoms and signs of hypersensitivity have occurred. Cardiac arrest, basilar artery ischemia, severe shock, convulsions, thrombophlebitis at the injection site and rare cases of death have been reported. Extravasation of the solution at the injection site causes intense pain at the site and a dull aching pain in the injected arm. (See WARNING.) Generalized hives and itching, bronchospasm and anaphylaxis have been reported. A strong taste may develop after injection.

Dosage and Administration: Parenteral drug products should be inspected visually for particulate matter and discoloration prior to administration, whenever solution and container permit. Do not mix or dilute with other solutions or drugs in syringe. Flush intravenous cannulas before and after drugs are injected to avoid physical incompatibility reactions. Inject the contents of the ampule or prefilled syringe rapidly into the antecubital vein, *after taking precautions to avoid extravasation.* A syringe, filled with fluorescein, is attached to transparent tubing and a 25 gauge scalp vein needle for injection. Insert the needle and draw the patient's blood to the hub of the syringe so that a *small* air bubble separates the patient's blood in the tubing from the fluorescein. With the room lights on, slowly inject the blood back into the vein while watching the skin over the needle tip. If the needle has extravasated, the patient's blood will be seen to bulge the skin and the injection should be stopped before any fluorescein is injected. When assured that extravasation has not occurred, the room light may be turned off and the fluorescein injection completed. Luminescence appears in the retina and choroidal vessels in 9 to 14 seconds and can be observed by standard viewing equipment. If potential allergy is suspected, an intradermal skin test may be performed prior to intravenous administration, i.e., 0.05 mL injected intradermally to be evaluated 30 to 60 minutes following injection. For children, the dose is calculated on the basis of 35 mg for each ten pounds of body weight.

How Supplied: 5 mL of 10% in pre-filled syringe; 10% in 5 mL ampule and 25% in 2 mL ampule.

10% NDC 0065-0092-05
10% NDC 0065-0093-05 syringe
25% NDC 0065-0094-02

Storage: Store at 8°–27°C (46°–80°F).

Rx Only

Reference:

1. Schatz, Burton, Yannuzzi, Rabb. Interpretation of Fundus Fluorescein Angiography, Page 38, C. V. Mosby Co., Saint Louis, 1978.

IOPIDINE® ℞

(apraclonidine hydrochloride ophthalmic solution),
1% As Base
Sterile

Description: IOPIDINE® Ophthalmic Solution contains apraclonidine hydrochloride, an alpha adrenergic agonist, in a sterile isotonic solution for topical application to the eye.

Apraclonidine hydrochloride is a white to off-white powder and is highly soluble in water. Its chemical name is 2-[(4-amino-2,6 dichlorophenyl)imino] imidazolidine monohydrochloride with an empirical formula of $C_9H_{11}Cl_3N_4$ and a molecular weight of 281.6. Each mL of IOPIDINE Ophthalmic Solution contains: Active: apraclonidine hydrochloride 11.5 mg equivalent to apraclonidine base 10 mg. Preservative: benzalkonium chloride 0.01%. Inactive: sodium chloride, sodium acetate, sodium hydroxide and/or hydrochloric acid (pH 4.4–7.8) and purified water.

Clinical Pharmacology: Apraclonidine is a relatively selective, alpha adrenergic agonist and does not have significant membrane stabilizing (local anesthetic) activity. When instilled into the eye, IOPIDINE (apraclonidine hydrochloride ophthalmic solution) has the action of reducing intraocular pressure. Ophthalmic apraclonidine has minimal effect on cardiovascular parameters.

Optic nerve head damage and visual field loss may result from an acute elevation in intraocular pressure that can occur after argon or Nd:YAG laser surgical procedures. Elevated intraocular pressure, whether acute or chronic in duration, is a major risk factor in the pathogenesis of visual field loss. The higher the peak or spike of intraocular pressure, the greater the likelihood of visual field loss and optic nerve damage especially in patients with previously compromised optic nerves. The onset of action with IOPIDINE Ophthalmic Solution can usually be noted within one hour and the maximum intraocular pressure reduction usually occurs three to five hours after application of a single dose. The precise mechanism of the ocular hypotensive action of IOPIDINE Ophthalmic Solution is not completely established at this time. Aqueous fluorophotometry studies in man suggest that its predominant action may be related to a reduction of aqueous formation. Controlled clinical studies of patients requiring argon laser trabeculoplasty, argon laser iridotomy or Nd:YAG posterior capsulotomy showed that IOPIDINE Ophthalmic Solution controlled or prevented the postsurgical intraocular pressure rise typically observed in patients after undergoing those procedures. After surgery, the mean intraocular pressure was 1.2 to 4 mmHg below the corresponding presurgical baseline pressure before IOPIDINE Ophthalmic Solution treatment. With placebo treatment, postsurgical pressures were 2.5 to 8.4 mmHg higher than their corresponding presurgical baselines. Overall, only 2% of patients treated with IOPIDINE Ophthalmic Solution had severe intraocular pressure elevations (spike ≥ 10 mmHg) during the first three hours after laser surgery, whereas 23% of placebo-treated patients responded with severe pressure spikes (Table 1). Of the patients that experienced a pressure spike after surgery, the peak intraocular pressure was above 30 mmHg in most patients (Table 2) and was above 50 mmHg in seven placebo-treated patients and one IOPIDINE Ophthalmic Solution-treated patient.

[See tables 1 & 2 above]

Table 1

Incidence of Intraocular Pressure Spikes ≥ 10 mmHg

			Treatment			
			Apraclonidine		Placebo	
Study	Laser Procedure	P-Value	[a]N	(%)	[a]N	(%)
1	Trabeculoplasty	<0.05	0/40	(0%)	6/35	(17%)
2	Trabeculoplasty	=0.06	2/41	(5%)	8/42	(19%)
1	Iridotomy	<0.05	0/11	(0%)	4/10	(40%)
2	Iridotomy	=0.05	0/17	(0%)	4/19	(21%)
1	Nd:YAG Capsulotomy	<0.05	3/80	(4%)	19/83	(23%)
2	Nd:YAG Capsulotomy	<0.05	0/83	(0%)	22/81	(27%)

[a]N = Number Spikes/Number Eyes.

Table 2

Magnitude of Postsurgical Intraocular Pressure in Trabeculoplasty, Iridotomy and Nd:YAG Capsulotomy Patients With Severe Pressure Spikes ≥ 10 mmHg

	Maximum Postsurgical Intraocular Pressure (mmHg)				
Treatment	Total Spikes	20–29 mmHg	30–39 mmHg	40–49 mmHg	>50 mmHg
IOPIDINE	8	1	4	2	1
Placebo	78	16	47	8	7

Indications and Usage: IOPIDINE (apraclonidine hydrochloride ophthalmic solution) is indicated to control or prevent postsurgical elevations in intraocular pressure that occur in patients after argon laser trabeculoplasty, argon laser iridotomy or Nd:YAG posterior capsulotomy.

Contraindication: IOPIDINE® Ophthalmic Solution is contraindicated for patients receiving monoamine oxidase inhibitor therapy and for patients with hypersensitivity to any component of this medication or to clonidine.

WARNINGS: For topical ophthalmic use only.

Precautions:

General: Since IOPIDINE Ophthalmic Solution is a potent depressor of intraocular pressure, patients who develop exaggerated reductions in intraocular pressure should be closely monitored. Although the acute administration of two drops of IOPIDINE® Ophthalmic Solution has minimal effect on heart rate or blood pressure in clinical studies evaluating patients undergoing anterior segment laser surgery, the preclinical pharmacologic profile of this drug suggests that caution should be observed in treating patients with severe cardiovascular disease including hypertension.

The possibility of a vasovagal attack occurring during laser surgery should be considered and caution used in patients with history of such episodes.

Topical ocular administration of two drops of 0.5%, 1% and 1.5% IOPIDINE Ophthalmic Solution to New Zealand Albino rabbits three times daily for one month resulted in sporadic and transient instances of minimal corneal cloudiness in the 1.5% group only. No histopathological changes were noted in those eyes. No adverse ocular effects were observed in cynomolgus monkeys treated with two drops of 1.5% IOPIDINE Ophthalmic Solution applied three times daily for three months. No corneal changes were observed in 320 humans given at least one dose of 1% IOPIDINE Ophthalmic Solution.

Drug Interactions:

Interactions with other agents have not been investigated.

Carcinogenesis, Mutagenesis, Impairment of Fertility: No significant change in tumor incidence or type was observed following two years of oral administration of apraclonidine HCl to rats and mice at dosages of 1 and 0.6 mg/kg/day, up to 50 and 30 times, respectively, the maximum dose recommended for human topical ocular use. Apraclonidine HCl was not mutagenic in a series of *in vitro* mutagenicity tests, including the Ames test, a mouse lymphoma forward mutation assay, a chromosome aberration assay in cultured Chinese hamster ovary (CHO) cells, a sister chromatid exchange assay in CHO cells, and a cell transformation assay. An *in vivo* mouse micronucleus assay conducted with apraclonidine HCl also provided no evidence of mutagenicity. Reproduction and fertility studies in rats showed no adverse effect on male or female fertility at a dose of 0.5 mg/kg/day (25 times the maximum recommended human dose).

Pregnancy: Pregnancy Category C: Apraclonidine HCl has been shown to have an embryocidal effect in rabbits when given in an oral dose of 3 mg/kg/day (150 times the maximum recommended human dose). Dose related maternal toxicity was observed in pregnant rats at 0.3 mg/kg/day (15 times the maximum recommended human dose). There are no adequate and well controlled studies in pregnant women. IOPIDINE 1.0% Ophthalmic Solution should be used during pregnancy only if the potential benefit justifies the potential risk to the fetus.

Nursing Mothers: It is not known if topically applied IOPIDINE Ophthalmic Solution is excreted in human milk. A decision should be made to discontinue nursing temporarily for the one day on which IOPIDINE® Ophthalmic Solution is used.

Pediatric Use: Safety and effectiveness in pediatric patients have not been established.

Adverse Reactions: The following adverse events, occuring in less than 2% of patients, were reported in association with the use of IOPIDINE Ophthalmic Solution in laser surgery: ocular injection, upper lid elevation, irregular heart rate, nasal decongestion, ocular inflammation, conjunctival blanching, and mydriasis. The following adverse events were observed in investigational studies dosing IOPIDINE Ophthalmic Solution once or twice daily for up to 28 days in nonlaser studies:

Ocular: Conjunctival blanching, upper lid elevation, mydriasis, burning, discomfort, foreign body sensation, dryness, itching, hypotony, blurred or dimmed vision, allergic response, conjunctival microhemorrhage.

Gastrointestinal: Abdominal pain, diarrhea, stomach discomfort, emesis.

Cardiovascular: Bradycardia, vasovagal attack, palpitations, orthostatic episode.

Central Nervous System: Insomnia, dream disturbances, irritability, decreased libido.

Other: Taste abnormalities, dry mouth, nasal burning or dryness, headache, head cold sensation, chest heaviness or burning, clammy or sweaty palms, body heat sensation, shortness

Continued on next page

Iopidine—Cont.

of breath, increased pharyngeal secretion, extremity pain or numbness, fatigue, paresthesia, pruritus not associated with rash.

Overdosage: While no instances of accidental or intentional ingestion of ophthalmic apraclonidine are known, overdose with the oral form of clonidine has been reported to cause hypotension, transient hypertension, asthenia, vomiting, irritability, diminished or absent reflexes, lethargy, somnolence, sedation or coma, pallor, hypothermia, bradycardia, conduction defects, arrhythmias, dryness of the mouth, miosis, apnea, respiratory depression, hypoventilation, and seizure. Treatment of an oral overdose includes supportive and symptomatic therapy, a patent airway should be maintained. Hemodialysis is of limited value since a maximum of 5% of circulating drug is removed.

Dosage and Administration: One drop of IOPIDINE Ophthalmic Solution should be instilled in the scheduled operative eye one hour before initiating anterior segment laser surgery and a second drop should be instilled to the same eye immediately upon completion of the laser surgical procedure. Use a separate container for each single-drop dose and discard each container after use.

How Supplied: IOPIDINE (apraclonidine hydrochloride ophthalmic solution), 1% as base, is a sterile, isotonic, aqueous solution containing apraclonidine hydrochloride.

Supplied as follows: 0.1 mL in plastic ophthalmic dispensers, packaged two per pouch. These dispensers are enclosed in a foil overwrap as an added barrier to evaporation.

0.1 mL: **NDC** 0065-0660-10

Storage: Store at 2° to 25°C (34° to 77°F). Protect from light.

Rx Only

U.S. Patents Nos. 4,517,199; 5,212,196

IOPIDINE® 0.5% ℞

(Apraclonidine Ophthalmic Solution)
0.5% As Base

Description: IOPIDINE® 0.5% Ophthalmic Solution contains apraclonidine hydrochloride, an alpha adrenergic agonist, in a sterile isotonic solution for topical application to the eye. Apraclonidine hydrochloride is a white to off-white powder and is highly soluble in water. Its chemical name is 2-[(4-amino-2,6 dichlorophenyl) imino]imidazolidine monohydrochloride with an empirical formula of $C_9H_{11}Cl_3N_4$ and a molecular weight of 281.57.

Each mL of IOPIDINE 0.5% Ophthalmic Solution contains: Active: apraclonidine hydrochloride 5.75 mg equivalent to apraclonidine base 5 mg; **Preservative**: benzalkonium chloride 0.01%. **Inactive**: sodium chloride, sodium acetate, sodium hydroxide and/or hydrochloric acid (pH 4.4–7.8) and purified water.

Clinical Pharmacology: Apraclonidine hydrochloride is a relatively selective alpha-2-adrenergic agonist. When instilled in the eye, IOPIDINE 0.5% Ophthalmic Solution, has the action of reducing elevated, as well as normal, intraocular pressure (IOP), whether or not accompanied by glaucoma. Ophthalmic apraclonidine has minimal effect on cardiovascular parameters.

Elevated IOP presents a major risk factor in glaucomatous field loss. The higher the level of IOP, the greater the likelihood of optic nerve damage and visual field loss. IOPIDINE 0.5% Ophthalmic Solution has the action of reducing IOP. The onset of action of apraclonidine can usually be noted within one hour, and maximum IOP reduction occurs about three hours after instillation. Aqueous fluorophotometry studies demonstrate that Apraclonidine's predominant mechanism of action is reduction of aqueous flow via stimulation of the alpha-adrenergic system.

Repeated dose-response and comparative studies (0.125% - 1.0% apraclonidine) demonstrate that 0.5% apraclonidine is at the top of the dose/response IOP reduction curve.

The clinical utility of IOPIDINE 0.5% Ophthalmic Solution is most apparent for those glaucoma patients on maximally tolerated medical therapy. Patients on maximally tolerated medical therapy with uncontrolled IOP and scheduled to undergo laser trabeculoplasty or trabeculectomy surgery were enrolled into a double-masked, placebo-controlled, multi-center clinical trial to determine if IOPIDINE 0.5% Ophthalmic Solution, dosed three times daily (TID), could delay the need for surgery for up to three months.

All patients enrolled into this trial had advanced glaucoma and were undergoing maximally tolerated medical therapy, i.e., patients were using combinations of a topical beta blocker, sympathomimetics, parasympathomimetics and oral carbonic anhydrase inhibitors. Patients were considered to be treatment failures in this study if, in the opinion of the investigators, their IOP was uncontrolled by the masked study medication or there was evidence of further optic nerve damage or visual field loss, and surgery was indicated. Of 171 patients receiving masked medication, 84 were treated with IOPIDINE 0.5% Ophthalmic Solution and 87 were treated with placebo (Apraclonidine vehicle).

Apraclonidine treatment resulted in a significantly greater percentage of treatment successes compared to patients treated with placebo. In this placebo-controlled maximum therapy trial, 14.3% of patients treated with IOPIDINE 0.5% Ophthalmic Solution were discontinued due to adverse events, primarily allergic-like reactions (12.9%).

The IOP lowering efficacy of IOPIDINE 0.5% Ophthalmic Solution diminishes over time in some patients. This loss of effect, or tachyphylaxis, appears to be an individual occurrence with a variable time of onset and should be closely monitored.

An unpredictable decrease of IOP control in some patients and incidence of ocular allergic responses and systemic side effects may limit the utility of IOPIDINE 0.5% Ophthalmic Solution. However, patients on maximally tolerated medical therapy may still benefit from the additional IOP reduction provided by the short-term use of IOPIDINE 0.5% Ophthalmic Solution.

Topical use of IOPIDINE 0.5% Ophthalmic Solution leads to systemic absorption. Studies of IOPIDINE 0.5% Ophthalmic Solution dosed one drop three times a day in both eyes for 10 days in normal volunteers yielded mean peak and trough concentrations of 0.9 ng/mL and 0.5 ng/mL, respectively. The half-life of IOPIDINE® 0.5% (Apraclonidine Ophthalmic Solution) was calculated to be 8 hours.

IOPIDINE 0.5% Ophthalmic Solution, because of its alpha adrenergic activity, is a vasoconstrictor. Single dose ocular blood flow studies in monkeys, using the microsphere technique, demonstrated a reduced blood flow for the anterior segment; however, no reduction in blood flow was observed in the posterior segment of the eye after a topical dose of IOPIDINE 0.5% Ophthalmic Solution. Ocular blood flow studies have not been conducted in humans.

Indications and Usage: IOPIDINE 0.5% Ophthalmic Solution is indicated for short-term adjunctive therapy in patients on maximally tolerated medical therapy who require additional IOP reduction. Patients on maximally tolerated medical therapy who are treated with IOPIDINE 0.5% Ophthalmic Solution to delay surgery should have frequent followup examinations and treatment should be discontinued if the intraocular pressure rises significantly.

The addition of IOPIDINE 0.5% Ophthalmic Solution to patients already using two aqueous suppressing drugs (i.e., beta-blocker plus carbonic anhydrase inhibitor) as part of their maximally tolerated medical therapy may not provide additional benefit. This is because IOPIDINE 0.5% Ophthalmic Solution is an aqueous suppressing drug and the addition of a third aqueous suppressant may not significantly reduce IOP.

The IOP lowering efficacy of IOPIDINE 0.5% Ophthalmic Solution diminishes over time in some patients. This loss of effect, or tachyphylaxis, appears to be an individual occurrence with a variable time of onset and should be closely monitored. The benefit for most patients is less than one month.

Contraindications: IOPIDINE 0.5% Ophthalmic Solution is contraindicated in patients with hypersensitivity to Apraclonidine or any other component of this medication, as well as systemic clonidine. It is also contraindicated in patients receiving monoamine oxidase inhibitors (MAO inhibitors).

Warnings: Not for injection or oral ingestion. Topical ophthalmic use only.

Precautions: General: Glaucoma patients on maximally tolerated medical therapy who are treated with IOPIDINE 0.5% Ophthalmic Solution to delay surgery should have their visual fields monitored periodically.

Although the topical use of IOPIDINE 0.5% Ophthalmic Solution has not been studied in renal failure patients, structurally related clonidine undergoes a significant increase in half-life in patients with severe renal impairment. Close monitoring of cardiovascular parameters in patients with impaired renal function is advised if they are candidates for topical Apraclonidine therapy. Close monitoring of cardiovascular parameters in patients with impaired liver function is also advised as the systemic dosage form of clonidine is partly metabolized in the liver.

While the topical administration of IOPIDINE 0.5% Ophthalmic Solution had minimal effect on heart rate or blood pressure in clinical studies evaluating glaucoma patients, the preclinical pharmacology profile of this drug suggest that caution should be observed in treating patients with severe, uncontrolled cardiovascular disease, including hypertension.

IOPIDINE 0.5% Ophthalmic Solution should be used with caution in patients with coronary insufficiency, recent myocardial infarction, cerebrovascular disease, chronic renal failure, Raynaud's disease, or thromboangitis obliterans. Caution and monitoring of depressed patients are advised since Apraclonidine has been infrequently associated with depression. Apraclonidine can cause dizziness and somnolence. Patients who engage in hazardous activities requiring mental alertness should be warned of the potential for a decrease in mental alertness while using Apraclonidine. Topical ocular administration of two drops of 0.5, 1.0 and 1.5% Apraclonidine Ophthalmic Solution to New Zealand albino rabbits three times daily for one month resulted in sporadic and transient instances of minimal corneal edema in the 1.5% group only; no histopathological changes were noted in thoses eyes.

Use of IOPIDINE 0.5% Ophthalmic Solution can lead to an allergic-like reaction characterized wholly or in part by the symptoms of hyperemia, pruritus, discomfort, tearing, foreign body sensation, and edema of the lids and conjunctiva. If ocular allergic-like symptoms occur, IOPIDINE® 0.5% (Apraclonidine Ophthalmic Solution) therapy should be discontinued.

Patient Information: Do not touch dropper tip to any surface as this may contaminate the contents.

Drug Interactions: Apraclonidine should not be used in patients receiving MAO inhibitors. (See CONTRAINDICATIONS). Although no specific drug interactions with topical glaucoma drugs or systemic medications were identified in clinical studies of IOPIDINE 0.5% Ophthalmic Solution, the possibility of an additive or potentiating effect with CNS depressants (alcohol, barbiturates, opiates, sedatives, anesthetics) should be considered. Tricyclic antidepressants have been reported to blunt the hypotensive effect of systemic clonidine. It is not known whether the concurrent use of these agents with Apraclonidine can lead to a reduction in IOP lowering effect. No data on the level of circulating catecholamines after Apraclonidine withdrawal are available. Caution, however, is advised in patients taking tricyclic antidepressants which can affect the metabolism and uptake of circulating amines.

An additive hypotensive effect has been reported with the combination of systemic clonidine and neuroleptic therapy. Systemic clonidine may inhibit the production of catecholamines in response to insulin-induced hypoglycemia and mask the signs and symptoms of hypoglycemia.

Since Aproclonidine may reduce pulse and blood pressure, caution in using drugs such as beta-blockers (ophthalmic and systemic), antihypertensives, and cardiac glycosides is advised. Patients using cardiovascular drugs concurrently with IOPIDINE 0.5% Ophthalmic Solution should have pulse and blood pressures frequently monitored. Caution should be exercised with simultaneous use of clonidine and other similar pharmacologic agents.

Carcinogenesis, Mutagenesis, Impairment of Fertility: No significant change in tumor incidence or type was observed following two years of oral administration of apraclonidine HCl to rats and mice at dosages of 1.0 and 0.6 mg/kg, up to 20 and 12 times, respectively, the maximum dose recommended for human topical ocular use.

Apraclonidine HCl was not mutagenic in a series of *in vitro* mutagenicity tests, including the Ames test, a mouse lymphoma forward mutation assay, a chromosome aberration assay in cultured Chinese hamster ovary (CHO) cells, a sister chromatid exchange assay in (CHO) cells, and a cell transformation assay. An *in vivo* mouse micronucleus assay conducted with apraclonidine HCl also provided no evidence of mutagenicity.

Reproduction and fertility studies in rats showed no adverse effect on male or female fertility at a dose of 0.5 mg/kg (5 to 10 times the maximum recommended human dose).

Pregnancy: Pregnancy Category C: Apraclonidine HCl has been shown to have an embryocidal effect in rabbits when given in an oral dose of 3.0 mg/kg (60 times the maximum recommended human dose). Dose related maternal toxicity was observed in pregnant rats at 0.3 mg/kg (6 times the maximum recommended human dose). There are no adequate and well controlled studies in pregnant women. IOPIDINE 0.5% Ophthalmic Solution should be used during pregnancy only if the potential benefit justifies the potential risk to the fetus.

Nursing Mothers: It is not known whether this drug is excreted in human milk. Because many drugs are excreted in human milk, caution should be exercised when IOPIDINE 0.5% Ophthalmic Solution is administered to a nursing woman.

Pediatric Use: Safety and effectiveness in pediatric patients have not been established.

Adverse Reactions: Use of IOPIDINE 0.5% Ophthalmic Solution can lead to an allergic-like reaction characterized wholly or in part by the symptoms of hyperemia, pruritus, discomfort, tearing, foreign body sensation, and edema of the lids and conjunctiva. If ocular allergic-like symptoms occur, IOPIDINE 0.5% Ophthalmic Solution therapy should be discontinued.

In clinical studies the overall discontinuation rate related to IOPIDINE 0.5% Ophthalmic Solution was 15%. The most commonly reported events leading to discontinuation included (in decreasing order of frequency) hyperemia, pruritus, tearing, discomfort, lid edema, dry mouth, and foreign body sensation. The following adverse reactions (incidences) were reported in clinical studies of IOPIDINE 0.5% (Apraclonidine Ophthalmic Solution) as being possibly, probably, or definitely related to therapy:

Ocular

Hyperemia (13%), pruritus (10%), discomfort (6%), tearing (4%). The following adverse reactions were reported in less than 3% of the patients: lid edema, blurred vision, foreign body sensation, dry eye, conjunctivitis, discharge, blanching. The following adverse reactions were reported in less than 1% of the patients: lid margin crusting, conjunctival follicles, conjunctival edema, edema, abnormal vision, pain, lid disorder, keratitis, blepharitis, photophobia, corneal staining, lid erythema, blepharoconjunctivitis, irritation, corneal erosion, corneal infiltrate, keratopathy, lid scales, lid retraction.

Nonocular

Body As A Whole: The following adverse reactions were reported in less than 3% of the patients: headache, asthenia. The following adverse reactions (incidences) were reported in less than 1% of the patients: chest pain, abnormal coordination, malaise, facial edema.

Cardiovascular: The following adverse reactions were reported in less than 1% of the patients: peripheral edema, arrhythmia. Although no reports of bradycardia related to IOPIDINE 0.5% Ophthalmic Solution were available from clinical studies, the possibility of its occurrence based on Apraclonidine's alpha-2-agonist effect should be considered (See Clinical Pharmacology Section).

Central Nervous System

The following adverse reactions were reported in less than 1% of the patients: somnolence, dizziness, nervousness, depression, insomnia, paresthesia.

Digestive System: Dry mouth (10%). The following adverse reactions were reported in less than 1% of the patients: constipation, nausea. Musculoskeletal: Myalgia (0.2%).

Respiratory System: Dry nose (2%). The following adverse reactions were reported in less than 1% of the patients: rhinitis, dyspnea, pharyngitis, asthma.

Skin: The following adverse reactions were reported in less than 1% of the patients: contact dermatitis, dermatitis.

Special Senses: Taste perversion (3%), parosmia (0.2%).

Overdosage: While no instances of accidental or intentional ingestion of ophthalmic apraclonidine are known, overdose with the oral form of clonidine has been reported to cause hypotension, transient hypertension, asthenia, vomiting, irritability, diminished or absent reflexes, lethargy, somnolence, sedation or coma, pallor, hypothermia, bradycardia, conduction defects, arrhythmias, dryness of the mouth, miosis, apnea, respiratory depression, hypoventilation, and seizure. Treatment of an oral overdose includes supportive and symptomatic therapy; a patent airway should be maintained. Hemodialysis is of limited value, since a maximum of 5% of circulating drug is removed.

Dosage and Administration: One to two drops of IOPIDINE 0.5% Ophthalmic Solution should be instilled in the affected eye(s) three times daily. Since IOPIDINE 0.5% Ophthalmic Solution will be used with other ocular glaucoma therapies, an approximate 5 minute interval between instillation of each medication should be practiced to prevent washout of the previous dose. NOT FOR INJECTION INTO THE EYE. NOT FOR ORAL INGESTION.

How Supplied: IOPIDINE 0.5% Ophthalmic Solution as base in a sterile, isotonic, aqueous solution containing apraclonidine hydrochloride.

Supplied in plastic ophthalmic DROP-TAINER® dispenser as follows:

5 mL NDC 0065-0665-05
10 mL NDC 0065-0665-10

Storage: Store between 2–27°C (36–80°F). Protect from freezing and light.

U.S. Patent No. 4,517,199

Rx Only

ISOPTO® CARBACHOL ℞
(carbachol)
Sterile Ophthalmic Solution

Description: ISOPTO® CARBACHOL is a cholinergic prepared as a sterile topical ophthalmic solution.

Chemical name: 2- [(Aminocarbonyl)oxy]-*N,N,N* -trimethylethanaminium chloride.

Each mL contains: Active: Carbachol 0.75%, 1.5%, 2.25%, or 3.0%. **Preservative:** Benzalkonium Chloride 0.005%. **Vehicle:** Hydroxypropyl Methylcellulose 1.0%. **Inactive:** Boric Acid, Sodium Chloride, Sodium Borate, Purified Water.

Clinical Pharmacology: A cholinergic (parasympathomimetic) agent. Carbachol has a double action, it not only stimulates the motor endplate of the muscle cell, as do all cholinesters, but it also partially inhibits cholinesterase.

Indications and Usage: For lowering intraocular pressure in the treatment of glaucoma.

Contraindications: Miotics are contraindicated where constriction is undesirable such as acute iritis. Contraindicated in those persons showing hypersensitivity to any component of this preparation.

Warnings: For topical use only. Not for injection. Carbachol should be used with caution in the presence of corneal abrasion to avoid excessive penetration which can produce systemic toxicity; and in patients with acute cardiac failure, bronchial asthma, active peptic ulcer, hyperthyroidism, gastrointestinal spasm, urinary tract obstruction, Parkinson's disease, recent myocardial infarct, systemic hypertension or hypotension. As with all miotics, retinal detachment has been reported when used in certain susceptible individuals.

Precautions: General: Avoid overdosage.

Information for Patients: The miosis usually causes difficulty in dark adaptation. Patient should be advised to exercise caution in night driving and other hazardous occupations in poor light. Do not touch dropper tip to any surface, as this may contaminate the solution.

Carcinogenesis, Mutagenesis, Impairment of Fertility. There have been no long-term studies done using carbachol in animals to evaluate carcinogenic potential.

Pregnancy. Pregnancy Category C. Animal reproduction studies have not been conducted with carbachol. It is also not known whether carbachol can cause fetal harm when administered to a pregnant woman or can affect reproduction capacity. Carbachol should be given to a pregnant woman only if clearly needed.

Nursing Mothers. It is not known whether this drug is excreted in human milk. Because many drugs are excreted in human milk, caution should be exercised when carbachol is administered to a nursing woman.

Continued on next page

Isopto Carbachol—Cont.

Adverse Reactions: Transient symptoms of stinging and burning may occur. This preparation is capable of producing systemic symptoms of a cholinesterase inhibitor even when the epithelium is intact. Transient ciliary and conjunctival injection, headache, and ciliary spasm with resultant temporary decrease of visual acuity may occur. Salivation, syncope, cardiac arrhythmia, gastrointestinal cramping, vomiting, asthma, hypotension, diarrhea, frequent urge to urinate, increased sweating, and irritation of eyes may occur.
Overdosage: Atropine should be administered parenterally (for dosage refer to Goodman & Gilman or other pharmacology reference).
Dosage and Administration: Instill two drops topically in the eye(s) up to three times daily or as indicated by physician.
How Supplied: 15mL and 30mL in plastic DROP-TAINER® Dispensers.

0.75%: 15 mL NDC 0998-0221-15
1.5%: 15 mL NDC 0998-0223-15
30 mL NDC 0998-0223-30
2.25%: 15 mL NDC 0998-0224-15
3%: 15 mL NDC 0998-0225-15
30 mL NDC 0998-0225-30

Storage: Store at 46°–80°F (8°–27°C).
Rx Only.

ISOPTO® CARPINE ℞
(pilocarpine hydrochloride)
Sterile Ophthalmic Solution

Description: ISOPTO® CARPINE (Pilocarpine Hydrochloride) is a cholinergic prepared as a sterile topical ophthalmic solution.
Chemical name:
2(3*H*)-Furanone, 3-ethyldihydro-
4-[(1-methyl-1*H* -imidazol-5-yl)-
methyl]-, monohydrochloride,
(3*S*-*cis*)-.

Each mL contains: Active: Pilocarpine Hydrochloride 1%, 2%, 4%, 6%, or 8%. **Preservative:** Benzalkonium Chloride 0.01%. **Vehicle:** 0.5% Hydroxypropyl Methylcellulose 2910. **Inactive:** Boric Acid, Sodium Citrate, Sodium Chloride (present in 1% only); Hydrochloric Acid and/or Sodium Hydroxide (to adjust pH); Purified Water.
Clinical Pharmacology: Pilocarpine is a direct acting cholinergic parasympathomimetic agent which acts through direct stimulation of muscarinic neuro receptors and smooth muscle such as the iris and secretory glands. Pilocarpine produces miosis through contraction of the iris sphincter, causing increased tension on the scleral spur and opening of the trabecular mesh work spaces to facilitate outflow of aqueous humor. Outflow resistance is thereby reduced, lowering intraocular pressure.
Indications and Usage: Pilocarpine Hydrochloride is a miotic (parasympathomimetic) used to control intraocular pressure. It may be used in combination with other miotics, beta blockers, carbonic anhydrase inhibitors, sympathomimetics, or hyperosmotic agents.
Contraindications: Miotics are contraindicated where constriction is undesirable such as in acute iritis, in those persons showing hypersensitivity to any of their components, and in pupillary block glaucoma.
Warnings: For topical use only. NOT FOR INJECTION.
Precautions: General. The miosis usually causes difficulty in dark adaptation. Patient should be advised to exercise caution in night driving and other hazardous occupations in poor illumination.
Carcinogenesis, Mutagenesis, Impairment of Fertility: There have been no long-term studies done using pilocarpine in animals to evaluate carcinogenic potential.
Pregnancy: Pregnancy Category C. Animal reproduction studies have not been conducted with pilocarpine. It is also not known whether pilocarpine can cause fetal harm when administered to a pregnant woman or can affect reproduction capacity. Pilocarpine should be given to a pregnant woman only if clearly needed.
Nursing Mothers: It is not known whether this drug is excreted in human milk. Because many drugs are excreted in human milk, caution should be exercised when pilocarpine is administered to a nursing woman.
Information for Patients: Do not touch dropper tip to any surface, as this may contaminate the solution.
Adverse Reactions: Transient symptoms of stinging and burning may occur. Ciliary spasm, conjunctival vascular congestion, temporal or supraorbital headache, and induced myopia may occur. This is especially true in younger individuals who have recently started administration. Reduced visual acuity in poor illumination is frequently experienced by older individuals and individuals with lens opacity. As with all miotics, rare cases of retinal detachment have been reported when used in certain susceptible individuals. Lens opacity may occur with prolonged use of pilocarpine.
Overdosage: Systemic toxicity following topical ocular administration of pilocarpine is rare, but occasional patients are peculiarly sensitive and develop sweating and gastrointestinal overactivity following suggested dosage and administration. Overdosage can produce sweating, salivation, nausea, tremors and slowing of the pulse and a decrease in blood pressure. In moderate overdosage, spontaneous recovery is to be expected and is aided by intravenous fluids to compensate for dehydration. For cases demonstrating severe poisoning, atropine is the pharmacologic antagonist to pilocarpine.[1]
A topical ocular overdose of an ophthalmic product containing pilocarpine may be flushed from the eye(s) with warm tap water.
Dosage and Administration: Two drops topically in the eye(s) up to three or four times daily as directed by a physician. Under selected conditions, more frequent instillations may be indicated. Individuals with heavily pigmented irides may require higher strengths.
How Supplied: In 15mL and 30mL plastic DROP-TAINER® dispensers.

1%—15mL: NDC 0998-0203-15
30mL: NDC 0998-0203-30
2%—15mL: NDC 0998-0204-15
30mL: NDC 0998-0204-30
4%—15mL: NDC 0998-0206-15
30mL: NDC 0998-0206-30
6%—15mL: NDC 0998-0208-15
8%—15mL: NDC 0998-0209-15

Storage: Store at 8° to 27°C (46° to 80°F).
Rx Only

[1] Grant, W. M., Toxicology Of The Eye, 3rd Edition (1986). Charles Thomas Publishing, Springfield, Il.

MAXITROL® ℞
(neomycin and polymyxin B sulfates and dexamethasone ophthalmic suspension and ointment)
Sterile

NAPHCON® A OTC
Eye Drops
Relieves Itching & Redness
EYE ALLERGY RELIEF

Temporary relief of the minor eye symptoms of itching and redness caused by ragweed, pollen, grass, animal hair and dander.
Description: Active: Pheniramine Maleate 0.3%, Naphazoline Hydrochloride 0.025%. **Preservative:** Benzalkonium Chloride 0.01%. **Inactive:** Sodium Chloride, Boric Acid, Sodium Borate, Edetate Disodium 0.01%, Sodium Hydroxide and/or Hydrochloric Acid (to adjust pH), Purified Water. The sterile ophthalmic solution has a pH of about 6 and a tonicity of about 270 mOsm/Kg.
Directions: Instill 1 or 2 drops in the affected eye(s) up to 4 times daily.
Warnings: To avoid contamination, do not touch tip of container to any surface. Replace cap after using.
If solution changes color or becomes cloudy, do not use.
If you experience eye pain, changes in vision, continued redness or irritation of the eye, or if the condition worsens, or persists for more than 72 hours, discontinue use and consult a physician. Overuse of this product may produce increased redness of the eye.
If you are sensitive to any ingredient in this product, do not use. Do not use this product if you have heart disease, high blood pressure, difficulty in urination due to enlargement of the prostate gland or narrow angle glaucoma unless directed by a physician.
Accidental oral ingestion in infants and children may lead to coma and marked reduction in body temperature. Before using in children under 6 years of age, consult your physician.
Keep this and all drugs out of reach of children. In case of accidental ingestion, seek professional assistance or contact a Poison Control Center immediately.
Remove contact lenses before using.
Store at 36°–80°F (2°–27°C).
Protect from light.
Use before the expiration date marked on the carton or bottle.
Keep this and all drugs out of reach of children.

NATACYN® ℞
(natamycin ophthalmic suspension, USP) 5% Sterile

Description: NATACYN® (natamycin ophthalmic suspension, USP) 5% is a sterile, antifungal drug for topical ophthalmic administration.
Chemical name:
Stereoisomer of 22-[(3-amino-3,6-dideoxy-β-D-mannopyranosyl)oxy]-1,3,26-trihydroxy-12-methyl-10-oxo-6,11,28-trioxatricyclo[22.3.1.0^{5,7}] octacosa-8,14,16,18,20-pentaene-25-carboxylic acid.
Other: Pimaricin

Each mL of the suspension contains: **Active:** Natamycin 5% (50mg). **Preservative:** Benzalkonium Chloride 0.02%. **Inactive:** Sodium Hydroxide and/or Hydrochloric Acid (neutralized to adjust the pH), Purified Water.
Clinical Pharmacology: Natamycin is a tetraene polyene antibiotic derived from *Streptomyces natalensis.* It possesses *in vitro* activity against a variety of yeast and filamentous fungi, including *Candida, Aspergillus, Cephalosporium, Fusarium* and *Penicillium.* The mechanism of action appears to be through binding of the molecule to the sterol moiety of the fungal cell membrane. The polyenesterol

complex alters the permeability of the membrane to produce depletion of essential cellular constituents. Although the activity against fungi is dose-related, natamycin is predominantly fungicidal.* Natamycin is not effective *in vitro* against gram-positive or gram-negative bacteria. Topical administration appears to produce effective concentrations of natamycin within the corneal stroma but not in intraocular fluid. Systemic absorption should not be expected following topical administration of NATACYN (natamycin ophthalmic suspension, USP) 5%. As with other polyene antibiotics, absorption from the gastrointestinal tract is very poor. Studies in rabbits receiving topical natamycin revealed no measurable compound in the aqueous humor or sera, but the sensitivity of the measurement was no greater than 2 mg/mL.

Indications and Usage: NATACYN (natamycin ophthalmic suspension, USP) 5% is indicated for the treatment of fungal blepharitis, conjunctivitis, and keratitis caused by susceptible organisms including *Fusarium solani* keratitis. As in other forms of suppurative keratitis, initial and sustained therapy of fungal keratitis should be determined by the clinical diagnosis, laboratory diagnosis by smear and culture of corneal scrapings and drug response. Whenever possible, the *in vitro* activity of natamycin against the responsible fungus should be determined. The effectiveness of natamycin as a single agent in fungal endophthalmitis has not been established.

Contraindications: NATACYN (natamycin ophthalmic suspension, USP) 5% is contraindicated in individuals with a history of hypersensitivity to any of its components.

Precautions: General. For topical eye use only—NOT FOR INJECTION. Failure of improvement of keratitis following 7–10 days of administration of the drug suggests that the infection may be caused by a microorganism not susceptible to natamycin.

Continuation of therapy should be based on clinical re-evaluation and additional laboratory studies.

Adherence of the suspension to areas of epithelial ulceration or retention of the suspension in the fornices occurs regularly. There have only been a limited number of cases in which natamycin has been used; therefore, it is possible that adverse reactions of which we have no knowledge at present may occur. For this reason, patients on this drug should be monitored at least twice weekly. Should suspicion of drug toxicity occur, the drug should be discontinued.

Information for Patients: Do not touch dropper tip to any surface, as this may contaminate the suspension.

Carcinogenesis, Mutagenesis, Impairment of Fertility: There have been no long term studies done using natamycin in animals to evaluate carcinogenesis, mutagenesis, or impairment of fertility.

Pregnancy: Pregnancy Category C. Animal reproduction studies have not been conducted with natamycin. It is also not known whether natamycin can cause fetal harm when administered to a pregnant woman or can affect reproduction capacity. NATACYN (natamycin ophthalmic suspension, USP) 5% should be given to a pregnant woman only if clearly needed.

Nursing Mothers: It is not known whether these drugs are excreted in human milk. Because many drugs are excreted in human milk, caution should be exercised when natamycin is administered to a nursing woman.

Pediatric Use: Safety and effectiveness in pediatric patients have not been establised.

Adverse Reactions: One case of conjunctival chemosis and hyperemia, thought to be allergic in nature, has been reported.

Dosage and Administration: SHAKE WELL BEFORE USING. The preferred initial dosage in fungal keratitis is one drop of NATACYN (natamycin ophthalmic suspension, USP) 5% instilled in the conjunctival sac at hourly or two-hourly intervals. The frequency of application can usually be reduced to one drop 6 to 8 times daily after the first 3 to 4 days. Therapy should generally be continued for 14 to 21 days or until there is resolution of active fungal keratitis. In many cases, it may be helpful to reduce the dosage gradually at 4 to 7 day intervals to assure that the replicating organism has been eliminated. Less frequent initial dosage (4 to 6 daily applications) may be sufficient in fungal blepharitis and conjunctivitis.

How Supplied: 15 mL in glass bottles with sterile dropper assembly. **NDC** 0065-0645-15.

Storage: May be stored in refrigerator [(36°–46° F) (2°–8°C)] or at room temperature [(46°–75° F) (8°–24°C)]. *Do not freeze.* Avoid exposure to light and excessive heat.

Rx Only

* Laupen, J.O.; McLellan, W.L.; El Nakeeb, M.A.: "Antibiotics and Fungal Physiology," Antimicrobial Agents and Chemotherapy, 1965:1006, 1965.

References:

1. Barckhausen, B.: Die Behandlung der Probleminfektionen das vorderen Augenabschnittes in der Praxis. Landarzt 46:842, 1970.
2. Cuendet, J.F.; Nouri, A.: Traitement local en ophthalmologie par un nouvel antibiotique fungicide, la "pimaricine". Ophthalmologica 145:297, 1963.
3. Forster, R.K.; Rebell, G.: "The Diagnosis and Management of Keratomycoses", Arch. Ophth. 93:1134, 1975.
4. Francois, J.; de Vos, El: Traitement des mycoses oculaires par la pimaricine. Bull. Soc. Belge Ophthal. 131:382, 1962.
5. Jones, D.B.; Sexton, R.; Rebell, G.: "Mycotic keratitis in South Florida: A Review of Thirty-nine Cases." Transactions ophthal. Soc. U.K. 89:781, 1969.
6. Jones, D.B.; Forster, R.K.; Rebell, G.: "*Fusarium solani* keratitis treated with Natamycin (pimaricin), 18 consecutive cases." Arch. Ophth. 88:147, 1972.
7. L'Editeur: Traitement des mycoses oculaires. Presse med. 77:147, 1969.
8. Vozza, R.; Bagolini, B.: Su di un caso di grave ulcerazione bilaterale delle palpebra de Candida albicans. Bol. Oculist. 43:433, 1964.

Manufactured Under License From Gist-Brocades, N.V., Delft, Holland

---

PATANOL® ℞

(olopatadine hydrochloride ophthalmic solution) 0.1%

Description: PATANOL® (olopatadine hydrochloride ophthalmic solution) 0.1% is a sterile ophthalmic solution containing olopatadine, a relatively selective H_1-receptor antagonist and inhibitor of histamine release from the mast cell for topical administration to the eyes. Olopatadine hydrochloride is a white, crystalline, water-soluble powder with a molecular weight of 373.88.

Chemical Name: 11-[(Z)-3-(Dimethylamino) propylidene]-6-11-dihydrodibenz[b,e] oxepin-2-acetic acid hydrochloride

Each mL of PATANOL contains: **Active:** 1.11 mg olopatadine hydrochloride equivalent to 1 mg olopatadine. **Preservative:** benzalkonium chloride 0.01%. **Inactives:** dibasic sodium phosphate; sodium chloride; hydrochloric acid/ sodium hydroxide (adjust pH); and purified water.

It has a pH of approximately 7 and an osmolality of approximately 300 mOsm/kg.

Clinical Pharmacology: Olopatadine is an inhibitor of the release of histamine from the mast cell and a relatively selective histamine H_1-antagonist that inhibits the *in vivo* and *in vitro* type 1 immediate hypersensitivity reaction. Olopatadine is devoid of effects on alpha-adrenergic, dopamine, muscarinic type 1 and 2, and serotonin receptors. Following topical ocular administration in man, olopatadine was shown to have low systemic exposure. Two studies in normal volunteers (totaling 24 subjects) dosed bilaterally with olopatadine 0.15% ophthalmic solution once every 12 hours for 2 weeks demonstrated plasma concentrations to be generally below the quantitation limit of the assay (<0.5 ng/mL). Samples in which olopatadine was quantifiable were typically found within 2 hours of dosing and ranged from 0.5 to 1.3 ng/mL. The half-life in plasma was approximately 3 hours, and elimination was predominantly through renal excretion. Approximately 60–70% of the dose was recovered in the urine as parent drug. Two metabolites, the mono-desmethyl and the N-oxide, were detected at low concentrations in the urine.

Results from conjunctival antigen challenge studies demonstrated that PATANOL, when subjects were challenged with antigen both initially and up to 8 hours after dosing, was significantly more effective than its vehicle in preventing ocular itching associated with allergic conjunctivitis.

Indications And Usage: PATANOL (olopatadine hydrochloride ophthalmic solution) 0.1% is indicated for the temporary prevention of itching of the eye due to allergic conjunctivitis.

Contraindications: PATANOL® is contraindicated in persons with a known hypersensitivity to olopatadine hydrochloride or any components of PATANOL.

Warnings: PATANOL is for topical use only and not for injection or oral use.

Precautions:

Information for Patients: To prevent contaminating the dropper tip and solution, care should be taken not to touch the eyelids or surrounding areas with the dropper tip of the bottle. Keep bottle tightly closed when not in use. Patients should be advised not to wear a contact lens if their eye is red. PATANOL® should not be used to treat contact lens related irritation. The preservative in PATANOL, benzalkonium chloride, may be absorbed by soft contact lenses. Patients who wear soft contact lenses and **whose eyes are not red,** should be instructed to wait at least ten minutes after instilling PATANOL before they insert their contact lenses.

Carcinogenesis, Mutagenesis, Impairment of Fertility: Olopatadine administered orally was not carcinogenic in mice and rats in doses up to 500 mg/kg/day and 200 mg/kg/day, respectively. Based on a 40 µl drop size, these doses were 78,125 and 31,250 times higher than the maximum recommended ocular human dose (MROHD). No mutagenic potential was observed when olopatadine was tested in an *in vitro* bacterial reverse mutation (Ames) test, an *in vitro* mammalian chromosome aberration assay or an *in vivo* mouse micronucleus test. Olopatadine administered to male and female rats at oral doses of 62,500 times MROHD level resulted in a slight decrease in the fertility index and reduced implantation rate; no effects on reproductive function were observed at doses of 7,800 times the maximum recommended ocular human use level.

Pregnancy: Pregnancy Category C: Olopatadine was found not to be teratogenic in rats and rabbits. However, rats treated at 600 mg/kg/day, or 93,750 times the MROHD and rabbits treated at 400 mg/kg/day, or 62,500 times the MROHD, during organogenesis showed a decrease in live fetuses. There are, however, no adequate and well controlled studies in preg-

Continued on next page

Patanol—Cont.

nant women. Because animal studies are not always predictive of human responses, this drug should be used in pregnant women only if the potential benefit to the mother justifies the potential risk to the embryo or fetus.

Nursing Mothers: Olopatadine has been identified in the milk of nursing rats following oral administration. It is not known whether topical ocular administration could result in sufficient systemic absorption to produce detectable quantities in the human breast milk. Nevertheless, caution should be exercised when PATANOL® is administered to a nursing mother.

Pediatric Use: Safety and effectiveness in pediatric patients below the age of 3 years have not been established.

Adverse Reactions: Headaches were reported at an incidence of 7%. The following adverse experiences were reported in less than 5% of patients: Asthenia, burning or stinging, cold syndrome, dry eye, foreign body sensation, hyperemia, keratitis, lid edema, pharyngitis, pruritus, rhinitis, sinusitis, and taste perversion. Some of these events were similar to the underlying disease being studied.

Dosage And Administration: The recommended dose is one to two drops in each affected eye two times per day at an interval of 6 to 8 hours.

How Supplied: PATANOL (olopatadine hydrochloride ophthalmic solution) 0.1% is supplied as follows: 5 mL in plastic DROP-TAINER® dispenser.

5 mL: NDC 0065-0271-05

Storage:

Store at 39°F to 86°F (4°C to 30°C).

U.S. Patents Nos. 4,871,865; 4,923,892; 5,116,863; 5,641,805.

Rx Only.

PILOPINE HS® GEL ℞

(pilocarpine hydrochloride ophthalmic gel) 4%

Description: PILOPINE HS® (pilocarpine hydrochloride ophthalmic gel) 4% is a sterile topical ophthalmic aqueous gel which contains more than 90% water and employs CARBOPOL 940, a synthetic high molecular weight cross-linked polymer of acrylic acid, to impart a high viscosity. The active ingredient, Pilocarpine Hydrochloride, is a cholinergic.

Chemical name:

2(3*H*)-Furanone, 3-ethyldihydro-4-[(1-methyl-1*H*-imidazol-5-yl)-methyl]-, monohydrochloride, (3*S-cis*)-.

PILOPINE HS Gel—Each Gram Contains: Active: Pilocarpine Hydrochloride 4% (40 mg). **Preservative**: Benzalkonium Chloride 0.008%. **Inactive:** Carbopol 940, Edetate Disodium, Hydrochloric Acid and/or Sodium Hydroxide (to adjust pH) and Purified Water.

Clinical Pharmacology: Pilocarpine is a direct acting cholinergic parasympathomimetic agent which acts through direct stimulation of muscarinic neuro receptors and smooth muscle such as the iris and secretory glands. Pilocarpine produces miosis through contraction of the iris sphincter, causing increased tension on the scleral spur and opening of the trabecular meshwork spaces to facilitate outflow of aqueous humor. Outflow resistance is thereby reduced, lowering intraocular pressure.

Indications and Usage: Pilocarpine Hydrochloride is a miotic (parasympathomimetic) used to control intraocular pressure. It may be used in combination with other miotics, beta blockers, carbonic anhydrase inhibitors, sympathomimetics or hyperosmotic agents.

Contraindications: Miotics are contraindicated where constriction is undesirable, such as in acute iritis, and in those persons showing hypersensitivity to any of their components.

Warnings: For topical use only.

Precautions: General: The miosis usually causes difficulty in dark adaptation. Patient should be advised to exercise caution in night driving and other hazardous occupations in poor illumination.

Information For Patients: Do not touch tube tip to any surface, as this may contaminate the gel.

Carcinogenesis, Mutagenesis, Impairment of Fertility: There have been no long-term studies done using Pilocarpine Hydrochloride in animals to evaluate carcinogenic potential.

Pregnancy: Pregnancy Category C. Animal reproduction studies have not been conducted with Pilocarpine Hydrochloride. It is also not known whether Pilocarpine Hydrochloride can cause fetal harm when administered to a pregnant woman or can affect reproduction capacity. PILOPINE HS® Gel should be given to a pregnant woman only if clearly needed.

Nursing Mothers: It is not known whether this drug is excreted in human milk. Because many drugs are excreted in human milk, caution should be exercised when Pilocarpine Hydrochloride is administered to a nursing woman.

Pediatric Use: Safety and effectiveness in pediatric patients have not been established.

Adverse Reactions: The following adverse experiences associated with pilocarpine therapy have been reported: lacrimation, burning or discomfort, temporal or periorbital headache, ciliary spasm, conjunctival vascular congestion, superficial keratitis and induced myopia. Systemic reactions following topical administration are extremely rare, but occasional patients are peculiarly sensitive to develop sweating and gastrointestinal overactivity following suggested dosage and administration. Ocular reactions usually occur during initiation of therapy and often will not persist with continued therapy. Reduced visual acuity in poor illumination is frequently experienced in older individuals and in those with lens opacity. A subtle corneal granularity was observed in about 10% of patients treated with PILOPINE HS Gel. Cases of retinal detachment have been reported during treatment with miotic agents; especially in young myopic patients. Lens opacity may occur with prolonged use of pilocarpine.

Overdosage: Overdosage can produce sweating, salivation, nausea, tremors, and slowing of the pulse and a decrease in blood pressure. Bronchial constriction may develop in asthmatic patients. In moderate overdosage, spontaneous recovery is to be expected and is aided by intravenous fluids to compensate for dehydration. For cases demonstrating severe poisoning, atropine is the pharmacologic antagonist to pilocarpine.

A topical ocular overdose of an ophthalmic product containing pilocarpine may be flushed from the eye(s) with warm tap water.

Dosage and Administration: Apply a one-half inch ribbon in the lower conjunctival sac of the affected eye(s) once a day at bedtime.

How Supplied: PILOPINE HS Gel is supplied as a 4% sterile aqueous gel in 4 gram tubes with ophthalmic tip.

4 gram: NDC 0065-0215-35

Storage: Store at room temperature 2°–27°C (36°–80°F). Avoid excessive heat. Do not freeze.

Rx Only.

Reference:

1. Grant, W.M., Toxicology Of the Eye, 4th Edition (1993), Charles Thomas Publishing, Springfield, IL.

Patented: U.S. Patent No. 4,271,143

TEARS NATURALE® II OTC

Lubricant Eye Drops

TEARS NATURALE FREE®

Lubricant Eye Drops

Description: TEARS NATURALE II is the only lubricant eye drop preserved with safe, nonsensitizing POLYQUAD 0.001%. *In vitro* studies have shown that POLYQUAD substantially avoids the damaging effects of epithelial cell toxicity possible with other tear substitute preservatives and allows epithelial cell growth. POLYQUAD has been shown to be 99% reaction-free in normal subjects and 97% reaction-free in subjects known to be preservative sensitive. TEARS NATURALE FREE is a preservative-free version of TEARS NATURALE II.

With their unique mucin like polymeric formulation, and with their natural pH, low viscosity, and isotonicity, TEARS NATURALE II and TEARS NATURALE FREE provide dry eye patients with comfort and prompt relief of dry eye symptoms.

Sterile-For Topical Eye Use Only

Ingredients: TEARS NATURALE II: Each mL contains: **Active**: DUASORB®, a water soluble polymeric system containing Dextran 70 0.1% and Hydroxypropyl Methylcellulose 2910 0.3%.

Preservative: POLYQUAD® (Polyquaternium-1) 0.001%.

Inactives: Sodium Borate, Potassium Chloride, Sodium Chloride, Purified Water. May contain Hydrochloric Acid and/or Sodium Hydroxide to adjust pH.

TEARS NATURALE FREE: Each mL contains: **Active**: DUASORB®, a water soluble polymeric system containing Dextran 70 0.1% and Hydroxypropyl Methylcellulose 2910 0.3%.

Inactives: Sodium Borate, Potassium Chloride, Sodium Chloride, Purified Water. May contain Hydrochloric Acid and/or Sodium Hydroxide to adjust pH.

Indications: For the temporary relief of burning and irritation due to dryness of the eye and for use as a protectant against further irritation. For the temporary relief of discomfort due to minor irritations of the eye or to exposure to wind or sun.

Warnings: If you experience eye pain, changes in vision, continued redness or irritation of the eye, or if the condition worsens or persists for more than 72 hours, discontinue use and consult a doctor.

If solution changes color or becomes cloudy, do not use.

To avoid contamination, do not touch tip of container to any surface. Replace cap after using. Keep this and all drugs out of the reach of children. In case of accidental ingestion, seek professional assistance or contact a Poison Control Center immediately.

Directions: TEARS NATURALE II: Instill 1 or 2 drops in the affected eye(s) as needed. TEARS NATURALE FREE: Make sure container is intact before use. To open, completely TWIST off tab. DO NOT pull off. Instill 1 or 2 drops in the affected eye(s) as needed. To close, align cap at right angle (90°) to vial and firmly press down. Improved vial design reduces chance of leakage. **DISCARD 12 HOURS AFTER OPENING.**

How Supplied: TEARS NATURALE II Lubricant Eye Drops are supplied in 15 mL and 30 mL plastic DROP-TAINER® bottles.

15 mL NDC 0065-0418-15

30 mL NDC 0065-0418-30

TEARS NATURALE FREE Lubricant Eye Drops are supplied in boxes of 35 0.03 fl. oz. re-closable vials.

NDC 0065-0416-32

Storage: Store at room temperature.

TOBRADEX® ℞
(tobramycin and dexamethasone ophthalmic suspension and ointment)
Sterile

Description: TOBRADEX® (tobramycin and dexamethasone ophthalmic suspension and ointment) are sterile, multiple dose antibiotic and steroid combinations for topical ophthalmic use.
Tobramycin
Chemical name:
O -3-Amino-3-deoxy-α-D-glucopyranosyl-(1→4)-*O* -[2,6-diamino-2,3,6-trideoxy-α-D-*ribo* -hexopyranosyl-(1→6)]-2-deoxy-L-streptamine
Dexamethasone
Chemical Name:
9-Fluoro-11β,17,21-trihydroxy-16α-methylpregna-1,4-diene-3,20-dione
Each mL of TOBRADEX® Suspension contains: Actives: Tobramycin 0.3% (3 mg) and Dexamethasone 0.1% (1 mg). Preservative: Benzalkonium Chloride 0.01%. Inactives: Tyloxapol, Edetate Disodium, Sodium Chloride, Hydroxyethyl Cellulose, Sodium Sulfate, Sulfuric Acid and/or Sodium Hydroxide (to adjust pH) and Purified Water.
Each gram of TOBRADEX® Ointment contains: Actives: Tobramycin 0.3% (3 mg) and Dexamethasone 0.1% (1 mg). Preservative: Chlorobutanol 0.5%. Inactives: Mineral Oil and White Petrolatum.

Clinical Pharmacology: Corticoids suppress the inflammatory response to a variety of agents and they probably delay or slow healing. Since corticoids may inhibit the body's defense mechanism against infection, a concomitant antimicrobial drug may be used when this inhibition is considered to be clinically significant. Dexamethasone is a potent corticoid.
The antibiotic component in the combination (tobramycin) is included to provide action against susceptible organisms. *In vitro* studies have demonstrated that tobramycin is active against susceptible strains of the following microorganisms:
Staphylococci, including *S. aureus* and *S. epidermidis* (coagulase-positive and coagulase-negative), including penicillin-resistant strains.
Streptococci, including some of the Group A-beta-hemolytic species, some nonhemolytic species, and some *Streptococcus pneumoniae. Pseudomonas aeruginosa, Escherichia coli, Klebsiella pneumoniae, Enterobacter aerogenes, Proteus mirabilis, Morganella morganii,* most *Proteus vulgaris* strains, *Haemophilus influenzae* and *H. aegyptius, Moraxella lacunata, Acinetobacter calcoaceticus* and some *Neisseria* species.
Bacterial susceptibility studies demonstrate that in some cases microorganisms resistant to gentamicin remain susceptible to tobramycin.
No data are available on the extent of systemic absorption from TOBRADEX® Ophthalmic Suspension or Ointment; however, it is known that some systemic absorption can occur with ocularly applied drugs. If the maximum dose of TOBRADEX Ophthalmic Suspension is given for the first 48 hours (two drops in each eye every 2 hours) and complete systemic absorption occurs, which is highly unlikely, the daily dose of dexamethasone would be 2.4 mg. The usual physiologic replacement dose is 0.75 mg daily. If TOBRADEX Ophthalmic Suspension is given after the first 48 hours as two drops in each eye every 4 hours, the administered dose of dexamethasone would be 1.2 mg daily. The administered dose for TOBRADEX Ophthalmic Ointment in both eyes four times daily would be 0.4 mg of dexamethasone daily.

Indications and Usage: TOBRADEX® Ophthalmic Suspension and Ointment are indicated for steroid-responsive inflammatory ocular conditions for which a corticosteroid is indicated and where superficial bacterial ocular infection or a risk of bacterial ocular infection exists.
Ocular steroids are indicated in inflammatory conditions of the palpebral and bulbar conjunctiva, cornea and anterior segment of the globe where the inherent risk of steroid use in certain infective conjunctivitides is accepted to obtain a diminution in edema and inflammation. They are also indicated in chronic anterior uveitis and corneal injury from chemical, radiation or thermal burns, or penetration of foreign bodies.
The use of a combination drug with an anti-infective component is indicated where the risk of superficial ocular infection is high or where there is an expectation that potentially dangerous numbers of bacteria will be present in the eye.
The particular anti-infective drug in this product is active against the following common bacterial eye pathogens:
Staphylococci, including *S. aureus* and *S. epidermidis* (coagulase-positive and coagulase-negative), including penicillin-resistant strains.
Streptococci, including some of the Group A-beta-hemolytic species, some nonhemolytic species, and some *Streptococcus pneumoniae. Pseudomonas aeruginosa, Escherichia coli, Klebsiella pneumoniae, Enterobacter aerogenes, Proteus mirabilis, Morganella morganii,* most *Proteus vulgaris* strains, *Haemophilus influenzae,* and *H. aegyptius, Moraxella lacunata, Acinetobacter calcoaceticus* and some *Neisseria* species.

Contraindications: Epithelial herpes simplex keratitis (dendritic keratitis), vaccinia, varicella, and many other viral diseases of the cornea and conjunctiva. Mycobacterial infection of the eye. Fungal diseases of ocular structures. Hypersensitivity to a component of the medication.

Warnings: NOT FOR INJECTION INTO THE EYE. Sensitivity to topically applied aminoglycosides may occur in some patients. If a sensitivity reaction does occur, discontinue use.
Prolonged use of steroids may result in glaucoma, with damage to the optic nerve, defects in visual acuity and fields of vision, and posterior subcapsular cataract formation. Intraocular pressure should be routinely monitored even though it may be difficult in children and uncooperative patients. Prolonged use may suppress the host response and thus increase the hazard of secondary ocular infections. In those diseases causing thinning of the cornea or sclera, perforations have been known to occur with the use of topical steroids. In acute purulent conditions of the eye, steroids may mask infection or enhance existing infection.

Precautions: General. The possibility of fungal infections of the cornea should be considered after long-term steroid dosing. As with other antibiotic preparations, prolonged use may result in overgrowth of nonsusceptible organisms, including fungi. If superinfection occurs, appropriate therapy should be initiated. When multiple prescriptions are required, or whenever clinical judgement dictates, the patient should be examined with the aid of magnification, such as slit lamp biomicroscopy and, where appropriate, fluorescein staining.
Cross-sensitivity to other aminoglycoside antibotics may occur; if hypersensitivity develops with this product, discontinue use and institute appropriate therapy.
Information for Patients: Do not touch dropper or tube tip to any surface, as this may contaminate the contents.
Carcinogenesis, Mutagenesis, Impairment of Fertility. No studies have been conducted to evaluate the carcinogenic or mutagenic potential. No impairment of fertility was noted in studies of subcutaneous tobramycin in rats at doses of 50 and 100 mg/kg/day.
Pregnancy Category C. Corticosteroids have been found to be teratogenic in animal studies. Ocular administration of 0.1% dexamethasone resulted in 15.6% and 32.3% incidence of fetal anomalies in two groups of pregnant rabbits. Fetal growth retardation and increased mortality rates have been observed in rats with chronic dexamethasone therapy. Reproduction studies have been performed in rats and rabbits with tobramycin at doses up to 100 mg/kg/day parenterally and have revealed no evidence of impaired fertility or harm to the fetus. There are no adequate and well controlled studies in pregnant women. TOBRADEX® Ophthalmic Suspension and Ointment should be used during pregnancy only if the potential benefit justifies the potential risk to the fetus.
Nursing Mothers. Systemically administered corticosteroids appear in human milk and could suppress growth, interfere with endogenous corticosteroid production, or cause other untoward effects. It is not known whether topical administration of corticosteroids could result in sufficient systemic absorption to produce detectable quantities in human milk. Because many drugs are excreted in human milk, caution should be exercised when TOBRADEX® Ophthalmic Suspension or Ointment is administered to a nursing woman.
Pediatric Use. Safety and effectiveness in pediatric patients have not been established.

Adverse Reactions: Adverse reactions have occurred with steroid/anti-infective combination drugs which can be attributed to the steroid component, the anti-infective component, or the combination. Exact incidence figures are not available. The most frequent adverse reactions to topical ocular tobramycin (TOBREX®) are hypersensitivity and localized ocular toxicity, including lid itching and swelling, and conjunctival erythema. These reactions occur in less than 4% of patients. Similar reactions may occur with the topical use of other aminoglycoside antibiotics. Other adverse reactions have not been reported; however, if topical ocular tobramycin is administered concomitantly with systemic aminoglycoside antibiotics, care should be taken to monitor the total serum concentration. The reactions due to the steroid component are: elevation of intraocular pressure (IOP) with possible development of glaucoma, and infrequent optic nerve damage; posterior subcapsular cataract formation; and delayed wound healing.
Secondary Infection. The development of secondary infection has occurred after use of combinations containing steroids and antimicrobials. Fungal infections of the cornea are particularly prone to develop coincidentally with long-term applications of steroids. The possibility of fungal invasion must be considered in any persistent corneal ulceration where steroid treatment has been used. Secondary bacterial ocular infection following suppression of host responses also occurs.

Overdosage: Clinically apparent signs and symptoms of an overdose of TOBRADEX Ophthalmic Suspension or Ointment (punctate keratitis, erythema, increased lacrimation, edema and lid itching) may be similar to adverse reaction effects seen in some patients.

Dosage and Administration: **Suspension:** One or two drops instilled into the conjunctival sac(s) every four to six hours. During the initial 24 to 48 hours, the dosage may be increased to one or two drops every two (2) hours. Frequency should be decreased gradually as warranted by improvement in clinical signs. Care should be taken not to discontinue therapy prematurely. **Ointment:** Apply a small

Continued on next page

Tobradex—Cont.

amount (approximately $^1/_2$ inch ribbon) into the conjunctival sac(s) up to three or four times daily.
Not more than 20 mL or 8 g should be prescribed initially and the prescription should not be refilled without further evaluation as outlined in PRECAUTIONS above.
How Supplied: Sterile ophthalmic suspension in 2.5 mL (NDC 0065-0647-25), 5 mL (NDC 0065-0647-05) and 10 mL (NDC 0065-0647-10) DROP-TAINER® dispensers. Sterile ophthalmic ointment in 3.5 g ophthalmic tube (NDC 0065-0648-35).
Storage: Store at 8° to 27°C (46° to 80°F). Store suspension upright and shake well before using.
Rx Only.
U.S. Patent No. 5,149,694

TOBREX® ℞
(tobramycin 0.3%)
Ophthalmic Ointment

Description: TOBREX® (tobramycin 0.3%) is a sterile topical ophthalmic antibiotic formulation prepared specifically for topical therapy of external ophthalmic infections.
Each gram of TOBREX Ophthalmic Ointment contains: **Active:** Tobramycin 0.3% (3 mg). **Preservative:** Chlorobutanol 0.5%. **Inactives:** Mineral Oil, White Petrolatum.
Tobramycin is a water-soluble aminoglycoside antibiotic active against a wide variety of gram-negative and gram-positive ophthalmic pathogens.
Chemical name:
0-{3-amino-3-deoxy-α-D-gluco-pyranosyl-(1→4) }-0-(2,6-diamino-2,3,6-trideoxy-α-D-ribohexo-pyranosyl-(1→6)}-2-deoxystreptamine.
Clinical Pharmacology: *In Vitro Data: In vitro* studies have demonstrated tobramycin is active against susceptible strains of the following microorganisms:
Staphylococci, including *S. aureus* and *S. epidermidis* (coagulase- positive and coagulase-negative), including penicillin-resistant strains.
Streptococci, including some of the Group A–beta-hemolytic species, some nonhemolytic species, and some *Streptococcus pneumoniae. Pseudomonas aeruginosa, Escherichia coli, Klebsiella pneumoniae, Enterobacter aerogenes, Proteus mirabilis, Morganella morganii,* most *Proteus vulgaris* strains, *Haemophilus influenzae* and *H. aegyptius, Moraxella lacunata, Acinetobacter calcoaceticus* and some *Neisseria* species. Bacterial susceptibility studies demonstrate that in some cases, microorganisms resistant to gentamicin retain susceptibility to tobramycin.
Indications and Usage: TOBREX® is a topical antibiotic indicated in the treatment of external infections of the eye and its adnexa caused by susceptible bacteria. Appropriate monitoring of bacterial response to topical antibiotic therapy should accompany the use of TOBREX. Clinical studies have shown tobramycin to be safe and effective for use in children.
Contraindications: TOBREX Ophthalmic Ointment is contraindicated in patients with known hypersensitivity to any of its components.
Warnings: NOT FOR INJECTION INTO THE EYE. Sensitivity to topically applied aminoglycosides may occur in some patients. If a sensitivity reaction to TOBREX occurs, discontinue use. Remove contact lenses before applying ointment.
Precautions: General. As with other antibiotic preparations, prolonged use may result in overgrowth of nonsusceptible organisms, including fungi. If superinfection occurs, appropriate therapy should be initiated. Ophthalmic ointments may retard corneal wound healing. Cross-sensitivity to other aminoglycoside antibiotics may occur; if hypersensitivity develops with this product, discontinue use and institute appropriate therapy.
Information For Patients: Do not touch tube tip to any surface, as this may contaminate the ointment.
Pregnancy Category B. Reproduction studies in three types of animals at doses up to thirty-three times the normal human systemic dose have revealed no evidence of impaired fertility or harm to the fetus due to tobramycin. There are, however, no adequate and well-controlled studies in pregnant women. Because animal studies are not always predictive of human response, this drug should be used during pregnancy only if clearly needed.
Nursing Mothers: Because of the potential for adverse reactions in nursing infants from TOBREX®, a decision should be made whether to discontinue nursing the infant or discontinue the drug, taking into account the importance of the drug to the mother.
Adverse Reactions: The most frequent adverse reactions to TOBREX Ophthalmic Ointment are hypersensitivity and localized ocular toxicity, including lid itching and swelling, and conjunctival erythema. These reactions occur in less than three of 100 patients treated with TOBREX. Similar reactions may occur with the topical use of other aminoglycoside antibiotics. Other adverse reactions have not been reported from TOBREX therapy; however, if topical ocular tobramycin is administered concomitantly with systemic aminoglycoside antibiotics, care should be taken to monitor the total serum concentration.
In clinical trials, TOBREX Ophthalmic Ointment produced significantly fewer adverse reactions (3.7%) than did GARAMYCIN® Ophthalmic Ointment (10.6%).
Overdosage: Clinically apparent signs and symptoms of an overdose of TOBREX Ophthalmic Ointment (punctate keratitis, erythema, increased lacrimation, edema and lid itching) may be similar to adverse reaction effects seen in some patients.
Dosage and Administration: In mild to moderate disease, apply a half-inch ribbon into the affected eye(s) two or three times per day. In severe infections, instill a half-inch ribbon into the affected eye(s) every three to four hours until improvement, following which treatment should be reduced prior to discontinuation.
How Supplied: 3.5g STERILE ointment in ophthalmic tube (NDC 0065-0644-35), containing tobramycin 0.3% (3 mg/g).
Storage: Store at 8°–27°C (46°–80°F).
Rx Only

TOBREX® ℞
(tobramycin 0.3%)
Ophthalmic Solution

Description: TOBREX® (tobramycin 0.3%) is a sterile topical ophthalmic antibiotic formulation prepared specifically for topical therapy of external ophthalmic infections.
Each mL of TOBREX solution contains: **Active:** Tobramycin 0.3% (3 mg). **Preservative:** Benzalkonium Chloride 0.01% (0.1 mg). **Inactives:** Boric Acid, Sodium Sulfate, Sodium Chloride, Tyloxapol, Sodium Hydroxide and/or Sulfuric Acid (to adjust pH) and Purified Water.
Tobramycin is a water-soluble aminoglycoside antibiotic active against a wide variety of gram-negative and gram-positive ophthalmic pathogens.
Chemical name:
0-{3-amino-3-deoxy-α-D-gluco-pyranosyl-(1→4) }-0-{2,6-diamino-2,3,6-trideoxy-α-D-ribohexo-pyranosyl-(1→6)}-2-deoxystreptamine.
Clinical Pharmacology: *In Vitro Data: In vitro* studies have demonstrated tobramycin is active against susceptible strains of the following microorganisms: Staphylococci, including *S. aureus* and *S. epidermidis* (coagulase-positive and coagulase-negative), including penicillin-resistant strains.
Streptococci, including some of the Group A-beta-hemolytic species, some nonhemolytic species, and some *Streptococcus pneumoniae. Pseudomonas aeruginosa, Escherichia coli, Klebsiella pneumoniae, Enterobacter aerogenes. Proteus mirabilis, Morganella morganii,* most *Proteus vulgaris* strains, *Haemophilus influenza* and *H. aegyptius, Moraxella lacunata, Acinetobacter calcoaceticus* and some *Neisseria* species. Bacterial susceptibility studies demonstrate that in some cases, microorganisms resistant to gentamicin retain susceptibility to tobramycin.
Indications and Usage: TOBREX is a topical antibiotic indicated in the treatment of external infections of the eye and its adnexa caused by susceptible bacteria. Appropriate monitoring of bacterial response to topical antibiotic therapy should accompany the use of TOBREX. Clinical studies have shown tobramycin to be safe and effective for use in children.
Contraindications: TOBREX Ophthalmic Solution is contraindicated in patients with known hypersensitivity to any of its components.
Warnings: NOT FOR INJECTION INTO THE EYE. Sensitivity to topically applied aminoglycosides may occur in some patients. If a sensitivity reaction to TOBREX® occurs, discontinue use. Remove contact lenses before using.
Precautions: General. As with other antibiotic preparations, prolonged use may result in overgrowth of nonsuceptible organisms, including fungi. If superinfection occurs, appropriate therapy should be initiated. Cross-sensitivity to other aminoglycoside antibiotics may occur; if hypersenstivity develops with this product, discontinue use and institute appropriate therapy.
Information For Patients: Do not touch dropper tip to any surface, as this may contaminate the solution.
Pregnancy Category B: Reproduction studies in three types of animals at doses up to thirty-three times the normal human systemic dose have revealed no evidence of impaired fertility or harm to the fetus due to tobramycin. There are, however, no adequate and well-controlled studies in pregnant women. Because animal studies are not always predictive of human response, this drug should be used during pregnancy only if clearly needed.
Nursing Mothers. Because of the potential for adverse reactions in nursing infants from TOBREX, a decision should be made whether to discontinue nursing the infant or discontinue the drug, taking into account the importance of the drug to the mother.
Adverse Reactions: The most frequent adverse reactions to TOBREX Ophthalmic Solution are hypersensitivity and localized ocular toxicity, including lid itching and swelling, and conjunctival erythema. These reactions occur in less than three of 100 patients treated with TOBREX. Similar reactions may occur with the topical use of other aminoglycoside antibiotics. Other adverse reactions have not been reported from TOBREX therapy; however, if topical ocular tobramycin is administered concomitantly with systemic aminoglycoside antibiotics, care should be taken to monitor the total serum concentration.

Overdosage: Clinically apparent signs and symptoms of an overdose of TOBREX Ophthalmic Solution (punctate keratitis, erythema, increased lacrimation, edema and lid itching) may be similar to adverse reaction effects seen in some patients.
Dosage and Administration: In mild to moderate disease, instill one or two drops into the affected eye(s) every four hours. In severe infections, instill two drops into the eye(s) hourly until improvement, following which treatment should be reduced prior to discontinuation.
How Supplied: 5 mL sterile solution in DROP-TAINER® dispenser (**NDC** 0065-0643-05), containing tobramycin 0.3% (3 mg/mL).
Storage: Store at 8°–27°C (46°–80°F).
Rx Only

VEXOL® 1% ℞

(rimexolone ophthalmic suspension)

Description: VEXOL® 1% Ophthalmic Suspension is a sterile, multi-dose topical ophthalmic suspension containing the corticosteroid, rimexolone. Rimexolone is a white, water-insoluble powder with an empirical formula of $C_{24}H_{34}O_3$ and a molecular weight of 370.53. Its chemical name is 11β-Hydroxy-16α, 17α-dimethyl-17-propionylandrosta-1,4-diene-3-one.
Each mL Contains: Active ingredient: rimexolone 10 mg (1%).
Preservative: benzalkonium chloride 0.01%.
Inactive ingredients: mannitol, carbomer 934P, polysorbate 80, sodium chloride, edetate disodium, sodium hydroxide and/or hydrochloric acid (to adjust pH) and purified water.
The pH of the suspension is 6.0 to 8.0 and the tonicity is 260 to 320 mOsmol/kg.
Clinical Pharmacology: Corticosteroids suppress the inflammatory response to a variety of inciting agents of a mechanical, chemical, or immunological nature. They inhibit edema, cellular infiltration, capillary dilatation, fibroblastic proliferation, deposition of collagen and scar formation associated with inflammation.
Placebo-controlled clinical studies demonstrated that VEXOL® 1% Ophthalmic Suspension is efficacious for the treatment of anterior chamber inflammation following cataract surgery.
In two controlled clinical trials, VEXOL® 1% Ophthalmic Suspension demonstrated clinical equivalence to 1% prednisolone acetate in reducing uveitic inflammation.
In a controlled 6-week study of steroid responsive subjects, the time to raise intraocular pressure was similar for VEXOL® 1% Ophthalmic Suspension and 0.1% fluorometholone given four times daily.
As with other topically administered ophthalmic drugs, VEXOL® 1% (Rimexolone Ophthalmic Suspension) is absorbed systemically. Studies in normal volunteers dosed bilaterally once every hour during waking hours for one week have demonstrated serum concentrations ranging from less than 80 pg/mL to 470 pg/mL. The mean serum concentrations were approximately 130 pg/mL. Serum concentrations were at or near steady state after 5 to 7 hourly doses. After decreasing the dosing frequency to once every two hours while awake during the second week of administration, mean serum concentrations were approximately 100 pg/mL. The serum half-life of rimexolone could not be reliably estimated due to the large number of samples below the quantitation limit of the assay (80 pg/mL). However, based on the time required to reach steady-state, the half-life appears to be short (1–2 hours).
Based upon *in vivo* and *in vitro* preclinical metabolism studies, and on *in vitro* results with human liver preparations, rimexolone undergoes extensive metabolism. Following IV administration of radio-labelled rimexolone to rats, greater than 80% of the dose is excreted via the feces as rimexolone and metabolites. Metabolites have been shown to be less active than parent drug, or inactive in human glucocorticoid receptor binding assays.
Indications and Usage: VEXOL® 1% Ophthalmic Suspension is indicated for the treatment of postoperative inflammation following ocular surgery and in the treatment of anterior uveitis.
Contraindications: VEXOL® 1% is contraindicated in epithelial herpes simplex keratitis (dendritic keratitis), vaccinia, varicella, and most other viral diseases of the cornea and conjunctiva; mycobacterial infection of the eye; fungal diseases of the eye; acute purulent untreated infections which, like other diseases caused by microorganisms, may be masked or enhanced by the presence of the steroid; and in those persons with hypersensitivity to any component of the formulation.
Warnings: Not for injection. Use in the treatment of herpes simplex infection requires great caution and frequent slit-lamp examinations. Prolonged use may result in ocular hypertension/glaucoma, damage to the optic nerve, defects in visual acuity and visual fields, and posterior subcapsular cataract formation. Prolonged use may also result in secondary ocular infections due to suppression of host response. Acute purulent infections of the eye may be masked or exacerbated by the presence of corticosteroid medication. In those diseases causing thinning of the cornea or sclera, perforation has been known to occur with topical steroids. It is advisable that the intraocular pressure be checked frequently.
Precautions: General: Fungal infections of the cornea are particularly prone to develop coincidentally with long-term local steroid application. Fungal invasion must be considered in any persistent corneal ulceration where a steroid has been or is in use.
For ophthalmic use only. The initial prescription and renewal of the medication order beyond 14 days should be made by a physician only after examination of the patient with the aid of magnification, such as slit lamp biomicroscopy and where appropriate, fluorescein staining. If signs and symptoms fail to improve after two days, the patient should be reevaluated.
If this product is used for 10 days or longer, intraocular pressure should be monitored even though it may be difficult in children and uncooperative patients (see WARNINGS).
Information for Patients: Do not touch dropper tip to any surface, as this may contaminate the suspension.
Carcinogenesis, mutagenesis, impairment of fertility: Rimexolone has been shown to be non-mutagenic in a battery of *in vitro* and *in vivo* mutagenicity assays. Fertility and reproductive capability were not impaired in a study in rats with plasma levels (42 ng/mL) approximately 200 times those obtained in clinical studies after topical administration (<0.2 ng/mL). Long-term studies have not been conducted in animals or humans to evaluate the carcinogenic potential of rimexolone.
Pregnancy: Pregnancy Category C. Rimexolone has been shown to be teratogenic and embryotoxic in rabbits following subcutaneous administration at the lowest dose tested (0.5 mg/kg/day, approximately 2 times the recommended human ophthalmic dose).
Corticosteroids are recognized to cause fetal resorptions and malformations in animals. There are no adequate and well-controlled studies in pregnant women. VEXOL® 1% (Rimexolone Ophthalmic Suspension) should be used in pregnant women only if the potential benefits to the mother justifies the potential risk to the fetus.
Nursing Mothers: It is not known whether topical ophthalmic administration of corticosteroids could result in sufficient systemic absorption to produce detectable quantities in human breast milk. Nevertheless, caution should be exercised when topical corticosteroids are administered to a nursing woman; a decision should be made whether to discontinue nursing or discontinue therapy, taking into consideration the importance of the drug to the mother.
Pediatric Use: Safety and effectiveness in pediatric patients have not been established.
Adverse Reactions: Reactions associated with ophthalmic steroids include elevated intraocular pressure, which may be associated with optic nerve damage, visual acuity and field defects, posterior subcapsular cataract formation, secondary ocular infection from pathogens including herpes simplex, and perforation of the globe where there is thinning of the cornea or sclera.
Ocular adverse reactions occurring in 1–5% of patients in clinical studies of VEXOL® 1% (Rimexolone Ophthalmic Suspension) included blurred vision, discharge, discomfort, ocular pain, increased intraocular pressure, foreign body sensation, hyperemia and pruritus. Other ocular adverse reactions occurring in less than 1% of patients included sticky sensation, increased fibrin, dry eye, conjunctival edema, corneal staining, keratitis, tearing, photophobia, edema, irritation, corneal ulcer, browache, lid margin crusting, corneal edema, infiltrate, and corneal erosion.
Non-ocular adverse reactions occurred in less than 2% of patients. These included headache, hypotension, rhinitis, pharyngitis, and taste perversion.
Dosage And Administration: Post-Operative Inflammation: Apply one–two drops of VEXOL® 1% Ophthalmic Suspension into the conjunctival sac of the affected eye four times daily beginning 24 hours after surgery and continuing throughout the first 2 weeks of the postoperative period.
Anterior Uveitis: Apply one–two drops of VEXOL® 1% Ophthalmic Suspension into the conjunctival sac of the affected eye every hour during waking hours for the first week, one drop every two hours during waking hours of the second week, and then taper until uveitis is resolved.
How Supplied: 2.5 mL, 5 mL and 10 mL in plastic DROP-TAINER® dispensers.
2.5 mL: NDC 0065-0626-20
5 mL: NDC 0065-0626-06
10 mL: NDC 0065-0626-10
Storage: Store upright between 4° and 30°C (40° and 86°F).
Shake Well Before Using.
Rx Only
U.S. Patent No. 4,686,214

Refer to Section 4
for information on
Contact Lenses.

Allergan, Inc.
2525 DUPONT DRIVE
P.O. BOX 19534
IRVINE, CA 92623-9534

Direct Inquiries to:
(714) 246-4500

ACULAR® ℞

(ketorolac tromethamine ophthalmic solution) 0.5%
Sterile

Description: ACULAR® (ketorolac tromethamine ophthalmic solution) is a member of the pyrrolo-pyrrole group of nonsteroidal anti-inflammatory drugs (NSAIDs) for ophthalmic use. Its chemical name is (±)-5-benzoyl-2, 3-dihydro-1*H*-pyrrolizine-1-carboxylic acid compound with 2-amino-2-(hydroxymethyl)-1,3-propanediol (1:1).

ACULAR® is supplied as a sterile isotonic aqueous 0.5% solution, with a pH of 7.4. ACULAR® is a racemic mixture of R-(+)- and S-(−)- ketorolac tromethamine. Ketorolac tromethamine may exist in three crystal forms. All forms are equally soluble in water. The pKa of ketorolac is 3.5. This white to off-white crystalline substance discolors on prolonged exposure to light. The molecular weight of ketorolac tromethamine is 376.41. The osmolality of ACULAR® is 290 mOsm/kg. Each mL of ACULAR® ophthalmic solution contains: Active: ketorolac tromethamine 0.5%. Preservative: benzalkonium chloride 0.01%. Inactives: edetate disodium 0.1%; octoxynol 40; sodium chloride; hydrochloric acid and/or sodium hydroxide to adjust the pH; and purified water.

Animal Pharmacology: Ketorolac tromethamine prevented the development of increased intraocular pressure induced in rabbits with topically applied arachidonic acid. Ketorolac did not inhibit rabbit lens aldose reductase *in vitro*.

Ketorolac tromethamine ophthalmic solution did not enhance the spread of ocular infections induced in rabbits with *Candida albicans, Herpes simplex* virus type one, or *Pseudomonas aeruginosa*.

Clinical Pharmacology: Ketorolac tromethamine is a nonsteroidal anti-inflammatory drug which, when administered systemically, has demonstrated analgesic, anti-inflammatory, and anti-pyretic activity. The mechanism of its action is thought to be due, in part, to its ability to inhibit prostaglandin biosynthesis. Ketorolac tromethamine given systemically does not cause pupil constriction.

Prostaglandins have been shown in many animal models to be mediators of certain kinds of intraocular inflammation. In studies performed in animal eyes, prostaglandins have been shown to produce disruption of the blood-aqueous humor barrier, vasodilation, increased vascular permeability, leukocytosis, and increased intraocular pressure. Prostaglandins also appear to play a role in the miotic response produced during ocular surgery by constricting the iris sphincter independently of cholinergic mechanisms.

Two drops (0.1 mL) of 0.5% ACULAR® ophthalmic solution instilled into the eyes of patients 12 hours and 1 hour prior to cataract extraction achieved measurable levels in 8 of 9 patients' eyes (mean ketorolac concentration 95 ng/mL aqueous humor, range 40 to 170 ng/mL). Ocular administration of ketorolac tromethamine reduces prostaglandin E_2 (PGE_2) levels in aqueous humor. The mean concentration of PGE_2 was 80 pg/mL in the aqueous humor of eyes receiving vehicle and 28 pg/mL in the eyes receiving ACULAR® 0.5% ophthalmic solution.

One drop (0.05 mL) of 0.5% ACULAR® ophthalmic solution was instilled into one eye and one drop of vehicle into the other eye TID in 26 normal subjects. Only 5 of 26 subjects had a detectable amount of ketorolac in their plasma (range 10.7 to 22.5 ng/mL) at Day 10 during topical ocular treatment. When ketorolac tromethamine 10 mg is administered systemically every 6 hours, peak plasma levels at steady state are around 960 ng/mL.

Two controlled clinical studies showed that ACULAR® ophthalmic solution was significantly more effective than its vehicle in relieving ocular itching caused by seasonal allergic conjunctivitis.

Two controlled clinical studies showed that patients treated for two weeks with ACULAR® ophthalmic solution were less likely to have measurable signs of inflammation (cell and flare) than patients treated with its vehicle.

Results from clinical studies indicated that ACULAR® has no significant effect upon intraocular pressure; however, changes in intraocular pressure may occur following cataract surgery.

ACULAR® ophthalmic solution has been safely administered in conjunction with other ophthalmic medications such as antibiotics, beta blockers, carbonic anhydrase inhibitors, cycloplegics, and mydriatics.

Indications and Usage: ACULAR® is indicated for the temporary relief of ocular itching due to seasonal allergic conjunctivitis. ACULAR® is also indicated for the treatment of postoperative inflammation in patients who have undergone cataract extraction.

Contraindications: ACULAR® ophthalmic solution is contraindicated in patients with previously demonstrated hypersensitivity to any of the ingredients in the formulation.

Warnings: There is the potential for cross-sensitivity to acetylsalicylic acid, phenylacetic acid derivatives, and other nonsteroidal anti-inflammatory agents. Therefore, caution should be used when treating individuals who have previously exhibited sensitivities to these drugs.

With some nonsteroidal anti-inflammatory drugs, there exists the potential for increased bleeding time due to interference with thrombocyte aggregation. There have been reports that ocularly applied nonsteroidal anti-inflammatory drugs may cause increased bleeding of ocular tissues (including hyphemas) in conjunction with ocular surgery.

Precautions:

General: It is recommended that ACULAR® ophthalmic solution be used with caution in patients with known bleeding tendencies or who are receiving other medications which may prolong bleeding time.

Information for Patients: ACULAR® should not be administered while wearing contact lenses.

Carcinogenesis, Mutagenesis, and Impairment of Fertility: An 18-month study in mice at oral doses of ketorolac tromethamine equal to the parenteral MRHD (Maximum Recommended Human Dose) and a 24-month study in rats at oral doses 2.5 times the parenteral MRHD, showed no evidence of tumorigenicity. Ketorolac tromethamine was not mutagenic in Ames test, unscheduled DNA synthesis and repair, and in forward mutation assays. Ketorolac did not cause chromosome breakage in the *in vivo* mouse micronucleus assay. At 1590 ug/mL (approximately 1000 times the average human plasma levels) and at higher concentrations, ketorolac tromethamine increased the incidence of chromosomal aberrations in Chinese hamster ovarian cells.

Impairment of fertility did not occur in male or female rats at oral doses of 9 mg/kg and 16 mg/kg respectively.

Pregnancy: Teratogenic Effects: Pregnancy Category C. Reproduction studies have been performed in rabbits, using daily oral doses at 3.6 mg/kg and in rats at 10 mg/kg during organogenesis. Results of these studies did not reveal evidence of teratogenicity to the fetus. Oral doses of ketorolac tromethamine at 1.5 mg/kg, which was half of the human oral exposure, administered after gestation day 17 caused dystocia and higher pup mortality in rats. There are no adequate and well-controlled studies in pregnant women. Ketorolac tromethamine should be used during pregnancy only if the potential benefit justifies the potential risk to the fetus.

Nonteratogenic Effects: Because of the known effects of prostaglandin-inhibiting drugs on the fetal cardiovascular system (closure of the ductus arteriosus), the use of ACULAR® ophthalmic solution during late pregnancy should be avoided.

Nursing Mothers: Caution should be exercised when ACULAR® is administered to a nursing woman.

Pediatric Use: Safety and efficacy in pediatric patients below the age of 12 have not been established.

Adverse Reactions: In controlled clinical studies, the most frequent adverse events reported with the use of ACULAR® ophthalmic solution have been transient stinging and burning on instillation. These events were reported by approximately 40% of patients treated with ACULAR® ophthalmic solution. In all development studies conducted, other adverse events occurring less than 5% of the time during treatment with ACULAR® included ocular irritation, allergic reactions, superficial ocular infections, and superficial keratitis.

Other adverse events reported rarely with the use of ACULAR® ophthalmic solution include: eye dryness, corneal infiltrates, corneal ulcer, and visual disturbance (blurry vision).

Dosage and Administration: The recommended dose of ACULAR® ophthalmic solution is one drop (0.25 mg) four times a day for relief of ocular itching due to seasonal allergic conjunctivitis.

For the treatment of postoperative inflammation in patients who have undergone cataract extraction, one drop of ACULAR® ophthalmic solution should be applied to the affected eye(s) four times daily beginning 24 hours after cataract surgery and continuing through the first 2 weeks of the postoperative period.

How Supplied: ACULAR® (ketorolac tromethamine ophthalmic solution) is available for topical ophthalmic administration as a 0.5% sterile solution, and is supplied in white opaque plastic bottles with controlled dropper tip in the following sizes:

3 mL—NDC 0023-2181-03
5 mL—NDC 0023-2181-05
10 mL—NDC 0023-2181-10

Store at controlled room temperature 15–30°C (59–86°F) with protection from light.

Rx only

U.S. Patent Nos. 4,089,969; 4,454,151; 5,110,493

ALLERGAN
Irvine, CA 92612

Shown in Product Identification Guide, page 103

ACULAR® PF ℞
(ketorolac tromethamine ophthalmic solution) 0.5%
Preservative-Free

Description: ACULAR® PF (ketorolac tromethamine ophthalmic solution) Preservative-Free is a member of the pyrrolo-pyrrole group of nonsteroidal anti-inflammatory drugs (NSAIDs) for ophthalmic use. Ketorolac tromethamine's chemical name is (±)-5-benzoyl-2,3-dihydro-1H pyrrolizine-1-carboxylic acid compound with 2-amino-2-(hydroxymethyl)-1,3-propanediol (1:1)
ACULAR® PF is a racemic mixture of R-(+) and S-(-)-ketorolac tromethamine. Ketorolac tromethamine may exist in three crystal forms. All forms are equally soluble in water. The pKa of ketorolac is 3.5. This white to off-white crystalline substance discolors on prolonged exposure to light. The molecular weight of ketorolac tromethamine is 376.41. The osmolality of ACULAR® PF is 290 mOsmol/kg. Each ml of ACULAR® PF contains: Active ingredient: ketorolac tromethamine 0.5%. Inactives: sodium chloride; hydrochloric acid and/or sodium hydroxide to adjust the pH to 7.4; and purified water.
Clinical Pharmacology: Ketorolac tromethamine is a nonsteroidal anti-inflammatory drug which, when administered systemically, has demonstrated analgesic, anti-inflammatory, and anti-pyretic activity. The mechanism of its action is thought to be due to its ability to inhibit prostaglandin biosynthesis. Ketorolac tromethamine given systemically does not cause pupil constriction.
One drop (0.05 mL) of ketorolac tromethamine (preserved) was instilled into one eye and one drop of vehicle into the other eye TID in 26 normal subjects. Only 5 of 26 subjects had a detectable amount of ketorolac in their plasma (range 10.7 to 22.5 ng/mL) at day 10 during topical ocular treatment. When ketorolac tromethamine 10 mg is administered systemically every 6 hours, peak plasma levels at steady state are around 960 ng/mL.
In two double-masked, multi-centered, parallel-group studies, 340 patients who had undergone incisional refractive surgery received ACULAR® PF or its vehicle QID for up to 3 days. Significant differences favored ACULAR® PF for the treatment of ocular pain and photophobia.
Results from clinical studies indicate that ketorolac tromethamine has no significant effect upon intraocular pressure.
Indications and Usage: ACULAR® PF ophthalmic solution is indicated for the reduction of ocular pain and photophobia following incisional refractive surgery.
Contraindications: ACULAR® PF is contraindicated in patients with previously demonstrated hypersensitivity to any of the ingredients in the formulation.
Warnings: There is the potential for cross-sensitivity to acetylsalicylic acid, phenylacetic acid derivatives, and other nonsteroidal anti-inflammatory agents. Therefore, caution should be used when treating individuals who have previously exhibited sensitivities to these drugs.
With some nonsteroidal anti-inflammatory drugs, there exists the potential for increased bleeding time due to interference with thrombocyte aggregation. There have been reports that ocularly applied nonsteroidal anti-inflammatory drugs may cause increased bleeding of ocular tissues (including hyphemas) in conjunction with ocular surgery.
Precautions
General: It is recommended that ACULAR® PF be used with caution in surgical patients with known bleeding tendencies or who are receiving other medications which may prolong bleeding time.
Wound healing may be delayed with the use of ACULAR® PF.
Information for Patients: ACULAR® PF should not be administered while wearing contact lenses.
The solution from one individual single-use vial is to be used immediately after opening for administration to one or both eyes, and the remaining contents should be discarded immediately after administration. To avoid contamination, do not touch tip of unit-dose vial to eye or any other surface.
Carcinogenesis, Mutagenesis, and Impairment of Fertility: An 18-month study in mice at oral doses of ketorolac tromethamine equal to the parenteral MRHD (Maximum Recommended Human Dose) and a 24-month study in rats at oral doses 2.5 times the parenteral MRHD, showed no evidence of tumorigenicity.
Ketorolac tromethamine was not mutagenic in the Ames test, unscheduled DNA synthesis and repair, and forward mutation assays. Ketorolac did not cause chromosome breakage in the *in vivo* mouse micronucleus assay. At 1590 µg/mL (approximately 1000 times the average human plasma levels) and at higher concentrations, ketorolac tromethamine increased the incidence of chromosomal aberrations in Chinese hamster ovarian cells. Impairment of fertility did not occur in male or female rats at oral doses of 9 mg/kg and 16 mg/kg, respectively.
Pregnancy: Teratogenic Effects: Pregnancy Category C: Reproduction studies have been performed in rabbits, using daily oral doses at 3.6 mg/kg and in rats at 10 mg/kg during organogenesis. Results of these studies did not reveal evidence of teratogenicity to the fetus. Oral doses of ketorolac tromethamine at 1.5 mg/kg, which was half of the human oral exposure, administered after gestation day 17 caused dystocia and higher pup mortality in rats. There are no adequate and well-controlled studies in pregnant women. Ketorolac tromethamine should be used during pregnancy only if the potential benefit justifies the potential risk to the fetus.
Nonteratogenic Effects: Because of the known effects of prostaglandin-inhibiting drugs on the fetal cardiovascular system (closure of the ductus arteriosus), the use of ACULAR® PF during late pregnancy should be avoided.
Nursing Mothers: Caution should be exercised when ACULAR® PF is administered to a nursing woman.
Pediatric Use: Safety and efficacy in pediatric patients below the age of 12 years have not been established.
Adverse Reactions: The most frequent adverse events reported with the use of ketorolac tromethamine ophthalmic solutions have been transient stinging and burning on instillation. These events were reported by approximately 20% of patients participating in clinical trials.
Other adverse events occurring 1%–10% of the time during treatment with ketorolac tromethamine ophthalmic solutions included ocular irritation, allergic reactions, superficial ocular infections, superficial keratitis, ocular inflammation, corneal edema, and iritis.
Other adverse events reported rarely with the use of ketorolac tromethamine ophthalmic solutions include: eye dryness, corneal infiltrates, corneal ulcer, visual disturbance (blurry vision), and headaches.
Dosage And Administration: The recommended dose of ACULAR® PF Preservative-Free is one drop (0.25 mg) four times a day in the operated eye as needed for pain and photophobia for up to 3 days after incisional refractive surgery.
How Supplied: ACULAR® PF (ketorolac tromethamine ophthalmic solution) 0.5% Preservative-Free is available as a sterile solution supplied in single-use vials as follows:
ACULAR® PF 12 Single-Use Vials 0.4 mL each - NDC 0023-9055-04. Store ACULAR® PF between 15°C–30°C (59°F–86°F) with protection from light.
Rx only
U.S. Patent Nos. 4,089,969; 4,454,151; 5,110,493

November 1997
Shown in Product Identification Guide, page 103

ALBALON® ℞
(naphazoline hydrochloride ophthalmic solution) 0.1%
with LIQUIFILM® (polyvinyl alcohol) 1.4%
sterile

Description: Naphazoline hydrochloride, an ocular vasoconstrictor, is an imidazoline derivative sympathomimetic amine. It occurs as a white, odorless crystalline powder having a bitter taste and is freely soluble in water and in alcohol.
Chemical Name: 2-(1-Naphthylmethyl)-2-imidazoline monohydrochloride
Contains: Active: naphazoline HCl 0.1%. Preservative: benzalkonium chloride 0.004%. Inactives: LIQUIFILM® (polyvinyl alcohol) 1.4%; edetate disodium; citric acid, monohydrate; sodium citrate, dihydrate; sodium chloride; sodium hydroxide to adjust the pH; and purified water. It has a pH of 5.5 to 7.0.
Clinical Pharmacology: Naphazoline constricts the vascular system of the conjunctiva. It is presumed that this effect is due to direct stimulation action of the drug upon the alpha-adrenergic receptors in the arterioles of the conjunctiva, resulting in decreased conjunctival congestion. Naphazoline belongs to the imidazoline class of sympathomimetics.
Indications and Usage: ALBALON® ophthalmic solution is indicated for use as a topical ocular vasoconstrictor.
Contraindications: ALBALON® ophthalmic solution is contraindicated in the presence of an anatomically narrow angle or in narrow-angle glaucoma or in persons who have shown hypersensitivity to any component of this preparation.
Warnings: Patients under therapy with MAO inhibitors may experience a severe hypertensive crisis if given a sympathomimetic drug. Use in children, especially infants, may result in CNS depression leading to coma and marked reduction in body temperature.
Precautions:
General: Use with caution in the presence of hypertension, cardiovascular abnormalities, hyperglycemia (diabetes), hyperthyroidism, infection or injury.
Patient Information: Patients should be advised to discontinue the drug and consult a physician if relief is not obtained within 48 hours of therapy, if irritation, blurring or redness persists or increases, or if symptoms of systemic absorption occur, i.e., dizziness, headache, nausea, decrease in body temperature, or drowsiness.
To prevent contaminating the dropper tip and solution, do not touch the eyelids or the surrounding area with the dropper tip of the bottle. If solution changes color or becomes cloudy, do not use.
Drug Interactions: Concurrent use of maprotiline or tricyclic antidepressants and naphaz-

Continued on next page

Albalon—Cont.

oline may potentiate the pressor effect of naphazoline. Patients under therapy with MAO inhibitors may experience a severe hypertensive crisis if given a sympathomimetic drug. (See **Warnings**).

Pregnancy: Pregnancy Category C: Animal reproduction studies have not been conducted with naphazoline. It is also not known whether naphazoline can cause fetal harm when administered to a pregnant woman or can affect reproduction capacity. Naphazoline should be given to a pregnant woman only if clearly needed.

Nursing Mothers: It is not known whether naphazoline is excreted in human milk. Because many drugs are excreted in human milk, caution should be exercised when naphazoline is administered to a nursing woman.

Pediatric Use: Safety and effectiveness in pediatric patients have not been established. See "**Warnings**" AND "**Contraindications**."

Adverse Reactions:

Ocular: Mydriasis, increased redness, irritation, discomfort, blurring, punctate keratitis, lacrimation, increased intraocular pressure.

Systemic: Dizziness, headache, nausea, sweating, nervousness, drowsiness, weakness, hypertension, cardiac irregularities, and hyperglycemia.

Dosage and Administration: Instill one or two drops in the conjunctival sac(s) every three to four hours as needed.

How Supplied: ALBALON® (naphazoline hydrochloride ophthalmic solution) 0.1% with LIQUIFILM® (polyvinyl alcohol) 1.4% is supplied sterile in plastic dropper bottles in the following sizes:

5 mL—NDC 11980-154-05
15 mL—NDC 11980-154-15

Note: Store at room temperature.

Rx only

ALPHAGAN® ℞

(brimonidine tartrate ophthalmic solution) 0.2%

Description: ALPHAGAN® (brimonidine tartrate ophthalmic solution) 0.2% is a relatively selective alpha-2 adrenergic agonist for ophthalmic use. The chemical name of brimonidine tartrate is 5-bromo-6-(2-imidazolidinylideneamino) quinoxaline L-tartrate. It is an off-white, pale yellow to pale pink powder. In solution, ALPHAGAN® has a clear, greenish-yellow color. It has a molecular weight of 442.24 as the tartrate salt and is water soluble (34 mg/mL). The molecular formula is $C_{11}H_{10}BrN_5 \cdot C_4H_6O_6$.

ALPHAGAN® (brimonidine tartrate ophthalmic solution) 0.2% is a sterile ophthalmic solution. Each mL of ALPHAGAN® Solution contains: **Active:** brimonidine tartrate 2 mg (equivalent to 1.32 mg as brimonidine free base). **Preservative:** benzalkonium chloride (0.05 mg). **Inactives:** polyvinyl alcohol; sodium chloride; sodium citrate; citric acid; and purified water. Hydrochloric acid and/or sodium hydroxide may be added to adjust pH (6.3–6.5).

Clinical Pharmacology:

Mechanism of Action: ALPHAGAN® is an alpha adrenergic receptor agonist. It has a peak ocular hypotensive effect occurring at two hours post-dosing. Fluorophotometric studies in animals and humans suggest that brimonidine tartrate has a dual mechanism of action by reducing aqueous humor production and increasing uveoscleral outflow.

Pharmacokinetics: After ocular administration of a 0.2% solution, plasma concentrations peaked within 1 to 4 hours and declined with a systemic half-life of approximately 3 hours. In humans, systemic metabolism of brimonidine is extensive. It is metabolized primarily by the liver. Urinary excretion is the major route of elimination of the drug and its metabolites. Approximately 87% of an orally-administered radioactive dose was eliminated within 120 hours, with 74% found in the urine.

Clinical Studies: Elevated IOP presents a major risk factor in glaucomatous field loss. The higher the level of IOP, the greater the likelihood of optic nerve damage and visual field loss. ALPHAGAN® has the action of lowering intraocular pressure with minimal effect on cardiovascular and pulmonary parameters. In comparative clinical studies with timolol 0.5%, lasting up to one year, the IOP lowering effect of ALPHAGAN® was approximately 4–6 mm Hg compared with approximately 6 mm Hg for timolol. In these studies, both patient groups were dosed BID, however, due to the duration of action of ALPHAGAN®, it is recommended that ALPHAGAN® be dosed TID. Eight percent of subjects were discontinued from studies due to inadequately controlled intraocular pressure, which in 30% of these patients occurred during the first month of therapy. Approximately 20% were discontinued due to adverse experiences.

Indications and Usage: ALPHAGAN® is indicated for lowering intraocular pressure in patients with open-angle glaucoma or ocular hypertension. The IOP lowering efficacy of ALPHAGAN® Ophthalmic Solution diminishes over time in some patients. This loss of effect appears with a variable time of onset in each patient and should be closely monitored.

Contraindications: ALPHAGAN® is contraindicated in patients with hypersensitivity to brimonidine tartrate or any component of this medication. It is also contraindicated in patients receiving monoamine oxidase (MAO) inhibitor therapy.

Precautions:

General: Although ALPHAGAN® had minimal effect on blood pressure of patients in clinical studies, caution should be exercised in treating patients with severe cardiovascular disease. ALPHAGAN® has not been studied in patients with hepatic or renal impairment; caution should be used in treating such patients. ALPHAGAN® should be used with caution in patients with depression, cerebral or coronary insufficiency, Raynaud's phenomenon, orthostatic hypotension or thromboangiitis obliterans. During the studies there was a loss of effect in some patients. The IOP-lowering efficacy observed with ALPHAGAN® Ophthalmic Solution during the first month may not always reflect the long-term level of IOP reduction. Patients prescribed IOP-lowering medication should be routinely monitored for IOP.

Information for Patients: The preservative in ALPHAGAN®, benzalkonium chloride, may be absorbed by soft contact lenses. Patients wearing soft contact lenses should be instructed to wait at least 15 minutes after instilling ALPHAGAN® to insert soft contact lenses.

As with other drugs in this class, ALPHAGAN® may cause fatigue and/or drowsiness in some patients. Patients who engage in hazardous activities should be cautioned of the potential for a decrease in mental alertness.

Drug Interactions: Although specific drug interaction studies have not been conducted with ALPHAGAN®, the possibility of an additive or potentiating effect with CNS depressants (alcohol, barbiturates, opiates, sedatives or anesthetics) should be considered. ALPHAGAN® did not have significant effects on pulse and blood pressure in clinical studies. However, since alpha-agonists, as a class, may reduce pulse and blood pressure, caution in using concomitant drugs such as beta-blockers (ophthalmic and systemic), antihypertensives and/or cardiac glycosides is advised. Tricyclic antidepressants have been reported to blunt the hypotensive effect of systemic clonidine. It is not known whether the concurrent use of these agents with ALPHAGAN® can lead to an interference in IOP lowering effect. No data on the level of circulating catecholamines after ALPHAGAN® is instilled are available. Caution, however, is advised in patients taking tricyclic antidepressants which can affect the metabolism and uptake of circulating amines.

Carcinogenesis, Mutagenesis, Impairment of Fertility: No compound-related carcinogenic effects were observed in 21 month and 2 year studies in mice and rats given oral doses of 2.5 mg/kg/day (as the free base) and 1.0 mg/kg/day, respectively (77 and 118 times, respectively, the human plasma drug concentration following the recommended ophthalmic dose). ALPHAGAN® was not mutagenic or cytogenic in a series of *in vitro* and *in vivo* studies including the Ames test, host-mediated assay, chromosomal aberration assay in Chinese Hamster Ovary (CHO) cells, cytogenic studies in mice and dominant lethal assay.

Pregnancy: Teratogenic Effects: Pregnancy Category B: Reproduction studies performed in rats with oral doses of 0.66 mg base/kg revealed no evidence of impaired fertility or harm to the fetus due to ALPHAGAN®. Dosing at this level produced 100 times the plasma drug concentration level seen in humans following multiple ophthalmic doses. There are no studies of ALPHAGAN® in pregnant women, however in animal studies, brimonidine crossed the placenta and entered into the fetal circulation to a limited extent. ALPHAGAN® should be used during pregnancy only if the potential benefit to the mother justifies the potential risk to the fetus.

Nursing Mothers: It is not known whether ALPHAGAN® is excreted in human milk, although in animal studies, brimonidine tartrate has been shown to be excreted in breast milk. A decision should be made whether to discontinue nursing or to discontinue the drug, taking into account the importance of the drug to the mother.

Pediatric Use: Safety and effectiveness in pediatric patients have not been established. Symptoms of bradycardia, hypotension, hypothermia, hypotonia and apnea have been reported in neonates receiving brimonidine.

Adverse Reactions: Adverse events occurring in approximately 10–30% of the subjects, in descending order of incidence, included oral dryness, ocular hyperemia, burning and stinging, headache, blurring, foreign body sensation, fatigue/drowsiness, conjunctival follicles, ocular allergic reactions, and ocular pruritus. Events occurring in approximately 3–9% of the subjects, in descending order included corneal staining/erosion, photophobia, eyelid erythema, ocular ache/pain, ocular dryness, tearing, upper respiratory symptoms, eyelid edema, conjunctival edema, dizziness, blepharitis, ocular irritation, gastrointestinal symptoms, asthenia, conjunctival blanching, abnormal vision and muscular pain. The following adverse reactions were reported in less than 3% of the patients: lid crusting, conjunctival hemorrhage, abnormal taste, insomnia, conjunctival discharge, depression, hypertension, anxiety, palpitations, nasal dryness and syncope.

Overdosage: No information is available on overdosage in humans. Treatment of an oral overdose includes supportive and symptomatic therapy; a patent airway should be maintained.

Dosage and Administration: The recommended dose is one drop of ALPHAGAN® in the affected eye(s) three times daily, approximately 8 hours apart.

How Supplied: ALPHAGAN® (brimonidine tartrate ophthalmic solution) 0.2% is supplied sterile in white opaque plastic dropper bottles as follows:

5 mL	NDC 0023-8665-05
10 mL	NDC 0023-8665-10
15 mL	NDC 0023-8665-15

Note: Store at or below 25° C (77° F).

Rx only.

ALLERGAN

Shown in Product Identification Guide, page 103

BETAGAN® ℞
(levobunolol HCl)
Liquifilm®
sterile ophthalmic solution
with C CAP® Compliance Cap Q.D. and B.I.D.

Description: BETAGAN® (levobunolol HCl) Liquifilm® sterile ophthalmic solution is a noncardioselective beta-adrenoceptor blocking agent for ophthalmic use.

Chemical Name: (-)-5-[3-(tert-Butylamino)2-hydroxypropoxy]-3,4-dihydro-1(2H)-naphthalenone hydrochloride.

BETAGAN® 0.25% and 0.5% contains: Active: levobunolol HCl 0.25% or 0.5%. Preservative: benzalkonium chloride (0.004%). Inactives: Liquifilm® (polyvinyl alcohol) 1.4%; edetate disodium; sodium metabisulfite; sodium phosphate, dibasic; potassium phosphate, monobasic; sodium chloride; hydrochloric acid or sodium hydroxide to adjust the pH; and purified water.

Clinical Pharmacology: Levobunolol HCl is a noncardioselective beta-adrenoceptor blocking agent, equipotent at both $beta_1$ and $beta_2$ receptors. Levobunolol HCl is greater than 60 times more potent than its dextro isomer in its beta-blocking activity, yet equipotent in its potential for direct myocardial depression. Accordingly, the levo isomer, levobunolol HCl, is used. Levobunolol HCl does not have significant local anesthetic (membrane-stabilizing) or intrinsic sympathomimetic activity.

Beta-adrenergic receptor blockade reduces cardiac output in both healthy subjects and patients with heart disease. In patients with severe impairment of myocardial function, beta-adrenergic receptor blockade may inhibit the stimulatory effect of the sympathetic nervous system necessary to maintain adequate cardiac function.

Beta-adrenergic receptor blockade in the bronchi and bronchioles results in increased airway resistance from unopposed para-sympathetic activity. Such an effect in patients with asthma or other bronchospastic conditions is potentially dangerous.

BETAGAN® (levobunolol HCl) has been shown to be an active agent in lowering elevated as well as normal intraocular pressure (IOP) whether or not accompanied by glaucoma. Elevated IOP presents a major risk factor in glaucomatous field loss. The higher the level of IOP, the greater the likelihood of optic nerve damage and visual field loss.

The onset of action with one drop of BETAGAN® can be detected within one hour after treatment, with maximum effect seen between 2 and 6 hours.

A significant decrease in IOP can be maintained for up to 24 hours following a single dose.

In two separate, controlled studies (one three month and one up to 12 months duration) BETAGAN® 0.25% b.i.d. controlled the IOP of approximately 64% and 70% of the subjects. The overall mean decrease from baseline was 5.4 mm Hg and 5.1 mm Hg respectively. In an open-label study, BETAGAN® 0.25% q.d. controlled the IOP of 72% of the subjects while achieving an overall mean decrease of 5.9 mm Hg.

In controlled clinical studies of approximately two years duration, intraocular pressure was well-controlled in approximately 80% of subjects treated with BETAGAN® 0.5% b.i.d. The mean IOP decrease from baseline was between 6.87 mm Hg and 7.81 mm Hg. No significant effects on pupil size, tear production or corneal sensitivity were observed. BETAGAN® at the concentrations tested, when applied topically, decreased heart rate and blood pressure in some patients. The IOP-lowering effect of BETAGAN® was well maintained over the course of these studies.

In a three month clinical study, a single daily application of 0.5% BETAGAN® controlled the IOP of 72% of subjects achieving an overall mean decrease in IOP of 7.0 mm Hg.

The primary mechanism of the ocular hypotensive action of levobunolol HCl in reducing IOP is most likely a decrease in aqueous humor production. BETAGAN® reduces IOP with little or no effect on pupil size or accommodation in contrast to the miosis which cholinergic agents are known to produce. The blurred vision and night blindness often associated with miotics would not be expected and have not been reported with the use of BETAGAN®. This is particularly important in cataract patients with central lens opacities who would experience decreased visual acuity with pupillary constriction.

Indications and Usage: BETAGAN® has been shown to be effective in lowering intraocular pressure and may be used in patients with chronic open-angle glaucoma or ocular hypertension.

Contraindications: BETAGAN® is contraindicated in those individuals with bronchial asthma or with a history of bronchial asthma, or severe chronic obstructive pulmonary disease (see WARNINGS); sinus bradycardia; second and third degree atrioventricular block; overt cardiac failure (see WARNINGS); cardiogenic shock; or hypersensitivity to any component of these products.

Warnings: As with other topically applied ophthalmic drugs, BETAGAN® may be absorbed systemically. The same adverse reactions found with systemic administration of beta-adrenergic blocking agents may occur with topical administration. For example, severe respiratory reactions and cardiac reactions, including death due to bronchospasm in patients with asthma, and rarely death in association with cardiac failure, have been reported with topical application of beta-adrenergic blocking agents (see CONTRAINDICATIONS).

Cardiac Failure: Sympathetic stimulation may be essential for support of the circulation in individuals with diminished myocardial contractility, and its inhibition by beta-adrenergic receptor blockade may precipitate more severe failure.

In Patients Without a History of Cardiac Failure: Continued depression of the myocardium with beta-blocking agents over a period of time can, in some cases, lead to cardiac failure. At the first sign or symptom of cardiac failure, BETAGAN® should be discontinued.

Obstructive Pulmonary Disease:
PATIENTS WITH CHRONIC OBSTRUCTIVE PULMONARY DISEASE (e.g., CHRONIC BRONCHITIS, EMPHYSEMA) OF MILD OR MODERATE SEVERITY, BRONCHOSPASTIC DISEASE OR A HISTORY OF BRONCHOSPASTIC DISEASE (OTHER THAN BRONCHIAL ASTHMA OR A HISTORY OF BRONCHIAL ASTHMA, IN WHICH BETAGAN® IS CONTRAINDICATED, See CONTRAINDICATIONS), SHOULD IN GENERAL NOT RECEIVE BETA BLOCKERS, INCLUDING BETAGAN®. However, if BETAGAN® is deemed necessary in such patients, then it should be administered cautiously since it may block bronchodilation produced by endogenous and exogenous catecholamine stimulation of $beta_2$ receptors.

Major Surgery: The necessity or desirability of withdrawal of beta-adrenergic blocking agents prior to major surgery is controversial. Beta-adrenergic receptor blockade impairs the ability of the heart to respond to beta-adrenergically mediated reflex stimuli. This may augment the risk of general anesthesia in surgical procedures. Some patients receiving beta-adrenergic receptor blocking agents have been subject to protracted severe hypotension during anesthesia. Difficulty in restarting and maintaining the heartbeat has also been reported. For these reasons, in patients undergoing elective surgery, gradual withdrawal of beta-adrenergic receptor blocking agents may be appropriate.

If necessary during surgery, the effects of beta-adrenergic blocking agents may be reversed by sufficient doses of such agonists as isoproterenol, dopamine, dobutamine or levarterenol (See OVERDOSAGE).

Diabetes Mellitus: Beta-adrenergic blocking agents should be administered with caution in patients subject to spontaneous hypoglycemia or to diabetic patients (especially those with labile diabetes) who are receiving insulin or oral hypoglycemic agents. Beta-adrenergic receptor blocking agents may mask the signs and symptoms of acute hypoglycemia.

Thyrotoxicosis: Beta-adrenergic blocking agents may mask certain clinical signs (e.g., tachycardia) of hyperthyroidism. Patients suspected of developing thyrotoxicosis should be managed carefully to avoid abrupt withdrawal of beta-adrenergic blocking agents, which might precipitate a thyroid storm.

These products contain sodium metabisulfite, a sulfite that may cause allergic-type reactions including anaphylactic symptoms and life-threatening or less severe asthmatic episodes in certain susceptible people. The overall prevalence of sulfite sensitivity in the general population is unknown and probably low. Sulfite sensitivity is seen more frequently in asthmatic than in nonasthmatic people.

Precautions:

General: BETAGAN® should be used with caution in patients with known hypersensitivity to other beta-adrenoceptor blocking agents. Use with caution in patients with known diminished pulmonary function.

BETAGAN® should be used with caution in patients who are receiving a beta-adrenergic blocking agent orally, because of the potential for additive effects on systemic beta-blockade or on intraocular pressure. Patients should not typically use two or more topical ophthalmic beta-adrenergic blocking agents simultaneously.

Because of the potential effects of beta-adrenergic blocking agents on blood pressure and pulse rates, these medications must be used cautiously in patients with cerebrovascular insufficiency. Should signs or symptoms develop that suggest reduced cerebral blood flow while using BETAGAN®, alternative therapy should be considered.

In patients with angle-closure glaucoma, the immediate objective of treatment is to reopen the angle. This requires, in most cases, constricting the pupil with a miotic. BETAGAN® has little or no effect on the pupil. When BETAGAN® is used to reduce elevated intraocular pressure in angle-closure glaucoma, it should be followed with a miotic and not alone.

Muscle Weakness: Beta-adrenergic blockade has been reported to potentiate muscle weakness consistent with certain myasthenic symp-

Continued on next page

Betagan—Cont.

toms (e.g., diplopia, ptosis and generalized weakness).

Drug Interactions: Although BETAGAN® used alone has little or no effect on pupil size, mydriasis resulting from concomitant therapy with BETAGAN® and epinephrine may occur. Close observation of the patient is recommended when a beta-blocker is administered to patients receiving catecholamine-depleting drugs such as reserpine, because of possible additive effects and the production of hypotension and/or marked bradycardia, which may produce vertigo, syncope, or postural hypotension.

Patients receiving beta-adrenergic blocking agents along with either oral or intravenous calcium antagonists should be monitored for possible atrioventricular conduction disturbances, left ventricular failure and hypotension. In patients with impaired cardiac function, simultaneous use should be avoided altogether.

The concomitant use of beta-adrenergic blocking agents with digitalis and calcium antagonists may have additive effects on prolonging atrioventricular conduction time.

Phenothiazine-related compounds and beta-adrenergic blocking agents may have additive hypotensive effects due to the inhibition of each other's metabolism.

Risk of anaphylactic reaction: While taking beta-blockers, patients with a history of severe anaphylactic reaction to a variety of allergens may be more reactive to repeated challenge, either accidental, diagnostic, or therapeutic. Such patients may be unresponsive to the usual doses of epinephrine used to treat allergic reaction.

Animal Studies: No adverse ocular effects were observed in rabbits administered BETAGAN® topically in studies lasting one year in concentrations up to 10 times the human dose concentration.

Carcinogenesis, mutagenesis, impairment of fertility: In a lifetime oral study in mice, there were statistically significant ($p \leq 0.05$) increases in the incidence of benign leiomyomas in female mice at 200 mg/kg/day (14,000 times the recommended human dose for glaucoma), but not at 12 or 50 mg/kg/day (850 and 3,500 times the human dose). In a two-year oral study of levobunolol HCl in rats, there was a statistically significant ($p \leq 0.05$) increase in the incidence of benign hepatomas in male rats administered 12,800 times the recommended human dose for glaucoma. Similar differences were not observed in rats administered oral doses equivalent to 350 times to 2,000 times the recommended human dose for glaucoma.

Levobunolol did not show evidence of mutagenic activity in a battery of microbiological and mammalian *in vitro* and *in vivo* assays.

Reproduction and fertility studies in rats showed no adverse effect on male or female fertility at doses up to 1,800 times the recommended human dose for glaucoma.

Pregnancy Category C: Fetotoxicity (as evidenced by a greater number of resorption sites) has been observed in rabbits when doses of levobunolol HCl equivalent to 200 and 700 times the recommended dose for the treatment of glaucoma were given. No fetotoxic effects have been observed in similar studies with rats at up to 1,800 times the human dose for glaucoma. Teratogenic studies with levobunolol in rats at doses up to 25 mg/kg/day (1,800 times the recommended human dose for glaucoma) showed no evidence of fetal malformations. There were no adverse effects on postnatal development of offspring. It appears when results from studies using rats and studies with other beta-adrenergic blockers are examined, that the rabbit may be a particularly sensitive species. There are no adequate and well controlled studies in pregnant women. BETAGAN® should be used during pregnancy only if the potential benefit justifies the potential risk to the fetus.

Nursing Mothers: It is not known whether this drug is excreted in human milk. Systemic beta-blockers and topical timolol maleate are known to be excreted in human milk. Caution should be exercised when BETAGAN® is administered to a nursing woman.

Pediatric Use: Safety and effectiveness in pediatric patients have not been established.

Adverse Reactions: In clinical trials, the use of BETAGAN® has been associated with transient ocular burning and stinging in up to 1 in 3 patients, and with blepharoconjunctivitis in up to 1 in 20 patients. Decreases in heart rate and blood pressure have been reported (see CONTRAINDICATIONS and WARNINGS).

The following adverse effects have been reported rarely with the use of BETAGAN®: iridocyclitis, headache, transient ataxia, dizziness, lethargy, urticaria and pruritus.

Decreased corneal sensitivity has been noted in a small number of patients. Although levobunolol has minimal membrane-stabilizing activity, there remains a possibility of decreased corneal sensitivity after prolonged use.

The following additional adverse reactions have been reported either with BETAGAN® or ophthalmic use of other beta-adrenergic receptor blocking agents:

BODY AS A WHOLE: Headache, asthenia, chest pain. **CARDIOVASCULAR:** Bradycardia, arrhythmia, hypotension, syncope, heart block, cerebral vascular accident, cerebral ischemia, congestive heart failure, palpitation, cardiac arrest. **DIGESTIVE:** Nausea, diarrhea. **PSYCHIATRIC:** Depression, confusion, increase in signs and symptoms of myasthenia gravis, paresthesia. **SKIN:** Hypersensitivity, including localized and generalized rash, alopecia, Stevens-Johnson Syndrome. **RESPIRATORY:** Bronchospasm (predominantly in patients with pre-existing bronchospastic disease), respiratory failure, dyspnea, nasal congestion. **UROGENITAL: Impotence. ENDOCRINE:** Masked symptoms of hypoglycemia in insulin-dependent diabetics (see WARNINGS). **SPECIAL SENSES:** Signs and symptoms of keratitis, blepharoptosis, visual disturbances including refractive changes (due to withdrawal of miotic therapy in some cases), diplopia, ptosis. Other reactions associated with the oral use of non-selective adrenergic receptor blocking agents should be considered potential effects with ophthalmic use of these agents.

Overdosage: No data are available regarding overdosage in humans. Should accidental ocular overdosage occur, flush eye(s) with water or normal saline. If accidentally ingested, efforts to decrease further absorption may be appropriate (gastric lavage). The most common signs and symptoms to be expected with overdosage with administration of a systemic beta-adrenergic blocking agent are symptomatic bradycardia, hypotension, bronchospasm, and acute cardiac failure. Should these symptoms occur, discontinue BETAGAN® therapy and initiate appropriate supportive therapy. The following supportive measures should be considered:

1. Symptomatic bradycardia: Use atropine sulfate intravenously in a dosage of 0.25 mg to 2 mg to induce vagal blockade. If bradycardia persists, intravenous isoproterenol hydrochloride should be administered cautiously. In refractory cases, the use of a transvenous cardiac pacemaker should be considered.
2. Hypotension: Use sympathomimetic pressor drug therapy, such as dopamine, dobutamine or levarterenol. In refractory cases, the use of glucagon hydrochloride may be useful.
3. Bronchospasm: Use isoproterenol hydrochloride. Additional therapy with aminophylline may be considered.
4. Acute cardiac failure: Conventional therapy with digitalis, diuretics and oxygen should be instituted immediately. In refractory cases, the use of intravenous aminophylline is suggested. This may be followed, if necessary, by glucagon hydrochloride, which may be useful.
5. Heart block (second or third degree): Use isoproterenol hydrochloride or a transvenous cardiac pacemaker.

Dosage and Administration: The recommended starting dose is one to two drops of BETAGAN® 0.5% in the affected eye(s) once a day. Typical dosing with BETAGAN® 0.25% is one to two drops twice daily. In patients with more severe or uncontrolled glaucoma, BETAGAN® 0.5% can be administered b.i.d. As with any new medication, careful monitoring of patients is advised. Dosages above one drop of BETAGAN® 0.5% b.i.d. are not generally more effective. If the patient's IOP is not at a satisfactory level on this regimen, concomitant therapy with dipivefrin and/or epinephrine, and/or pilocarpine and other miotics, and/or systemically administered carbonic anhydrase inhibitors, such as acetazolamide, can be instituted. Patients should not typically use two or more topical ophthalmic beta-adrenergic blocking agents simultaneously.

How Supplied: BETAGAN® (levobunolol HCl) Liquifilm® sterile ophthalmic solution is supplied in white opaque plastic dropper bottles as follows:

BETAGAN 0.25%:
C CAP® Compliance Cap
B.I.D. (twice daily)
5 mL—NDC 11980-469-25
10 mL—NDC 11980-469-20

BETAGAN 0.5%:
Standard Cap
2 mL—NDC 11980-252-02
C CAP® Compliance Cap
Q.D. (once daily)
5 mL—NDC 11980-252-65
10 mL—NDC 11980-252-60
15 mL—NDC 11980-252-61
C CAP® Compliance Cap
B.I.D. (twice daily)
5 mL—NDC 11980-252-25
10 mL—NDC 11980-252-20
15 mL—NDC 11980-252-21

NOTE: Protect from light. Store at controlled room temperature 15°–30°C (59°–86°F).

Rx only

C CAP® Compliance Cap Patient Instructions

Instructions for use:

1. On the first usage, make sure the number "1" or the correct day of the week appears in the window. If not, click the cap to the right station.
2. Remove the cap and apply medication.
3. Replace the cap. Hold the C CAP® between your thumb and forefinger. Now rotate the bottle until the cap clicks to the next station.
4. When it's time to take your next dose, repeat steps 2 and 3.

Don't try to catch up on missed doses by applying more than one dose at a time. Each time you replace the cap, turn it until you hear the click. The number in the window specifies your next dosage.

Shown in Product Identification Guide, page 103

BLEPH®–10 ℞
(sulfacetamide sodium ophthalmic solution, USP) 10%

BLEPH®–10
(sulfacetamide sodium ophthalmic ointment, USP) 10%

Description: BLEPH®-10 (sulfacetamide sodium ophthalmic solution and ointment USP) 10% are sterile topical antibacterial agents for ophthalmic use.
Chemical Name: N-Sulfanilylacetamide monosodium salt monohydrate.
Contains:
BLEPH®-10 solution: Active: Sulfacetamide sodium 10% (100 mg/mL). Preservative: benzalkonium chloride (0.005%). Inactives: polyvinyl alcohol 1.4%; sodium thiosulfate; sodium phosphate dibasic; sodium phosphate monobasic; edetate disodium; polysorbate 80; hydrochloric acid and/or sodium hydroxide to adjust the pH; and purified water.
BLEPH®-10 ointment:
Active: Sulfacetamide sodium 10% (100 mg/g). Preservative: phenylmercuric acetate (0.0008%). Inactives: white petrolatum, mineral oil, and petrolatum (and) lanolin alcohol.
Clinical Pharmacology:
Microbiology: The sulfonamides are bacteriostatic agents and the spectrum of activity is similar for all. Sulfonamides inhibit bacterial synthesis of dihydrofolic acid by preventing the condensation of the pteridine with aminobenzoic acid through competitive inhibition of the enzyme dihydropteroate synthetase. Resistant strains have altered dihydropteroate synthetase with reduced affinity for sulfonamides or produce increased quantities of aminobenzoic acid.
Topically applied sulfonamides are considered active against susceptible strains of the following common bacterial eye pathogens: *Escherichia coli, Staphylococcus aureus, Streptococcus pneumoniae, Streptococcus* (viridans group), *Haemophilus influenzae, Klebsiella* species, and *Enterobacter* species.
Topically applied sulfonamides do not provide adequate coverage against *Neisseria* species, *Serratia marcescens* and *Pseudomonas aeruginosa.* A significant percentage of staphylococcal isolates are completely resistant to sulfa drugs.
Indications and Usage: BLEPH®-10 solution and ointment are indicated for the treatment of conjunctivitis and other superficial ocular infections due to the following susceptible microorganisms. BLEPH®-10 solution is also indicated as an adjunctive in systemic sulfonamide therapy of trachoma:
Escherichia coli, Staphylococcus aureus, Streptococcus pneumoniae, Streptococcus (viridans group), *Haemophilus influenzae, Klebsiella* species, and *Enterobacter* species.
Topically applied sulfonamides do not provide adequate coverage against *Neisseria* species, *Serratia marcescens* and *Pseudomonas aeruginosa.* A significant percentage of staphylococcal isolates are completely resistant to sulfa drugs.
Contraindications: BLEPH®-10 solution and ointment are contraindicated in individuals who have a hypersensitivity to sulfonamides or to any ingredient of the preparations.
Warnings: FOR TOPICAL EYE USE ONLY—NOT FOR INJECTION.
FATALITIES HAVE OCCURRED, ALTHOUGH RARELY, DUE TO SEVERE REACTIONS TO SULFONAMIDES INCLUDING STEVENS-JOHNSON SYNDROME, TOXIC EPIDERMAL NECROLYSIS, FULMINANT HEPATIC NECROSIS, AGRANULOCYTOSIS, APLASTIC ANEMIA AND OTHER BLOOD DYSCRASIAS. Sensitizations may recur when a sulfonamide is readministered, irrespective of the route of administration. Sensitivity reactions have been reported in individuals with no prior history of sulfonamide hypersensitivity. At the first sign of hypersensitivity, skin rash or other serious reaction, discontinue use of these preparations.
Precautions:
General: Prolonged use of topical antibacterial agents may give rise to overgrowth of nonsusceptible organisms including fungi. Bacterial resistance to sulfonamides may also develop.
The effectiveness of sulfonamides may be reduced by the para-aminobenzoic acid present in purulent exudates.
Ophthalmic ointments may retard corneal wound healing.
Sensitization may recur when a sulfonamide is readministered irrespective of the route of administration, and cross-sensitivity between different sulfonamides may occur.
At the first sign of hypersensitivity, increase in purulent discharge, or aggravation of inflammation or pain, the patient should discontinue use of the medication and consult a physician (see **Warnings**).
Information for patients: To avoid contamination, do not touch tip of container to the eye, eyelid or any surface.
Drug interactions: Sulfacetamide preparations are incompatible with silver preparations.
Carcinogenesis, Mutagenesis, Impairment of Fertility: No studies have been conducted in animals or in humans to evaluate the possibility of these effects with ocularly administered sulfacetamide. Rats appear to be especially susceptible to the goitrogenic effects of sulfonamides, and long-term oral administration of sulfonamides has resulted in thyroid malignancies in these animals.
Pregnancy: Pregnancy Category C. Animal reproduction studies have not been conducted with sulfonamide ophthalmic preparations. Kernicterus may occur in the newborn as a result of treatment of a pregnant woman at term with orally administered sulfonamides. There are no adequate and well controlled studies of sulfonamide ophthalmic preparations in pregnant women and it is not known whether topically applied sulfonamides can cause fetal harm when administered to a pregnant woman. This product should be used in pregnancy only if the potential benefit justifies the potential risk to the fetus.
Nursing mothers: Systematically administered sulfonamides are capable of producing kernicterus in infants of lactating women. Because of the potential for the development of kernicterus in neonates, a decision should be made whether to discontinue nursing or discontinue the drug taking into account the importance of the drug to the mother.
Pediatric Use: Safety and effectiveness in children below the age of two months have not been established.
Adverse Reactions: Bacterial and fungal corneal ulcers have developed during treatment with sulfonamide ophthalmic preparations.
The most frequently reported reactions are local irritation, stinging and burning. Less commonly reported reactions include non-specific conjunctivitis, conjunctival hyperemia, secondary infections and allergic reactions.
Fatalities have occurred, although rarely, due to severe reactions to sulfonamides including Stevens-Johnson syndrome, toxic epidermal necrolysis, fulminant hepatic necrosis, agranulocytosis, aplastic anemia, and other blood dyscrasias (see **Warnings**).
Dosage and Administration: For conjunctivitis and other superficial ocular infections:
BLEPH®-10 solution:
Instill one or two drops into the conjunctival sac(s) of the affected eye(s) every two to three hours initially. Dosages may be tapered by increasing the time interval between doses as the condition responds. The usual duration of treatment is seven to ten days.
For trachoma:
Instill two drops into the conjunctival sac(s) of the affected eye(s) every two hours. Topical administration must be accompanied by systemic administration.
BLEPH®-10 ointment:
Apply a small amount (approximately one-half inch ribbon) into the conjunctival sac(s) of the affected eye(s) every three to four hours and at bedtime. Dosages may be tapered by increasing the time interval between doses as the condition responds. The ointment may be used as adjunct to the solution. The usual duration of treatment is seven to ten days.
How Supplied: BLEPH®-10 (sulfacetamide sodium ophthalmic solution, USP) 10% is supplied sterile in plastic bottles in the following sizes:

2.5 mL—NDC 11980-011-03
5 mL—NDC 11980-011-05
15 mL—NDC 11980-011-15

Note: Store between 8°–25°C (46°–77°F). Protect from light. Sulfonamide solutions, on long standing, will darken in color and should be discarded.
BLEPH®-10 (sulfacetamide sodium ophthalmic ointment, USP) 10% is supplied sterile in ophthalmic ointment tubes in the following size:

3.5 g—NDC 0023-0311-04

Note: Store away from heat, 40°C (104°F).
Caution: Rx only

BLEPHAMIDE® ℞
(sulfacetamide sodium—prednisolone acetate ophthalmic suspension)
sterile

Description: BLEPHAMIDE® ophthalmic suspension is a topical anti-inflammatory/anti-infective combination product for ophthalmic use.
Chemical Names: Sulfacetamide sodium: N-sulfanilylacetamide monosodium salt monohydrate.
Prednisolone acetate: 11β, 17, 21-trihydroxypregna-1, 4-diene-3, 20-dione 21-acetate.
Contains: Actives: sulfacetamide sodium 10.0%, prednisolone acetate (microfine suspension) 0.2%. Preservative: benzalkonium chloride (0.004%). Inactives: polyvinyl alcohol 1.4%; polysorbate 80; edetate disodium; sodium phosphate, dibasic; potassium phosphate, monobasic; sodium thiosulfate; hydrochloric acid and/or sodium hydroxide to adjust the pH; and purified water.
Clinical Pharmacology: Corticosteroids suppress the inflammatory response to a variety of agents and they probably delay or slow healing. Since corticosteroids may inhibit the body's defense mechanism against infection, a concomitant antibacterial drug may be used when this inhibition is considered to be clinically significant in a particular case.
When a decision to administer both a corticosteroid and an antibacterial is made, the administration of such drugs in combination has the advantage of greater patient compliance and convenience, with the added assurance that the appropriate dosage of both drugs is administered. When both types of drugs are in the same formulation, compatibility of ingredients is assured and the correct volume of drug is delivered and retained. The relative potency of corticosteroids depends on the molecular structure, concentration and release from the vehicle.
Microbiology: Sulfacetamide sodium exerts a bacteriostatic effect against susceptible bac-

Continued on next page

Blephamide Suspension—Cont.

teria by restricting the synthesis of folic acid required for growth through competition with p-aminobenzoic acid.

Some strains of these bacteria may be resistant to sulfacetamide or resistant strains may emerge *in vivo*.

The anti-infective component in these products is included to provide action against specific organisms susceptible to it. Sulfacetamide sodium is active *in vitro* against susceptible strains of the following microorganisms: *Escherichia coli, Staphylococcus aureus, Streptococcus pneumoniae, Streptococcus* (*viridans* group), *Haemophilus influenzae, Klebsiella* species, and *Enterobacter* species. This product does not provide adequate coverage against: *Neisseria* species, *Pseudomonas* species, and *Serratia marcescens* (see **Indications and Usage**).

Indications and Usage: A steroid/anti-infective combination is indicated for steroid-responsive inflammatory ocular conditions for which a corticosteroid is indicated and where superficial bacterial infection or a risk of bacterial ocular infection exists.

Ocular steroids are indicated in inflammatory conditions of the palpebral and bulbar conjunctiva, cornea, and anterior segment of the globe where the inherent risk of corticosteroid use in certain infective conjunctivitides is accepted to obtain a diminution in edema and inflammation. They are also indicated in chronic anterior uveitis and corneal injury from chemical, radiation, or thermal burns or penetration of foreign bodies.

The use of a combination drug with an anti-infective component is indicated where the risk of superficial ocular infection is high or where there is an expectation that potentially dangerous numbers of bacteria will be present in the eye.

The particular anti-bacterial drug in this product is active against the following common bacterial eye pathogens: *Escherichia coli, Staphylococcus aureus, Streptococcus pneumoniae, Streptococcus* (viridans group), *Haemophilus influenzae, Klebsiella* species, and *Enterobacter* species. This product does not provide adequate coverage against *Neisseria* species, *Pseudomonas* species, and *Serratia marcescens.*

A significant percentage of staphylococcal sulates are completely resistant to sulfa drugs.

Contraindications: BLEPHAMIDE® ophthalmic suspension is contraindicated in most viral diseases of the cornea and conjunctiva including epithelial herpes simplex keratitis (dendritic keratitis), vaccinia, and varicella, and also in mycobacterial infection of the eye and fungal diseases of ocular structures.

This product is also contraindicated in individuals with known or suspected hypersensitivity to any of the ingredients of this preparation, to other sulfonamides and to other corticosteroids. See **Warnings**. (Hypersensitivity to the antimicrobial component occurs at a higher rate than for other components.)

Warnings:

NOT FOR INJECTION INTO THE EYE.

Prolonged use of corticosteroids may result in ocular hypertension/glaucoma with damage to the optic nerve, defects in visual acuity and fields of vision, and in posterior subcapsular cataract formation.

Acute anterior uveitis may occur in susceptible individuals, primarily Blacks.

Prolonged use of BLEPHAMIDE® ophthalmic suspension may suppress the host response and thus increase the hazard of secondary ocular infections. In those diseases causing thinning of the cornea or sclera, perforation has been known to occur with the use of topical corticosteroids. In acute purulent conditions of the eye, corticosteroids may mask infection or enhance existing infection.

If the product is used for 10 days or longer, intraocular pressure should be routinely monitored even though it may be difficult in children and uncooperative patients. Corticosteroids should be used with caution in the presence of glaucoma. Intraocular pressure should be checked frequently.

A significant percentage of staphylococcal isolates are completely resistant to sulfonamides.

The use of steroids after cataract surgery may delay healing and increase the incidence of filtering blebs.

The use of ocular corticosteroids may prolong the course and may exacerbate the severity of many viral infections of the eye (including herpes simplex). Employment of corticosteroid medication in the treatment of herpes simplex requires great caution.

Topical steroids are not effective in mustard gas keratitis and Sjögren's keratoconjunctivitis.

Fatalities have occurred, although rarely, due to severe reactions to sulfonamides including Stevens-Johnson syndrome, toxic epidermal necrolysis, fulminant hepatic necrosis, agranulocytosis, aplastic anemia and other blood dyscrasias. Sensitization may recur when a sulfonamide is readministered, irrespective of the route of administration.

If signs of hypersensitivity or other serious reactions occur, discontinue use of this preparation. Cross-sensitivity among corticosteroids has been demonstrated (see **Adverse Reactions**).

Precautions:

General: The initial prescription and renewal of the medication order beyond 20 milliliters of the suspension should be made by a physician only after examination of the patient with the aid of magnification, such as slit lamp biomicroscopy and, where appropriate, fluorescein staining. If signs and symptoms fail to improve after two days, the patient should be re-evaluated.

The possibility of fungal infections of the cornea should be considered after prolonged corticosteroid dosing. Use with caution in patients with severe dry eye. Fungal cultures should be taken when appropriate.

The p-amino benzoic acid present in purulent exudates competes with sulfonamides and can reduce their effectiveness.

Information for Patients: If inflammation or pain persists longer than 48 hours or becomes aggravated, the patient should be advised to discontinue use of the medication and consult a physician (see **Warnings**).

Contact lenses should not be worn during the use of this product.

This product is sterile when packaged. To prevent contamination, care should be taken to avoid touching the applicator tip to eyelids or to any other surface. The use of this bottle by more than one person may spread infection. Keep bottle tightly closed when not in use. Protect from light. Sulfonamide solutions darken on prolonged standing and exposure to heat and light. Do not use if solution has darkened. Yellowing does not affect activity. Keep out of the reach of children.

Laboratory Tests: Eyelid cultures and tests to determine the susceptibility of organisms to sulfacetamide may be indicated if signs and symptoms persist or recur in spite of the recommended course of treatment with BLEPHAMIDE® ophthalmic suspension.

Drug Interactions: BLEPHAMIDE® ophthalmic suspension is incompatible with silver preparations. Local anesthetics related to p-amino benzoic acid may antagonize the action of the sulfonamides.

Carcinogenesis, Mutagenesis, Impairment of Fertility: Prednisolone has been reported to be noncarcinogenic. Long-term animal studies for carcinogenic potential have not been performed with sulfacetamide.

One author detected chromosomal nondisjunction in the yeast *Saccharomyces cerevisiae* following application of sulfacetamide sodium. The significance of this finding to topical ophthalmic use of sulfacetamide sodium in the human in unknown.

Mutagenic studies with prednisolone have been negative. Studies on reproduction and fertility have not been performed with sulfacetamide. A long-term chronic toxicity study in dogs showed that high oral doses of prednisolone prevented estrus. A decrease in fertility was seen in male and female rats that were mated following oral dosing with another glucocorticosteroid.

Pregnancy: Teratogenic Effects: Pregnancy Category C. Animal reproduction studies have not been conducted with sulfacetamide sodium. Prednisolone has been shown to be teratogenic in rabbits, hamsters, and mice. In mice, prednisolone has been shown to be teratogenic when given in doses 1 to 10 times the human ocular dose. Dexamethasone, hydrocortisone and prednisolone were ocularly applied to both eyes of pregnant mice five times per day on days 10 through 13 of gestation. A significant increase in the incidence of cleft palate was observed in the fetuses of the treated mice. There are no adequate well-controlled studies in pregnant women dosed with corticosteroids.

Kernicterus may be precipitated in infants by sulfonamides being given systemically during the third trimester of pregnancy. It is not known whether sulfacetamide sodium can cause fetal harm when administered to a pregnant woman or whether it can affect reproductive capacity.

BLEPHAMIDE® ophthalmic suspension should be used during pregnancy only if the potential benefit justifies the potential risk to the fetus.

Nursing Mothers: It is not known whether topical administration of corticosteroids could result in sufficient systemic absorption to produce detectable quantities in human milk. Systemically administered corticosteroids appear in human milk and could suppress growth, interfere with endogenous corticosteroid production, or cause other untoward effects. Systemically administered sulfonamides are capable of producing kernicterus in infants of lactating women. Because of the potential for serious adverse reactions in nursing infants from sulfacetamide sodium and prednisolone acetate ophthalmic suspensions, a decision should be made whether to discontinue nursing or to discontinue the medication.

Pediatric Use: Safety and effectiveness in pediatric patients below the age of six have not been established.

Adverse Reactions: Adverse reactions have occurred with corticosteroid/anti-bacterial combination drugs which can be attributed to the corticosteroid component, the antibacterial component, or the combination. Exact incidence figures are not available since no denominator of treated patients is available.

Reactions occurring most often from the presence of the anti-bacterial ingredient are allergic sensitizations. Fatalities have occurred, although rarely, due to severe reactions to sulfonamides including Stevens-Johnson syndrome, toxic epidermal necrolysis, fulminant hepatic necrosis, agranulocytosis, aplastic anemia, and other blood dyscrasias (See **Warnings**).

Sulfacetamide sodium may cause local irritation.

The reactions due to the corticosteroid component in decreasing order of frequency are: elevation of intraocular pressure (IOP) with possible development of glaucoma and infrequent

optic nerve damage, posterior subcapsular cataract formation, and delayed wound healing.
Although systemic effects are extremely uncommon, there have been rare occurrences of systemic hypercorticoidism after use of topical corticosteroids.
Corticosteroid-containing preparations can also cause acute anterior uveitis or perforation of the globe. Mydriasis, loss of accommodation and ptosis have occasionally been reported following local use of corticosteroids.
Secondary Infection: The development of secondary infection has occurred after use of combinations containing corticosteroids and antibacterials. Fungal and viral infections of the cornea are particularly prone to develop coincidentally with long-term applications of corticosteroid. The possibility of fungal invasion must be considered in any persistent corneal ulceration where corticosteroid treatment has been used.
Secondary bacterial ocular infection following suppression of host responses also occurs.
SHAKE WELL BEFORE USING. Two drops should be instilled into the conjunctival sac every four hours during the day and at bedtime.
Not more than 20 milliliters should be prescribed initially, and the prescription should not be refilled without further evaluation as outlined in **Precautions** above.
BLEPHAMIDE® dosage may be reduced, but care should be taken not to discontinue therapy prematurely. In chronic conditions withdrawal of treatment should be carried out by gradually decreasing the frequency of application.
If signs and symptoms fail to improve after two days, the patient should be re-evaluated (see **Precautions**).
How Supplied: BLEPHAMIDE® ophthalmic suspension is supplied in plastic dropper bottles in the following sizes:

5 mL—NDC 11980-022-05
10 mL—NDC 11980-022-10

Note: Protect from freezing. **Shake well before using.**
Storage: Store BLEPHAMIDE® at 8°–24°C (46°–75°F) in an upright position.
PROTECT FROM LIGHT
Sulfonamide solutions darken on prolonged standing and exposure to heat and light. Do not use if solution has darkened.
Yellowing does not affect activity.
KEEP OUT OF REACH OF CHILDREN
Rx only.

Shown in Product Identification Guide, page 103

BLEPHAMIDE® ℞
(sulfacetamide sodium and prednisolone acetate ophthalmic ointment USP) 10%/0.2% sterile

Description: BLEPHAMIDE® (sulfacetamide sodium and prednisolone acetate ophthalmic ointment USP) is a sterile topical ophthalmic ointment combining an antibacterial and a corticosteroid.
Contains: Actives: sulfacetamide sodium 10% and prednisolone acetate 0.2%. Preservative: phenylmercuric acetate (0.0008%). Inactives: mineral oil; white petrolatum; and petrolatum (and) lanolin alcohol.
Chemical Names: Sulfacetamide sodium: N-sulfanilylacetamide monosodium salt monohydrate.
Prednisolone acetate: 11β, 17, 21-trihydroxypregna-1,4-diene-3, 20-dione, 21-acetate.
Clinical Pharmacology: Corticosteroids suppress the inflammatory response to a variety of agents and they probably delay or slow healing. Since corticosteroids may inhibit the body's defense mechanism against infection, a concomitant antibacterial drug may be used when this inhibition is considered to be clinically significant in a particular case.
When a decision to administer both a corticosteroid and an antibacterial is made, the administration of such drugs in combination has the advantage of greater patient compliance and convenience, with the added assurance that the appropriate dosage of both drugs is administered, plus assured compatibility of ingredients when both types of drugs are in the same formulation and, particularly, that the correct volume of drug is delivered and retained.
The relative potency of corticosteroids depends on the molecular structure, concentration and release from the vehicle.
Microbiology: Sulfacetamide exerts a bacteriostatic effect against susceptible bacteria by restricting the synthesis of folic acid required for growth through competition with p-amino benzoic acid.
Some strains of these bacteria may be resistant to sulfacetamide or resistant strains may emerge *in vivo.*
The anti-infective component in BLEPHAMIDE® ointment is included to provide action against specific organisms susceptible to it. Sulfacetamide sodium is active *in vitro* against susceptible strains of the following microorganisms: *Escherichia coli, Staphylococcus aureus, Streptococcus pneumoniae, Streptococcus* (viridans group), *Haemophilus influenzae, Klebsiella* species, and *Enterobacter* species. This product does not provide adequate coverage against: *Neisseria* species, *Pseudomonas* species, and *Serratia marcescens* (see **Indications and Usage**).
Indications and Usage: BLEPHAMIDE® ophthalmic ointment is indicated for steroid-responsive inflammatory ocular conditions for which a corticosteroid is indicated and where superficial bacterial ocular infection or a risk of bacterial ocular infection exists.
Ocular corticosteroids are indicated in inflammatory conditions of the palpebral and bulbar conjunctiva, cornea, and anterior segment of the globe where the inherent risk of corticosteroid use in certain infective conjunctivitides is accepted to obtain diminution in edema and inflammation. They are also indicated in chronic anterior uveitis and corneal injury from chemical, radiation or thermal burns or penetration of foreign bodies.
The use of a combination drug with an anti-infective component is indicated where the risk of superficial ocular infection is high or where there is an expectation that potentially dangerous numbers of bacteria will be present in the eye.
The particular antibacterial drug in this product is active against the following common bacterial eye pathogens: *Escherichia coli, Staphylococcus aureus, Streptococcus pneumoniae, Streptococcus* (viridans group), *Haemophilus influenzae, Klebsiella* species, and *Enterobacter* species.
The product does not provide adequate coverage against: *Neisseria* species, *Pseudomonas* species, and *Serratia marcescens.*
A significant percentage of staphylococcal isolates are completely resistant to sulfa drugs.
Contraindications: BLEPHAMIDE® ophthalmic ointment is contraindicated in most viral diseases of the cornea and conjunctiva including epithelial herpes simplex keratitis (dendritic keratitis), vaccinia, and varicella, and also in mycobacterial infection of the eye and fungal diseases of ocular structures.
This product is also contraindicated in individuals with known or suspected hypersensitivity to any of the ingredients of this preparation, to other sulfonamides and to other corticosteroids. See **Warnings**. (Hypersensitivity to the antimicrobial component occurs at a higher rate than for other components).
Warnings:
NOT FOR INJECTION INTO THE EYE.
Prolonged use of corticosteroids may result in ocular hypertension/glaucoma with damage to the optic nerve, defects in visual acuity and fields of vision, and in posterior subcapsular cataract formation.
Acute anterior uveitis may occur in susceptible individuals, primarily Blacks.
Prolonged use of BLEPHAMIDE® ophthalmic ointment may suppress the host response and thus increase the hazard of secondary ocular infections. In those diseases causing thinning of the cornea or sclera, perforation has been known to occur with the use of topical corticosteroids. In acute purulent conditions of the eye, corticosteroids may mask infection or enhance existing infection.
If the product is used for 10 days or longer, intraocular pressure should be routinely monitored even though it may be difficult in children and uncooperative patients. Corticosteroids should be used with caution in the presence of glaucoma. Intraocular pressure should be checked frequently.
A significant percentage of staphylococcal isolates are completely resistant to sulfonamides.
The use of steroids after cataract surgery may delay healing and increase the incidence of filtering blebs.
The use of ocular corticosteroids may prolong the course and may exacerbate the severity of many viral infections of the eye (including herpes simplex). Employment of corticosteroid medication in the treatment of herpes simplex requires great caution.
Topical steroids are not effective in mustard gas keratitis and Sjogren's keratoconjunctivitis.
Fatalities have occurred, although rarely, due to severe reactions to sulfonamides including Stevens-Johnson syndrome, toxic epidermal necrolysis, fulminant hepatic necrosis, agranulocytosis, aplastic anemia and other blood dyscrasias. Sensitization may recur when a sulfonamide is readministered, irrespective of the route of administration.
If signs of hypersensitivity or other serious reactions occur, discontinue use of this preparation. Cross-sensitivity among corticosteroids has been demonstrated (see **Adverse Reactions**).
Precautions:
General: The initial prescription and renewal of the medication order beyond 8 g of ointment should be made by a physician only after examination of the patient with the aid of magnification, such as slit lamp biomicroscopy and, where appropriate, fluorescein staining. If signs and symptoms fail to improve after two days, the patient should be re-evaluated. The possibility of fungal infections of the cornea should be considered after prolonged corticosteroid dosing. Use with caution in patients with severe dry eye. Fungal cultures should be taken when appropriate.
The p-amino benzoic acid present in purulent exudates competes with sulfonamides and can reduce their effectiveness. Ophthalmic ointments may retard corneal healing.
Information for Patients: If inflammation or pain persists longer than 48 hours or becomes aggravated, the patient should be advised to discontinue use of the medication and consult a physician (see **Warnings**).
This product is sterile when packaged. To prevent contamination, care should be taken to avoid touching the tube tip to eyelids or to any other surface. The use of this tube by more

Continued on next page

Blephamide Ointment—Cont.

than one person may spread infection. Keep tube tightly closed when not in use. Keep out of the reach of children.

Laboratory Tests: Eyelid cultures and tests to determine the susceptibility of organisms to sulfacetamide may be indicated if signs and symptoms persist or recur in spite of the recommended course of treatment with BLEPHAMIDE® ophthalmic ointment.

Drug Interactions: BLEPHAMIDE® ophthalmic ointment is incompatible with silver preparations. Local anesthetics related to p-amino benzoic acid may antagonize the action of the sulfonamides.

Carcinogenesis, Mutagenesis, Impairment of Fertility: Prednisolone has been reported to be noncarcinogenic. Long-term animal studies for carcinogenic potential have not been performed with sulfacetamide.

One author detected chromosomal nondisjunction in the yeast *Saccharomyces cerevisiae* following application of sulfacetamide sodium. The significance of this finding to topical ophthalmic use of sulfacetamide sodium in the human is unknown.

Mutagenic studies with prednisolone have been negative. Studies on reproduction and fertility have not been performed with sulfacetamide. A long-term chronic toxicity study in dogs showed that high oral doses of prednisolone prevented estrus. A decrease in fertility was seen in male and female rats that were mated following oral dosing with another glucocorticosteroid.

Pregnancy: Teratogenic Effects: Pregnancy Category C. Animal reproduction studies have not been conducted with sulfacetamide sodium. Prednisolone has been shown to be teratogenic in rabbits, hamsters, and mice. In mice, prednisolone has been shown to be teratogenic when given in doses 1 to 10 times the human ocular dose. Dexamethasone, hydrocortisone and prednisolone were ocularly applied to both eyes of pregnant mice five times per day on days 10 through 13 of gestation. A significant increase in the incidence of cleft palate was observed in the fetuses of the treated mice. There are no adequate well-controlled studies in pregnant women dosed with corticosteroids.

Kernicterus may be precipitated in infants by sulfonamides being given systemically during the third trimester of pregnancy. It is not known whether sulfacetamide sodium can cause fetal harm when administered to a pregnant woman or whether it can affect reproductive capacity.

BLEPHAMIDE® ophthalmic ointment should be used during pregnancy only if the potential benefit justifies the potential risk to the fetus.

Nursing Mothers: It is not known whether topical administration of corticosteroids could result in sufficient systemic absorption to produce detectable quantities in human milk. Systemically administered corticosteroids appear in human milk and could suppress growth, interfere with endogenous corticosteroid production, or cause other untoward effects. Systemically administered sulfonamides are capable of producing kernicterus in infants of lactating women. Because of the potential for serious adverse reactions in nursing infants from sulfacetamide sodium and prednisolone acetate ophthalmic ointments, a decision should be made whether to discontinue nursing or to discontinue the medication.

Pediatric Use: Safety and effectiveness in children below the age of six have not been established.

Adverse Reactions: Adverse reactions have occurred with corticosteroid/antibacterial combination drugs which can be attributed to the corticosteroid component, the antibacterial component, or the combination. Exact incidence figures are not available since no denominator of treated patients is available.

Reactions occurring most often from the presence of the antibacterial ingredient are allergic sensitizations. Fatalities have occurred, although rarely, due to severe reactions to sulfonamides including Stevens-Johnson syndrome, toxic epidermal necrolysis, fulminant hepatic necrosis, agranulocytosis, aplastic anemia, and other blood dyscrasias (See **Warnings**).

Sulfacetamide sodium may cause local irritation.

The reactions due to the corticosteroid component in decreasing order of frequency are: elevation of intraocular pressure (IOP) with possible development of glaucoma and infrequent optic nerve damage, posterior subcapsular cataract formation, and delayed wound healing.

Although systemic effects are extremely uncommon, there have been rare occurrences of systemic hypercorticoidism after use of topical steroids.

Corticosteroid-containing preparations can also cause acute anterior uveitis or perforation of the globe. Mydriasis, loss of accommodation and ptosis have occasionally been reported following local use of corticosteroids.

Secondary Infection: The development of secondary infection has occurred after use of combinations containing corticosteroids and antibacterials. Fungal and viral infections of the cornea are particularly prone to develop coincidentally with long-term applications of corticosteroid. The possibility of fungal invasion must be considered in any persistent corneal ulceration where corticosteroid treatment has been used.

Secondary bacterial ocular infection following suppression of host responses also occurs.

Dosage and Administration: A small amount, approximately $^1/_2$ inch ribbon of ointment, should be applied in the conjunctival sac three or four times daily and once or twice at night.

Not more than 8 g should be prescribed initially.

The dosing of BLEPHAMIDE® ophthalmic ointment may be reduced, but care should be taken not to discontinue therapy prematurely. In chronic conditions, withdrawal of treatment should be carried out by gradually decreasing the frequency of application.

If signs and symptoms fail to improve after two days, the patient should be re-evaluated (see **Precautions**).

How Supplied: BLEPHAMIDE® (sulfacetamide sodium and prednisolone acetate ophthalmic ointment USP) 10%/0.2% is supplied sterile in 3.5 gram ointment tubes:

NDC 0023-0313-04.

Note: Store away from heat.

Rx only

Shown in Product Identification Guide, page 103

CELLUVISC® OTC
(carboxymethylcellulose sodium) 1%
Lubricant Eye Drops
Preservative-Free

Soothing Relief For Dry, Irritated Eyes.

Due to its thicker formula, CELLUVISC® is an ideal eye drop for persistent dry eye conditions. CELLUVISC® restores the moisture your eyes crave with a gentle protecting and lubricating formula that has some of the healthy qualities as natural tears. So, you can enjoy long-lasting relief from the irritating, scratchy feeling of dry, irritated eyes.

To avoid the use of potentially irritating preservatives found in bottled eye drops, CELLUVISC® comes in preservative-free, air-tight, single-use containers. So you can apply CELLUVISC® as often as necessary without the risk of preservative-induced irritation.

Contains: Active: Carboxymethylcellulose sodium 1%. Inactives: calcium chloride, potassium chloride, purified water, sodium chloride, and sodium lactate.

Indications: For the temporary relief of burning, irritation and discomfort due to dryness of the eye or exposure to wind or sun. Also may be used as a protectant against further irritation.

Warnings: To avoid contamination, do not touch tip of container to any surface. Do not reuse. Once opened, discard. If you experience eye pain, changes in vision, continued redness or irritation of the eye, or if the condition worsens or persists for more than 72 hours, discontinue use and consult a doctor. If solution changes color or becomes cloudy, do not use. Keep this and all drugs out of the reach of children. In case of accidental ingestion, seek professional assistance or contact a poison control center immediately.

Directions: Instill 1 or 2 drops in the affected eye(s) as needed.

Note: Use only if single-use container is intact. Do not touch unit-dose tip to eye. Celluvisc® may cause temporary blurring due to its viscosity.

How Supplied: Celluvisc® (carboxymethylcellulose sodium) 1% Lubricant Ophthalmic Solution is supplied in sterile, preservative-free, disposable, single-use containers of 0.01 fluid ounces each, in the following size:

30 single-use containers—NDC 0023-4554-30.

Shown in Product Identification Guide, page 103

CHLOROPTIC® ℞
(chloramphenicol) 1.0%
S.O.P.®
sterile ophthalmic ointment

> **Warning:** Bone marrow hypoplasia including aplastic anemia and death have been reported following topical application of chloramphenicol. Chloramphenicol should not be used when less potentially dangerous agents would be expected to provide effective treatment.

Description: Chloroptic® (chloramphenicol ophthalmic ointment, USP) is a sterile topical anti-infective product for ophthalmic use.

Contains:

Active: chloramphenicol .... 1% (10 mg/g)

Preservative: chlorobutanol (chloral deriv.) .... 0.5% (5 mg/g)

Inactives: white petrolatum; mineral oil; polyoxyl 40 stearate; polyethylene glycol 300 and petrolatum (and) lanolin alcohol.

Clinical Pharmacology: Chloramphenicol is a broad-spectrum antibiotic originally isolated from *Streptomyces venezuelae*. It is primarily bacteriostatic and acts by inhibition of protein synthesis by interfering with the transfer of activated amino acids from soluble RNA to ribosomes. It has been noted that chloramphenicol is found in measurable amounts in the aqueous humor following topical application to the eye. Development of resistance to chloramphenicol can be regarded as minimal for staphylococci and many other species of bacteria.

Indications and Usage: Chloramphenicol should be used only in those serious infections for which less potentially dangerous drugs are ineffective or contraindicated (See Boxed Warning). Bacteriological studies should be performed to determine the causative organisms and their sensitivity to chloramphenicol.

Chloroptic® ointment is indicated for the treatment of surface ocular infections involving the conjunctiva and/or cornea caused by chloramphenicol-susceptible organisms.
Chloramphenicol is active against the following common bacterial eye pathogens: *Staphylococcus aureus,* streptococci, including *Streptococcus pneumoniae, Escherichia coli, Haemophilus influenzae, Klebsiella/Enterobacter* species, *Moraxella lacunata* (Morax-Axenfeld bacillus), and *Neisseria* species. This product does not provide adequate coverage against: *Pseudomonas aeruginosa* or *Serratia marcescens.*
Contraindications: This product is contraindicated in persons sensitive to any of the components.
Warnings: SEE BOXED WARNING
Precautions: General: The prolonged use of antibiotics may occasionally result in overgrowth of nonsusceptible organisms, including fungi. If new infections appear while using this medication or clinical improvement is not observed within 1 week, the drug should be discontinued and appropriate measures should be taken.
In all serious infections the topical use of chloramphenicol should be supplemented by appropriate systemic medication.
Ophthalmic ointments may retard corneal wound healing.
Information for Patients: Do not touch tube tip to any surface as this may contaminate the ointment.
Carcinogenesis, mutagenesis and impairment of fertility: No long-term studies have been conducted in animals or in humans to evaluate the carcinogenic potential or effects on fertility with chloramphenicol. However, there is some clinical evidence that aplastic anemia due to chloramphenicol may be associated with subsequent development of leukemia.
Pregnancy: Pregnancy Category C: Chloramphenicol has been shown to be embryocidal and teratogenic in rat, mouse, rabbit and chicken embryos/fetuses (See below). There are no adequate and well-controlled studies in pregnant women. Chloramphenicol should be used during pregnancy only if the potential benefit justifies the potential risk to the fetus.
Embryotoxic effects: Significantly lower numbers of live fetuses and an increase in the number of early embryonic resorptions occurred after pregnant **rats** were treated orally with 500 mg/kg (equivalent to 7500 times the recommended maximum daily adult topical ophthalmic dose of 1% ophthalmic ointment) from days 5 to 15 of their pregnancy. Similar findings were seen with groups receiving higher oral doses (1000 mg/kg or 2000 mg/kg) at various dosing intervals. Female mice receiving 1000 mg/kg orally from days 6 to 12 of their pregnancy showed a significant increase in the number of resorptions. Female **rabbits** receiving the same oral dosing (1000 mg/kg) from days 8 to 11 had an increase in the number of resorptions of embryos without placentation. Chloramphenicol (2.5 mg) injected into **chicken eggs** resulted in a 20% embryo mortality rate one day after administration, which increased to 100% embryo mortality on the 11th day of incubation.
Teratogenicity: When given to female **rats** orally at 2000 mg/kg from days 6 to 8 of pregnancy, 36% of the fetuses exhibited either an omphalocele or an umbilical hernia, with costal fusions. Fetuses of the **rats** treated with 1000 mg/kg orally from days 7 to 12 of pregnancy or 2000 mg/kg from days 11 to 13, and of **mice** treated with 1000 mg/kg from days 6 to 12, had a higher incidence of missing ossification of the phalangeal nuclei of the forelegs and hindlegs and of the 5th sternebra. This correlated with a decrease in the average weight of the fetuses. **Rabbit** fetuses displayed more frequent absence of the phalangeal nuclei of the forelegs than control when pregnant rabbits received 500 mg/kg orally on days 6 to 15 of pregnancy. More frequent missing ossification of the phalangeal nulcei of the forelegs and hindlegs and an increase in the number of unevenly ossified vertebrae was seen in the fetuses of rabbits when pregnant females were given 1000 mg/kg from days 6 to 9 of pregnancy. Teratogenic effects of chloramphenicol (0.5 mg) when injected into **chicken eggs**, included malformations of the beak, eyes and legs.
Nursing Mothers: Because of the potential for serious, adverse reactions in nursing infants from chloramphenicol, a decision should be made whether to discontinue nursing or to discontinue the drug, taking into account the importance of the drug to the mother.
Pediatric Use: Safety and effectiveness in pediatric patients have not been established.
Adverse Reactions: Blood dyscrasias have been reported in association with the use of chloramphenicol (See WARNINGS).
Allergic or inflammatory reactions due to individual hypersensitivity and occasional burning or stinging may occur with the use of Chloroptic Ophthalmic Ointment.
Dosage and Administration: A small amount (approximately 1/2 inch) of ointment should be placed in the lower conjunctival sac every three hours. Administration should be continued day and night for the first 48 hours, after which the interval between applications may be increased. Treatment should be continued for approximately 7 days. Treatment should be continued for at least 48 hours after the eye appears normal. Treatment should not be continued for more than three weeks without re-evaluation by the prescribing physician.
How Supplied: Chloroptic® (chloramphenicol ophthalmic ointment, USP) 1% is supplied sterile in ophthalmic ointment tubes in the following size:

3.5g—NDC 0023-0301-04

Note: Store between 15°–25°C (59°–77°F).
Rx only.

CHLOROPTIC®* ℞
(chloramphenicol 0.5%)
sterile ophthalmic solution

Description:
Contains: Active: chloramphenicol 0.5% (5 mg/mL). Preservative: chlorobutanol (chloral derivative) 0.5%. Inactives: polyethylene glycol 300; polyoxyl 40 stearate; sodium hydroxide or hydrochloric acid to adjust the pH and purified water.
Actions: CHLOROPTIC® (chloramphenicol) has a wide spectrum of antimicrobial activity and is effective against many gram-negative and gram-positive organisms such as *Escherichia coli, Haemophilus influenzae, Staphylococcus aureus, Streptococcus hemolyticus,* and *Moraxella lacunata* (Morax-Axenfeld bacillus).
Indications: For the treatment of superficial ocular infections involving the conjunctiva and/or cornea caused by chloramphenicol-susceptible organisms.
Contraindications: Contraindicated in patients who are hypersensitive to chloramphenicol.
Warnings: As with other antibiotics, prolonged use may result in overgrowth of nonsusceptible organisms. If superinfection occurs, or if clinical improvement is not noted within a reasonable period, discontinue use and institute appropriate therapy. Sensitivity reactions such as stinging, itching, angioneurotic edema, urticaria, vesicular and maculopapular dermatitis may also occur in some patients. Occasionally one sees hematopoietic toxicity with the use of systemic chloramphenicol, and rarely with topical administration. This type of blood dyscrasia is generally a dose-related toxic effect on bone marrow and is usually reversible on cessation of the drug. Rare cases of aplastic anemia have been reported with prolonged (months to years) or frequent intermittent (over months and years) use of topical chloramphenicol.
Adverse Reactions: The most serious reaction reported following prolonged or frequent intermittent use of topical chloramphenicol is bone marrow aplasia.
Dosage and Administration: One or two drops 4 to 6 times a day for the first 72 hours, depending upon the severity of the condition. Intervals between applications may be increased after the first two days. Since the action of the drug is primarily bacteriostatic, therapy should be continued for 48 hours after an apparent cure has been attained.
How Supplied: CHLOROPTIC® (chloramphenicol) sterile ophthalmic solution is supplied in plastic dropper bottles in the following sizes:

2.5 mL—NDC 11980-109-03
7.5 mL—NDC 11980-109-08

Refrigerate until dispensed.
Rx only

*U.S. Patent 3,702,364

EPIFRIN® ℞
(epinephrine, USP)
sterile ophthalmic solution

Description: EPIFRIN® (epinephrine, USP) sterile ophthalmic solution is a topical sympathomimetic agent for ophthalmic use.
Chemical Name: 1,2-Benzenediol,4-[1-hydroxy-2-(methylamino)ethyl]-, (R)-.
Contains:
Active: epinephrine, USP 0.5%, 1%, 2%
Preservative: benzalkonium chloride
Inactives: sodium metabisulfite; edetate disodium; hydrochloric acid; and purified water.
Clinical Pharmacology: Epinephrine is an adrenergic agonist that stimulates α- and β-adrenergic receptors. The capacity of EPIFRIN® (epinephrine, USP) to decrease the aqueous inflow in open-angle glaucoma has been well documented. Studies have also shown that prolonged topical epinephrine therapy offers significant improvement in the coefficient of aqueous outflow.
EPIFRIN® is effective alone in reducing intraocular pressure and is particularly useful in combination with miotics or beta-adrenergic blocking agents for the difficult-to-control patients. The addition of EPIFRIN® to the patient's regimen often provides better control of intraocular pressure than the original agent alone.
Indications and Usage: EPIFRIN® is indicated for the treatment of chronic simple glaucoma.
Contraindications: EPIFRIN® should not be used in patients who have had an attack of narrow-angle glaucoma, since dilation of the pupil may trigger an acute attack. Do not use if hypersensitive to any ingredient.
Warnings:

1. EPIFRIN® should be used with caution in patients with a narrow angle, since dilation of the pupil may trigger an acute attack of narrow-angle glaucoma.
2. Use with caution in patients with hypertensive cardiovascular disease or coronary artery disease.
3. Epinephrine has been reported to produce reversible macular edema in some aphakic patients and should be used with caution in these patients.

Continued on next page

Epifrin—Cont.

Contains sodium metabisulfite, a sulfite that may cause allergic-type reactions, including anaphylactic symptoms and life-threatening or less severe asthmatic episodes in certain susceptible people. The overall prevalence of sulfite sensitivity in the general population is unknown and probably low. Sulfite sensitivity is seen more frequently in asthmatic than in nonasthmatic people.

Precautions:

General: Epinephrine in any form is relatively uncomfortable upon instillation. However, discomfort lessens as the concentration of epinephrine decreases. EPIFRIN® is not for injection.

Carcinogenesis, mutagenesis and impairment of fertility: No studies have been conducted in animals or in humans to evaluate the potential of these effects.

Pregnancy Category C: Animal reproduction studies have not been conducted with epinephrine. It is also not known whether epinephrine can cause fetal harm when administered to a pregnant woman or if it can affect reproduction capacity. Epinephrine should be given to a pregnant woman only if clearly needed.

Pediatric Use: Safety and effectiveness in pediatric patients have not been established.

Adverse Reactions: Undesirable reactions to topical epinephrine include eye pain or ache, browache, headache, conjunctival hyperemia and allergic lid reactions.

Adrenochrome deposits in the conjunctiva and cornea after prolonged epinephrine therapy have been reported. Topical epinephrine has been reported to produce reversible macular edema in some aphakic patients.

Overdosage: Accidental ingestion will not cause problems because pharmacologically active concentrations of epinephrine cannot be achieved orally in man. Should accidental overdosage in the eye(s) occur, flush eye(s) with water or normal saline.

Dosage and Administration: The usual dosage is 1 drop in the affected eye(s) once or twice daily. However, the dosage should be adjusted to meet the needs of the individual patients. This is made easier with EPIFRIN® (epinephrine, USP) sterile ophthalmic solution available in three strengths.

How Supplied: EPIFRIN® is available on prescription only in plastic dropper bottles in the following concentrations and sizes:

0.5%	15 mL—NDC 11980-119-15
1%	15 mL—NDC 11980-122-15
2%	15 mL—NDC 11980-058-15

Note: Protect from light and excessive heat. If the solution discolors or a precipitate forms, it should be discarded.

FML FORTE® ℞
(fluorometholone) 0.25%
LIQUIFILM®
sterile ophthalmic suspension

Description: FML FORTE® LIQUIFILM® sterile ophthalmic suspension is a topical anti-inflammatory product for ophthalmic use.

Chemical Name: Fluorometholone: 9-Fluoro-11β, 17-dihydroxy-6α-methylpregna-1,4-diene-3,20-dione.

Contains: Active: fluorometholone 0.25%. Preservative: benzalkonium chloride 0.005%. Inactives: LIQUIFILM® (polyvinyl alcohol) 1.4%; edetate disodium; sodium chloride; sodium phosphate, monobasic; sodium phosphate, dibasic; polysorbate 80; sodium hydroxide to adjust the pH; and purified water.

Clinical Pharmacology: Corticosteroids inhibit the inflammatory response to a variety of inciting agents and probably delay or slow healing. They inhibit the edema, fibrin deposition, capillary dilation, leukocyte migration, capillary proliferation, fibroblast proliferation, deposition of collagen, and scar formation associated with inflammation.

There is no generally accepted explanation for the mechanism of action of ocular corticosteroids. However, corticosteroids are thought to act by the induction of phospholipase A_2 inhibitory proteins, collectively called lipocortins. It is postulated that these proteins control the biosynthesis of potent mediators of inflammation such as prostaglandins and leukotrienes by inhibiting the release of their common precursor, arachidonic acid. Arachidonic acid is released from membrane phospholipids by phospholipase A_2.

Corticosteroids are capable of producing a rise in intraocular pressure. In clinical studies of documented steroid-responders, fluorometholone demonstrated a significantly longer average time to produce a rise in intraocular pressure than dexamethasone phosphate; however, in a small percentage of individuals a significant rise in intraocular pressure occurred within one week. The ultimate magnitude of the rise was equivalent for both drugs.

Indications and Usage: FML FORTE® suspension is indicated for the treatment of corticosteroid-responsive inflammation of the palpebral and bulbar conjunctiva, cornea and anterior segment of the globe.

Contraindications: FML FORTE® suspension is contraindicated in most viral diseases of the cornea and conjunctiva, including epithelial herpes simplex keratitis (dendritic keratitis), vaccinia, and varicella, and also in mycobacterial infection of the eye and fungal diseases of ocular structures. FML FORTE® suspension is also contraindicated in individuals with known or suspected hypersensitivity to any of the ingredients of this preparation and to other corticosteroids.

Warnings: Prolonged use of corticosteroids may result in glaucoma, with damage to the optic nerve, defects in visual acuity and fields of vision, and in posterior subcapsular cataract formation. Prolonged use may also suppress the host immune response and thus increase the hazard of secondary ocular infections.

Various ocular diseases and long-term use of topical corticosteroids have been known to cause corneal and scleral thinning. Use of topical corticosteroids in the presence of thin corneal or scleral tissue may lead to perforation.

Acute purulent infections of the eye may be masked or activity enhanced by the presence of corticosteroid medication.

If this product is used for 10 days or longer, intraocular pressure should be routinely monitored even though it may be difficult in children and uncooperative patients. Steroids should be used with caution in the presence of glaucoma. Intraocular pressure should be checked frequently.

The use of steroids after cataract surgery may delay healing and increase the incidence of bleb formation.

Use of ocular steroids may prolong the course and may exacerbate the severity of many viral infections of the eye (including herpes simplex). Employment of a corticosteroid medication in the treatment of patients with a history of herpes simplex requires great caution; frequent slit lamp microscopy is recommended.

Corticosteroids are not effective in mustard gas keratitis and Sjögren's keratoconjunctivitis.

Precautions:

General: The initial prescription and renewal of the medication order beyond 20 milliliters of FML FORTE® suspension should be made by a physician only after examination of the patient with the aid of magnification, such as slit lamp biomicroscopy and, where appropriate, fluorescein staining. If signs and symptoms fail to improve after two days, the patient should be re-evaluated.

As fungal infections of the cornea are particularly prone to develop coincidentally with long-term local corticosteroid applications, fungal invasion should be suspected in any persistent corneal ulceration where a corticosteroid has been used or is in use. Fungal cultures should be taken when appropriate.

If this product is used for 10 days or longer, intraocular pressure should be monitored (see **Warnings**).

Information for Patients: If inflammation or pain persists longer than 48 hours or becomes aggravated, the patient should be advised to discontinue use of the medication and consult a physician.

This product is sterile when packaged. To prevent contamination, care should be taken to avoid touching the bottle tip to eyelids or to any other surface. The use of this bottle by more than one person may spread infection. Keep bottle tightly closed when not in use. Keep out of reach of children.

Carcinogenesis, mutagenesis, impairment of fertility: No studies have been conducted in animals or in humans to evaluate the possibility of these effects with fluorometholone.

Pregnancy: Teratogenic effects. Pregnancy Category C: Fluorometholone has been shown to be embryocidal and teratogenic in rabbits when administered at low multiples of the human ocular dose. Fluorometholone was applied ocularly to rabbits daily on days 6–18 of gestation, and dose-related fetal loss and fetal abnormalities including cleft palate, deformed rib cage, anomalous limbs and neural abnormalities such as encephalocele, craniorachischisis, and spina bifida were observed. There are no adequate and well-controlled studies of fluorometholone in pregnant women, and it is not known whether fluorometholone can cause fetal harm when administered to a pregnant woman. Fluorometholone should be used during pregnancy only if the potential benefit justifies the potential risk to the fetus.

Nursing Mothers: It is not known whether topical ophthalmic adminstration of corticosteroids could result in sufficient systemic absorption to produce detectable quantities in human milk. Systemically administered corticosteroids appear in human milk and could suppress growth, interfere with endogenous corticosteroids production, or cause other untoward effects. Because of the potential for serious adverse reactions in nursing infants from fluorometholone, a decision should be made whether to discontinue nursing or to discontinue the drug, taking into account the importance of the drug to the mother.

Pediatric Use: Safety and effectiveness in infants below the age of two years have not been established.

Adverse Reactions: Adverse reactions include, in decreasing order of frequency, elevation of intraocular pressure (IOP) with possible development of glaucoma and infrequent optic nerve damage, posterior subcapsular cataract formation, and delayed wound healing.

Although systemic effects are extremely uncommon, there have been rare occurrences of systemic hypercorticoidism after use of topical steroids.

Corticosteroid-containing preparations have also been reported to cause acute anterior uveitis and perforation of the globe. Keratitis, conjunctivitis, corneal ulcers, mydriasis, conjunctival hyperemia, loss of accommodation and ptosis have occasionally been reported following local use of corticosteroids.

The development of secondary ocular infection (bacterial, fungal and viral) has occurred. Fungal and viral infections of the cornea are particularly prone to develop coincidentally with long-term applications of steroids. The possibility of fungal invasion should be considered in any persistent corneal ulceration where steroid treatment has been used (see **Warnings**). Other adverse events reported with the use of FML FORTE® include transient burning and stinging upon instillation, ocular irritation, taste perversion, and visual disturbance (blurry vision).

Dosage and Administration: Instill one drop into the conjunctival sac two to four times daily. Care should be taken not to discontinue therapy prematurely. If signs and symptoms fail to improve after two days, the patient should be re-evaluated (see **Precautions**).

The dosing of FML FORTE® suspension may be reduced, but care should be taken not to discontinue therapy prematurely. In chronic conditions, withdrawal of treatment should be carried out by gradually decreasing the frequency of applications.

How Supplied: FML FORTE® (fluorometholone) 0.25% LIQUIFILM® sterile ophthalmic suspension is supplied in plastic dropper bottles in the following sizes:

2 mL—NDC 11980-228-02
5 mL—NDC 11980-228-05
10 mL—NDC 11980-228-10
15 mL—NDC 11980-228-15

Note: Store at or below 25°C (77°F); protect from freezing. **Shake well before using.**

Rx only

FML® ℞
(fluorometholone) 0.1%

LIQUIFILM®
sterile ophthalmic suspension

Description: FML® (fluorometholone) 0.1% LIQUIFILM® sterile ophthalmic suspension is a topical anti-inflammatory agent for ophthalmic use.

Chemical Name: Fluorometholone: 9-Fluoro-11β,17-dihydroxy-6α-methylpregna-1,4-diene-3,20-dione.

Contains:
Active: fluorometholone 0.1%. Inactives: benzalkonium chloride 0.004%; LIQUIFILM® (polyvinyl alcohol) 1.4%; edetate disodium; sodium chloride; sodium phosphate, monobasic; sodium phosphate, dibasic; polysorbate 80; sodium hydroxide to adjust the pH, and purified water.

Clinical Pharmacology: Corticosteroids inhibit the inflammatory response to a variety of inciting agents and probably delay or slow healing. They inhibit the edema, fibrin deposition, capillary dilation, leukocyte migration, capillary proliferation, fibroblast proliferation, deposition of collagen, and scar formation associated with inflammation.

There is no generally accepted explanation for the mechanism of action of ocular corticosteroids. However, corticosteroids are thought to act by the induction of phospholipase A_2 inhibitory proteins, collectively called lipocortins. It is postulated that these proteins control the biosynthesis of potent mediators of inflammation such as prostaglandins and leukotrienes by inhibiting the release of their common precursor arachidonic acid. Arachidonic acid is released from membrane phospholipids by phospholipase A_2.

Corticosteroids are capable of producing a rise in intraocular pressure. In clinical studies on patients' eyes treated with both dexamethasone and fluorometholone 0.1% suspensions, fluorometholone demonstrated a lower propensity to increase intraocular pressure than did dexamethasone.

Indications and Usage: FML® suspension is indicated for the treatment of corticosteroid-responsive inflammation of the palpebral and bulbar conjunctiva, cornea and anterior segment of the globe.

Contraindications: FML® suspension is contraindicated in most viral diseases of the cornea and conjunctiva, including epithelial herpes simplex keratitis (dendritic keratitis), vaccinia, and varicella, and also in mycobacterial infection of the eye and fungal diseases of ocular structures. FML® suspension is also contraindicated in individuals with known or suspected hypersensitivity to any of the ingredients of this preparation and to other corticosteroids.

Warnings: Prolonged use of corticosteroids may result in glaucoma with damage to the optic nerve, defects in visual acuity and fields of vision, and in posterior subcapsular cataract formation. Prolonged use may also suppress the host immune response and thus increase the hazard of secondary ocular infections.

Various ocular diseases and long-term use of topical corticosteroids have been known to cause corneal and scleral thinning. Use of topical corticosteroids in the presence of thin corneal or scleral tissue may lead to perforation.

Acute purulent infections of the eye may be masked or activity enhanced by presence of corticosteroid medication.

If this product is used for 10 days or longer, intraocular pressure should be routinely monitored even though it may be difficult in children and uncooperative patients. Steroids should be used with caution in the presence of glaucoma. Intraocular pressure should be checked frequently.

The use of steroids after cataract surgery may delay healing and increase the incidence of bleb formation.

Use of ocular steroids may prolong the course and may exacerbate the severity of many viral infections of the eye (including herpes simplex). Employment of a corticosteroid medication in the treatment of patients with a history of herpes simplex requires great caution; frequent slit lamp microscopy is recommended.

Corticosteroids are not effective in mustard gas keratitis and Sjögren's keratoconjunctivitis.

Precautions:

General: The initial prescription and renewal of the medication order beyond 20 milliliters of FML® suspension should be made by a physician only after examination of the patient with the aid of magnification, such as slit lamp biomicroscopy and, where appropriate, fluorescein staining. If signs and symptoms fail to improve after two days, the patient should be re-evaluated.

As fungal infections of the cornea are particularly prone to develop coincidentally with long-term local corticosteroid applications, fungal invasion should be suspected in any persistent corneal ulceration where a corticosteroid has been used or is in use. Fungal cultures should be taken when appropriate.

If this product is used for 10 days or longer, intraocular pressure should be monitored (see **Warnings**).

Information for Patients: If inflammation or pain persists longer than 48 hours or becomes aggravated, the patient should be advised to discontinue use of the medication and consult a physician.

This product is sterile when packaged. To prevent contamination, care should be taken to avoid touching the bottle tip to eyelids or to any other surface. The use of this bottle by more than one person may spread infection. Keep bottle tightly closed when not in use. Keep out of the reach of children.

Carcinogenesis, mutagenesis, impairment of fertility: No studies have been conducted in animals or in humans to evaluate the possibility of these effects with fluorometholone.

Pregnancy: Teratogenic effects. Pregnancy Category C: Fluorometholone has been shown to be embryocidal and teratogenic in rabbits when administered at low multiples of the human ocular dose. Fluorometholone was applied ocularly to rabbits daily on days 6–18 of gestation, and dose-related fetal loss and fetal abnormalities including cleft palate, deformed rib cage, anomalous limbs and neural abnormalities such as encephalocele, craniorachischisis, and spina bifida were observed. There are no adequate and well-controlled studies of fluorometholone in pregnant women, and it is not known whether fluorometholone can cause fetal harm when administered to a pregnant woman. Fluorometholone should be used during pregnancy only if the potential benefit justifies the potential risk to the fetus.

Nursing Mothers: It is not known whether topical ophthalmic administration of corticosteroids could result in sufficient systemic absorption to produce detectable quantities in human milk. Systemically administered corticosteroids appear in human milk and could suppress growth, interfere with endogenous corticosteroid production, or cause other untoward effects. Because of the potential for serious adverse reactions in nursing infants from fluorometholone, a decision should be made whether to discontinue nursing or to discontinue the drug, taking into account the importance of the drug to the mother.

Pediatric Use: Safety and effectiveness in infants below the age of 2 years have not been established.

Adverse Reactions: Adverse reactions include, in decreasing order of frequency, elevation of intraocular pressure (IOP) with possible development of glaucoma and infrequent optic nerve damage, posterior subcapsular cataract formation, and delayed wound healing.

Although systemic effects are extremely uncommon, there have been rare occurrences of systemic hypercorticoidism after use of topical steroids.

Corticosteroid-containing preparations have also been reported to cause acute anterior uveitis and perforation of the globe. Keratitis, conjunctivitis, corneal ulcers, mydriasis, conjunctival hyperemia, loss of accommodation and ptosis have occasionally been reported following local use of corticosteroids.

The development of secondary ocular infection (bacterial, fungal and viral) has occurred. Fungal and viral infections of the cornea are particularly prone to develop coincidentally with long-term applications of steroids. The possibility of fungal invasion should be considered in any persistent corneal ulceration where steroid treatment has been used (see **Warnings**).

Transient burning and stinging upon instillation and other minor symptoms of ocular irritation have been reported with the use of FML® suspension. Other adverse events reported with the use of FML® suspension include: allergic reactions, visual disturbance (blurry vision) and taste perversion.

Dosage and Administration: Instill one drop into the conjunctival sac two to four times daily. During the initial 24 to 48 hours, the dosage may be increased to one application every four hours. Care should be taken not to discontinue therapy prematurely.

If signs and symptoms fail to improve after two days, the patient should be re-evaluated (see **Precautions**).

The dosing of FML® suspension may be reduced, but care should be taken not to discontinue therapy prematurely. In chronic conditions, withdrawal of treatment should be carried out by gradually decreasing the frequency of applications.

Continued on next page

FML—Cont.

How Supplied: FML® (fluorometholone) 0.1% LIQUIFILM® sterile ophthalmic suspension is supplied in plastic dropper bottles in the following sizes:

1 mL—NDC 11980-211-01
5 mL—NDC 11980-211-05
10 mL—NDC 11980-211-10
15 mL—NDC 11980-211-15

Note: Store at or below 25°C (77°F); protect from freezing. **Shake well before using.**
Rx only

FML® ℞
(fluorometholone ophthalmic ointment) 0.1% sterile

Description: FML® (fluorometholone ophthalmic ointment) 0.1% is a topical anti-inflammatory agent for ophthalmic use.
Chemical Name: Fluorometholone: 9-Fluoro-11β, 17-dihydroxy-6α-methylpregna-1,4-diene-3,20-dione.
Contains: Active: fluorometholone 0.1%. Preservative: phenylmercuric acetate (0.0008%). Inactives: white petrolatum; mineral oil; and petrolatum (and) lanolin alcohol.
Clinical Pharmacology: Corticosteroids inhibit the inflammatory response to a variety of inciting agents and probably delay or slow healing. They inhibit the edema, fibrin deposition, capillary dilation, leukocyte migration, capillary proliferation, fibroblast proliferation, deposition of collagen and scar formation associated with inflammation.
There is no generally accepted explanation for the mechanism of action of ocular corticosteroids. However, corticosteroids are thought to act by the induction of phospholipase A_2 inhibitory proteins, collectively called lipocortins. It is postulated that these proteins control the biosynthesis of potent mediators of inflammation such as prostaglandins and leukotrienes by inhibiting the release of their common precursor arachidonic acid. Arachidonic acid is released from membrane phospholipids by phospholipase A_2.
Corticosteroids are capable of producing a rise in intraocular pressure. In clinical studies of documented steroid-responders, fluorometholone demonstrated a significantly longer average time to produce a rise in intraocular pressure than dexamethasone phosphate; however, in a small percentage of individuals, a significant rise in intraocular pressure occurred within one week. The ultimate magnitude of the rise was equivalent for both drugs.
Indications and Usage: FML® ophthalmic ointment is indicated for the treatment of steroid-responsive inflammation of the palpebral and bulbar conjunctiva, cornea and anterior segment of the globe.
Contraindications: FML® ophthalmic ointment is contraindicated in most viral diseases of the cornea and conjunctiva, including epithelial herpes simplex keratitis (dendritic keratitis), vaccinia, and varicella and also in mycobacterial infection of the eye and fungal diseases of ocular structures. FML® ointment is also contraindicated in individuals with known or suspected hypersensitivity to any of the ingredients of this preparation and to other corticosteroids.
Warnings: Prolonged use of corticosteroids may result in glaucoma with damage to the optic nerve, defects in visual acuity and fields of vision, and in posterior subcapsular cataract formation. Prolonged use may also suppress the host immune response and thus increase the hazard of secondary ocular infections.
Various ocular diseases and long-term use of topical corticosteroids have been known to cause corneal and scleral thinning. Use of topical corticosteroids in the presence of thin corneal or scleral tissue may lead to perforation. Acute purulent infections of the eye may be masked or activity enhanced by the presence of corticosteroid medication.
If this product is used for 10 days or longer, intraocular pressure should be routinely monitored even though it may be difficult in children and uncooperative patients. Steroids should be used with caution in the presence of glaucoma. Intraocular pressure should be checked frequently.
The use of steroids after cataract surgery may delay healing and increase the incidence of bleb formation.
Use of ocular steroids may prolong the course and may exacerbate the severity of many viral infections of the eye (including herpes simplex). Employment of a corticosteroid medication in the treatment of patients with a history of herpes simplex requires great caution; frequent slit lamp microscopy is recommended.
Corticosteroids are not effective in mustard gas keratitis and Sjögren's keratoconjunctivitis.
Precautions:
General: The initial prescription and renewal of the medication order beyond 8 grams of FML® ophthalmic ointment should be made by a physician only after examination of the patient with the aid of magnification, such as slit lamp biomicroscopy and, where appropriate, fluorescein staining. If signs and symptoms fail to improve after two days, the patient should be re-evaluated.
As fungal infections of the cornea are particularly prone to develop coincidentally with long-term local corticosteroid applications, fungal invasion should be suspected in any persistent corneal ulceration where a corticosteroid has been used or is in use. Fungal cultures should be taken when appropriate.
If this product is used for 10 days or longer, intraocular pressure should be monitored (see **Warnings**).
Ophthalmic ointments may retard corneal healing.
Information for Patients: If inflammation or pain persists longer than 48 hours or becomes aggravated, the patient should be advised to discontinue use of the medication and consult a physician.
This product is sterile when packaged. To prevent contamination, care should be taken to avoid touching the tube tip to eyelids or to any other surface. The use of this tube by more than one person may spread infection. Keep tube tightly closed when not in use. Keep out of the reach of children.
Carcinogenesis, mutagenesis, impairment of fertility: No studies have been conducted in animals or in humans to evaluate the possibility of these effects with fluorometholone.
Pregnancy: Teratogenic effects. Pregnancy Category C: Fluorometholone has been shown to be embryocidal and teratogenic in rabbits when administered at low multiples of the human ocular dose. Fluorometholone was applied ocularly to rabbits daily on days 6–18 of gestation, and dose-related fetal loss and fetal abnormalities including cleft palate, deformed rib cage, anamalous limbs and neural abnormalities such as encephalocele, craniorachischisis, and spina bifida were observed. There are no adequate and well-controlled studies of fluorometholone in pregnant women, and it is not known whether fluorometholone can cause fetal harm when administered to a pregnant woman. Fluorometholone should be used during pregnancy only if the potential benefit justifies the potential risk to the fetus.
Nursing Mothers: It is not known whether topical ophthalmic administration of corticosteroids could result in sufficient systemic absorption to produce detectable quantities in human milk. Systemically administered corticosteroids appear in human milk and could suppress growth, interfere with endogenous corticosteroid production, or cause other untoward effects. Because of the potential for serious adverse reactions in nursing infants from fluorometholone, a decision should be made whether to discontinue nursing or to discontinue the drug, taking into account the importance of the drug to the mother.
Pediatric Use: Safety and effectiveness in infants below the age of 2 years have not been established.
Adverse Reactions: Adverse reactions include, in decreasing order of frequency, elevation of intraocular pressure (IOP) with possible development of glaucoma and infrequent optic nerve damage, posterior subcapsular cataract formation, and delayed wound healing.
Although systemic effects are extremely uncommon, there have been rare occurrences of systemic hypercorticoidism after use of topical steroids.
Corticosteroid-containing preparations have also been reported to cause acute anterior uveitis and perforation of the globe. Keratitis, conjunctivitis, corneal ulcers, mydriasis, conjunctival hyperemia, loss of accommodation and ptosis have occasionally been reported following local use of corticosteroids.
The development of secondary ocular infection (bacterial, fungal and viral) has occurred. Fungal and viral infections of the cornea are particularly prone to develop coincidentally with long-term applications of steroids. The possibility of fungal invasion should be considered in any persistent corneal ulceration where steroid treatment has been used (see **Warnings**).
Dosage and Administration: A small amount (approximately 1/2 inch ribbon) of ointment should be applied to the conjunctival sac one to three times daily. During the initial 24 to 48 hours, the frequency of dosing may be increased to one application every four hours. Care should be taken not to discontinue therapy prematurely.
If signs and symptoms fail to improve after two days, the patient should be re-evaluated (see **Precautions**).
The dosing of FML® ophthalmic ointment may be reduced, but care should be taken not to discontinue therapy prematurely. In chronic conditions, withdrawal of treatment should be carried out by gradually decreasing the frequency of applications.
How Supplied: FML® (fluorometholone ophthalmic ointment) 0.1% is supplied in ophthalmic ointment tubes in the following size:

3.5 g—NDC 0023-0316-04

Note: Store at or below 25°C (77°F). Avoid exposure to temperatures above 40°C (104°F).
Rx only

FML-S® ℞
(fluorometholone, sulfacetamide sodium) LIQUIFILM®
sterile ophthalmic suspension

Description: FML-S® LIQUIFILM sterile ophthalmic suspension is a topical anti-inflammatory/anti-infective combination product for ophthalmic use.
Chemical Names: Fluorometholone: 9-Fluoro-11β, 17-dihydroxy-6α-methylpregna-1,4-diene-3, 20-dione.
Sulfacetamide sodium: N-Sulfanilylacetamide monosodium salt monohydrate.
Contains: Actives: fluorometholone 0.1%, sulfacetamide sodium 10%. Preservative: benzalkonium chloride (0.006%). Inactives: Liquifilm® (polyvinyl alcohol) 1.4%; edetate disodium;

polysorbate 80; povidone; sodium chloride; sodium phosphate, dibasic; sodium phosphate, monobasic; sodium thiosulfate; hydrochloric acid and/or sodium hydroxide to adjust the pH; and purified water.

Clinical Pharmacology: Corticosteroids suppress the inflammatory response to a variety of agents and they probably delay or slow healing. Corticosteroids and their derivatives are capable of producing a rise in intraocular pressure. Since corticosteroids may inhibit the body's defense mechanism against infection, a concomitant antimicrobial drug may be used when this inhibition is considered to be clinically significant in a particular case.

In clinical studies of documented steroid-responders, fluorometholone demonstrated a significantly longer average time to produce a rise in intraocular pressure than dexamethasone phosphate; however, in a small percentage of individuals, a significant rise in intraocular pressure occurred within one week. The ultimate magnitude of the rise was equivalent for both drugs.

The anti-infective component in FML-S® is included to provide action against specific organisms susceptible to it. Sulfacetamide sodium is active *in-vitro* against susceptible strains of the following microorganisms: *Escherichia coli, Staphylococcus aureus, Streptococcus pneumoniae, Streptococcus* (viridans group), *Haemophilus influenzae, Klebsiella* species, and *Enterobacter* species. Some strains of these bacteria may be resistant to sulfacetamide or resistant strains may emerge *in vivo.*

When a decision to administer both a corticosteroid and an antimicrobial is made, the administration of such drugs in combination has the advantage of greater patient compliance and convenience, with the added assurance that the appropriate dosage of both drugs is administered. When both types of drugs are in the same formulation, compatibility of ingredients is assured and the correct volume of drug is delivered and retained.

The relative potency of corticosteroid formulations depends on the molecular structure, concentration, and release from the vehicle.

Indications and Usage: FML-S® is indicated for steroid-responsive inflammatory ocular conditions for which a corticosteroid is indicated and where superficial bacterial ocular infection or a risk of bacterial ocular infection exists.

Ocular steroids are indicated in inflammatory conditions of the palpebral and bulbar conjunctiva, cornea, and anterior segment of the globe where the inherent risk of steroid use in certain infective conjunctivitides is accepted to obtain a diminution in edema and inflammation. They are also indicated in chronic anterior uveitis and corneal injury from chemical, radiation or thermal burns or penetration of foreign bodies.

The use of a combination drug with an anti-infective component is indicated where the risk of superficial ocular infection is high or where there is an expectation that potentially dangerous numbers of bacteria will be present in the eye.

The anti-infective drug in this product, sulfacetamide, is active against the following common bacterial eye pathogens: *Escherichia coli, Staphylococcus aureus, Streptococcus pneumoniae, Streptococcus* (viridans group), *Haemophilus influenzae, Klebsiella* species, and *Enterobacter* species.

The product does not provide adequate coverage against: *Neisseria* species and *Serratia marcescens.* A significant percentage of Staphylococcal isolates are completely resistant to sulfa drugs.

Contraindications: FML-S® suspension is contraindicated in most viral diseases of the cornea and conjunctiva, including epithelial herpes simplex keratitis (dendritic keratitis), vaccinia, and varicella, and also in mycobacterial infection of the eye and fungal diseases of ocular structures. FML-S® suspension is also contraindicated in individuals with known or suspected hypersensitivity to any of the ingredients of this preparation, to sulfonamides and to other corticosteroids.

Warnings:

NOT FOR INJECTION INTO THE EYE.

Prolonged use of steroids may result in glaucoma, with damage to the optic nerve, defects in visual acuity and fields of vision, and in posterior subcapsular cataract formation. If used for longer than 10 days, intraocular pressure should be routinely monitored even though it may be difficult in children and uncooperative patients.

Prolonged use of steroids may suppress the host immune response in ocular tissues and thus increase the hazard of secondary ocular infections. Various ocular diseases and long-term use of topical corticosteroids have been known to cause corneal and scleral thinning. Use of topical corticosteroids in the presence of thin corneal or scleral tissue may lead to perforation. In acute purulent conditions of the eye, corticosteroids may mask infection or enhance existing infection.

Use of ocular steroids may prolong the course and may exacerbate the severity of many viral infections of the eye.

Employment of a corticosteroid medication in the treatment of patients with a history of herpes simplex requires great caution.

FATALITIES HAVE OCCURRED, ALTHOUGH RARELY, DUE TO SEVERE REACTIONS TO SULFONAMIDES INCLUDING STEVENS-JOHNSON SYNDROME, TOXIC EPIDERMAL NECROLYSIS, FULMINANT HEPATIC NECROSIS, AGRANULOCYTOSIS, APLASTIC ANEMIA, AND OTHER BLOOD DYSCRASIAS. Sensitizations may recur when a sulfonamide is readministered, irrespective of the route of administration. If signs of hypersensitivity or other serious reactions occur, discontinue use of this preparation (see **Adverse Reactions**).

Cross-sensitivity among corticosteroids has been demonstrated.

A significant percentage of staphylococcal isolates are completely resistant to sulfa drugs.

Precautions:

General: The initial prescription and renewal of the medication order beyond 20 milliliters should be made only by a physician after evaluation of the patient's intraocular pressure, examination of the patient with the aid of magnification, such as slit lamp biomicroscopy and, where appropriate, fluorescein staining.

Keep this and all drugs out of the reach of children.

Drug Interactions: Sulfacetamide preparations are incompatible with silver preparations.

Carcinogenesis, mutagenesis, impairment of fertility: No studies have been conducted in animals or in humans to evaluate the possibility of these effects with fluorometholone or sulfacetamide.

Pregnancy: Pregnancy Category C: Animal studies have not been conducted with FML-S® Liquifilm Ophthalmic Suspension. Fluorometholone has been shown to be embryocidal and teratogenic in rabbits when administered at low multiples of the human dose. Fluorometholone was applied ocularly to rabbits daily on days 6–18 of gestation, and dose-related fetal loss and fetal abnormalities including cleft palate, deformed rib cage, anomalous limbs and neural abnormalities such as encephalocele, craniorachischisis, and spina bifida were observed. Kernicterus may be precipitated in infants by sulfonamides being given systemically during the third trimester of pregnancy. There are no adequate and well-controlled studies of FML-S® Liquifilm Ophthalmic Suspension in pregnant women, and it is not known whether FML-S® can cause fetal harm when administered to a pregnant woman. FML-S® Liquifilm Ophthalmic Suspension should be used during pregnancy only if the potential benefit justifies the potential risk to the fetus.

Nursing Mothers: It is not known whether topical administration of corticosteroids could result in sufficient systemic absorption to produce detectable quantities in breast milk. Systemically administered corticosteroids appear in breast milk and could suppress growth, interfere with endogenous corticosteroid production, or cause other untoward effects. Systemically administered sulfonamides are capable of producing kernicterus in infants of lactating women. Because of the potential for serious adverse reactions in nursing infants from FML-S, a decision should be made whether to discontinue nursing or to discontinue the medication.

Pediatric Use: Safety and effectiveness in pediatric patients have not been established.

Adverse Reactions: Adverse reactions have occurred with corticosteroid/anti-infective combination drugs which can be attributed to the corticosteroid component, the anti-infective component, or the combination. Exact incidence figures are not available since no denominator of treated patients is available.

Reactions occurring most often from the presence of the anti-infective ingredient are allergic sensitizations. Fatalities have occurred, although rarely, due to severe reactions to sulfonamides including Stevens-Johnson syndrome, toxic epidermal necrolysis, fulminant hepatic necrosis, agranulocytosis, aplastic anemia, and other blood dyscrasias (see **Warnings**). Sulfacetamide sodium may cause local irritation.

The reactions due to the corticosteroid component in decreasing order of frequency are: elevation of intraocular pressure (IOP) with possible development of glaucoma, and infrequent optic nerve damage; posterior subcapsular cataract formation; and delayed wound healing.

Secondary Infection: The development of secondary infection has occurred after use of combinations containing corticosteroids and antimicrobials. Fungal infections of the cornea are particularly prone to develop coincidentally with long-term application of corticosteroids. When signs of chronic ocular inflammation persist following prolonged corticosteroid dosing, the possibility of fungal infections of the cornea should be considered.

Secondary bacterial ocular infection following suppression of host responses also occurs.

Dosage and Administration: One drop of FML-S® should be instilled into the conjunctival sac four times daily. Care should be taken not to discontinue therapy prematurely.

Not more than 20 milliliters should be prescribed initially and the prescription should not be refilled without further evaluation as outlined in **Precautions** above.

How Supplied: FML-S® (fluorometholone, sulfacetamide sodium) Liquifilm® Sterile Ophthalmic Suspension is supplied in plastic dropper bottles in the following sizes:

5 mL—NDC 11980-422-05
10 mL—NDC 11980-422-10

Note: Store at controlled room temperature 15°–30°C (59°–86°F). Protect from freezing and light. **SHAKE WELL BEFORE USING.** Do not use suspension if it is dark brown.

Rx only

Continued on next page

GENOPTIC® ℞
(gentamicin sulfate ophthalmic solution, USP) 0.3%
Sterile
and

GENOPTIC® ℞
(gentamicin sulfate ophthalmic ointment, USP)
Sterile
Each gram contains gentamicin sulfate, USP equivalent to 3.0 mg gentamicin

Description: GENOPTIC® is a sterile, topical anti-infective agent for ophthalmic use. Gentamicin sulfate is a water-soluble antibiotic of the aminoglycoside group.
Gentamicin is obtained from cultures of *Micromonospora purpurea.* It is a mixture of the sulfate salts of gentamicin C_1, C_2, and C_{1A}. All three components appear to have similar antimicrobial activities. Gentamicin sulfate occurs as a white to buff powder and is soluble in water and insoluble in alcohol.
GENOPTIC® Solution:
Contains: Each mL contains—Active: gentamicin sulfate equivalent to 3 mg (0.3%) gentamicin base. Preservative: benzalkonium chloride. Inactives: Liquifilm® (polyvinyl alcohol) 14 mg (1.4%); edetate disodium; sodium phosphate, dibasic; sodium chloride; hydrochloric acid and/or sodium hydroxide to adjust the pH; and purified water. The solution is an aqueous, buffered solution with a pH of 7.2–7.5.
GENOPTIC® Ointment:
Contains: Each gram contains gentamicin sulfate, USP (equivalent to 3.0 mg gentamicin) in a base of white petrolatum, with methylparaben (0.5 mg) and propylparaben (0.1 mg) as preservatives.
Clinical Pharmacology: Microbiology: Gentamicin sulfate is active *in vitro* against many strains of the following microorganisms: *Staphylococcus aureus, Staphylococcus epidermidis, Streptococcus pyogenes, Streptococcus pneumoniae, Enterobacter aerogenes, Escherichia coli, Haemophilus influenzae, Klebsiella pneumoniae, Neisseria gonorrhoeae, Pseudomonas aeruginosa,* and *Serratia marcescens.*
Indications and Usage: GENOPTIC® Ointment and Solution are indicated in the topical treatment of ocular bacterial infections including conjunctivitis, keratitis, keratoconjunctivitis, corneal ulcers, blepharitis, blepharoconjunctivitis, acute meibomianitis, and dacryocystitis, caused by susceptible strains of the following microorganisms: *Staphylococcus aureus, Staphylococcus epidermidis, Streptococcus pyogenes, Streptococcus pneumoniae, Enterobacter aerogenes, Escherichia coli, Haemophilus influenzae, Klebsiella pneumoniae, Neisseria gonorrhoeae, Pseudomonas aeruginosa, and Serratia marcescens.*
Contraindications: GENOPTIC® is contraindicated in patients with known hypersensitivity to any of the components.
Warnings
NOT FOR INJECTION INTO THE EYE.
Gentamicin sulfate ophthalmic ointment and solution are not for injection. They should never be injected subconjunctivally, nor should they be directly introduced into the anterior chamber of the eye.
Precautions:
General: Prolonged use of topical antibiotics may give rise to overgrowth of nonsusceptible organisms, including fungi. Bacterial resistance to gentamicin may also develop. If purulent discharge, inflammation or pain becomes aggravated, the patient should discontinue use of the medication and consult a physician.
If irritation or hypersensitivity to any component of the drug develops, the patient should discontinue use of this preparation, and appropriate therapy should be instituted.
Ophthalmic ointments may retard corneal healing.
Information for Patients: To avoid contamination, do not touch tip of container to the eye, eyelid or any surface.
Carcinogenesis, Mutagenesis, Impairment of Fertility: There are no published carcinogenicity or impairment of fertility studies on gentamicin. Aminoglycoside antibiotics have been found to be non-mutagenic.
Pregnancy: Pregnancy Category C. Gentamicin has been shown to depress body weights, kidney weights and median glomerular counts in newborn rats when administered systemically to pregnant rats in daily doses approximately 500 times the maximum recommended ophthalmic human dose. There are no adequate and well-controlled studies in pregnant women. Gentamicin should be used during pregnancy only if the potential benefit justifies the potential risk to the fetus.
Adverse Reactions: Bacterial and fungal corneal ulcers have developed during treatment with gentamicin ophthalmic preparations.
The most frequently reported adverse reactions are ocular burning and irritation upon drug instillation, non-specific conjunctivitis, conjunctival epithelial defects and conjunctival hyperemia.
Other adverse reactions which have occurred rarely are allergic reactions, thrombocytopenic purpura and hallucinations.
GENOPTIC® Solution:
Dosage and Administration: Instill one or two drops into the affected eye(s) every four hours. In severe infections, dosage may be increased to as much as two drops every hour.
How Supplied: GENOPTIC® (gentamicin sulfate ophthalmic solution, USP) 0.3% is supplied sterile in plastic dropper bottles in the following sizes:
1 mL—NDC 11980-117-01
5 mL—NDC 11980-117-05
Note: Store at or below 25°C (77°F). Avoid exposure to excessive heat (104°F/40°C or above).
GENOPTIC® Ointment:
Dosage and Administration: Apply a small amount (about $^1/_2$ inch) to the affected eye two to three times a day.
How Supplied: GENOPTIC® (gentamicin sulfate ophthalmic ointment, USP) 0.3% is supplied sterile in a 3.5 gram tube (NDC 0023-0320-04).
Note: Store between 2° and 30°C (36° and 86°F).
Rx only.

HMS® ℞
(medrysone) 1.0%

LIQUIFILM®
sterile ophthalmic suspension

Description: HMS® (medrysone) 1.0% LIQUIFILM® sterile ophthalmic suspension is a topical anti-inflammatory agent for ophthalmic use.
Chemical Name: 11β-Hydroxy-6α-methylpregn-4-ene-3, 20-dione.
Contains: Active: medrysone 1.0%. Preservative: benzalkonium chloride 0.004%. Inactives: LIQUIFILM® (polyvinyl alcohol) 1.4%. edetate disodium; sodium chloride; potassium chloride; sodium phosphate, monobasic; sodium phosphate, dibasic; hydroxypropyl methylcellulose; sodium hydroxide to adjust the pH; and purified water.
Clinical Pharmacology: HMS® (medrysone) is a synthetic corticosteroid with topical anti-inflammatory and anti-allergic activity. Corticosteroids inhibit the inflammatory response to inciting agents of mechanical, chemical, or immunological nature of edema, fibrin deposition, capillary dilation and leukocyte migration, capillary proliferation, deposition of collagen and scar formation. HMS® (medrysone) has less anti-inflammatory potency than 0.1% dexamethasone. Data from 2 uncontrolled studies[1-2] indicate that in patients with increased intraocular pressure and in those susceptible to a rise in intraocular pressure, there is less effect on pressure with HMS® than with dexamethasone or betamethasone.
Indications and Usage: HMS® (medrysone) is indicated for the treatment of allergic conjunctivitis, vernal conjunctivitis, episcleritis, and epinephrine sensitivity.
Contraindications: HMS® (medrysone) is contraindicated in the following conditions:
Acute superficial herpes simplex
Viral diseases of the conjunctiva and cornea
Ocular tuberculosis
Fungal diseases of the eye
Hypersensitivity to any of the components of the drug
Warnings:
Acute purulent infections of the eye may be masked, enhanced or activated by the presence of corticosteroid medication.
Corneal or scleral perforation occasionally has been reported with prolonged use of topical corticosteroids. In high dosages, they have been associated with corneal thinning.
Prolonged use of topical corticosteroids may increase intraocular pressure, with resultant glaucoma, damage to the optic nerve, and defects in visual acuity and fields of vision. However, data from 2 uncontrolled studies[1-2] indicate that in patients with increased intraocular pressure and in those susceptible to a rise in intraocular pressure upon application of topical corticosteroids, there is less effect on pressure with HMS® than with dexamethasone or betamethasone.
Prolonged use of topical corticosteroids may rarely be associated with development of posterior subcapsular cataracts.
Systemic absorption and systemic side effects may result with the use of topical corticosteroids.
HMS® is not recommended for use in iritis and uveitis as its therapeutic effectiveness has not been demonstrated in these conditions.
Corticosteroid medication in the presence of stromal herpes simplex requires great caution; frequent slit-lamp microscopy is suggested.
Prolonged use may aid in the establishment of secondary ocular infections from fungi and viruses liberated from ocular tissue.
Precautions:
General: With prolonged use of HMS®, the intraocular pressure and the lens should be examined periodically. In persistent corneal ulceration where a corticosteroid has been used, or is in use, fungal infection should be suspected.
Carcinogenesis, mutagenesis, impairment of fertility: No studies have been conducted in animals or in humans to evaluate the potential of these effects.
Pregnancy Category C: Medrysone has been shown to be embryocidal in rabbits when given in doses 10 and 30 times the human dose. Medrysone was ocularly applied to both eyes of pregnant rabbits 2 drops 4 times per day on day 6 through 18 of gestation. A significant increase in early resorptions was observed in the treated rabbits. There are no adequate or well-controlled studies in pregnant women. Medrysone should be used during pregnancy only if the potential benefit justifies the potential risk to the fetus.
Pediatric Use: Safety and effectiveness in pediatric patients have not been established.
Adverse Reactions: Adverse reactions include occasional transient stinging and burning on instillation. Increased intraocular pressure, which may be associated with optic nerve damage and defects in the visual fields,

and posterior subcapsular cataract formation have been reported rarely with the use of HMS®.

Overdosage: Overdosage will not ordinarily cause acute problems. If accidentally ingested, drink fluids to dilute.

Dosage and Administration: Shake well before using. Instill one drop in the conjunctival sac up to every four hours.

How Supplied: HMS® (medrysone) 1.0% LIQUIFILM® sterile ophthalmic suspension is supplied in plastic dropper bottles in the following sizes:

5 mL—NDC 11980-074-05
10 mL—NDC 11980-074-10

Note: Protect from freezing.

Rx only

References:

1. Becker B, Kolker AE. Intraocular pressure response to topical corticosteroids. In: Leopold IH, ed. Ocular therapy, complications and management. St. Louis: CV Mosby, 1967.
2. Spaeth G. Hydroxymethylprogesterone. *Arch Ophthalmol.* 1966;75:783–787.

OCUFEN® ℞
(flurbiprofen sodium ophthalmic solution) 0.03%
sterile

Description: OCUFEN® (flurbiprofen sodium ophthalmic solution) 0.03% is a sterile topical nonsteroidal anti-inflammatory product for ophthalmic use.

Chemical Name: Sodium (±)-2-(2-fluoro-4-biphenyl)-propionate dihydrate.

Contains: Active: flurbiprofen sodium 0.03%. Preservative: thimerosal 0.005%. Inactives: polyvinyl alcohol 1.4%; edetate disodium; potassium chloride; sodium chloride; sodium citrate; citric acid; hydrochloric acid and/or sodium hydroxide to adjust the pH; and purified water.

Clinical Pharmacology: Flurbiprofen sodium is one of a series of phenylalkanoic acids that have shown analgesic, antipyretic, and anti-inflammatory activity in animal inflammatory diseases. Its mechanism of action is believed to be through inhibition of the cyclooxygenase enzyme that is essential in the biosynthesis of prostaglandins.

Prostaglandins have been shown in many animal models to be mediators of certain kinds of intraocular inflammation. In studies performed on animal eyes, prostaglandins have been shown to produce disruption of the blood-aqueous humor barrier, vasodilatation, increased vascular permeability, leukocytosis, and increased intraocular pressure.

Prostaglandins also appear to play a role in the miotic response produced during ocular surgery by constricting the iris sphincter independently of cholinergic mechanisms. In clinical studies, OCUFEN® has been shown to inhibit the miosis induced during the course of cataract surgery.

Results from clinical studies indicate that flurbiprofen sodium has no significant effect upon intraocular pressure.

Indications and Usage: OCUFEN® is indicated for the inhibition of intraoperative miosis.

Contraindications: OCUFEN® is contraindicated in individuals who are hypersensitive to any components of the medication.

Warnings: With nonsteroidal anti-inflammatory drugs, there exists the potential for increased bleeding due to interference with thrombocyte aggregation. There have been reports that OCUFEN® may cause increased bleeding of ocular tissues (including hyphemas) in conjunction with ocular surgery. There exists the potential for cross-sensitivity to acetylsalicylic acid and other nonsteroidal anti-inflammatory drugs. Therefore, caution should be used when treating individuals who have previously exhibited sensitivities to these drugs.

Precautions:

General: Wound healing may be delayed with the use of OCUFEN®. It is recommended that OCUFEN® (flurbiprofen sodium ophthalmic solution) 0.03% be used with caution in surgical patients with known bleeding tendencies or who are receiving other medications which may prolong bleeding time.

Drug Interactions: Interaction of OCUFEN® with other topical ophthalmic medications has not been fully investigated. Although clinical studies with acetylcholine chloride and animal studies with acetylcholine chloride or carbachol revealed no interference, and there is no known pharmacological basis for an interaction, there have been reports that acetylcholine chloride and carbachol have been ineffective when used in patients treated with OCUFEN®.

Carcinogenesis, mutagenesis, impairment of fertility: Long-term studies in mice and/or rats have shown no evidence of carcinogenicity or impairment of fertility with flurbiprofen.

Long-term mutagenicity studies in animals have not been performed.

Pregnancy: Pregnancy Category C. Flurbiprofen has been shown to be embryocidal, delay parturition, prolong gestation, reduce weight, and/or slightly retard growth of fetuses when given to rats in daily oral doses of 0.4 mg/kg (approximately 67 times the human daily topical dose) and above. There are no adequate and well-controlled studies in pregnant women. OCUFEN® should be used during pregnancy only if the potential benefit justifies the potential risk to the fetus.

Nursing Mothers: It is not known whether this drug is excreted in human milk. Because many drugs are excreted in human milk and because of the potential for serious adverse reactions in nursing infants from flurbiprofen sodium, a decision should be made whether to discontinue nursing or to discontinue the drug, taking into account the importance of the drug to the mother.

Pediatric use: Safety and effectiveness in pediatric patients have not been established.

Adverse Reactions: Transient burning and stinging upon instillation and other minor symptoms of ocular irritation have been reported with the use of OCUFEN®. Other adverse reactions reported with the use of OCUFEN® include: fibrosis, miosis, and mydriasis.

Increased bleeding tendency of ocular tissues in conjunction with ocular surgery has also been reported.

Overdosage: Overdosage will not ordinarily cause acute problems. If accidentally ingested, drink fluids to dilute.

Dosage and Administration: A total of four (4) drops of OCUFEN® should be administered by instilling 1 drop approximately every ½ hour beginning 2 hours before surgery.

How Supplied: OCUFEN® (flurbiprofen sodium ophthalmic solution) 0.03% is supplied in plastic dropper bottles in the following size:

2.5 mL—NDC 11980-801-03

Note: Store at room temperature.

Caution: Rx only

OCUFLOX® ℞
(ofloxacin ophthalmic solution) 0.3%
sterile

Description: OCUFLOX® (ofloxacin ophthalmic solution) 0.3% is a sterile ophthalmic solution. It is a fluorinated carboxyquinolone anti-infective for topical ophthalmic use.

Structural Formula:

ofloxacin

ofloxacin

$C_{18}H_{20}FN_3O_4$ Mol Wt. 361.37

Chemical Name: (±)-9-Fluoro-2,3-dihydro-3-methyl-10-(4-methyl-1-piperazinyl)-7-oxo-7H-pyrido[1,2,3-de]-1,4 benzoxazine-6-carboxylic acid.

Contains:

Active:	ofloxacin 0.3% (3 mg/mL);
Preservative:	benzalkonium chloride (0.005%);
Inactives:	sodium chloride and purified water. May also contain hydrochloric acid and/or sodium hydroxide to adjust pH.

OCUFLOX® solution is unbuffered and formulated with a pH of 6.4 (range—6.0 to 6.8). It has an osmolality of 300 mOsm/kg. Ofloxacin is a fluorinated 4-quinolone which differs from other fluorinated 4-quinolones in that there is a six member (pyridobenzoxazine) ring from positions 1 to 8 of the basic ring structure.

Clinical Pharmacology: Pharmacokinetics: Serum, urine and tear concentrations of ofloxacin were measured in 30 healthy women at various time points during a ten-day course of treatment with OCUFLOX® solution. The mean serum ofloxacin concentration ranged from 0.4 ng/mL to 1.9 ng/mL. Maximum ofloxacin concentration increased from 1.1 ng/mL on day one to 1.9 ng/mL on day 11 after QID dosing for 10 ½ days. Maximum serum ofloxacin concentrations after ten days of topical ophthalmic dosing were more than 1000 times lower than those reported after standard oral doses of ofloxacin.

Tear ofloxacin concentrations ranged from 5.7 to 31 μg/g during the 40 minute period following the last dose on day 11. Mean tear concentration measured four hours after topical ophthalmic dosing was 9.2 μg/g.

Corneal tissue concentrations of 4.4 μg/mL were observed four hours after beginning topical ocular application of two drops of OCUFLOX® every 30 minutes. Ofloxacin was excreted in the urine primarily unmodified.

Microbiology: Ofloxacin has in vitro activity against a broad range of gram-positive and gram-negative aerobic and anaerobic bacteria. Ofloxacin is bactericidal at concentrations equal to or slightly greater than inhibitory concentrations. Ofloxacin is thought to exert a bactericidal effect on susceptible bacterial cells by inhibiting DNA gyrase, an essential bacterial enzyme which is a critical catalyst in the duplication, trascription, and repair of bacterial DNA.

Cross-resistance has been observed between ofloxacin and other fluoroquinolones. There is generally no cross-resistance between ofloxacin and other classes of antibacterial agents such as beta-lactams or aminoglycosides.

Ofloxacin has been shown to be active against most strains of the following organisms both in vitro and clinically, in conjunctival and/or corneal ulcer infections as described in the **INDICATIONS AND USAGE** section.

Continued on next page

Ocuflox—Cont.

AEROBES, GRAM-POSITIVE:
Staphylococcus aureus
Staphylococcus epidermidis
Streptococcus pneumoniae
AEROBES, GRAM-NEGATIVE:
Enterobacter cloacae
Haemophilus influenzae
Proteus mirabilis
Pseudomonas aeruginosa
*Serratia marcescens**
ANAEROBIC SPECIES:
Propionibacterium acnes
*Efficacy for this organism was studied in fewer than 10 infections.

The safety and effectiveness of OCUFLOX® in treating ophthalmologic infections due to the following organisms have not been established in adequate and well-controlled clinical trials. OCUFLOX® has been shown to be active in vitro against most strains of these organisms but the clinical significance of ophthalmologic infections is unknown.

AEROBES, GRAM-POSITIVE:
Enterococcus faecalis
Listeria monocytogenes
Staphylococcus capitis
Staphylococcus hominus
Staphylococcus simulans
Streptococcus pyogenes
AEROBES, GRAM-NEGATIVE:
Acinetobacter calcoaceticus var. *anitratus*
Acinetobacter calcoaceticus var. *lwoffii*
Citrobacter diversus
Citrobacter freundii
Enterobacter aerogenes
Enterobacter agglomerans
Escherichia coli
Haemophilus parainfluenzae
Klebsiella oxytoca
Klebsiella pneumoniae
Moraxella (Branhamella) catarrhalis
Moraxella lacunata
Morganella morganii
Neisseria gonorrhoeae
Pseudomonas acidovorans
Pseudomonas fluorescens
Shigella sonnei
OTHER:
Chalmydia trachomatis

Clinical Studies:
Conjunctivitis: In a randomized, double-masked, multicenter clinical trial, OCUFLOX® solution was superior to its vehicle after 2 days of treatment in patients with conjunctivitis and positive conjunctival cultures. Clinical outcomes for the trial demonstrated a clinical improvement rate of 86% (54/63) for the ofloxacin treated group versus 72% (48/67) for the placebo treated group after 2 days of therapy. Microbiological outcomes for the same clinical trial demonstrated an eradication rate for causative pathogens of 65% (41/63) for the ofloxacin treated group versus 25% (17/67) for the vehicle treated group after 2 days of therapy. Please note that microbiologic eradication does not always correlate with clinical outcome in anti-infective trials.
Corneal Ulcers: In a randomized, double-masked, multi-center clinical trial of 140 subjects with positive cultures, OCUFLOX® treated subjects had an overall clinical success rate (complete re-epithelialization and no progression of the infiltrate for two consecutive visits) of 82% (61/74) compared to 80% (53/66) for the fortified antibiotic group, consisting of 1.5% tobramycin and 10% cefazolin solutions. The median time to clinical success was 11 days for the ofloxacin group and 10 days for the fortified treatment group.

Indications and Usage: OCUFLOX® solution is indicated for the treatment of infections caused by susceptible strains of the following bacteria in the conditions listed below:

CONJUNCTIVITIS:

Gram-positive bacteria:
Staphylococcus aureus
Staphylococcus epidermidis
Streptococcus pneumoniae

Gram-negative bacteria:
Enterobacter cloacae
Haemophilus influenzae
Proteus mirabilis
Pseudomonas aeruginosa

CORNEAL ULCERS:

Gram-positive bacteria:
Staphylococcus aureus
Staphylococcus epidermidis
Streptococcus pneumoniae

Gram-negative bacteria:
Pseudomonas aeruginosa
*Serratia marcescens**

Anaerobic species:
Propionibacterium acnes

*Efficacy for this organism was studied in fewer than 10 infections.

Contraindications:
OCUFLOX® solution is contraindicated in patients with a history of hypersensitivity to ofloxacin, to other quinolones, or to any of the components in this medication.

Warnings: NOT FOR INJECTION
OCUFLOX® solution should not be injected subconjunctivally, nor should it be introduced directly into the anterior chamber of the eye.
Serious and occasionally fatal hypersensitivity (anaphylactic) reactions, some following the first dose, have been reported in patients receiving systemic quinolones, including ofloxacin. Some reactions were accompanied by cardiovascular collapse, loss of consciousness, angioedema (including laryngeal, pharyngeal or facial edema), airway obstruction, dyspnea, urticaria, and itching. A rare occurrence of Stevens-Johnson syndrome, which progressed to toxic epidermal necrolysis, has been reported in a patient who was receiving topical ophthalmic ofloxacin. If an allergic reaction to ofloxacin occurs, discontinue the drug. Serious acute hypersensitivity reactions may require immediate emergency treatment. Oxygen and airway management, including intubation should be administered as clinically indicated.

Precautions: General: As with other anti-infectives, prolonged use may result in overgrowth of nonsusceptible organisms, including fungi. If superinfection occurs discontinue use and institute alternative therapy. Whenever clinical judgment dictates, the patient should be examined with the aid of magnification, such as slit lamp biomicroscopy and, where appropriate, fluorescein staining. Ofloxacin should be discontinued at the first appearance of a skin rash or any other sign of hypersensitivity reaction.
The systemic administration of quinolones, including ofloxacin, has led to lesions or erosions of the cartilage in weight-bearing joints and other signs of arthropathy in immature animals of various species. Ofloxacin, administered systemically at 10 mg/kg/day in young dogs (equivalent to 110 times the maximum recommended daily *adult ophthalmic* dose) has been associated with these types of effects.
Information for Patients: Avoid contaminating the applicator tip with material from the eye, fingers or other source.
Systemic quinolones, including ofloxacin, have been associated with hypersensitivity reactions, even following a single dose. Discontinue use immediately and contact your physician at the first sign of a rash or allergic reaction.
Drug Interactions: Specific drug interaction studies have not been conducted with OCUFLOX® ophthalmic solution. However, the systemic administration of some quinolones has been shown to elevate plasma concentrations of theophylline, interfere with the metabolism of caffeine, and enhance the effects of the oral anticoagulant warfarin and its derivatives, and has been associated with transient elevations in serum creatinine in patients receiving cyclosporine concomitantly.
Carcinogenesis, Mutagenesis, Impairment of Fertility: Long term studies to determine the carcinogenic potential of ofloxacin have not been conducted.
Ofloxacin was not mutagenic in the Ames test, in vitro and in vivo cytogenic assay, sister chromatid exchange assay (Chinese hamster and human cell lines), unscheduled DNA synthesis (UDS) assay using human fibroblasts, the dominant lethal assay, or mouse micronucleus assay. Ofloxacin was positive in the UDS test using rat hepatocyte, and in the mouse lymphoma assay.
In fertility studies in rats, ofloxacin did not affect male or female fertility or morphological or reproductive performance at oral dosing up to 360 mg/kg/day (equivalent to 4000 times the maximum recommended daily ophthalmic dose).
Pregnancy: Teratogenic Effects. Pregnancy Category C: Ofloxacin has been shown to have an embryocidal effect in rats and in rabbits when given in doses of 810 mg/kg/day (equivalent to 9000 times the maximum recommended daily ophthalmic dose) and 160 mg/kg/day (equivalent to 1800 times the maximum recommended daily ophthalmic dose). These dosages resulted in decreased fetal body weight and increased fetal mortality in rats and rabbits, respectively. Minor fetal skeletal variations were reported in rats receiving doses of 810 mg/kg/day. Ofloxacin has not been shown to be teratogenic at doses as high as 810 mg/kg/day and 160 mg/kg/day when administered to pregnant rats and rabbits, respectively.
Nonteratogenic Effects: Additional studies in rats with doses up to 360 mg/kg/day during late gestation showed no adverse effect on late fetal development, labor, delivery, lactation, neonatal viability, or growth of the newborn.
There are, however, no adequate and well-controlled studies in pregnant women. OCUFLOX® solution should be used during pregnancy only if the potential benefit justifies the potential risk to the fetus.
Nursing Mothers: In nursing women a single 200 mg dose resulted in concentrations of ofloxacin in milk which were similar to those found in plasma. It is not known whether ofloxacin is excreted in human milk following topical ophthalmic administration. Because of the potential for serious adverse reactions from ofloxacin in nursing infants, a decision should be made whether to discontinue nursing or to discontinue the drug, taking into account the importance of the drug to the mother.
Pediatric Use: Safety and effectiveness in infants below the age of one year have not been established.
Quinolones, including ofloxacin, have been shown to cause arthropathy in immature animals after oral administration; however, topical ocular administration of ofloxacin to immature animals has not shown any arthropathy. There is no evidence that the ophthalmic dosage form of ofloxacin has any effect on weight bearing joints.

Adverse Reactions: Ophthalmic Use: The most frequently reported drug-related adverse reaction was transient ocular burning or discomfort. Other reported reactions include stinging, redness, itching, chemical conjunctivitis/keratitis, periocular/facial edema, foreign body sensation, photophobia, blurred vision, tearing, dryness, and eye pain. Rare reports of dizziness have been received.

Dosage and Administration: The recommended dosage regimen for the treatment of **bacterial conjunctivitis** is:

Days 1 and 2
Instill one to two drops every two to four hours in the affected eye(s).
Days 3 through 7
Instill one to two drops four times daily.

The recommended daily dosage regimen for the treatment of **bacterial corneal ulcer** is:

Days 1 and 2
Instill one to two drops instilled into the affected eye every 30 minutes, while awake. Awaken at approximately four and six hours after retiring and instill one to two drops.
Days 3 through 7 to 9
Instill one to two drops hourly, while awake.
Days 7 to 9 through treatment completion
Instill one to two drops, four times daily.

How Supplied: OCUFLOX® (ofloxacin ophthalmic solution) 0.3% is supplied sterile in plastic dropper bottles of the following sizes:
1 mL—NDC 11980-779-01
5 mL—NDC 11980-779-05
10 mL—NDC 11980-779-10
Note: Store at 15–25°C (59–77°F)
Rx only
May 1996
Allergan America, Hormigueros, Puerto Rico 00660
Licensed from: Daiichi Pharmaceutical Co., Ltd., Tokyo, Japan and Santen Pharmaceutical Co., Ltd., Osaka, Japan
U.S. PAT. NOS. 4,382,892; 4,551,456
 70829 10B

Shown in Product Identification Guide, page 103

OPHTHETIC® ℞
(proparacaine HCl) 0.5%
sterile ophthalmic solution

Description: OPHTHETIC® (proparacaine HCl) 0.5% sterile ophthalmic solution is a topical local anesthetic for ophthalmic use.
Chemical Name:
Benzoic acid, 3-amino-4-propoxy-,2-(diethylamino)ethyl ester, monohydrochloride.
Contains:
Active: proparacaine 0.5%
Preservative: benzalkonium chloride (0.01%)
Inactives: glycerin, sodium chloride and purified water. pH may be adjusted with hydrochloric acid and/or sodium hydroxide.
Clinical Pharmacology: OPHTHETIC® sterile ophthalmic solution is a rapidly-acting topical anesthetic, with induced anesthesia lasting 15 minutes or longer.
Indications and Usage: OPHTHETIC® sterile ophthalmic solution is indicated for procedures in which a topical ophthalmic anesthetic is indicated: corneal anesthesia of short duration, e.g., tonometry, gonioscopy, removal of corneal foreign bodies, and for short corneal and conjunctival procedures.
Contraindications: OPHTHETIC® sterile ophthalmic solution should be considered contraindicated in patients with known hypersensitivity to any of the ingredients of this preparation.
Warnings: Prolonged use of a topical ocular anesthetic is not recommended. It may produce permanent corneal opacification with accompanying visual loss.
Precautions:
Carcinogenesis, Mutagenesis, Impairment of Fertility: Long-term studies in animals have not been performed to evaluate carcinogenic potential, mutagenicity, or possible impairment of fertility in males or females.
Pregnancy: Pregnancy Category C: Animal reproduction studies have not been conducted with OPHTHETIC® (proparacaine hydrochloride) ophthalmic solution. It is also not known whether proparacaine hydrochloride can cause fetal harm when administered to a pregnant woman or can affect reproduction capacity. Proparacaine hydrochloride should be administered to a pregnant woman only if clearly needed.
Nursing Mothers: It is not known whether this drug is excreted in human milk. Because many drugs are excreted in human milk, caution should be exercised when proparacaine hydrochloride is administered to a nursing mother.
Pediatric Use: Safety and effectiveness in pediatric patients have not been established.
Adverse Reactions: Occasional temporary stinging, burning, and conjunctival redness may occur with the use of proparacaine. A rare, severe, immediate-type, apparently hyperallergic corneal reaction, characterized by acute, intense and diffuse epithelial keratitis, a gray, ground glass appearance, sloughing of large areas of necrotic epithelium, corneal filaments and sometimes, iritis with descemetitis has been reported.
Allergic contact dermatitis from proparacaine with drying and fissuring of the fingertips has also been reported.
Dosage and Administration:
Usual Dosage: Removal of foreign bodies and sutures, and for tonometry: 1 to 2 drops (in single instillations) in each eye before operating.
Deep Ophthalmic Anesthesia: 1 drop in each eye every 5 to 10 minutes for 5–7 doses.
Note: OPHTHETIC® should be clear to straw-color. If the solution becomes darker, discard the solution.
How Supplied:
OPHTHETIC® sterile ophthalmic solution is supplied in plastic dropper bottles in the following size:
15 mL—NDC 11980-048-15
Bottle must be stored in unit carton to protect contents from light. Store bottles under refrigeration at 2°C to 8°C (36°F to 46°F).
Rx only

OPTICROM® ℞
(cromolyn sodium ophthalmic solution, USP) 4%
Sterile

Prescribing Information
Description: OPTICROM® (cromolyn sodium ophthalmic solution, USP) 4% is a clear, colorless, sterile solution intended for topical ophthalmic use.
Cromolyn sodium is represented by the following structural formula:

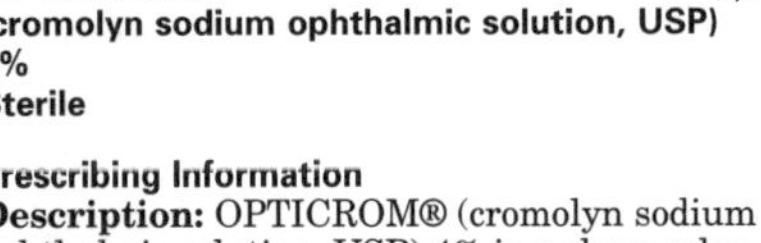

NaOOC … O … OH … OCH_2CHCH_2O … COONa

$C_{23}H_{14}Na_2O_{11}$ Mol. Wt 512.34

Chemical Name: Disodium 5-5′ - [(2-hydroxy trimethylene) dioxy] bis [4-oxo-4*H*-1-benzopyran-2-carboxylate].
Pharmacologic Category: Mast cell stabilizer
Each mL contains: **Active**: Cromolyn sodium 40 mg (4%); **Preservative**: Benzalkonium chloride 0.01%; **Inactives**: Edetate disodium 0.1% and purified water. It has a pH of 4.0 to 7.0.
Clinical Pharmacology: *In vitro* and *in vivo* animal studies have shown that cromolyn sodium inhibits the degranulation of sensitized mast cells which occurs after exposure to specific antigens. Cromolyn sodium acts by inhibiting the release of histamine and SRS-A (slow-reacting substance of anaphylaxis) from the mast cell.
Another activity demonstrated *in vitro* is the capacity of cromolyn sodium to inhibit the degranulation of non-sensitized rat mast cells by phospholipase A and the subsequent release of chemical mediators. Another study showed that cromolyn sodium did not inhibit the enzymatic activity of released phospholipase A on its specific substrate.
Cromolyn sodium has no intrinsic vasoconstrictor, antihistamine, or anti-inflammatory activity.
Cromolyn sodium is poorly absorbed. When multiple doses of cromolyn sodium ophthalmic solution are instilled into normal rabbit eyes, less than 0.07% of the administered dose of cromolyn sodium is absorbed into the systemic circulation (presumably by way of the eye, nasal passages, buccal cavity, and gastro intestinal tract). Trace amounts (less than 0.01%) of the cromolyn sodium dose penetrate into the aqueous humor and clearance from this chamber is virtually complete within 24 hours after treatment is stopped.
In normal volunteers, analysis of drug excretion indicates that approximately 0.03% of cromolyn sodium is absorbed following administration to the eye.
Indications and Usage: OPTICROM® is indicated in the treatment of vernal keratoconjunctivitis, vernal conjunctivitis, and vernal keratitis.
Contraindications: OPTICROM® is contraindicated in those patients who have shown hypersensitivity to cromolyn sodium or to any of the other ingredients.
Precautions: General: Patients may experience a transient stinging or burning sensation following application of OPTICROM®.
The recommended frequency of administration should not be exceeded (see **Dosage and Administration**).
Information for Patients: Patients should be advised to follow the patient instructions listed on the Information for Patients sheet.
Users of contact lenses should refrain from wearing lenses while exhibiting the signs and symptoms of vernal keratoconjunctivitis, vernal conjunctivitis, or vernal keratitis. Do not wear contact lenses during treatment with OPTICROM®.
Carcinogenesis, Mutagenesis, and Impairment of Fertility: Long term studies of cromolyn sodium in mice (12 months intraperitoneal administration at doses up to 150 mg/kg three days per week), hamsters (intraperitoneal administration at doses up to 52.6 mg/kg three days per week for 15 weeks followed by 17.5 mg/kg three days per week for 37 weeks), and rats (18 months subcutaneous administration at doses up to 75 mg/kg six days per week) showed no neoplastic effects. The average daily maximum dose levels administered in these studies were 192.9 mg/m^2 for mice, 47.2 mg/m^2 for hamsters and 385.8 mg/m^2 for rats. These doses correspond to approximately 6.8, 1.7, and 14 times the maximum daily human dose of 28 mg/m^2.
Cromolyn sodium showed no mutagenic potential in the Ames *Salmonella*/microsome plate assays, mitotic gene conversion in *Saccharomyces cerevisiae* and in an *in vitro* cytogenetic study in human peripheral lymphocytes.
No evidence of impaired fertility was shown in laboratory reproduction studies conducted

Continued on next page

Opticrom—Cont.

subcutaneously in rats at the highest doses tested, 175 mg/kg/day (1050 mg/m^2) in males and 100 mg/kg/day (600 mg/m^2) in females. These doses are approximately 37 and 21 times the maximum daily human dose, respectively, based on mg/m^2.

Pregnancy. Teratogenic Effects: Pregnancy Category B. Reproduction studies with cromolyn sodium administered subcutaneously to pregnant mice and rats at maximum daily doses of 540 mg/kg (1620 mg/m^2) and 164 mg/kg (984 mg/m^2), respectively, and intravenously to rabbits at a maximum daily dose of 485 mg/kg (5820 mg/m^2) produced no evidence of fetal malformation. These doses represent approximately 57, 35, and 205 times the maximum daily human dose, respectively, on a mg/m^2 basis. Adverse fetal effects (increased resorption and decreased fetal weight) were noted only at the very high parenteral doses that produced maternal toxicity. There are, however, no adequate and well-controlled studies in pregnant women. Because animal reproduction studies are not always predictive of human response, this drug should be used during pregnancy only if clearly needed.

Nursing Mothers: It is not known whether this drug is excreted in human milk. Because many drugs are excreted in human milk, caution should be exercised when OPTICROM® is administered to a nursing woman.

Pediatric Use: Safety and effectiveness in children below the age of 4 years have not been established.

Adverse Reactions: The most frequently reported adverse reaction attributed to the use of OPTICROM®, on the basis of reoccurrence following readministration, is transient ocular stinging or burning upon instillation.

The following adverse reactions have been reported as infrequent events. It is unclear whether they are attributed to the drug:

Conjunctival injection; watery eyes; itchy eyes; dryness around the eye; puffy eyes; eye irritation; and styes.

Immediate hypersensitivity reactions have been reported rarely and include dyspnea, edema, and rash.

Dosage and Administration: The dose is 1–2 drops in each eye 4–6 times a day at regular intervals. One drop contains approximately 1.6 mg cromolyn sodium.

Patients should be advised that the effect of OPTICROM® therapy is dependent upon its administration at regular intervals, as directed.

Symptomatic response to therapy (decreased itching, tearing, redness, and discharge) is usually evident within a few days, but longer treatment for up to six weeks is sometimes required. Once symptomatic improvement has been established, therapy should be continued for as long as needed to sustain improvement.

If required, corticosteroids may be used concomitantly with OPTICROM®.

How Supplied: OPTICROM® (cromolyn sodium ophthalmic solution, USP) 4% is supplied as 10 mL of solution in an opaque polyethylene eye drop bottle.

10 mL **NDC** 0023-6422-10

Store at Controlled Room Temperature 20–25°C (68–77°F). Protect from light - store in original carton. Keep tightly closed and out of the reach of children.

Rx only

ALLERGAN

POLY-PRED® ℞

(prednisolone acetate, neomycin sulfate, polymyxin B sulfate)
Liquifilm®
sterile ophthalmic suspension

Description: POLY-PRED® Liquifilm® sterile ophthalmic suspension is a topical anti-inflammatory/anti-infective combination product for ophthalmic use.

Chemical Name: Prednisolone acetate: 11β, 17, 21-Trihydroxypregna-1, 4-diene-3, 20-dione 21-acetate.

Neomycin sulfate is the sulfate salt of neomycin B and neomycin C which are produced by the growth of *Streptomyces fradiae* (Fam. *Streptomycetaceae*). It has a potency equivalent to not less than 600 micrograms per milligram of neomycin base, calculated on an anhydrous basis.

Polymyxin B sulfate is the sulfate salt of polymyxin B_1 and polymyxin B_2 which are produced by the growth of *Bacillus polymyxa* (Prazmowski) Migula (Fam. *Bacillaceae*). It has a potency of not less than 6,000 polymyxin B units per milligram, calculated on an anhydrous basis.

Contains: Actives: prednisolone acetate (microfine suspension) 0.5%, neomycin sulfate equivalent to 0.35% neomycin base, polymyxin B sulfate 10,000 units/mL. Preservative: thimerosal 0.001%. Inactives: Liquifilm® (polyvinyl alcohol) 1.4%; polysorbate 80; propylene glycol; sodium acetate; and purified water.

Clinical Pharmacology: Corticosteroids suppress the inflammatory response to a variety of agents and they probably delay or slow healing. Since corticosteroids may inhibit the body's defense mechanism against infection, a concomitant antimicrobial drug may be used when this inhibition is considered to be clinically significant in a particular case.

The anti-infective components in POLY-PRED® are included to provide action against specific organisms susceptible to them. Neomycin sulfate and polymyxin B sulfate are considered active against the following microorganisms: *Staphylococcus aureus; Escherichia coli; Haemophilus influenzae; Klebsiella / Enterobacter* species; *Neisseria* species; and *Pseudomonas aeruginosa.*

When a decision to administer both a corticosteroid and an antimicrobial is made, the administration of such drugs in combination has the advantage of greater patient compliance and convenience, with the added assurance that the appropriate dosage of both drugs is administered. When both types of drugs are in the same formulation, compatibility of ingredients is assured and the correct volume of drug is delivered and retained.

The relative potency of corticosteroids depends on the molecular structure, concentration and release from the vehicle.

Indications and Usage: A steroid/anti-infective combination is indicated for steroid-responsive inflammatory ocular conditions for which a corticosteroid is indicated and where bacterial infection or a risk of bacterial ocular infection exists.

Ocular steroids are indicated in inflammatory conditions of the palpebral and bulbar conjunctiva, cornea, and anterior segment of the globe where the inherent risk of steroid use in certain infective conjunctivitides is accepted to obtain a diminution in edema and inflammation. They are also indicated in chronic anterior uveitis and corneal injury from chemical, radiation or thermal burns or penetration of foreign bodies.

The use of a combination drug with an anti-infective component is indicated where the risk of infection is high or where there is an expectation that potentially dangerous numbers of bacteria will be present in the eye.

The particular anti-infective drugs in this product are active against the following common bacterial eye pathogens: *Staphylococcus aureus; Escherichia coli; Haemophilus influenzae; Klebsiella / Enterobacter* species; *Neisseria* species; and *Pseudomonas aeruginosa.*

The product does not provide adequate coverage against: *Serratia marcescens;* Streptococci, including *Streptococcus pneumoniae.*

Contraindications: Epithelial herpes simplex keratitis (dendritic keratitis), vaccinia, varicella, and many other viral diseases of the cornea and conjunctiva. Mycobacterial infection of the eye. Fungal diseases of the ocular structures. Hypersensitivity to a component of the medication. (Hypersensitivity to the antibiotic component occurs at a higher rate than for other components.)

The use of these combinations is always contraindicated after uncomplicated removal of a corneal foreign body.

Warnings: Prolonged use may result in glaucoma, with damage to the optic nerve, defects in visual acuity and fields of vision, and in posterior subcapsular cataract formation. Prolonged use may suppress the host response and thus increase the hazard of secondary ocular infections. In those diseases causing thinning of the cornea or sclera, perforations have been known to occur with the use of topical steroids. In acute purulent conditions of the eye, steroids may mask infection or enhance existing infection. If these products are used for 10 days or longer, intraocular pressure should be routinely monitored even though it may be difficult in children and uncooperative patients.

Employment of a steroid medication in the treatment of herpes simplex requires great caution.

There exists a potential for neomycin sulfate to cause cutaneous sensitization. The exact incidence of this reaction is unknown.

Precautions: The initial prescription and renewal of the medication order beyond 20 milliliters should be made by a physician only after examination of the patient with the aid of magnification, such as slit lamp biomicroscopy and, where appropriate, fluorescein staining.

The possibility of persistent fungal infections of the cornea should be considered after prolonged steroid dosing.

Adverse Reactions: Adverse reactions have occurred with steroid/anti-infective combination drugs which can be attributed to the steroid component, the anti-infective component, or the combination. Exact incidence figures are not available since no denominator of treated patients is available.

Reactions occurring most often from the presence of the anti-infective ingredients are allergic sensitizations. The reactions due to the steroid component in decreasing order of frequency are: elevation of intraocular pressure (IOP) with possible development of glaucoma, and infrequent optic nerve damage; posterior subcapsular cataract formation; and delayed wound healing.

Secondary Infection: The development of secondary infection has occurred after use of combinations containing steroids and antimicrobials. Fungal infections of the cornea are particularly prone to develop coincidentally with long-term applications of steroid. The possibility of fungal invasion must be considered in any persistent corneal ulceration where steroid treatment has been used.

Secondary bacterial ocular infection following suppression of host responses also occurs.

Dosage and Administration: TO TREAT THE EYE: 1 or 2 drops every 3 or 4 hours, or more frequently as required. Acute infections may require administration every 30 minutes, with frequency of administration reduced as the infection is brought under control. TO

TREAT THE LIDS: Instill 1 or 2 drops in the eye every 3 to 4 hours, close the eye and rub the excess on the lids and lid margins.

Not more than 20 milliliters should be prescribed initially and the prescription should not be refilled without further evaluation as outlined in the **Precautions** section above.

How Supplied: POLY-PRED® Liquifilm® sterile ophthalmic suspension is supplied in plastic dropper bottles in the following sizes:

5 mL—NDC 0023-0028-05
10 mL—NDC 0023-0028-10

Note: Store at or below 25°C (77°F). Protect from freezing. **Shake well before using.**

Rx only

POLYTRIM® ℞
(TRIMETHOPRIM SULFATE AND POLYMYXIN B SULFATE OPHTHALMIC SOLUTION) Sterile

Description: POLYTRIM® (trimethoprim sulfate and polymyxin B sulfate ophthalmic solution) is a sterile antimicrobial solution for topical ophthalmic use. It has pH of 4.0 to 6.2 and osmolality of 270 to 310 mOsm/kg.

Chemical Names: Trimethoprim sulfate, 2,4-Diamino-5-(3,4,5-trimethoxybenzyl) pyrimidine sulfate, is a white, odorless, crystalline powder with a molecular weight of 678.72.

Polymyxin B sulfate is the sulfate salt of polymyxin B_1 and B_2 which are produced by the growth of *Bacillus polymyxa* (Prazmowski) Migula (Fam. Bacillaceae). It has a potency of not less than 6,000 polymyxin B units per mg, calculated on an anhydrous basis.

Contains: Actives: trimethoprim sulfate equivalent to 1 mg/mL, polymyxin B sulfate 10,000 units/mL. Preservative: benzalkonium chloride 0.04 mg/mL. Inactives: sodium chloride, sulfuric acid and purified water. May also contain sodium hydroxide for pH adjustment.

Clinical Pharmacology: Trimethoprim is a synthetic antibacterial drug active against a wide variety of aerobic gram-positive and gram-negative ophthalmic pathogens. Trimethoprim blocks the production of tetrahydrofolic acid from dihydrofolic acid by binding to and reversibly inhibiting the enzyme dihydrofolate reductase. This binding is stronger for the bacterial enzyme than for the corresponding mammalian enzyme and therefore selectively interferes with bacterial biosynthesis of nucleic acids and proteins.

Polymyxin B, a cyclic lipopeptide antibiotic, is bactericidal for a variety of gram-negative organisms, especially *Pseudomonas aeruginosa.* It increases the permeability of the bacterial cell membrane by interacting with the phospholipid components of the membrane.

Blood samples were obtained from 11 human volunteers at 20 minutes, 1 hour and 3 hours following instillation in the eye of 2 drops of ophthalmic solution containing 1 mg trimethoprim and 10,000 units polymyxin B per mL. Peak serum concentrations were approximately 0.03 µg/mL trimethoprim and 1 unit/mL polymyxin B.

Microbiology: *In vitro* studies have demonstrated that the anti-infective components of POLYTRIM® are active against the following bacterial pathogens that are capable of causing external infections of the eye:

Trimethoprim: *Staphylococcus aureus* and *Staphylococcus epidermidis, Streptococcus pyogenes, Streptococcus faecalis, Streptococcus pneumoniae, Haemophilus influenzae, Haemophilus aegyptius, Escherichia coli, Klebsiella pneumoniae, Proteus mirabilis* (indole-negative), *Proteus vulgaris* (indole-positive), *Enterobacter aerogenes,* and *Serratia marcescens.*

Polymyxin B: *Pseudomonas aeruginosa, Escherichia coli, Klebsiella pneumoniae, Enterobacter aerogenes* and *Haemophilus influenzae.*

Indications and Usage: POLYTRIM® Ophthalmic Solution is indicated in the treatment of surface ocular bacterial infections, including acute bacterial conjunctivitis, and blepharoconjunctivitis, caused by susceptible strains of the following microorganisms: *Staphylococcus aureus, Staphylococcus epidermidis, Streptococcus pneumoniae, Streptococcus viridans, Haemophilus influenzae* and *Pseudomonas aeruginosa.**

*Efficacy for this organism in this organ system was studied in fewer than 10 infections.

Contraindications: POLYTRIM® Ophthalmic Solution is contraindicated in patients with known hypersensitivity to any of its components.

Warnings

NOT FOR INJECTION INTO THE EYE.

If a sensitivity reaction to POLYTRIM® occurs, discontinue use. POLYTRIM® Ophthalmic Solution is not indicated for the prophylaxis or treatment of ophthalmia neonatorum.

Precautions:

General: As with other antimicrobial preparations, prolonged use may result in overgrowth of nonsusceptible organisms, including fungi. If superinfection occurs, appropriate therapy should be initiated.

Information for Patients: Avoid contaminating the applicator tip with material from the eye, fingers, or other source. This precaution is necessary if the sterility of the drops is to be maintained.

If redness, irritation, swelling or pain persists or increases, discontinue use immediately and contact your physician. Patients should be advised not to wear contact lenses if they have signs and symptoms of ocular bacterial infections.

Carcinogenesis, Mutagenesis, Impairment of Fertility:

Carcinogenesis: Long-term studies in animals to evaluate carcinogenic potential have not been conducted with polymyxin B sulfate or trimethoprim.

Mutagenesis: Trimethoprim was demonstrated to be non-mutagenic in the Ames assay. In studies at two laboratories no chromosomal damage was detected in cultured Chinese hamster ovary cells at concentrations approximately 500 times human plasma levels after oral administration; at concentrations approximately 1000 times human plasma levels after oral administration in these same cells a low level of chromosomal damage was induced at one of the laboratories. Studies to evaluate mutagenic potential have not been conducted with polymyxin B sulfate.

Impairment of Fertility: Polymyxin B sulfate has been reported to impair the motility of equine sperm, but its effects on male or female fertility are unknown.

No adverse effects on fertility or general reproductive performance were observed in rats given trimethoprim in oral dosages as high as 70 mg/kg/day for males and 14 mg/kg/day for females.

Pregnancy: *Teratogenic Effects: Pregnancy Category C.* Animal reproduction studies have not been conducted with polymyxin B sulfate. It is not known whether polymyxin B sulfate can cause fetal harm when administered to a pregnant woman or can affect reproduction capacity.

Trimethoprim has been shown to be teratogenic in the rat when given in oral doses 40 times the human dose. In some rabbit studies, the overall increase in fetal loss (dead and resorbed and malformed conceptuses) was associated with oral doses 6 times the human therapeutic dose.

While there are no large well-controlled studies on the use of trimethoprim in pregnant women, Brumfitt and Pursell, in a retrospective study, reported the outcome of 186 pregnancies during which the mother received either placebo or oral trimethoprim in combination with sulfamethoxazole. The incidence of congenital abnormalities was 4.5% (3 of 66) in those who received placebo and 3.3% (4 of 120) in those receiving trimethoprim and sulfamethoxazole. There were no abnormalities in the 10 children whose mothers received the drug during the first trimester. In a separate survey, Brumfitt and Pursell also found no congenital abnormalities in 35 children whose mothers had received oral trimethoprim and sulfamethoxazole at the time of conception or shortly thereafter.

Because trimethoprim may interfere with folic acid metabolism, trimethoprim should be used during pregnancy only if the potential benefit justifies the potential risk to the fetus.

Nonteratogenic Effects: The oral administration of trimethoprim to rats at a dose of 70 mg/kg/day commencing with the last third of gestation and continuing through parturition and lactation caused no deleterious effects on gestation or pup growth and survival.

Nursing Mothers: It is not known whether this drug is excreted in human milk. Because many drugs are excreted in human milk, caution should be exercised when POLYTRIM® Ophthalmic Solution is administered to a nursing woman.

Pediatric Use: Safety and effectiveness in children below the age of 2 months have not been established (see **Warnings**).

Adverse Reactions: The most frequent adverse reaction to POLYTRIM® Ophthalmic Solution is local irritation consisting of increased redness, burning, stinging, and/or itching. This may occur on instillation, within 48 hours, or at any time with extended use. There are also multiple reports of hypersensitivity reactions consisting of lid edema, itching, increased redness, tearing, and/or circumocular rash. Photosensitivity has been reported in patients taking oral trimethoprim.

Dosage and Administration: In mild to moderate infections, instill one drop in the affected eye(s) every three hours (maximum of 6 doses per day) for a period of 7 to 10 days.

How Supplied: A sterile ophthalmic solution, each mL contains trimethoprim sulfate equivalent to 1 mg trimethoprim and polymyxin B sulfate 10,000 units in a plastic dropper bottle of 10 mL (NDC 0023-7824-10). 5 mL (NDC 0023-7824-05).

Note: Store at 15°–25°C (59°–77°F) and protect from light.

Rx only

PRED FORTE® ℞
(prednisolone acetate) 1%
sterile ophthalmic suspension

Description: PRED FORTE® (prednisolone acetate) 1% sterile ophthalmic suspension is a topical anti-inflammatory agent for ophthalmic use.

Chemical Name: 11β, 17, 21-Trihydroxypregna-1,4-diene-3,20-dione 21-acetate.

Contains: Active: prednisolone acetate (microfine suspension) 1.0%. Inactives: benzalkonium chloride; polysorbate 80; boric acid; sodium citrate; sodium bisulfite; sodium chloride; edetate disodium; hydroxypropyl methylcellulose; and purified water.

Clinical Pharmacology: Prednisolone acetate is a glucocorticoid that, on the basis of weight, has 3 to 5 times the anti-inflammatory potency of hydrocortisone. Glucocorticoids inhibit the edema, fibrin deposition, capillary dilation and phagocytic migration of the acute

Continued on next page

Pred Forte—Cont.

inflammatory response as well as capillary proliferation, deposition of collagen and scar formation.

Indications and Usage: PRED FORTE® is indicated for the treatment of steroid-responsive inflammation of the palpebral and bulbar conjunctiva, cornea and anterior segment of the globe.

Contraindications: PRED FORTE® is contraindicated in most viral diseases of the cornea and conjunctiva including epithelial herpes simplex keratitis (dendritic keratitis), vaccinia, and varicella, and also in mycobacterial infection of the eye and fungal diseases of ocular structures. PRED FORTE® suspension is also contraindicated in individuals with known or suspected hypersensitivity to any of the ingredients of this preparation and to other corticosteroids.

Warnings: Prolonged use of corticosteroids may result in glaucoma with damage to the optic nerve, defects in visual acuity, and fields of vision, and in posterior subcapsular cataract formation. Prolonged use may also suppress the host immune response and thus increase the hazard of secondary ocular infections.

Since PRED FORTE® contains no antimicrobial, if infection is present, appropriate measures must be taken to counteract the organisms involved.

Various ocular diseases and long-term use of topical corticosteroids have been known to cause corneal and scleral thinning. Use of topical corticosteroids in the presence of thin corneal or scleral tissue may lead to perforation. Acute purulent infections of the eye may be masked or activity enhanced by the presence of corticosteroid medication.

If this product is used for 10 days or longer, intraocular pressure should be routinely monitored even though it may be difficult in children and uncooperative patients. Steroids should be used with caution in the presence of glaucoma. Intraocular pressure should be checked frequently.

The use of steroids after cataract surgery may delay healing and increase the incidence of bleb formation.

Use of ocular steroids may prolong the course and may exacerbate the severity of many viral infections of the eye (including herpes simplex). Employment of a corticosteroid medication in the treatment of patients with a history of herpes simplex requires great caution; frequent slitlamp microscopy is recommended.

Corticosteroids are not effective in mustard gas keratitis and Sjögren's keratoconjunctivitis.

Contains sodium bisulfite, a sulfite that may cause allergic-type reactions, including anaphylactic symptoms and life-threatening or less severe asthmatic episodes in certain susceptible people. The overall prevalence of sulfite sensitivity in the general population is unknown and probably low. Sulfite sensitivity is seen more frequently in asthmatic than in nonasthmatic people.

Precautions:

General: The initial prescription and renewal of the medication order beyond 20 milliliters of PRED FORTE® should be made by a physician only after examination of the patient with the aid of magnification, such as slitlamp biomicroscopy, and, where appropriate, fluorescein staining. If signs and symptoms fail to improve after 2 days, the patient should be re-evaluated.

As fungal infections of the cornea are particularly prone to develop coincidentally with long-term local corticosteroid applications, fungal invasion should be suspected in any persistent corneal ulceration where a corticosteroid has been used or is in use. Fungal cultures should be taken when appropriate.

If this product is used for 10 days or longer, intraocular pressure should be monitored (see **Warnings**).

Information for patients: If inflammation or pain persists longer than 48 hours or becomes aggravated, the patient should be advised to discontinue use of the medication and consult a physician.

This product is sterile when packaged. To prevent contamination, care should be taken to avoid touching the bottle tip to eyelids or to any other surface. The use of this bottle by more than one person may spread infection. Keep bottle tightly closed when not in use. Keep out of the reach of children.

Carcinogenesis, mutagenesis, Impairment of fertility: No studies have been conducted in animals or in humans to evaluate the potential of these effects.

Pregnancy Category C: Prednisolone has been shown to be teratogenic in mice when given in doses 1–10 times the human dose. There are no adequate well-controlled studies in pregnant women. Prednisolone should be used during pregnancy only if the potential benefit justifies the potential risk to the fetus.

Dexamethasone, hydrocortisone and prednisolone were ocularly applied to both eyes of pregnant mice five times per day on days 10 through 13 of gestation. A significant increase in the incidence of cleft palate was observed in the fetuses of the treated mice.

Nursing Mothers: It is not known whether topical ophthalmic administration of corticosteroids could result in sufficient systemic absorption to produce detectable quantities in breast milk. Systemically administered corticosteroids appear in human milk and could suppress growth, interfere with endogenous corticosteroid production, or cause other untoward effects. Because of the potential for serious adverse reactions in nursing infants from prednisolone, a decision should be made whether to discontinue nursing or discontinue the drug, taking into account the importance of the drug to the mother.

Pediatric Use: Safety and effectiveness in pediatric patients have not been established.

Adverse Reactions: Adverse reactions include, in decreasing order of frequency, elevation of intraocular pressure (IOP) with possible development of glaucoma and infrequent optic nerve damage, posterior subcapsular cataract formation, and delayed would healing.

Although systemic effects are extremely uncommon, there have been rare occurrences of systemic hypercorticoidism after use of topical steroids.

Corticosteroid-containing preparations have also been reported to cause acute anterior uveitis and perforation of the globe. Keratitis, conjunctivitis, corneal ulcers, mydriasis, conjunctival hyperemia, loss of accommodation and ptosis have occasionally been reported following local use of corticosteroids.

The development of secondary ocular infection (bacterial, fungal, and viral) have occurred. Fungal and viral infections of the cornea are particularly prone to develop coincidentally with long-term applications of steroid. The possibility of fungal invasion should be considered in any persistent corneal ulceration where steroid treatment has been used (see **Warnings**).

Transient burning and stinging upon instillation and other minor symptoms of ocular irritation have been reported with the use of PRED FORTE® suspension. Other adverse events reported with the use of PRED FORTE® suspension include: visual disturbance (blurry vision) and allergic reactions.

Overdosage: Overdosage will not ordinarily cause acute problems. If accidentally ingested, drink fluids to dilute.

Dosage and Administration: Shake well before using. Instill one to two drops into the conjunctival sac two to four times daily. During the initial 24 to 48 hours, the dosing frequency may be increased if necessary. Care should be taken not to discontinue therapy prematurely. If signs and symptoms fail to improve after 2 days, the patient should be re-evaluated (see **Precautions**).

NOTE: Keep this and all medications out of the reach of children.

How Supplied: PRED FORTE® (prednisolone acetate) 1% sterile ophthalmic suspension is supplied in plastic dropper bottles in the following sizes:

1 mL—**NDC** 11980-180-01
5 mL—**NDC** 11980-180-05
10 mL—**NDC** 11980-180-10
15 mL—**NDC** 11980-180-15

Note: Protect from freezing.

Rx only

Shown in Product Identification Guide, page 103

PRED-G® ℞

(gentamicin and prednisolone acetate ophthalmic suspension, USP) 0.3%/1.0% sterile

Description: PRED-G® sterile ophthalmic suspension is a topical anti-inflammatory/anti-infective combination product for ophthalmic use.

Chemical Names: Prednisolone acetate: 11β, 17,21-Trihydroxypregna-1,4-diene-3,20-dione 21-acetate.

Gentamicin sulfate is the sulfate salt of gentamicin C_1, gentamicin C_2, and gentamicin C_{1A} which are produced by the growth of *Micromonospora purpurea.*

Contains: Actives: Gentamicin sulfate equivalent to 0.3% gentamicin base; prednisolone acetate (microfine suspension) 1.0%. Preservative: Benzalkonium chloride 0.005%. Inactives: Liquifilm® (polyvinyl alcohol) 1.4%; edetate disodium; hydroxypropyl methylcellulose, polysorbate 80; sodium citrate, dihydrate; sodium chloride; and purified water. May contain sodium hydroxide and/or hydrochloric acid to adjust the pH.

Clinical Pharmacology: Corticosteroids suppress the inflammatory response to a variety of agents and they probably delay or slow healing. Since corticosteroids may inhibit the body's defense mechanism against infection, a concomitant antimicrobial drug may be used when this inhibition is considered to be clinically significant in a particular case.

The anti-infective component in PRED-G® is included to provide action against specific organisms susceptible to it. Gentamicin sulfate is active *in vitro* against susceptible strains of the following microorganisms: *Staphylococcus aureus, Streptococcus pyogenes, Streptococcus pneumoniae, Enterobacter aerogenes, Escherichia coli, Haemophilus influenzae, Klebsiella pneumoniae, Neisseria gonorrhoeae, Pseudomonas aeruginosa, and Serratia marcescens.*

When a decision to administer both a corticosteroid and an antimicrobial is made, the administration of such drugs in combination has the advantage of greater patient compliance and convenience, with the added assurance that the appropriate dosage of both drugs is administered. When both types of drugs are in the same formulation, compatibility of ingredients is assured and the correct volume of drug is delivered and retained.

The relative potency of corticosteroids depends on the molecular structure, concentration, and release from the vehicle.

Indications and Usage: PRED-G® suspension is indicated for steroid-responsive inflammatory ocular conditions for which a corticosteroid is indicated and where superficial bacterial ocular infection or a risk of bacterial ocular infection exists.

Ocular steroids are indicated in inflammatory conditions of the palpebral and bulbar conjunctiva, cornea, and anterior segment of the globe where the inherent risk of steroid use in certain infective conjunctivitides is accepted to obtain a diminution in edema and inflammation. They are also indicated in chronic anterior uveitis and corneal injury from chemical, radiation, or thermal burns or penetration of foreign bodies.

The use of a combination drug with an anti-infective component is indicated where the risk of superficial ocular infection is high or where there is an expectation that potentially dangerous numbers of bacteria will be present in the eye.

The particular anti-infective drug in this product is active against the following common bacterial eye pathogens: *Staphylococcus aureus, Streptococcus pyogenes, Streptococcus pneumoniae, Enterobacter aerogenes, Escherichia coli, Haemophilus influenzae, Klebsiella pneumoniae, Neisseria gonorrhoeae, Pseudomonas aeruginosa, and Serratia marcescens.*

Contraindications: PRED-G® suspension is contraindicated in most viral diseases of the cornea and conjunctiva including epithelial herpes simplex keratitis (dendritic keratitis), vaccinia, and varicella, and also in mycobacterial infection of the eye and fungal diseases of the ocular structures. PRED-G® suspension is also contraindicated in individuals with known or suspected hypersensitivity to any of the ingredients of this preparation or to other corticosteroids.

Warnings: Prolonged use of corticosteroids may result in glaucoma with damage to the optic nerve, defects in visual acuity and fields of vision, and in posterior subcapsular cataract formation. Prolonged use of corticosteroids may suppress the host response and thus increase the hazard of secondary ocular infections.

Various ocular diseases and long-term use of topical corticosteroids have been known to cause corneal and scleral thinning. Use of topical corticosteroids in the presence of thin corneal or scleral tissue may lead to perforation. Acute purulent infections of the eye may be masked or enhanced by the presence of corticosteroid medication.

If this product is used for 10 days or longer, intraocular pressure should be routinely monitored even though it may be difficult in children and uncooperative patients. Steroids should be used with caution in the presence of glaucoma. Intraocular pressure should be checked frequently.

The use of steroids after cataract surgery may delay healing and increase the incidence of bleb formation.

Use of ocular steroids may prolong the course and may exacerbate the severity of many viral infections of the eye (including herpes simplex). Employment of a corticosteroid medication in the treatment of patients with a history of herpes simplex requires great caution; frequent slit lamp microscopy is recommended.

PRED-G® sterile ophthalmic suspension is not for injection. It should never be injected subconjunctivally, nor should it be directly introduced into the anterior chamber of the eye.

Precautions:

General: Ocular irritation and punctate keratitis have been associated with the use of PRED-G® suspension. The initial prescription and renewal of the medication order beyond 20 milliliters should be made by a physician only after examination of the patient's intraocular pressure, examination of the patient with the aid of magnification such as slit lamp biomicroscopy and, where appropriate, fluorescein staining.

As fungal infections of the cornea are particularly prone to develop coincidentally with long-term corticosteroid applications, fungal invasion should be suspected in any persistent corneal ulceration where a corticosteroid has been used or is in use. Fungal cultures should be taken when appropriate.

Information for Patients: If inflammation or pain persists longer than 48 hours or becomes aggravated, the patient should be advised to discontinue use of the medication and consult a physician.

This product is sterile when packaged. To prevent contamination, care should be taken to avoid touching the bottle tip to eyelids or to any other surface. The use of this bottle by more than one person may spread infection. Store at 15°–25°C (59°–77°F). Protect from freezing and from heat of 40°C (104°F) and above. Keep out of the reach of children. Shake well before using.

Carcinogenesis, mutagenesis, impairment of fertility: There are no published carcinogenicity or impairment of fertility studies on gentamicin. Aminoglycoside antibiotics have been found to be non-mutagenic.

There are no published mutagenicity or impairment of fertility studies on prednisolone. Prednisolone has been reported to be non-carcinogenic.

Pregnancy: Pregnancy Category C. Gentamicin has been shown to depress body weight, kidney weight, and median glomerular counts in newborn rats when administered systemically to pregnant rats in daily doses approximately 500 times the maximum recommended ophthalmic human dose. There are no adequate and well-controlled studies in pregnant women. Gentamicin should be used during pregnancy only if the potential benefit justifies the potential risk to the fetus.

Prednisolone has been shown to be teratogenic in mice when given in doses 1–10 times the human ocular dose. Dexamethasone, hydrocortisone and prednisolone were applied to both eyes of pregnant mice five times per day on days 10 through 13 of gestation. A significant increase in the incidence of cleft palate was observed in the fetuses of the treated mice. There are no adequate well-controlled studies in pregnant women. PRED-G® suspension should be used during pregnancy only if the potential benefit justifies the potential risk to the fetus.

Nursing Mothers: It is not known whether topical administration of corticosteroids could result in sufficient systemic absorption to produce detectable quantities in human milk. Systemically administered corticosteroids appear in human milk and could suppress growth, interfere with endogenous corticosteroid production, or cause other untoward effects. Because of the potential for serious adverse reactions in nursing infants from PRED-G® suspension, a decision should be made whether to discontinue nursing while the drug is being administered or to discontinue the medication.

Pediatric Use: Safety and effectiveness in pediatric patients have not been established.

Adverse Reactions: Adverse reactions have occurred with steroid/anti-infective combination drugs which can be attributed to the steroid component, the anti-infective component, or the combination. Exact incidence figures are not available since no denominator of treated patients is available.

Reactions occurring most often from the presence of the anti-infective ingredient are allergic sensitizations. The reactions due to the steroid component in decreasing order of frequency are: elevation of intraocular pressure (IOP) with possible development of glaucoma, and infrequent optic nerve damage; posterior subcapsular cataract formation; and delayed wound healing.

Burning, stinging and other symptoms of irritation have been reported with PRED-G®. Superficial punctate keratitis has been reported occasionally with onset occurring typically after several days of use.

Secondary Infection: The development of secondary infection has occurred after use of combinations containing steroids and antimicrobials. Fungal and viral infections of the cornea are particularly prone to develop coincidentally with long-term applications of steroid. The possibility of fungal invasion should be considered in any persistent corneal ulceration where steroid treatment has been used. (See **Warnings**).

Secondary bacterial ocular infection following suppression of host responses also occurs.

Dosage and Administration: Instill one drop into the conjunctival sac two to four times daily. During the initial 24 to 48 hours, the dosing frequency may be increased, if necessary, up to 1 drop every hour. Care should be taken not to discontinue therapy prematurely. If signs and symptoms fail to improve after two days, the patient should be re-evaluated. (See **Precautions**)

Not more than 20 milliliters should be prescribed initially and the prescription should not be refilled without further evaluation as outlined in **Precautions** above.

How Supplied: PRED-G® (gentamicin and prednisolone acetate ophthalmic suspension, USP) 0.3%/1.0% is supplied in sterile plastic dropper bottles in the following sizes:

2 mL—NDC 0023-0106-02
5 mL—NDC 0023-0106-05
10 mL—NDC 0023-0106-10

Note: Store at 15°–25°C (59°–77°F). Avoid excessive heat, 40° C (104° F) and above. Protect from freezing. **Shake well before using.**

RX only

PRED–G® ℞

(gentamicin and prednisolone acetate ophthalmic ointment, USP) 0.3%/0.6% sterile

Description: PRED-G® sterile ophthalmic ointment is a topical anti-inflammatory/anti-infective combination product for ophthalmic use.

Chemical Names: Prednisolone acetate: 11β,17,21-Trihydroxypregna-1,4-diene-3, 20-dione 21-acetate.

Gentamicin sulfate is the sulfate salt of gentamicin C_1, gentamicin C_2, and gentamicin C_{1A} which are produced by the growth of *Micromonospora purpurea.*

Contains: Actives: gentamicin sulfate equivalent to 0.3% gentamicin base, prednisolone acetate 0.6%. Preservative: chlorobutanol (chloral derivative) 0.5%. Inactives: white petrolatum; mineral oil; petrolatum (and) lanolin alcohol; and purified water.

Clinical Pharmacology: Corticosteroids suppress the inflammatory response to a variety of agents and they probably delay or slow healing. Since corticosteroids may inhibit the body's defense mechanism against infection, a concomitant antimicrobial drug may be used when this inhibition is considered to be clinically significant in a particular case.

The anti-infective component in PRED-G® is included to provide action against specific organisms susceptible to it. Gentamicin sulfate is active *in vitro* against susceptible strains of the following microorganisms: *Staphylococcus aureus, Streptococcus pyogenes, Streptococcus pneumoniae, Enterobacter*

Continued on next page

Pred-G —Cont.

aerogenes, Escherichia coli, Hemophilus influenzae, Klebsiella pneumoniae, Neisseria gonorrhoeae, Pseudomonas aeruginosa, and *Serratia marcescens.*

When a decision to administer both a corticosteroid and an antimicrobial is made, the administration of such drugs in combination has the advantage of greater patient compliance and convenience, with the added assurance that the appropriate dosage of both drugs is administered. When both types of drugs are in the same formulation, compatibility of ingredients is assured and the correct volume of drug is delivered and retained.

The relative potency of corticosteroids depends on the molecular structure, concentration, and release from the vehicle.

Indications and Usage: PRED-G® is indicated for steroid-responsive inflammatory ocular conditions for which a corticosteroid is indicated and where superficial bacterial ocular infection or a risk of bacterial ocular infection exists.

Ocular steroids are indicated in inflammatory conditions of the palpebral and bulbar conjunctiva, cornea, and anterior segment of the globe where the inherent risk of steroid use in certain infective conjunctivitides is accepted to obtain a diminution in edema and inflammation. They are also indicated in chronic anterior uveitis and corneal injury from chemical, radiation, or thermal burns or penetration of foreign bodies.

The use of a combination drug with an anti-infective component is indicated where the risk of superficial ocular infection is high or where there is an expectation that potentially dangerous numbers of bacteria will be present in the eye.

The particular anti-infective drug in this product is active against the following common bacterial eye pathogens: *Staphylococcus aureus, Streptococcus pyogenes, Streptococcus pneumoniae, Enterobacter aerogenes, Escherichia coli, Hemophilus influenzae, Klebsiella pneumoniae, Neisseria gonorrhoeae, Pseudomonas aeruginosa,* and *Serratia marcescens.*

Contraindications: Epithelial herpes simplex keratitis (dendritic keratitis), vaccinia, varicella, and many other viral diseases of the cornea and conjunctiva. Mycobacterial infection of the eye. Fungal diseases of the ocular structures. Hypersensitivity to a component of the medication. (Hypersensitivity to the antibiotic component occurs at a higher rate than for other components.)

PRED-G® is always contraindicated after uncomplicated removal of a corneal foreign body.

Warnings: Prolonged use may result in glaucoma with damage to the optic nerve, defects in visual acuity and fields of vision, and in posterior subcapsular cataract formation. Prolonged use may suppress the host immune response and thus increase the hazard of secondary ocular infections. In those diseases causing thinning of the cornea or sclera, perforations have been known to occur with the use of topical steroids. In acute purulent conditions of the eye, steroids may mask infection or enhance existing infection. If these products are used for 10 days or longer, intraocular pressure should be routinely monitored even though it may be difficult in children and uncooperative patients.

Employment of a steroid medication in the treatment of patients with a history of herpes simplex requires great caution. PRED-G® is contraindicated in patients with active herpes simplex keratitis.

Precautions:

General: Ocular irritation and punctate keratitis have been associated with the use of PRED-G®. The initial prescription and renewal of the medication order beyond 8 grams should be made by a physician only after examination of the patient's intraocular pressure, examination of the patient with the aid of magnification, such as slit lamp biomicroscopy and, where appropriate, fluorescein staining. The possibility of fungal infections of the cornea should be considered after prolonged steroid dosing.

Carcinogenesis, mutagenesis, impairment of fertility: There are no published carcinogenicity or impairment of fertility studies on gentamicin. Aminoglycoside antibiotics have been found to be non-mutagenic.

There are no published mutagenicity or impairment of fertility studies on prednisolone. Prednisolone has been reported to be non-carcinogenic.

Pregnancy: Pregnancy Category C: Gentamicin has been shown to depress newborn body weights, kidney weights, nephron counts and shows evidence of glomeruli and proximal tubule nephrotoxicity in rats when administered systemically in daily doses of approximately 500 times the maximum recommended ophthalmic dose in humans.

Prednisolone has been shown to be teratogenic in mice when given in doses 1–10 times the human dose. Dexamethasone, hydrocortisone and prednisolone were ocularly applied to both eyes of pregnant mice five times per day on days 10 through 13 of gestation. A significant increase in the incidence of cleft palate was observed in the fetuses of the treated mice. There are no adequate well-controlled studies in pregnant women. PRED-G® should be used during pregnancy only if the potential benefit justifies the potential risk to the fetus.

Nursing Mothers: It is not known whether topical administration of corticosteroids could result in sufficient systemic absorption to produce detectable quantities in breast milk. Systemically administered corticosteroids appear in breast milk and could suppress growth, interfere with endogenous corticosteroid production, or cause other untoward effects. Because of the potential for serious adverse reactions in nursing infants from PRED-G® a decision should be made whether to discontinue nursing or to discontinue the medication.

Pediatric Use: Safety and effectiveness in pediatric patients have not been established.

Adverse Reactions: Adverse reactions have occurred with steroid/anti-infective combination drugs which can be attributed to the steroid component, the anti-infective component, or the combination. Exact incidence figures are not available since no denominator of treated patients is available.

The most frequent reactions observed include ocular discomfort, irritation upon instillation of the medication and punctate keratitis. These reactions have resolved upon discontinuation of the medication.

Reactions occurring most often from the presence of the anti-infective ingredient are allergic sensitizations. The reactions due to the steroid component in decreasing order of frequency are: elevation of intraocular pressure (IOP) with possible development of glaucoma, and infrequent optic nerve damage; posterior subcapsular cataract formation; and delayed wound healing.

Secondary Infection: The development of secondary infection has occurred after use of combinations containing steroids and antimicrobials. Fungal infections of the cornea are particularly prone to develop coincidentally with long-term applications of steroid. The possibility of fungal invasion must be considered in any persistent corneal ulceration where steroid treatment has been used.

Secondary bacterial ocular infection following suppression of host responses also occurs.

Dosage and Administration: A small amount ($^1/_2$ inch ribbon) of ointment should be applied in the conjunctival sac one to three times daily. Care should be taken not to discontinue therapy prematurely.

Not more than 8 grams should be prescribed initially and the prescription should not be refilled without further evaluation as outlined in **Precautions** above.

How Supplied: PRED-G® (gentamicin and prednisolone acetate ophthalmic ointment, USP) 0.3%/0.6% is supplied in ophthalmic ointment tubes of the following size:

3.5 g—NDC 0023-0066-04

Note: Store at 15°–25°C (59°–77°F).

Rx only

PRED MILD® ℞

(prednisolone acetate) 0.12%
sterile ophthalmic suspension

Description: PRED MILD® (prednisolone acetate) 0.12% sterile ophthalmic suspension is a topical anti-inflammatory agent for ophthalmic use.

Chemical Name: 11β,17,21-Trihydroxypregna-1,4-diene-3,20-dione 21-acetate.

Contains: Active: prednisolone acetate (microfine suspension) 0.12%. Preservative: benzalkonium chloride. Inactives: polysorbate 80; boric acid; sodium citrate; sodium bisulfite; sodium chloride; edetate disodium; hydroxypropyl methylcellulose; and purified water.

Clinical Pharmacology: Prednisolone acetate is a glucocorticoid that, on the basis of weight, has 3 to 5 times the anti-inflammatory potency of hydrocortisone. Glucocorticoids inhibit the edema, fibrin deposition, capillary dilation and phagocytic migration of the acute inflammatory response as well as capillary proliferation, deposition of collagen and scar formation.

Indications and Usage: PRED MILD® is indicated for the treatment of mild to moderate noninfectious allergic and inflammatory disorders of the lid, conjunctiva, cornea and sclera (including chemical and thermal burns).

Contraindications: PRED MILD® suspension is contraindicated in acute untreated purulent ocular infections, in most viral diseases of the cornea and conjunctiva including epithelial herpes simplex keratitis (dendritic keratitis), vaccinia, and varicella, and also in mycobacterial infection of the eye and fungal diseases of ocular structures. PRED MILD® suspension is also contraindicated in individuals with known or suspected hypersensitivity to any of the ingredients of this preparation and to other corticosteroids.

Warnings: Prolonged use of corticosteroids may result in glaucoma with damage to the optic nerve, defects in visual acuity, and fields of vision, and in posterior subcapsular cataract formation. Prolonged use may also suppress the host immune response and thus increase the hazard of secondary ocular infections.

Since PRED MILD® contains no antimicrobial, if infection is present, appropriate measures must be taken to counteract the organisms involved.

Various ocular diseases and long-term use of topical corticosteroids have been known to cause corneal and scleral thinning. Use of topical corticosteroids in the presence of thin corneal or scleral tissue may lead to perforation. Acute purulent infections of the eye may be masked or activity enhanced by the presence of corticosteroid medication.

If this product is used for 10 days or longer, intraocular pressure should be routinely monitored even though it may be difficult in children and uncooperative patients. Steroids should be used with caution in the presence of glaucoma. Intraocular pressure should be checked frequently.

The use of steroids after cataract surgery may delay healing and increase the incidence of bleb formation.

Use of ocular steroids may prolong the course and may exacerbate the severity of many viral infections of the eye (including herpes simplex). Employment of a corticosteroid medication in the treatment of patients with a history of herpes simplex requires great caution; frequent slit lamp microscopy is recommended.

Corticosteroids are not effective in mustard gas keratitis and Sjögren's keratoconjunctivitis.

Contains sodium bisulfite, a sulfite that may cause allergic-type reactions, including anaphylactic symptoms and life-threatening or less severe asthmatic episodes in certain susceptible people. The overall prevalence of sulfite sensitivity in the general population is unknown and probably low. Sulfite sensitivity is seen more frequently in asthmatic than in nonasthmatic people.

Precautions:

General: The initial prescription and renewal of the medication order beyond 20 milliliters of PRED MILD® should be made by a physician only after examination of the patient with the aid of magnification, such as slit lamp biomicroscopy, and, where appropriate, fluorescein staining. If signs and symptoms fail to improve after 2 days, the patient should be re-evaluated.

As fungal infections of the cornea are particularly prone to develop coincidentally with long-term local corticosteroid applications, fungal invasion should be suspected in any persistent corneal ulceration where a corticosteroid has been used or is in use. Fungal cultures should be taken when appropriate.

If this product is used for 10 days or longer, intraocular pressure should be monitored (see **Warnings**).

Information for patients: If inflammation or pain persists longer than 48 hours or becomes aggravated, the patient should be advised to discontinue use of the medication and consult a physician.

This product is sterile when packaged. To prevent contamination, care should be taken to avoid touching the bottle tip to eyelids or to any other surface. The use of this bottle by more than one person may spread infection. Keep bottle tightly closed when not in use. Keep out of the reach of children.

Carcinogenesis, mutagenesis, Impairment of Fertility: No studies have been conducted in animals or in humans to evaluate the potential of these effects.

Pregnancy Category C: Prednisolone has been shown to be teratogenic in mice when given in doses 1–10 times the human dose. There are no adequate well-controlled studies in pregnant women. Prednisolone should be used during pregnancy only if the potential benefit justifies the potential risk to the fetus.

Dexamethasone, hydrocortisone and prednisolone were ocularly applied to both eyes of pregnant mice five times per day on days 10 through 13 of gestation. A significant increase in the incidence of cleft palate was observed in the fetuses of the treated mice.

Nursing Mothers: It is not known whether topical ophthalmic administration of corticosteroids could result in sufficient systemic absorption to produce detectable quantities in breast milk. Systemically administered corticosteroids appear in human milk and could suppress growth, interfere with endogenous corticosteroid production, or cause other untoward effects. Because of the potential for serious adverse reactions in nursing infants from prednisolone, a decision should be made whether to discontinue nursing or to discontinue the drug, taking into account the importance of the drug to the mother.

Pediatric use: Safety and effectiveness in pediatric patients have not been established.

Adverse Reactions: Adverse reactions include, in decreasing order of frequency, elevation of intraocular pressure (IOP) with possible development of glaucoma and infrequent optic nerve damage, posterior subcapsular cataract formation, and delayed would healing.

Although systemic effects are extremely uncommon, there have been rare occurrences of systemic hypercorticoidism after use of topical steroids.

Corticosteroid-containing preparations have also been reported to cause acute anterior uveitis and perforation of the globe. Keratitis, conjunctivitis, corneal ulcers, mydriasis, conjunctival hyperemia, loss of accommodation and ptosis have occasionally been reported following local use of corticosteroids.

The development of secondary ocular infection (bacterial, fungal, and viral) has occurred. Fungal and viral infections of the cornea are particularly prone to develop coincidentally with long-term applications of steroids. The possibility of fungal invasion should be considered in any persistent corneal ulceration where steroid treatment has been used (see **Warnings**).

Transient burning and stinging upon instillation and other minor symptoms of ocular irritation have been reported with the use of PRED MILD® suspension.

Overdosage: Overdosage will not ordinarily cause acute problems. If accidentally ingested, drink fluids to dilute.

Dosage and Administration: Shake well before using. Instill one to two drops into the conjunctival sac two to four times daily. During the initial 24 to 48 hours, the dosing frequency may be increased if necessary. Care should be taken not to discontinue therapy prematurely. If signs and symptoms fail to improve after 2 days, the patient should be re-evaluated (see **Precautions**).

How Supplied: PRED MILD® (prednisolone acetate) 0.12% sterile ophthalmic suspension is supplied in plastic dropper bottles in the following sizes:

5 mL—NDC 11980-174-05
10 mL—NDC 11980-174-10

Note: Store at controlled room temperature 15°–30°C (59°–86°F). Protect from freezing.

Rx only

PROPINE® ℞

(dipivefrin hydrochloride)
ophthalmic solution, USP, 0.1% sterile
with C CAP® Compliance Cap B.I.D.

Description: PROPINE® contains dipivefrin hydrochloride in a sterile, isotonic solution. Dipivefrin HCl is a white, crystalline powder, freely soluble in water.

Empirical Formula: $C_{19}H_{29}O_5N \cdot HCl$

Chemical Name: (±)-3,4-Dihydroxy-α-[(methylamino)methyl]benzyl alcohol 3,4-dipivalate hydrochloride.

Contains:

Active: dipivefrin HCl* 0.1%

Preservative: benzalkonium chloride 0.005%

Inactives: edetate disodium; sodium chloride; hydrochloric acid to adjust pH; and purified water.

*Licensed under U.S. Patent Nos. 3,839,584 and 3,809,714.

Clinical Pharmacology: PROPINE® (dipivefrin HCl) is a member of a class of drugs known as prodrugs. Prodrugs are usually not active in themselves and require biotransformation to the parent compound before therapeutic activity is seen. These modifications are undertaken to enhance absorption, decrease side effects and enhance stability and comfort, thus making the parent compound a more useful drug. Enhanced absorption makes the prodrug a more efficient delivery system for the parent drug because less drug will be needed to produce the desired therapeutic response.

PROPINE® is a prodrug of epinephrine formed by the diesterification of epinephrine and pivalic acid. The addition of pivaloyl groups to the epinephrine molecule enhances its lipophilic character and, as a consequence, its penetration into the anterior chamber.

PROPINE® is converted to epinephrine inside the human eye by enzyme hydrolysis. The liberated epinephrine, an adrenergic agonist, appears to exert its action by decreasing aqueous production and by enhancing outflow facility. The PROPINE® prodrug delivery system is a more efficient way of delivering the therapeutic effects of epinephrine, with fewer side effects than are associated with conventional epinephrine therapy.

The onset of action with one drop of PROPINE® occurs about 30 minutes after treatment, with maximum effect seen at about one hour.

Using a prodrug means that less drug is needed for therapeutic effect since absorption is enhanced with the prodrug. PROPINE® at 0.1% dipivefrin was judged less irritating than a 1% solution of epinephrine hydrochloride or bitartrate. In addition, only 8 of 455 patients (1.8%) treated with PROPINE® reported discomfort due to photophobia, glare or light sensitivity.

Indications: PROPINE® (dipivefrin HCl) is indicated as initial therapy for the control of intraocular pressure in chronic open-angle glaucoma. Patients responding inadequately to other antiglaucoma therapy may respond to addition of PROPINE®.

In controlled and open-label studies of glaucoma, PROPINE® demonstrated a statistically significant intraocular pressure-lowering effect. Patients using PROPINE® twice daily in studies with mean durations of 76–146 days experienced mean pressure reductions ranging from 20–24%.

Therapeutic response to PROPINE® twice daily is somewhat less than 2% epinephrine twice daily. Controlled studies showed statistically significant differences in lowering of intraocular pressure between PROPINE® and 2% epinephrine. In controlled studies in patients with a history of epinephrine intolerance, only 3% of patients treated with PROPINE® exhibited intolerance, while 55% of those treated with epinephrine again developed intolerance.

Therapeutic response to PROPINE® twice daily therapy is comparable to 2% pilocarpine 4 times daily. In controlled clinical studies comparing PROPINE® and 2% pilocarpine, there were no statistically significant differences in the maintenance of IOP levels for the two medications. PROPINE® does not produce miosis or accommodative spasm which cholinergic agents are known to produce. Night blindness often associated with miotic agents is not present with PROPINE® therapy. Patients with cataracts avoid the inability to see around lenticular opacities caused by constricted pupil.

Contraindications: PROPINE® should not be used in patients with narrow angles since any dilation of the pupil may predispose the patient to an attack of angle-closure glaucoma. This product is contraindicated in patients who are hypersensitive to any of its components.

Precautions: Aphakic Patients. Macular edema has been shown to occur in up to 30% of aphakic patients treated with epinephrine. Discontinuation of epinephrine generally results in reversal of the maculopathy.

Continued on next page

Propine—Cont.

Pregnancy: Pregnancy Category B. Reproduction studies have been performed in rats and rabbits at daily oral doses up to 10 mg/kg body weight (5 mg/kg in teratogenicity studies), and have revealed no evidence of impaired fertility or harm to the fetus due to dipivefrin HCl. There are, however, no adequate and well-controlled studies in pregnant women. Because animal reproduction studies are not always predictive of human response, this drug should be used during pregnancy only if clearly needed.
Nursing Mothers. It is not known whether this drug is excreted in human milk. Because many drugs are excreted in human milk, caution should be exercised when PROPINE® is administered to a nursing woman.
Pediatric Use: Safety and effectiveness in pediatric patients have not been established.
Animal Studies. Rabbit studies indicated a dose-related incidence of meibomian gland retention cysts following topical administration of both dipivefrin hydrochloride and epinephrine.
Adverse Reactions:
Cardiovascular Effects. Tachycardia, arrhythmias and hypertension have been reported with ocular administration of epinephrine.
Local Effects. The most frequent side effect reported with PROPINE® alone were injection in 6.5% of patients and burning and stinging in 6%. Follicular conjunctivitis, mydriasis, blurry vision, headache, and allergic reaction to PROPINE® have been reported. Epinephrine therapy can lead to adrenochrome deposits in the conjunctiva and cornea.
Dosage and Administration: Initial Glaucoma Therapy. The usual dosage of PROPINE® is one drop in the eye(s) every 12 hours.
Replacement with PROPINE®. When patients are being transferred to PROPINE® from antiglaucoma agents other than epinephrine, on the first day continue the previous medication and add one drop of PROPINE® in each eye every 12 hours. On the following day, discontinue the previously used antiglaucoma agent and continue with PROPINE®.
In transferring patients from conventional epinephrine therapy to PROPINE®, simply discontinue the epinephrine medication and institute the PROPINE® regimen.
Addition of PROPINE®. When patients on other antiglaucoma agents require additional therapy, add one drop of PROPINE® every 12 hours.
Concomitant Therapy. For difficult to control patients, the addition of PROPINE® to other agents such as pilocarpine, carbachol, echothiophate iodide or acetazolamide has been shown to be effective.
Note: Not for injection.
How Supplied: PROPINE® (dipivefrin HCl) ophthalmic solution, USP, 0.1%, is supplied sterile in plastic dropper bottles as follows:
C CAP® Compliance Cap B.I.D. (twice daily)
5 mL—NDC 11980-260-25
10 mL—NDC 11980-260-20
15 mL—NDC 11980-260-21
Note: Store in tight, light-resistant containers.
Rx only
C CAP® Compliance Cap Patient Instructions

Instructions for use:

1. On the first usage, make sure the number "1" appears in the window. If not, click the cap to the right station.
2. Remove the cap and apply medication.
3. Replace the cap. Hold the C CAP® between your thumb and forefinger. Now rotate the bottle until the cap clicks to the next station.
4. When it's time to take your next dose, repeat steps 2 and 3.

Important Notes: Don't try to catch up on missed doses by applying more than one dose at a time.
Each time you replace the cap, turn it until you hear the click.
The number in the window specifies your *next* dosage.

REFRESH PLUS®
(carboxymethylcellulose sodium) 0.5%
Lubricant Eye Drops
Preservative-Free

Immediate, Long-Lasting Relief.
Many things can make your eyes feel dry, scratchy, burning or uncomfortable. Air conditioners or heaters. Computer use. Reading. Some medications. Wind. Or a reduction in the amount of tears your body produces—tears which help to lubricate and nourish your eyes. REFRESH PLUS® restores the moisture your eyes crave with a special formula that has some of the healthy qualities as natural tears. Since REFRESH PLUS® is preservative-free, it also avoids the potential irritation to your eyes caused by the preservatives found in bottled eye drops. So you can apply REFRESH PLUS® as often as necessary without the risk of preservative-induced irritation.
Contains: Active: Carboxymethylcellulose sodium 0.5%. Inactives: calcium chloride, magnesium chloride, potassium chloride, purified water, sodium chloride, and sodium lactate. May also contain hydrochloric acid or sodium hydroxide to adjust pH.
Indications: For temporary relief of burning, irritation and discomfort due to dryness of the eye or due to exposure to wind or sun. Also may be used as a protectant against further irritation.
Warnings: To avoid contamination, do not touch tip of container to any surface. Do not reuse. Once opened, discard. If you experience eye pain, changes in vision, continued redness or irritation of the eye, or if the condition worsens or persists for more than 72 hours, discontinue use and consult a doctor. If solution changes color or becomes cloudy, do not use. Keep this and all drugs out of the reach of children. In case of accidental ingestion, seek professional assistance or contact a Poison Control Center immediately.
Directions: To open, firmly bend tab back and forth, then pull to remove. Instill 1 or 2 drops in the affected eye(s) and discard container.
Note: Use only if single-use container is intact. Do not touch unit-dose tip to eye.
How Supplied: In sterile, preservative-free, disposable, single-use containers of 0.01 fluid ounces each in the following sizes:
30 single-use containers—NDC 0023-5487-30
50 single-use containers—NDC 0023-5487-50.

Shown in Product Identification Guide, page 103

REFRESH PM® OTC
Lubricant Eye Ointment
Preservative-Free

SOOTHES, MOISTURIZES, AND PROTECTS!
Refresh P.M.® has been specially formulated to soothe, moisturize and protect dry, irritated eyes. Refresh P.M.® is convenient for use at bedtime.
Just as important, Refresh P.M.® is preservative-free to avoid the risk of preservative-induced irritation.
Contains: Actives: white petrolatum 56.8%, mineral oil 41.5%; Inactives: lanolin alcohols; purified water and sodium chloride.
Indications: For the temporary relief of burning, irritation discomfort due to dryness of the eye or due to exposure to wind or sun. Also may be used as a protectant against further irritation.
Warnings: To avoid contamination, do not touch tip of container to any surface. Replace cap after using. If you experience eye pain, changes in vision, continued redness or irritation of the eye, or if the condition worsens or persists for more than 72 hours, discontinue use and consult a doctor. Keep this and all drugs out of the reach of children. In case of accidental ingestion, seek professional assistance or contact a poison control center immediately.
Directions: Pull down the lower lid of the affected eye and apply a small amount (one-fourth inch) of ointment to the inside of the eyelid. Store away from heat. Protect from freezing.
Note: Use only if imprinted wrap on box is intact.
How Supplied: As a sterile eye lubricant in 3.5 g tube—NDC 0023-0667-04

Shown in Product Identification Guide, page 103

REFRESH TEARS® OTC
(carboxymethylcellulose sodium) 0.5%
Lubricant Eye Drops

REFRESH TEARS® provides soothing relief for dry, irritated eyes with a formula that resembles your body's own tears. REFRESH TEARS® contains a unique, mild, nonsensitizing preservative that, when used, ultimately changes into components of natural tears. Use REFRESH TEARS® for long-lasting relief of your dry, irritated eyes as often as needed.
Contains: Active: carboxymethylcellulose sodium 0.5%. Inactives: boric acid, calcium chloride, magnesium chloride, potassium chloride, purified water, Purite™ (stabilized oxychloro complex), and sodium chloride. May also contain sodium hydroxide to adjust pH.
Indications: For the temporary relief of burning, irritation, and discomfort due to dryness of the eye or due to exposure to wind or sun. Also may be used as a protectant against further irritation.
Warnings: To avoid contamination, do not touch tip of the container to any surface. Replace cap after using. If you experience eye pain, changes in vision, continued redness or irritation of the eye, or if the condition worsens or persists for more than 72 hours, discontinue use and consult a doctor. If solution changes color or becomes cloudy, do not use. Keep this and all drugs out of the reach of children. In case of accidental ingestion, seek professional assistance or contact a Poison Control Center immediately.
Directions: Instill 1 or 2 drops in the affected eye(s) as needed.
Note: Use only if imprinted tape seals on top and bottom flaps are intact and clearly legible.
How Supplied: REFRESH TEARS® (carboxymethylcellulose sodium) 0.5% Lubricant Eye Drops are supplied in the following sizes:
15-mL bottle – NDC 0023-0798-15.
30-mL bottle – NDC 0023-0798-30.

Shown in Product Identification Guide, page 103

Refer to Section 9
for information on
Intraocular Products.

Bausch & Lomb, Inc
1400 NORTH GOODMAN
ROCHESTER, NY 14609

Direct Inquiries to:
North American Vision Care
Customer Service
1-800-553-5340

Moisturizing
ALL CLEAR™ **OTC**
Redness Reliever/Lubricant Eye Drops

Description: Lubricant-Polyethylene Glycol 300 (0.2%), Redness reliever-Naphazoline Hydrochloride (0.012%). Preserved with Benzalkonium Chloride (0.01%). Also contains: Boric Acid, Edetate Disodium, Sodium Borate, Sodium Chloride.
Uses: Relieves redness of the eye due to minor eye irritations. For the temporary relief of burning and irritation due to dryness of the eye and for use as a protectant against further irritation or to relieve dryness of the eye.
Warnings:
- Remove contact lenses before using.
- To avoid contamination, do not touch tip of container to any surface.
- Replace cap after using.
- If solution changes color or becomes cloudy, do not use.
- If you experience eye pain, changes in vision, continued redness or irritation of the eye or if the condition worsens or persists for more than 72 hours, discontinue use and consult a doctor.
- If you have glaucoma, do not use this product except under the advice and supervision of a doctor.
- Overuse of this product may produce increased redness of the eye.
- Do not use in children under 6 years of age unless directed by a physician.
- Keep this and all drugs out of the reach of children.
- In case of accidental injection, seek professional assistance or contact a Poison Control Center immediately.
- Store at room temperature.
- Use before the expiration date marked on the carton and bottle.

How Supplied: 1 size, 0.5 oz multi-dose bottle

Shown in Product Identification Guide, page 104

Moisturizing
ALL CLEAR AR™ **OTC**
Lubricant Eye Drops/Redness Reliever

Description: Lubricant-Hydroxypropyl Methylcellulose (0.5%), Redness reliever–Naphazoline Hydrochloride (0.03%). Preserved with Benzalkonium Chloride (0.01%). Also contains: Boric Acid, Edetate Disodium, Purified Water, Sodium Borate, Sodium Chloride.
Uses: For the temporary relief of discomfort due to minor irritations of the eye or to exposure to wind or sun. For use as a lubricant to prevent further irritation or to relieve dryness of the eye. Also relieves redness of the eye due to minor eye irritations.
Warnings:
- Remove contact lenses before using.
- To avoid contamination, do not touch tip or container to any surface.
- Replace cap after using.
- If solution changes color or becomes cloudy, do not use.
- If you experience eye pain, changes in vision, continued redness or irritation of the eye, or if the condition worsens or persists for more than 72 hours, discontinue use and consult a doctor.
- If you have glaucoma, do not use this product except under the advice and supervision of a doctor.
- Overuse of the product may produce increased redness of the eye.
- Do not use in children under 8 years of age unless directed by a physician.
- Keep this and all drugs out of the reach of children.
- In case of accidental ingestion, seek professional assistance or contact a Poison Control Center immediately.
- Store at room temperature.
- Use before the expiration date marked on the carton and bottle.

How Supplied: 1 size, 0.5 oz multi-dose bottle

Shown in Product Identification Guide, page 104

COLLYRIUM for FRESH EYES **OTC**
[*ko-lir 'e-um*]
EYE WASH
A neutral borate solution

Description: Soothing Collyrium Eye Wash for Fresh Eyes is specially formulated to soothe, refresh, and cleanse irritated eyes. Collyrium Eye Wash is a neutral borate solution that contains boric acid, sodium borate, benzalkonium chloride as a preservative, and water.
Indications: Patients are advised of the following. Use Collyrium Eye Wash to cleanse the eye, loosen foreign material, air pollutants or chlorinated water.
Recommended Uses:
Home—For emergency flushing of foreign bodies or whenever a soothing eye rinse is necessary.
Hospitals, dispensaries and clinics—For emergency flushing of chemicals or foreign bodies from the eye.
Directions: Patients are advised of the following. Remove the eyecup from blister. Puncture bottle by twisting threaded eyecup down onto bottle; then remove it from the bottle. Rinse eyecup with clean water immediately before and after each use. Avoid contamination of rim and interior surfaces of eyecup. Fill eyecup one-half full with Collyrium Eye Wash. Apply cup tightly to the affected eye to prevent escape of the liquid and tilt head backward. Open eyelid wide and rotate eyeball to thoroughly wash eye. Rinse cup with clean water after use and recap by twisting threaded eyecup on the bottle for storage.
Warnings: Patients are advised of the following. Do not use if solution changes color or becomes cloudy, or with a wetting solution for contact lenses or other eye care products containing polyvinyl alcohol.
To avoid contamination do not touch tip of container to any surface. Replace cap after using. If you experience eye pain, changes in vision, continued redness, irritation of the eye, or if the condition worsens or persists, consult a doctor. Obtain immediate medical treatment for all open wounds in or near the eyes.
The Collyrium for Fresh Eyes bottle is sealed for your protection. Prior to first use, remove cap and squeeze bottle. If bottle leaks, do not use.
Keep this and all medication out of the reach of children.
Keep bottle tightly closed at Room Temperature, Approx. 77° F (25° C).
How Supplied: Bottles of 4 FL. OZ. (118 mL) with eyecup.
Manufactured by
Wyeth-Ayerst Laboratories
Rouses Point, NY 12979
Marketed by
Bausch & Lomb
Rochester, NY 14604

Shown in Product Identification Guide, page 104

COMPUTER EYE DROPS **OTC**
Lubricant Eye Drops

Description: Lubricant–Glycerin (1.0%). Preserved with Benzalkonium Chloride (0.01%). Also contains: Sodium Chloride, Potassium Chloride, Sodium Borate, Botic Acid, Edetate Disodium.
Uses: For use as a lubricant to prevent further irritation or to relieve dryness of the eye.
Warnings:
- To avoid contamination, do not touch tip of container to any surface.
- Replace cap after using.
- If solution changes color or becomes cloudy do not use.
- If you experience eye pain, changes in vision, continued redness or irritation of the eye, or if the condition worsens or persists for more than 72 hours discontinue use and consult a doctor.
- Keep this and all drugs out of the reach of children.
- Keep container tightly closed.
- In case of accidental ingestion, seek professional assistance or contact a Poison Control Center immediately.
- Remove contact lenses before using.
- Store at room temperature.
- Use before expiration date marked on the carton and bottle.

How Supplied: 1 size, 0.5 oz multi-dose bottle

EYE WASH **OTC**
Eye Irrigating Solution

Description: A sterile, isotonic solution that contains Boric Acid, Purified Water, Sodium Borate and Sodium Chloride; preserved with Edetate Disodium 0.025% and Sorbic Acid 0.1%.
Warnings:
- To avoid contamination, do not touch tip of container to any surface.
- Replace cap after using.
- If solution changes color or becomes cloudy, do not use.
- If you experience eye pain, changes in vision, continued redness or irritation of the eye, or if the condition worsens or persists, consult a doctor.
- Obtain immediate medical treatment for all open wounds in or near the eyes.
- Use only as directed. If you experience any chemical burns, consult a doctor immediately.
- Keep this and all drugs out of the reach of children.
- In case of accidental ingestion, seek professional assistance or contact a Poison Control Center immediately.
- Use before the expiration date marked on bottle and carton.
- Store at room temperature.

How Supplied: 1 size, 4.0 oz bottle

MOISTURE EYES™ **OTC**
Lubricant Eye Drops

Description: Lubricant–Propylene Glycol (1.0%), Glycerin (0.3%). Preserved with Benz-

Continued on next page

Moisture Eyes—Cont.

alkonium Chloride (0.01%). Also contains: Boric Acid, Sodium Chloride. Potassium Chloride, Sodium Borate, Edetate Disodium.
Uses: For the temporary relief of burning and irritation due to dryness of the eye. For use as a protectant against further irritation or to relieve dryness of the eye.
Warnings:
- To avoid contamination, do not touch tip of container to any surface.
- Replace cap after using.
- If solution changes color or becomes cloudy, do not use.
- If you experience eye pain, changes in vision, continued redness or irritation of the eye, or if the condition worsens or persists for more than 72 hours, discontinue use and consult a doctor.
- Keep this and all drugs out of the reach of children.
- Keep container tightly closed.
- In case of accidental ingestion, seek professional assistance or contact a Poison Control Center immediately.
- Remove contact lenses before using.
- Store at room temperature.
- Use before expiration date marked on the carton and bottle.

How Supplied: 2 sizes, 0.5 oz, 1.0 oz multi-dose bottles

Shown in Product Identification Guide, page 104

Preservative Free
MOISTURE EYES™ OTC
Lubricant Eye Drops
Artificial Tears

Description: Propylene Glycol (0.95%). Also contains: Boric Acid, Sodium Chloride, Potassium Chloride, Sodium Borate, Edetate Disodium.
Uses: For the temporary relief of burning and irritation due to dryness of the eye and for use as a lubricant to prevent further irritation or to relieve dryness of the eye.
Warnings:
- **Use only if single-use dispenser is intact.**
- To avoid contamination, do not touch tip of dispenser to any surface.
- Do not reuse.
- Once opened, discard.
- If the solution changes color or becomes cloudy, do not use.
- If you experience eye pain, changes in vision, continued redness or irritation of the eye, or if the condition worsens or persists for more than 72 hours, discontinue use and consult a doctor.
- Keep this and all drugs out of the reach of children.
- In case of accidental ingestion, seek professional assistance or contact a Poison Control Center immediately.

How Supplied: One size, 32 count, 0.2 oz vials

Shown in Product Identification Guide, page 104

Preservative Free
MOISTURE EYES™ PM OTC
Lubricant Eye Ointment
Soothing Nighttime Dry Eye Relief

Contains: While petrolatum (80%) and mineral oil (20%). Contains no preservatives.
Directions: Pull down the lower lid of the affected eye and apply a small amount of Moisture Eyes PM Ointment to the inside of the eyelid.
Uses: For use as a lubricant to prevent further irritation or to relieve redness of the eye.
Warnings:
- To avoid contamination, do not touch tip of container to any surface.
- Replace cap after using.
- If you experience eye pain, changes in vision, continued redness or irritation of the eye, or if the condition worsens or persists for more than 72 hours, discontinue use and consult a doctor.
- Not for use with contact lenses.
- Do not use if bottom ridge of cap is exposed prior to initial use.
- Use before expiration date on crimp of tube.
- Keep this and all drugs out of the reach of children.
- In case of accidental ingestion, seek professional assistance or a Poison Control Center immediately.
- Store at room temperature.

How Supplied: One size, 3.5 g tube
Manufactured for:
Bausch & Lomb, Rochester, NY 14692-0450
X050313 R. 7:97-7G DU31334 6324102

OPCON-A® OTC
Itching &
Redness Reliever Eyes Drops
Eye Allergy Relief
- Temporarily relieves minor eye symptoms of **itching and redness** caused by pollen, ragweed, grass, animal hair and dander.
- Clinically proven effective for relief of itchy, red eyes.
- Once available by prescription only. Opcon-A combines an antihistamine with a redness reliever for the temporary relief of itchy, red eyes.

Ingredients: (ACTIVE) pheniramine maleate (0.315%), naphazoline hydrochloride (0.02675%). **(INACTIVE)** hydroxypropyl methylcellulose (0.5%), sodium chloride and purified water with a boric acid and sodium borate buffer system preserved with benzalkonium chloride (0.01%) and edetate disodium (0.1%). The solution has a pH of 5.5–6.3 and tonicity of 270–335 mOsm/Kg.
Directions: Adults and children 6 years of age and older: Instill 1 or 2 drops in the affected eye(s) up to 4 times daily. After instilling drops in the eye, some users may experience a brief tingling sensation.
Indications: For the temporary relief of **redness and itching** of the eye due to pollen, ragweed, grass, animal hair and dander.
Warnings: To avoid contamination, do not touch tip of container to any surface. Replace cap after using. If solution changes color or becomes cloudy, do not use. If you experience eye pain, changes in vision, continued redness or irritation of the eye, or if the condition worsens or persists for more than 72 hours, discontinue use and consult a physician. Overuse of this product may produce increased redness of the eye.
If you are sensitive to any ingredient in this product, do not use. Do not use this product if you have heart disease, high blood pressure, difficulty in urination due to enlargement of the prostate gland or narrow angle glaucoma unless directed by a physician.
Do not use in children under 6 years of age unless directed by a physician. Keep this and all drugs out of the reach of children. In case of accidental ingestion, seek professional assistance or contact a Poison Control Center immediately. Accidental oral ingestion in infants and children may lead to coma and marked reduction in body temperature.
Remove contact lenses before using.
Store at room temperature (15–30°C) (59–86°F).
Protect from light.
Use before the expiration date marked on the carton or bottle.
Bausch & Lomb
Rochester, NY 14692-0450
REV 10/98

Shown in Product Identification Guide, page 104

Bausch & Lomb Pharmaceutical, Inc.
8500 HIDDEN RIVER PARKWAY
TAMPA, FL 33637

NDC 24208	PRODUCT	
-353-	**ALREX™** Loteprednol Etabonate Ophthalmic Suspension 0.2% -05 5 mL bottle -10 10 mL bottle	℞
-825-55	**ATROPINE SULFATE OPHTHALMIC OINTMENT USP, 1%-STERILE** 3.5 gram tubes	℞
-750-	**ATROPINE SULFATE OPHTHALMIC SOLUTION USP, 1%-STERILE** 5mL: -60 15mL: -06	℞
555-55	**BACITRACIN ZINC & Polymyxin B Sulfate Ophthalmic Ointment** 3.5 g tube	℞
300-10	**CROLOM®** Cromolyn Sodium Ophthalmic Solution USP, 4% (10 mL)	℞
-735-	**CYCLOPENTOLATE HYDROCHLORIDE OPHTHALMIC SOLUTION USP, 1% -STERILE** 2mL: -01 15mL: -06	℞
-720-02	**DEXAMETHASONE SODIUM PHOSPHATE** Ophthalmic Solution, USP, 0.1% Dexamethasone Phosphate Equivalent 5 mL bottle	℞
540-05	**DIPIVEFRIN HYDROCHLORIDE** Ophthalmic Solution USP, 0.1% 5 mL Bottle	℞
540-10	**DIPIVEFRIN HYDROCHLORIDE** Ophthalmic Solution USP, 0.1% 10 mL Bottle	℞
540-15	**DIPIVEFRIN HYDROCHLORIDE** Ophthalmic Solution USP, 0.1% 15 mL Bottle	℞
910-	**ERYTHROMYCIN OPHTHALMIC** Ointment USP, 0.5% -19 50 × 1 g tube -55 3.5 g tube	℞
732-05	**FLUORESCEIN SODIUM & BENOXINATE HCL OPHTHALMIC SOLUTION** USP, 0.25%/ 0.4% 5 ml	℞

288- **FLUOROMETHOLONE OPHTHALMIC** ℞
Suspension USP, 0.1%
-05 5 mL bottle
-10 10 mL bottle
-15 15 mL bottle

314-25 **FLURBIPROFEN** ℞
Sodium Ophthalmic Solution USP, 0.03%
2.5 ml

-580- **GENTAMICIN SULFATE** ℞
Ophthalmic Solution USP, 0.3%
5mL: -60
15mL: -64

-505- **LEVOBUNOLOL HYDROCHLORIDE OPHTHALMIC SOLUTION USP, 0.5%** ℞
5mL: -05
10mL: -10
15 mL: -15

-545- **LEVOBUNOLOL HYDROCHLORIDE OPHTHALMIC USP, 0.25%** ℞
5mL: -05
10mL: -10

-299- **LOTEMAX®** ℞
Loteprednol Etabonate Opthalmic Suspension 0.5%
-05 5 mL bottle
-10 10 mL bottle
-15 15 mL bottle

-280-15 **MUROCEL® SOLUTION** **OTC**
Methylcellulose Lubricant Ophthalmic Solution USP, 1%
15 mL

-278-05 **MUROCOLL® 2 SOLUTION** ℞
Phenylephrine Hydrochloride 10% and Scopolamine Hydrobromide 0.3% Ophthalmic Solution
5 mL

-385 **MURO 128® 5% OINTMENT** **OTC**
Sodium Chloride Hypertonicity Ophthalmic Ointment USP, 5%
3.5g -55
TWIN PACK 2× 3.5g: -56

-276-15 **MURO 128® 2% SOLUTION** **OTC**
Sodium Chloride Hypertonicity Ophthalmic Solution USP, 2%
15 mL

-277- **MURO 128® 5% SOLUTION** **OTC**
Sodium Chloride Hypertonicity Ophthalmic Solution USP, 5%
15 mL -15
30 mL -30

-725-06 **NAPHAZOLINE HYDROCHLORIDE OPHTHALMIC SOLUTION** ℞
USP, 0.1%
15mL

-785-55 **NEOMYCIN & POLYMYXIN B SULFATES, BACITRACIN ZINC AND HYDROCORTISONE OPHTHALMIC** ℞
Ointment USP
3.5 g tube

-780-55 **NEOMYCIN AND POLYMYXIN B SULFATES AND BACITRACIN ZINC OPHTHALMIC** ℞
Ointment USP, Sterile
3.5 gram tubes

-795-35 **NEOMYCIN AND POLYMYXIN B SULFATES AND DEXAMETHASONE OPHTHALMIC OINTMENT USP STERILE** ℞
3.5 gram tubes

830-60 **NEOMYCIN AND POLYMYXIN B SULFATES AND DEXAMETHASONE** ℞
Ophthalmic Suspension USP
5 mL Bottle

790-62 **NEOMYCIN AND POLYMYXIN B SULFATES AND GRAMICIDIN** ℞
Ophthalmic Solution USP
10 mL Bottle

955-60 **NEOMYCIN SULFATE AND DEXAMETHASONE SODIUM PHOSPHATE** ℞
Ophth. Sol.
5 mL bottle

-275- **OPTIPRANOLOL® SOLUTION** ℞
metipranolol ophthalmic solution
0.3%-Sterile
5 mL: -07
10 mL: -09

-740- **PHENYLEPHRINE HYDROCHLORIDE OPHTHALMIC SOLUTION USP, 2.5%-STERILE** ℞
2mL: -59
5mL: -02
15mL: -06

-806-15 **PILOCARPINE HYDROCHLORIDE OPHTHALMIC SOLUTION USP,** ℞
0.5%-Sterile
15mL

-676- **PILOCARPINE HYDROCHLORIDE OPHTHALMIC SOLUTION USP,** ℞
1%-Sterile
15mL: -15
TWIN PACK 2×15 mL: -30

-681- **PILOCARPINE HYDROCHLORIDE OPHTHALMIC SOLUTION USP,** ℞
2%-Sterile
15mL: -15
TWIN PACK 2×15 mL: -30

-811-15 **PILOCARPINE HYDROCHLORIDE OPHTHALMIC SOLUTION USP,** ℞
3%-Sterile
15mL

-686- **PILOCARPINE HYDROCHLORIDE OPHTHALMIC SOLUTION USP,** ℞
4%-Sterile
15mL: -15
TWIN PACK 2×15 mL: -30

-821-15 **PILOCARPINE HYDROCHLORIDE OPHTHALMIC SOLUTION USP,** ℞
6%-Sterile
15mL

715- **PREDNISOLONE SODIUM PHOSPHATE OPHTHALMIC SOLUTION USP, 1%** ℞
5 mL: -02
10 mL: -10
15 mL: -06

730-06 **PROPARACAINE HYDROCHLORIDE OPHTHALMIC SOLUTION USP,** ℞
0.5%
15 mL bottle

317-05 **SULFACETAMIDE SODIUM AND PREDNISOLONE SODIUM PHOSPHATE** ℞
Ophthalmic Solution 10%/0.23% (prednisolone phosphate)
5 mL Bottle

317-10 **SULFACETAMIDE SODIUM AND PREDNISOLONE SODIUM PHOSPHATE** ℞
Ophthalmic Solution 10%/0.23% (prednisolone phosphate)
10 mL Bottle

-670-04 **SULFACETAMIDE SODIUM OPHTHALMIC SOLUTION, USP 10%-STERILE** ℞
15mL:

-920-64 **TETRACAINE HYDRO-CHLORIDE OPHTHALMIC SOLUTION USP, 0.5%-STERILE** ℞
15mL bottle

-324- **TIMOLOL MALEATE OPHTHALMIC SOLUTION USP, 0.5%** ℞
-05 5 mL bottle
-10 10 mL bottle
-15 15 mL bottle

-330- **TIMOLOL MALEATE OPHTHALMIC SOLUTION USP, 0.25%** ℞
-05 5 mL bottle
-10 10 mL bottle
-15 15 mL bottle

-290-05 **TOBRAMYCIN OPHTHALMIC SOLUTION USP, 0.3%** ℞
5mL bottle

315-10 **TRIMETHOPRIM SULFATE AND POLYMYXIN B SULFATE OPHTHALMIC SOLUTION** ℞
10mL bottle

-590-64 **TROPICAMIDE OPHTHALMIC SOLUTION, USP 0.5%** ℞
15 mL bottle

-585- **TROPICAMIDE OPHTHALMIC SOLUTION, USP 1%** ℞
-59 2 mL bottle
-64 15 mL bottle

390-83 **FLUOR-I-STRIP®** ℞
9mg Fluorescein Sodium Ophthalmic Strips
Box of 300

Continued on next page

391-83	**FLUOR-I-STRIP® A.T.** 1 mg Fluorescein Sodium Ophthalmic Strips Box of 300	℞
377-11	**OCUCOAT®** Lubricating Eye Drops 15 mL bottle	OTC
384-48	**OCUCOAT PF®** Lubricating Eye Drops 28 × 0.5 mL Unit Dose	OTC
387-60	**OCUVITE®** Vitamin and Mineral Supplement Bottle of 60	OTC
387-62	**OCUVITE®** Vitamin and Mineral Supplement Bottle of 120	OTC
388-19	**OCUVITE® extra®** Vitamin and Mineral Supplement Bottle of 50	OTC
394-07	**REV-EYES®** Dapiprazole HCl Ophthalmic Solution 0.5% 25 mg Vial	℞

NDC 57782	**PRODUCT**	
070-25	**EYE WASH** Eye Irrigating Solution-Sterile 4 fl. oz. (120 mL)	OTC
-481-35	**LUBRITEARS® LUBRICANT EYE OINTMENT** (Lanolin Oil, Mineral Oil, White Petrolatum, Lubricant Eye Ointment) 3.5 gram tube	OTC
-755-15	**DRY EYES LUBRICANT EYE DROPS** Polyvinyl Alcohol 1.4% Lubricant Eye Drops-Sterile 15 mL	OTC
-761-35	**DRY EYES LUBRICANT EYE OINTMENT** Lanolin Oil, Mineral Oil, White Petrolatum, Lubricant Eye Ointment–Preservative Free $^1/_8$ oz. tube	OTC
322-15	**ARTIFICIAL TEARS LUBRICANT EYE DROPS** (Hydroxypropyl Methylcellulose 2910 Lubricant Eye Drops)	OTC

ALREX™ ℞

[*ăl rĕx*]

loteprednol etabonate
ophthalmic suspension 0.2%
STERILE OPHTHALMIC SUSPENSION

Description: ALREX™ (loteprednol etabonate ophthalmic suspension) contains a sterile, topical anti-inflammatory corticosteroid for ophthalmic use. Loteprednol etabonate is a white to off-white powder.

Loteprednol etabonate is represented by the following structural formula:

[See chemical structure at top of next column]

Chemical name:

chloromethyl 17α[(ethoxycarbonyl)oxy]-11β-hydroxy-3-oxoandrosta-1,4-diene-17β-carboxylate.

OCH_2Cl $C=O$ $OCO_2C_2H_5$ HO O

$C_{24}H_{31}ClO_7$ Mol. Wt. 466.96

Each mL contains:

ACTIVE: Loteprednol Etabonate 2 mg (0.2%); INACTIVES: Edetate Disodium, Glycerin, Povidone, Purified Water and Tyloxapol. Hydrochloric Acid and/or Sodium Hydroxide may be added to adjust the pH to 5.3–5.6. The suspension is essentially isotonic with a tonicity of 250 to 310 mOsmol/kg.

PRESERVATIVE ADDED: Benzalkonium Chloride 0.01%.

Clinical Pharmacology: Corticosteroids inhibit the inflammatory response to a variety of inciting agents and probably delay or slow healing. They inhibit the edema, fibrin deposition, capillary dilation, leukocyte migration, capillary proliferation, fibroblast proliferation, deposition of collagen, and scar formation associated with inflammation. There is no generally accepted explanation for the mechanism of action of ocular corticosteroids. However, corticosteroids are thought to act by the induction of phospholipase A_2 inhibitory proteins, collectively called lipocortins. It is postulated that these proteins control the biosynthesis of potent mediators of inflammation such as prostaglandins and leukotrienes by inhibiting the release of their common precursor arachidonic acid. Arachidonic acid is released from membrane phospholipids by phospholipase A_2. Corticosteroids are capable of producing a rise in intraocular pressure.

Loteprednol etabonate is structurally similar to other corticosteroids. However, the number 20 position ketone group is absent. It is highly lipid soluble which enhances its penetration into cells. Loteprednol etabonate is synthesized through structural modifications of prednisolone-related compounds so that it will undergo a predictable transformation to an inactive metabolite. Based upon *in vivo* and *in vitro* preclinical metabolism studies, loteprednol etabonate undergoes extensive metabolism to inactive carboxylic acid metabolites.

Results from a bioavailability study in normal volunteers established that plasma levels of loteprednol etabonate and Δ^1 cortienic acid etabonate (PJ 91), its primary, inactive metabolite, were below the limit of quantitation (1 ng/mL) at all sampling times. The results were obtained following the ocular administration of one drop in each eye of 0.5% loteprednol etabonate 8 times daily for 2 days or 4 times daily for 42 days. This study suggests that limited (<1 ng/mL) systemic absorption occurs with ALREX.

Clinical Studies:

In two double-masked, placebo-controlled six-week environmental studies of 268 patients with seasonal allergic conjunctivitis, ALREX, when dosed four times per day was superior to placebo in the treatment of the signs and symptoms of seasonal allergic conjunctivitis. ALREX provided reduction in bulbar conjunctival injection and itching, beginning approximately 2 hours after instillation of the first dose and throughout the first 14 days of treatment.

Indications and Usage: ALREX Ophthalmic Suspension is indicated for the temporary relief of the signs and symptoms of seasonal allergic conjunctivitis.

Contraindications: ALREX, as with other ophthalmic corticosteroids, is contraindicated in most viral diseases of the cornea and conjunctiva including epithelial herpes simplex keratitis (dendritic keratitis), vaccinia, and varicella, and also in mycobacterial infection of the eye and fungal diseases of ocular structures. ALREX is also contraindicated in individuals with known or suspected hypersensitivity to any of the ingredients of this preparation and to other corticosteroids.

Warnings: Prolonged use of corticosteroids may result in glaucoma with damage to the optic nerve, defects in visual acuity and fields of vision, and in posterior subcapsular cataract formation. Steroids should be used with caution in the presence of glaucoma.

Prolonged use of corticosteroids may suppress the host response and thus increase the hazard of secondary ocular infections. In those diseases causing thinning of the cornea or sclera, perforations have been known to occur with the use of topical steroids. In acute purulent conditions of the eye, steroids may mask infection or enhance existing infection.

Use of ocular steroids may prolong the course and may exacerbate the severity of many viral infections of the eye (including herpes simplex). Employment of a corticosteroid medication in the treatment of patients with a history of herpes simplex requires great caution.

Precautions:

General: For ophthalmic use only. The initial prescription and renewal of the medication order beyond 14 days should be made by a physician only after examination of the patient with the aid of magnification, such as slit lamp biomicroscopy and, where appropriate, fluorescein staining.

If signs and symptoms fail to improve after two days, the patient should be re-evaluated.

If this product is used for 10 days or longer, intraocular pressure should be monitored.

Fungal infections of the cornea are particularly prone to develop coincidentally with long-term local steroid application. Fungus invasion must be considered in any persistent corneal ulceration where a steroid has been used or is in use. Fungal cultures should be taken when appropriate.

Information for Patients: This product is sterile when packaged. Patients should be advised not to allow the dropper tip to touch any surface, as this may contaminate the suspension. If redness or itching becomes aggravated, the patient should be advised to consult a physician.

Patients should be advised not to wear a contact lens if their eye is red. ALREX should not be used to treat contact lens related irritation. The preservative in ALREX, benzalkonium chloride, may be absorbed by soft contact lenses. Patients who wear soft contact lenses **and whose eyes are not red**, should be instructed to wait at least ten minutes after instilling ALREX before they insert their contact lenses.

Carcinogenesis, mutagenesis, impairment of fertility: Long-term animal studies have not been conducted to evaluate the carcinogenic potential of loteprednol etabonate. Loteprednol etabonate was not genotoxic *in vitro* in the Ames test, the mouse lymphoma tk assay, or in a chromosome aberration test in human lymphocytes, or *in vivo* in the single dose mouse micronucleus assay. Treatment of male and female rats with up to 50 mg/kg/day and 25 mg/kg/day of loteprednol etabonate, respectively, (1500 and 750 times the maximum clinical dose, respectively) prior to and during mating did not impair fertility in either gender.

Pregnancy: Teratogenic effects: Pregnancy Category C. Loteprednol etabonate has been shown to be embryotoxic (delayed ossification) and teratogenic (increased incidence of meningocele, abnormal left common carotid artery, and limb flexures) when administered orally to rabbits during organogenesis at a dose of 3 mg/kg/day (85 times the maximum daily clinical dose), a dose which caused no maternal toxicity. The no-observed-effect-level (NOEL) for these effects was 0.5 mg/kg/day (15 times the maximum daily clinical dose). Oral treatment of rats during organogenesis resulted in teratogenicity (absent innominate artery at ≥5mg/kg/day doses, and cleft palate and umbilical hernia at ≥50 mg/kg/day) and embryotoxicity (increased post-implantation losses at 100 mg/kg/day and decreased fetal body weight and skeletal ossification with ≥50 mg/kg/day). Treatment of rats with 0.5 mg/kg/day (15 times the maximum clinical dose) during organogenesis did not result in any reproductive toxicity. Loteprednol etabonate was maternally toxic (significantly reduced body weight gain during treatment) when administered to pregnant rats during organogenesis at doses of ≥5 mg/kg/day.

Oral exposure of female rats to 50 mg/kg/day of loteprednol etabonate from the start of the fetal period through the end of lactation, a maternally toxic treatment regimen (significantly decreased body weight gain), gave rise to decreased growth and survival, and retarded development in the offspring during lactation; the NOEL for these effects was 5 mg/kg/day. Loteprednol etabonate had no effect on the duration of gestation or paturition when administered orally to pregnant rats at doses up to 50 mg/kg/day during the fetal period.

Nursing Mothers: It is not known whether topical ophthalmic administration of corticosteroids could result in sufficient systemic absorption to produce detectable quantities in human milk. Systemic steroids appear in human milk and could suppress growth, interfere with endogenous corticosteroid production, or cause other untoward effects. Caution should be exercised when ALREX is administered to a nursing woman.

Pediatric Use: Safety and effectiveness in pediatric patients have not been established.

Adverse Reactions: Reactions associated with ophthalmic steroids include elevated intraocular pressure, which may be associated with optic nerve damage, visual acuity and field defects, posterior subcapsular cataract formation, secondary ocular infection from pathogens including herpes simplex, and perforation of the globe where there is thinning of the cornea or sclera.

Ocular adverse reactions occurring in 5–15% of patients treated with loteprednol etabonate ophthalmic suspension (0.2%–0.5%) in clinical studies included abnormal vision/blurring, burning on instillation, chemosis, discharge, dry eyes, epiphora, foreign body sensation, itching, injection, and photophobia. Other ocular adverse reactions occurring in less than 5% of patients include conjunctivitis, corneal abnormalities, eyelid erythema, keratoconjunctivitis, ocular irritation/pain/discomfort, papillae, and uveitis. Some of these events were similar to the underlying ocular disease being studied.

Non-ocular adverse reactions occurred in less than 15% of patients. These include headache, rhinitis and pharyngitis.

In a summation of controlled, randomized studies of individuals treated for 28 days or longer with loteprednol etabonate, the incidence of significant elevation of intraocular pressure (≥10 mm Hg) was 2% (15/901) among patients receiving loteprednol etabonate, 7% (11/164) among patients receiving 1% prednisolone acetate and 0.5% (3/583) among patients receiving placebo. Among the smaller group of patients who were studied with ALREX, the incidence of clinically significant increases in IOP (≥10 mm Hg) was 1% (1/133) with ALREX and 1% (1/135) with placebo.

Dosage and Administration: SHAKE VIGOROUSLY BEFORE USING.

One drop instilled into the affected eye(s) four times daily.

How Supplied: ALREX™ (loteprednol etabonate ophthalmic suspension, 0.2%) is supplied in a plastic bottle with a controlled drop tip in the following sizes:

5 mL bottle (NDC 24208-353-05)-AB35307
10 mL bottle (NDC 24208-353-10)-AB35309

DO NOT USE IF NECKBAND IMPRINTED WITH "Protective Seal" AND YELLOW IS NOT INTACT.

Storage: Store upright between 15°–25°C (59°–77°F). DO NOT FREEZE.

KEEP OUT OF REACH OF CHILDREN

Rx only
Manufactured by
Bausch & Lomb Pharmaceuticals, Inc., Tampa, Florida 33637
under Agreement with Pharmos Corporation.
U.S. Patent No. 4,996,335
U.S. Patent No. 5,540,930

R.3/98
X050331 (Folded)
XM10033 (Flat)
Rev. 3/98–8C

Shown in Product Identification Guide, page 104

CROLOM® ℞
cromolyn sodium
ophthalmic solution USP, 4%
STERILE OPHTHALMIC SOLUTION

Description: Crolom® (Cromolyn Sodium Ophthalmic Solution USP, 4%) is a clear, colorless, sterile solution for topical ophthalmic use. Cromolyn sodium is represented by the following structural formula:

NaOOC ... COONa; OH; OCH_2CHCH_2O

$C_{23}H_{14}Na_2O_{11}$

Chemical Name: Disodium 5,5[1]-[(2-hydroxytrimethylene) dioxy] bis [4-oxo - 4*H*-1-benzopyran-2-carboxylate]

Pharmacologic Category: Mast cell stabilizer.

EACH mL CONTAINS: ACTIVE: Cromolyn Sodium 40 mg (4%); INACTIVES: Edetate Disodium 0.1% and Purified Water. Hydrochloric Acid and/or Sodium Hydroxide may be added to adjust pH (4.0–7.0). PRESERVATIVE: Benzalkonium Chloride 0.01%.

Clinical Pharmacology: *In vitro* and *in vivo* animal studies have shown that cromolyn sodium inhibits the degranulation of sensitized mast cells which occurs after exposure to specific antigens. Cromolyn sodium acts by inhibiting the release of histamine and SRS-A (slow-reacting substance of anaphylaxis) from the mast cell.

Another activity demonstrated *in vitro* is the capacity of cromolyn sodium to inhibit the degranulation of non-sensitized rat mast cells by phospholipase A and the subsequent release of chemical mediators. Another study showed that cromolyn sodium did not inhibit the enzymatic activity of released phospholipase A on its specific substrate.

Cromolyn sodium has no intrinsic vasoconstrictor, antihistaminic or anti-inflammatory activity.

Cromolyn sodium is poorly absorbed. When multiple doses of cromolyn sodium ophthalmic solution are instilled into normal rabbit eyes, less than 0.07% of the administered dose of cromolyn sodium is absorbed into the systemic circulation (presumably by way of the eye, nasal passages, buccal cavity and gastrointestinal tract). Trace amounts (less than 0.01%) of the cromolyn sodium dose penetrate into the aqueous humor, and clearance from this chamber is virtually complete within 24 hours after treatment is stopped.

In normal volunteers, analysis of drug excretion indicates that approximately 0.03% of cromolyn sodium is absorbed following administration to the eye.

A study on corneal epithelial wound healing in albino rabbits failed to demonstrate any significant difference in the rate of corneal re-epithelialization between cromolyn sodium ophthalmic solution, sterile saline solution, no treatment and an ophthalmic corticosteroid.

Indications And Usage: Cromolyn sodium ophthalmic solution is indicated in the treatment of vernal keratoconjunctivitis, vernal conjunctivitis, and vernal keratitis.

Symptomatic response to therapy (decreased itching, tearing, redness and discharge) is usually evident within a few days, but longer treatment for up to six weeks is sometimes required. Once symptomatic improvement has been established, therapy should be continued for as long as needed to sustain improvement.

If required, corticosteroids may be used concomitantly with cromolyn sodium ophthalmic solution.

Users of soft (hydrophilic) contact lenses should refrain from wearing lenses while under treatment with cromolyn sodium ophthalmic solution (see **Contraindications**). Wear can be resumed within a few hours after discontinuation of the drug.

Contraindications: Cromolyn sodium ophthalmic solution is contraindicated in those patients who have shown hypersensitivity to cromolyn sodium or to any of the other ingredients.

As with all ophthalmic preparations containing benzalkonium chloride, patients are advised not to wear soft contact lenses during treatment with cromolyn sodium ophthalmic solution.

Precautions: General: Patients may experience a transient stinging or burning sensation following spplication of cromolyn sodium ophthalmic solution.

The recommended frequency of administration should not be exceeded. The dose for adults and children is 1 or 2 drops in each eye 4 to 6 times a day at regular intervals.

Carcinogenesis, Mutagenesis, and Impairment of Fertility: Long-term studies in mice (12 months intraperitoneal treatment followed by six months observation), hamsters (12 months intraperitoneal treatment followed by 12 months observation) and rats (18 months subcutaneous treatment) showed no neoplastic effect of cromolyn sodium.

No evidence of chromosomal damage or cytotoxicity was obtained in various mutagenesis studies.

No evidence of impaired fertility was shown in laboratory animal reproduction studies.

Pregnancy: Teratogenic effects: Pregnancy Category B. Reproduction studies with cromolyn sodium administered parenterally to pregnant mice, rats and rabbits in doses up to 338 times the human clinical doses produced no evidence of fetal malformations. Adverse fetal effects (increased resorption and decreased fetal weight) were noted only at the very high parenteral doses that produced maternal toxicity. There are, however, no adequate and well controlled studies in pregnant women. Because animal reproduction studies are not always predictive of human response, this drug should be used during pregnancy only if clearly needed.

Continued on next page

Crolom—Cont.

Nursing Mothers: It is not known whether this drug is excreted in human milk. Because many drugs are excreted in human milk, caution should be exercised when cromolyn sodium ophthalmic solution is administered to a nursing woman.
Pediatic Use: Safety and effectiveness in children below the age of 4 years have not been established.
Adverse Reactions: The most frequently reported adverse reaction attributed to the use of cromolyn sodium ophthalmic solution, on the basis of reoccurrence following readministration, is transient ocular stinging or burning upon instillation.
The following adverse reactions have been reported as infrequent events. It is unclear whether they are attributable to the drug:
Conjunctival injection
Watery eyes
Itchy eyes
Dryness around the eye
Puffy eyes
Eye irritation
Styes
Dosage And Administration: The dose for adults and children is 1 or 2 drops in each eye 4 to 6 times a day at regular intervals.
One drop contains approximately 1.6 mg cromolyn sodium.
Patients should be advised that the effect of cromolyn sodium ophthalmic solution therapy is dependent upon its administration at regular intervals, as directed.
FOR OPHTHALMIC USE ONLY
How Supplied: Crolom® (Cromolyn Sodium Ophthalmic Solution USP, 4%) is supplied in a plastic bottle individually cartoned with a controlled drop tip in the following sizes:
10 mL bottle (NDC 24208-300-10)—AB30709

DO NOT USE IF IMPRINTED NECKBAND IS NOT INTACT.

Storage: Store between 15°–30°C (59°–86°F). Protect from light. Keep tightly closed. Replace cap immediately after use.
KEEP OUT OF REACH OF CHILDREN.
Rx only
Bausch & Lomb
Pharmaceuticals, Inc.
Tampa, Florida 33637

R.3/98

Shown in Product Identification Guide, page 104

FLUOR-I-STRIP® ℞

[floo-or 'a "strip]
(Fluorescein Sodium Ophthalmic Strips)
Composition(per strip):

Fluorescein Sodium 9 mg	diagnostic dye
Chlorobutanol (chloral derivative) 0.5%	preservative
Polysorbate 80	surface active agent
Potassium Chloride	
Boric Acid	buffering agents
Sodium Carbonate	

Description: FLUOR-I-STRIP is a specially prepared sterile ophthalmic strip for diagnostic use.
Indications: For staining the anterior segment of the eye when:
a) delineating a corneal injury, herpetic lesion or foreign body,
b) determining the site of an intraocular injury,
c) fitting contact lenses,
d) making the fluorescein test to ascertain postoperative closure of the sclerocorneal (also referred to as corneoscleral) wound in delayed anterior chamber reformation,
e) making the lacrimal drainage test.
Directions for Use: To open envelope, grasp pull-tabs firmly and separate slowly. Separate the two strips by tearing off white tab end. Moisten end of strip with a drop of sterile water. Place moistened strip at the fornix in the lower cul-de-sac close to the punctum. For best results, patient should close lid tightly over strip until desired amount of staining is obtained. Another method is to retract upper lid and touch tip of strip to the bulbar conjunctiva on the temporal side until an adequate amount of stain is available for a clearly defined end-point reading.
Warning: Never use fluorescein while the patient is wearing *soft contact lenses* because the lenses may become stained. Whenever fluorescein is used, flush the eyes with sterile, normal saline solution, and wait at least one hour before replacing the lenses.
Storage: Store at room temperature (approximately 25°C).
How Supplied: Boxes of 300 strips in individual envelopes (NDC 24208-390-83).
Manufactured by
Wyeth Ayerst Laboratories
Rouses Point, NY 12979
Marketed by
Bausch & Lomb Pharmaceuticals
Tampa, FL 33637

Shown in Product Identification Guide, page 104

FLUOR-I-STRIP® -A.T. ℞

[floo-or 'a "strip]
(Fluorescein Sodium Ophthalmic Strips)
For Applanation Tonometry
Composition(Per Strip):

Fluorescein Sodium 1 mg	diagnostic dye
Chlorobutanol (chloral derivative) 0.5%	preservative
Polysorbate 80	surface active agent
Boric Acid	
Potassium Chloride	buffering agents
Sodium Carbonate	

Description: FLUOR-I-STRIP-A.T. consists of sterile ophthalmic strips, specially prepared for diagnostic use in applanation tonometry.
Indications: For staining the anterior segment of the eye when:
a) delineating a corneal injury, herpetic lesion or foreign body,
b) determining the site of an intraocular injury,
c) fitting contact lenses,
d) making the fluorescein test to ascertain postoperative closure of the sclerocorneal (also referred to as corneoscleral) wound in delayed anterior chamber reformation,
e) making the lacrimal drainage test.
Directions for Use: To open envelope, grasp pull-tabs firmly and separate slowly. Separate the two strips by tearing off white tab end. Anesthetize the eyes. Retract upper lid and touch tip of strip to the bulbar conjunctiva on the temporal side until an adequate amount of stain is available for a clearly defined end-point reading.
Warning: Never use fluorescein while the patient is wearing *soft contact lenses* because the lenses may become stained. Whenever fluorescein is used, flush the eyes with sterile, normal saline solution, and wait at least one hour before replacing the lenses.
Storage: Store at room temperature (approximately 25°C).
How Supplied: Boxes of 300 strips, 2 in each envelope NDC 24208-391-83
Manufactured by
Wyeth-Ayerst Laboratories
Rouses Point, NY 12979
Marketed by
Bausch & Lomb Pharmaceuticals
Tampa, FL 33637

Shown in Product Identification Guide, page 104

LOTEMAX® ℞

[Lō tĕ max]
loteprednol etabonate ophthalmic suspension 0.5%
STERILE OPHTHALMIC SUSPENSION

Description: LOTEMAX™ (loteprednol etabonate ophthalmic suspension) contains a sterile, topical anti-inflammatory corticosteroid for ophthalmic use. Loteprednol etabonate is a white to off-white powder.
Loteprednol etabonate is represented by the following structural formula:

$C_{24}H_{31}ClO_7$ Mol. Wt. 466.96

Chemical name:
chloromethyl 17α-[(ethoxycarbol)oxy]-11β-hydroxy-3-oxoandrosta-1,4-diene-17β-carboxylate
Each mL contains:
ACTIVE: Loteprednol Etabonate 5 mg (0.5%);
INACTIVES: Edetate Disodium, Glycerin, Povidone, Purified Water and Tyloxapol. Hydrochloric Acid and/or Sodium Hydroxide may be added to adjust the pH to 5.3–5.6. The suspension is essentially isotonic with a tonicity of 250 to 310 mOsmol/kg.
PRESERVATIVE ADDED: Benzalkonium Chloride 0.01%.
Clinical Pharmacology: Corticosteroids inhibit the inflammatory response to a variety of inciting agents and probably delay or slow healing. They inhibit the edema, fibrin deposition, capillary dilation, leukocyte migration, capillary proliferation, fibroblast proliferation, deposition of collagen, and scar formation associated with inflammation. There is no generally accepted explanation for the mechanism of action of ocular corticosteroids. However, corticosteroids are thought to act by the induction of phospholipase A_2 inhibitory proteins, collectively called lipocortins. It is postulated that these proteins control the biosynthesis of potent mediators of inflammation such as prostaglandins and leukotrienes by inhibiting the release of their common precursor, arachidonic acid. Arachidonic acid is released from membrane phospholipids by phospholipase A_2. Corticosteroids are capable of producing a rise in intraocular pressure.
Loteprednol etabonate is structurally similar to other corticosteroids. However, the number 20 position ketone group is absent. It is highly lipid soluble which enhances its penetration into cells. Loteprednol etabonate is synthesized through structural modifications of prednisolone-related compounds so that it will undergo a predictable transformation to an inactive metabolite. Based upon *in vivo* and *in vitro* preclinical metabolism studies, loteprednol etabonate undergoes extensive metabolism to inactive carboxylic acid metabolites.

Results from a bioavailability study in normal volunteers established that plasma levels of loteprednol etabonate and Δ^1 cortienic acid etabonate (PJ 91), its primary, inactive metabolite, were below the limit of quantitation (1 ng/mL) at all sampling times. The results were obtained following the ocular administration of one drop in each eye of 0.5% loteprednol etabonate 8 times daily for 2 days or 4 times daily for 42 days. This study suggests that limited (<1 ng/mL) systemic absorption occurs with LOTEMAX.

Clinical Studies:

Post-operative Inflammation: Placebo-controlled clinical studies demonstrated that LOTEMAX is effective for the treatment of anterior chamber inflammation as measured by cell and flare.

Giant Papillary Conjunctivitis: Placebo-controlled clinical studies demonstrated that LOTEMAX was effective in reducing the signs and symptoms of giant papillary conjunctivitis after 1 week of treatment and continuing for up to 6 weeks while on treatment.

Seasonal Allergic Conjunctivitis: A placebo-controlled clinical study demonstrated that LOTEMAX was effective in reducing the signs and symptoms of allergic conjunctivitis during peak periods of pollen exposure.

Uveitis: Controlled clinical studies of patients with uveitis demonstrated the LOTEMAX was less effective than prednisolone acetate 1%. Overall, 72% of patients treated with LOTEMAX experienced resolution of anterior chamber cell by day 28, compared to 87% of patients treated with prednisolone acetate 1%. The incidence of patients with clinically significant increases in IOP (≥10 mmHg) was 1% with LOTEMAX and 6% with prednisolone acetate 1%.

Indications and Usage: LOTEMAX is indicated for the treatment of steroid responsive inflammatory conditions of the palpebral and bulbar conjunctiva, cornea and anterior segment of the globe such as allergic conjunctivitis, acne rosacea, superficial punctate keratitis, herpes zoster keratitis, iritis, cyclitis, selected infective conjunctivitides, when the inherent hazard of steroid use is accepted to obtain an advisable diminution in edema and inflammation.

LOTEMAX was less effective than prednisolone acetate 1% in two 28-day controlled clinical studies in acute anterior uveitis, where 72% of patients treated with LOTEMAX experienced resolution of anterior chamber cells, compared to 87% of patients treated with prednisolone acetate 1%. The incidence of patients with clinically significant increases in IOP (≥10 mmHg) was 1% with LOTEMAX and 6% with prednisolone acetate 1%. LOTEMAX should not be used in patients who require a more potent corticosteroid for this indication.

LOTEMAX is also indicated for the treatment of post-operative inflammation following ocular surgery.

Contraindications: LOTEMAX, as with other ophthalmic corticosteroids, is contraindicated in most viral diseases of the cornea and conjunctiva including epithelial herpes simplex keratitis (dendritic keratitis), vaccinia, and varicella, and also in mycobacterial infection of the eye and fungal diseases of ocular structures. LOTEMAX is also contraindicated in individuals with known or suspected hypersensitivity to any of the ingredients of this preparation and to other corticosteroids.

Warnings: Prolonged use of corticosteroids may result in glaucoma with damage to the optic nerve, defects in visual acuity and fields of vision, and in posterior subcapsular cataract formation. Steroids should be used with caution in the presence of glaucoma.

Prolonged use of corticosteroids may suppress the host response and thus increase the hazard of secondary ocular infections. In those diseases causing thinning of the cornea or sclera, perforations have been known to occur with the use of topical steroids. In acute purulent conditions of the eye, steroids may mask infection or enhance existing infection.

Use of ocular steroids may prolong the course and may exacerbate the severity of many viral infections of the eye (including herpes simplex). Employment of a corticosteroid medication in the treatment of patients with a history of herpes simplex requires great caution.

The use of steroids after cataract surgery may delay healing and increase the incidence of bleb formation.

Precautions:

General: For ophthalmic use only. The initial prescription and renewal of the medication order beyond 14 days should be made by a physician only after examination of the patient with the aid of magnification, such as slit lamp biomicroscopy and, where appropriate, fluorescein staining.

If signs and symptoms fail to improve after two days, the patient should be re-evaluated.

If this product is used for 10 days or longer, intraocular pressure should be monitored even though it may be difficult in children and uncooperative patients (see WARNINGS).

Fungal infections of the cornea are particularly prone to develop coincidentally with long-term local steroid application. Fungus invasion must be considered in any persistent corneal ulceration where a steroid has been used or is in use. Fungal cultures should be taken when appropriate.

Information for Patients: This product is sterile when packaged. Patients should be advised not to allow the dropper tip to touch any surface, as this may contaminate the suspension. If pain develops, redness, itching or inflammation becomes aggravated, the patient should be advised to consult a physician. As with all ophthalmic preparations containing benzalkonium chloride, patients should be advised not to wear soft contact lenses when using LOTEMAX®.

Carcinogenesis, mutagenesis, impairment of fertility: Long-term animal studies have not been conducted to evaluate the carcinogenic potential of loteprednol etabonate. Loteprednol etabonate was not gentoxic *in vitro* in the Ames test, the mouse lymphoma tk assay, or in a chromosome aberration test in human lymphocytes, or *in vivo* in the single dose mouse micronucleus assay. Treatment of male and female rats with up to 50 mg/kg/day and 25 mg/kg/day of loteprednol etabonate, respectively, (600 and 300 times the maximum clinical dose, respectively) prior to and during mating did not impair fertility in either gender.

Pregnancy: Teratogenic effects: Pregnancy Category C. Loteprednol etabonate has been shown to be embryotoxic (delayed ossification) and teratogenic (increased incidence of meningocele, abnormal left common carotid artery, and limb flexures) when administered orally to rabbits during organogenesis at a dose of 3 mg/kg/day (35 times the maximum daily clinical dose), a dose which caused no maternal toxicity. The no-observed-effect-level (NOEL) for these effects was 0.5 mg/kg/day (6 times the maximum daily clinical dose). Oral treatment of rats during organogenesis resulted in teratogenicity (absent innominate artery at ≥5mg/kg/day doses, and cleft palate and umbilical hernia at ≥50 mg/kg/day) and embryotoxicity (increased post-implantation losses at 100 mg/kg /day and decreased fetal body weight and skeletal ossification with ≥50 mg/kg/day). Treatment of rats with 0.5 mg/kg/day (6 times the maximum clinical dose) during organogenesis did not result in any reproductive toxicity. Loteprednol etabonate was maternally toxic (significantly reduced body weight gain during treatment) when administered to pregnant rats during organogenesis at doses of ≥5 mg/kg/day.

Oral exposure of female rats to 50 mg/kg/day of loteprednol etabonate from the start of the fetal period through the end of lactation, a maternally toxic treatment regimen (significantly decreased body weight gain), gave rise to decreased growth and survival, and retarded development in the offspring during lactation; the NOEL for these effects was 5 mg/kg/day. Loteprednol etabonate had no effect on the duration of gestation or parturition when administered orally to pregnant rats at doses up to 50 mg/kg/day during the fetal period.

Nursing Mothers: It is not known whether topical ophthalmic administration of corticosteroids could result in sufficient systemic absorption to produce detectable quantities in human milk. Systemic steroids appear in human milk and could suppress growth, interfere with endogenous corticosteroid production, or cause other untoward effects. Caution should be exercised when LOTEMAX is administered to a nursing women.

Pediatric Use: Safety and effectiveness in pediatric patients have not been established.

Adverse Reactions: Reactions associated with ophthalmic steroids include elevated intraocular pressure, which may be associated with optic nerve damage, visual acuity and field defects, posterior subcapsular cataract formation, secondary ocular infection from pathogens including herpes simplex, and perforation of the globe where there is thinning of the cornea or sclera.

Ocular adverse reactions occurring in 5–15% of patients treated with loteprednol etabonate ophthalmic suspension (0.2%–0.5%) in clinical studies included abnormal vision/blurring, burning on instillation, chemosis, discharge, dry eyes, epiphora, foreign body sensation, itching, injection, and photophobia. Other ocular adverse reactions occurring in less than 5% of patients include conjunctivitis, corneal abnormalities, eyelid erythema, keratoconjunctivitis, ocular irritation/pain/discomfort, papillae, and uveitis. Some of these events were similar to the underlying ocular disease being studied.

Non-ocular adverse reactions occurred in less than 15% of patients. These include headache, rhinitis and pharyngitis.

In a summation of controlled, randomized studies of individuals treated for 28 days or longer with loteprednol etabonate, the incidence of significant elevation of intraocular pressure (≥10 mmHg) was 2% (15/901) among patients receiving loteprednol etabonate, 7% (11/164) among patients receiving 1% prednisolone acetate and 0.5% (3/583) among patients receiving placebo.

Dosage and Administration: SHAKE VIGOROUSLY BEFORE USING.

Steroid Responsive Disease Treatment: Apply one to two drops of LOTEMAX into the conjunctival sac of the affected eye(s) four times daily. During the initial treatment within the first week, the dosing may be increased, up to 1 drop every hour, if necessary. Care should be taken not to discontinue therapy prematurely. If signs and symptoms fail to improve after two days, the patient should be re-evaluated (See PRECAUTIONS).

Post-Operative Inflammation: Apply one to two drops of LOTEMAX into the conjunctival sac of the operated eye(s) four times daily beginning 24 hours after surgery and continuing throughout the first 2 weeks of the post-operative period.

How Supplied: LOTEMAX™ (loteprednol etabonate ophthalmic suspension) is supplied in a plastic bottle with a controlled drop tip in the following sizes:

2.5 mL (NDC 24208-299-25)-AB29904

Continued on next page

Lotemax—Cont.

5 mL (NDC 24208-299-05)-AB29907
10 mL (NDC 24208-299-10)-AB29909
15 mL (NDC 24208-299-15)-AB29911

DO NOT USE IF NECKBAND IMPRINTED WITH "Protective Seal" AND YELLOW IS NOT INTACT.

Storage: Store upright between 15°–25°C (59°–77°F). DO NOT FREEZE.
KEEP OUT OF REACH OF CHILDREN.

Rx only

Manufactured by
Bausch & Lomb Pharmaceuticals, Inc., Tampa, Florida 33637
under Agreement with Pharmos Corporation.
U.S. Patent No. 4,996,335
U.S. Patent No. 5,540,930
©Bausch & Lomb Pharmaceuticals, Inc.

Rev. 3/98-8C

Shown in Product Identification Guide, page 104

MURO 128® 2% OTC
[*mŭ 'rō* 128]
Sodium Chloride Hypertonicity Ophthalmic Solution, 2%

MURO 128® 5% OTC
Sodium Chloride Hypertonicity Ophthalmic Solution, 5%
STERILE OPHTHALMIC SOLUTION

Description: Muro 128® 2% Solution is a sterile ophthalmic solution used to draw water out of the cornea of the eye.
Each mL Contains: ACTIVE: Sodium Chloride 2%; INACTIVES: Boric Acid, Hydroxypropyl Methylcellulose 2910, Propylene Glycol, Sodium Borate, Purified Water. Sodium Hydroxide and/or Hydrochloric Acid may be added to adjust pH.
PRESERVATIVES: Methylparaben 0.046%, Propylparaben 0.02%
Description: Muro 128® 5% Solution is a sterile ophthalmic solution used to draw water out of the cornea of the eye.
Each mL Contains: ACTIVE: Sodium Chloride 5% INACTIVES: Boric Acid, Hydroxypropyl Methylcellulose 2910, Propylene Glycol, Sodium Borate, Purified Water. Sodium Hydroxide and/or Hydrochloric Acid may be added to adjust pH.
PRESERVATIVES: Methylparaben 0.023%, Propylparaben 0.01%
Indication: For the temporary relief of corneal edema.
Warnings: Do not use this product except under the advice and supervision of a doctor.
If you experience eye pain, changes in vision, continued redness or irritation of the eye, or if the condition worsens or persists, consult a doctor.
To avoid contamination of the product, do not touch the tip of the container to any surface. Replace cap after using.
This product may cause temporary burning and irritation on being instilled into the eye.
If the solution changes color or becomes cloudy, do not use.
In case of accidental ingestion, seek professional assistance or contact a Poison Control Center immediately.
Directions: Instill 1 or 2 drops in the affected eye(s) every 3 or 4 hours, or as directed by a doctor.
FOR OPHTHALMIC USE ONLY
How Supplied: Muro 128 2% Solution is supplied in a plastic controlled drop tip bottle in the following size:
$^1/_2$ Fl. Oz. (15 mL) (NDC 24208-276-15)—Prod. No. AB15511
How Supplied: Muro 128 5% Solution is supplied in $^1/_2$ Fl. Oz. (15 mL) or 1 Fl. Oz. (30 mL) plastic controlled dropper tip bottles.
15 mL [NDC 24208-277-15]—Prod. No. AB15611
30 mL [NDC 24208-277-30]—Prod. No. AB15616

DO NOT USE IF IMPRINTED NECKBAND IS NOT INTACT

Storage: Store between 15°–30°C [59°–86°F]. KEEP TIGHTLY CLOSED. **STORE UPRIGHT AND IMMEDIATELY REPLACE CAP AFTER USE.**
KEEP OUT OF REACH OF CHILDREN.
Bausch & Lomb
Pharmaceuticals, Inc.
Tampa, FL 33637
MURO is a trademark of MURO Pharmaceutical, Inc.

R.1/97-7A

Shown in Product Identification Guide, page 104

MURO 128® OINTMENT OTC
[*mŭ 'rō* 128]
sodium chloride hypertonicity ophthalmic ointment, 5%
FOR CORNEAL EDEMA
STERILE OPHTHALMIC OINTMENT

Description: Muro 128® Ointment is a sterile ophthalmic ointment used to draw water out of the cornea of the eye.
Each Gram Contains: ACTIVE: Sodium Chloride 5% INACTIVES: Lanolin, Mineral Oil, White Petrolatum, Purified Water.
Indication: For the temporary relief of corneal edema.
Warnings: Do not use this product except under the advice and supervision of a doctor.
If you experience eye pain, changes in vision, continued redness or irritation of the eye, or if the condition worsens or persists, consult a doctor.
To avoid contamination of the product, do not touch the tip of the container to any surface. Replace cap after using.
This product may cause temporary burning and irritation on being instilled into the eye.
In case of accidental ingestion, seek professional assistance or contact a Poison Control Center immediately.
Directions: Pull down lower lid of the affected eye(s) and apply a small amount (approximately $^1/_4$ inch) of the ointment to the inside of the eyelid every 3 or 4 hours, or as directed by a doctor.
FOR OPHTHALMIC USE ONLY
How Supplied: Muro 128® Ointment is supplied in $^1/_8$ oz (3.5 g) tube.
[NDC 24208-385-55]—Prod. No. AB15834
TWIN PACK: 2 x $^1/_8$ oz (2 x 3.5 g)
[NDC 24208-385-56]—Prod. No. AB15899
NOTE: Tubes are filled by weight ($^1/_8$ oz/3.5g) not volume.
See Crimp of tube for Lot Number and Expiration Date.

DO NOT USE IF BOTTOM RIDGE OF TUBE CAP IS EXPOSED AND IMPRINTED SEAL ON BOX IS BROKEN OR MISSING.

KEEP OUT OF REACH OF CHILDREN.
Storage: Store between 15°–30°C (59°–86°F). DO NOT FREEZE.
KEEP TIGHTLY CLOSED.
Bausch & Lomb
Pharmaceuticals, Inc.
Tampa, FL 33637
MURO is a trademark of MURO Pharmaceutical, Inc.

R5/97

Shown in Product Identification Guide, page 104

OCUCOAT® and OCUCOAT PF® OTC
Lubricating Eye Drops

Description: Multidose: Dextran 70 (0.1%), hydroxypropyl methylcellulose 2910 (0.8%), monobasic sodium phosphate, dibasic sodium phosphate, potassium chloride, sodium chloride, dextrose and purified water. Preserved with benzalkonium chloride (0.01%). May also contain hydrochloric acid and/or sodium hydroxide to adjust the pH.
Unit Dose: Dextran 70 (0.1%), hydroxypropyl methylcellulose 2910 (0.8%), monobasic sodium phosphate, dibasic sodium phosphate, potassium chloride, sodium chloride, dextrose and purified water. May also contain hydrochloric acid and/or sodium hydroxide to adjust the pH.
Indications: For use as a lubricant to prevent further irritation or to relieve dryness of the eye.
Directions: Multidose: Carefully tilt container over the open eye. Without touching the eye or eyelid, squeeze one or two drops into the affected eye(s) as needed or as directed by a doctor.
Unit Dose: Detach a single-dose container from the strip. Be sure each container is intact before using it. Do not use if container is not intact.
To open, gently twist off the tip.
With thumb and finger on either side of the bubble, carefully tilt the container over the open eye. Without touching the tip to the eye or eyelid, squeeze one or two drops into the affected eye(s) as needed or as directed by a doctor.
Do not reuse. Once opened, discard.
Warnings: Keep this and all drugs out of the reach of children. In case of accidental ingestion, seek professional assistance or contact a Poison Control Center immediately.
If you experience eye pain, changes in vision, continued redness or irritation of the eye, or if the condition worsens or persists for more than 72 hours, discontinue use and consult a doctor.
If solution changes color or becomes cloudy, do not use.
To avoid contamination, do not touch tip of container to any surface.
For multidose units, replace cap immediately after using.
For unit dose units, discard after single use.
How Supplied:
OCUCOAT:
NDC 24208-377-11—15 mL (0.5 FL. OZ.) bottle
OCUCOAT PF:
NDC 24208-384-48—28 single-dose containers (0.5 mL each)
FOR OPHTHALMIC USE ONLY.
STORE AT ROOM TEMPERATURE.
Marketed by
Bausch & Lomb Pharmaceuticals, Inc.
Tampa, FL 33637

Shown in Product Identification Guide, page 104

OCUVITE® OTC
Vitamin and Mineral Supplement

Description: Each tablet contains:
For Adults—Percentage of US Recommended Daily Allowance (US RDA)
[See table at top of next page]
Inactive Ingredients: Dibasic Calcium Phosphate, FD&C Yellow No. 6, hydroxypropyl methylcellulose, magnesium stearate, microcrystalline cellulose, polysorbate 80, polyvinyl-

	Source	Amount	% Daily Value
Zinc	Zinc Oxide*	40 mg (elemental)	267%
Copper	Cupric Oxide	2 mg (elemental)	100%
Vitamin C	Ascorbic Acid	60 mg	100%
Vitamin E	dl-Alpha Tocopheryl Acetate	30 IU	100%
Vitamin A	Beta Carotene	5000 IU	100%
Selenium	Sodium Selenate	40 mcg (elemental)	**

* Zinc oxide is the most concentrated form of zinc and contains more elemental zinc than any other zinc salt (ie: zinc sulfate or zinc acetate).
** No US RDA established.

pyrrolidone, silica gel, sodium lauryl sulfate, stearic acid, titanium dioxide and triethyl citrate.
Indications: OCUVITE is specifically formulated to supplement the diets of people who may have or be at risk of deficiencies of the vitamins and minerals found in the OCUVITE formulation.
Recommended Intake: Adults. One tablet, one or two times daily or as directed by their doctor.
How Supplied: Peach, eye shaped, film coated tablet engraved LL on one side, 04 on the other side.
NDC 24208-38760—Bottle of 60
NDC 24208-38762—Bottle of 120
Store at Room Temperature.
MADE IN U.S.A.
Marketed by
Bausch & Lomb Pharmaceuticals
Tampa, FL 33637

Shown in Product Identification Guide, page 104

OCUVITE® extra® OTC
Vitamin and Mineral Supplement

Description: Each tablet contains:
[See table below]
Inactive Ingredients: Dibasic Calcium Phosphate, FD&C Yellow No. 6, Hydroxypropyl Methylcellulose, Magnesium Stearate, Microcrystalline Cellulose, Mineral Oil, Polysorbate 80, Polyvinylpyrrolidone, Silica Gel, Sodium Lauryl Sulfate, Stearic Acid, Titanium Dioxide and Triethyl Citrate.
Indications: OCUVITE EXTRA is specifically formulated to supplement the diets of people who may have or be at risk of deficiencies of the vitamins and minerals found in the OCUVITE EXTRA formulation.

	Source	Amount	% Daily Value
Zinc	Zinc Oxide*	40 mg (elemental)	267%
Copper	Cupric Oxide	2 mg (elemental)	100%
Vitamin C	Ascorbic Acid	200 mg	333%
Vitamin E	dl-Alpha Tocopheryl Acetate	50 IU	167%
Vitamin A	Beta Carotene	6000 IU	120%
Selenium	Sodium Selenate	40 mcg (elemental)	57%
Riboflavin		3 mg	176%
Niacinamide		40 mg	200%
Manganese		5 mg	250%
L-Glutathione		5 mg	†

* Zinc oxide is the most concentrated form of zinc and contains more elemental zinc than any other zinc salt (ie: zinc sulfate or zinc acetate).
† No US RDA established.

Recommended Intake: Adults: One tablet, one or two times daily or as directed by their doctor.
How Supplied: Orange, eye shaped, film coated tablet engraved OCUVITE on one side, 05 on the other side.
NDC 24208-388-19—Bottle of 50
Store at Room Temperature
MADE IN U.S.A.
Marketed by
Bausch & Lomb Pharmaceuticals
Tampa, FL 33637

Shown in Product Identification Guide, page 104

OPTIPRANOLOL® ℞
metipranolol ophthalmic solution 0.3%

Description: OPTIPRANOLOL® (metipranolol 0.3%) Sterile Ophthalmic Solution contains metipranolol, a non-selective beta-adrenergic receptor blocking agent. Metipranolol is a white, odorless, crystalline powder. The molecular weight is 309.40.
The empinic chemical formula of metipranolol is $C_{17}H_{27}NO_4$.
The chemical name of metipranolol is (±)-1-(4-Hydroxy-2, 3, 5-trimethylphenoxy)-3-(isopropylamino)-2-propanol-4-acetate.
The chemical structure of metipranolol is:

Each mL of OPTIPRANOLOL® contains 3 mg metipranolol. INACTIVES: povidone, glycerol, hydrochloric acid, sodium chloride, edetate disodium, and purified water. Sodium Hydroxide may be added to adjust pH. PRESERVATIVE: Benzalkonium chloride 0.004%.
Clinical Pharmacology: Metipranolol blocks $beta_1$ and $beta_2$ (non-selective) adrenergic receptors. It does not have significant intrinsic sympathomimetic activity, and has only weak local anesthetic (membrane-stabilizing) and myocardial depressant activity.
Orally administered beta-adrenergic blocking agents reduce cardiac output in both healthy subjects and patients with heart disease. In patients with severe impairment of myocardial function, beta-adrenergic receptor antagonists may inhibit the sympathetic stimulatory effect necessary to maintain adequate cardiac output.
Beta-adrenergic receptor blockade in the bronchi and bronchioles may result in significantly increased airway resistance from unopposed para-sympathetic activity. Such an effect is potentially dangerous in patients with asthma or other bronchospastic conditions (see CONTRAINDICATIONS and WARNINGS).
OPTIPRANOLOL® Ophthalmic Solution, when applied topically in the eye, has the action of reducing elevated as well as normal intraocular pressure (IOP), whether or not accompanied by glaucoma. Elevated intraocular pressure is a major risk factor in the pathogenesis of glaucomatous visual field loss. The higher the level of intraocular pressure, the greater the likelihood of glaucomatous visual field loss and optic nerve damage.
The primary mechanism of the ocular hypotensive action of metipranolol is most likely due to a reduction in aqueous humor production. A slight increase in outflow may be an additional mechanism. OPTIPRANOLOL® Ophthalmic Solution reduces IOP with little or no effect on pupil size or accommodation.
Animal Pharmacology: In rabbits administered metipranolol in one eye at 2 to 4 fold increased concentrations, multi-focal interstitial nephritis was observed in male animals, and lympho-hystiocytic and heterophilic interstitial pneumonia was observed in female animals. The clinical relevance of these findings in unknown.
Indications And Usage: OPTIPRANOLOL® Ophthalmic Solution is indicated in the treatment of ocular conditions where lowering intraocular pressure is likely to be of therapeutic benefit, including patients with ocular hypertension, and patients with chronic open angle glaucoma.
In controlled studies of patients with intraocular pressure greater than 24 mmHg at baseline, OPTIPRANOLOL® Ophthalmic Solution reduced the average intraocular pressure approximately 20–26%.
The onset of action of OPTIPRANOLOL® Ophthalmic Solution, as measured by a reduction in intraocular pressure, occurs within 30 minutes after a single administration. The maximum effect occurs at about 2 hours. A reduction in intraocular pressure can be demonstrated 24 hours after a single dose. Clinical studies in patients with glaucoma treated for up to two years indicate that an intraocular pressure lowering effect is maintained.
In clinical trials, OPTIPRANOLOL® Ophthalmic Solution was safely used during concomitant therapy with pilocarpine, epinephrine or acetazolamide.
Contraindications: Hypersensitivity to any component of this product.
OPTIPRANOLOL® Ophthalmic Solution is contraindicated in patients with bronchial asthma or a history of bronchial asthma, or severe chronic obstructive pulmonary disease;

Continued on next page

Optipranolol—Cont.

symptomatic sinus bradycardia; greater than a first degree atrioventricular block; cardiogenic shock; or overt cardiac failure.

Warnings: As with other topically applied ophthalmic drugs, this drug may be absorbed systemically. Thus, the same adverse reactions found with systemic administration of beta-adrenergic blocking agents may occur with topical administration. For example, severe respiratory reactions and cardiac reactions, including death due to bronchospasm in patients with asthma, and rarely, death in association with cardiac failure, have been reported following topical application of beta-adrenergic blocking agents (see CONTRAINDICATIONS).

Since OPTIPRANOLOL® Ophthalmic Solution had a minor effect on heart rate and blood pressure in clinical studies, caution should be observed in treating patients with a history of cardiac failure. Treatment with OPTIPRANOLOL® Ophthalmic Solution should be discontinued at the first evidence of cardiac failure.

OPTIPRANOLOL® Ophthalmic Solution, or other beta-blockers, should not, in general, be administered to patients with chronic obstructive pulmonary disease (e.g., chronic bronchitis, emphysema) of mild or moderate severity (see CONTRAINDICATIONS). However, if the drug is necessary in such patients, then it should be administered with caution since it may block bronchodilation produced by endogenous and exogenous catecholamine stimulation of $beta_2$ receptors.

Precautions: General: Because of potential effects of beta-adrenergic receptor blocking agents relative to blood pressure and pulse, these should be used with caution in patients with cerebrovascular insufficiency. If signs or symptoms suggesting reduced cerebral blood flow develop following initiation of therapy with OPTIPRANOLOL® Ophthalmic Solution, alternative therapy shoulld be considered.

Some authorities recommend gradual withdrawal of beta-adrenergic receptor blocking agents in patients undergoing elective surgery. If necessary during surgery, the effects of beta-adrenergic receptor blocking agents may be reversed by sufficient doses of such agonists as isoproterenol, dopamine, dobutamine or levarterenol.

While OPTIPRANOLOL® Ophthalmic Solution has demonstrated a low potential for systemic effect, it should be used with caution in patients with diabetes (especially labile diabetes,) because of possible masking of signs and symptoms of acute hypoglycemia.

Beta-adrenergic receptor blocking agents may mask certain signs and symptoms of hyperthyroidism, and their abrupt withdrawal might precipitate a thyroid storm.

Beta-adrenergic blockade has been reported to potentiate muscle weakness consistent with certain myasthenic symptoms (e.g., diplopia, ptosis, and generalized weakness).

Risk of anaphylactic reaction: While taking beta-blockers, patients with a history of severe anaphylactic reaction to a variety of allergens may be more reactive to repeated challenge, either accidental, diagnostic, or therapeutic. Such patients may be unresponsive to the usual doses of epinephrine used to treat allergic reaction.

Drug Interactions:

OPTIPRANOLOL® Ophthalmic Solution should be used with caution in patients who are receiving a beta-adrenergic blocking agent orally, because of the potential for additive effects on systemic beta-blockade.

Close observation of the patient is recommended when a beta-blocker is administered to patients receiving catecholamine-depleting drugs such as reserpine, because of possible additive effects and the production of hypotension and/or bradycardia.

Caution should be used in the coadministration of beta-adrenergic receptor blocking agents, such as metipranolol, and oral or intravenous calcium channel antagonists, because of possible precipitation of left ventricular failure, and hypotension. In patients with impaired cardiac function, who are receiving calcium channel antagonists, coadministration should be avoided.

The concomitant use of beta-adrenergic receptor blocking agents with digitalis and calcium channel antagonists may have additive effecets, prolonging atrioventricular conduction time.

Caution should be used in patients using concomitant adrenergic psychotropic drugs.

Ocular:

In patients with angle-closure glaucoma, the immediate treatment objective is to re-open the angle by constriction of the pupil with a miotic agent. OPTIPRANOLOL® Ophthalmic Solution has little or no effect on the pupil, therefore, when it is used to reduce intraocular pressure in angle-closure glaucoma, it should be used only with concomitant administration of a miotic agent.

Carcinogenesis, Mutagensis, Impairment of Fertility:

Lifetime studies with metipranolol have heen conducted in mice at oral doses of 5, 50, and 100 mg/kg/day and in rats at oral doses of up to 70 mg/kg/day. Metipranolol demonstrated no carcinogenic effect. In the mouse study, female animals receiving the low, but not the intermediate or high dose, had an increased number of pulmonary adenomas. The significance of this observation is unknown. In a variety of *in vitro* and *in vivo* bacterial and mammalian cell assays, metipranolol was nonmutagenic.

Reproduction and fertility studies of metipranolol in rats and mice showed no adverse effect on male fertility at oral doses of up to 50 mg/kg/day, and female fertility at oral doses of up to 25 mg/kg/day.

Pregnancy:

Pregnancy Category C:No drug related effects were reported for the segment II teratology study in fetal rats after administration, during organogenesis, to dams of up to 50 mg/kg/day. OPTIPRANOLOL® Ophthalmic Solution has been shown to increase fetal resorption, fetal death, and delayed development when administered orally to rabbits at 50 mg/kg during organogenesis.

There are no adequate and well-controlled studies in pregnant women. OPTIPRANOLOL® Ophthalmic Solution should be used during pregnancy only if the potential benefit justifies the potential risk to the fetus.

Nursing Mothers:

It is not known whether OPTIPRANOLOL® Ophthalmic Solution is excreted in human milk. Because many drugs are excreted in human milk, caution should be exercised when OPTIPRANOLOL® Ophthalmic Solution is administered to nursing women.

Pediatric Use:

Safety and effectiveness in children have not been established.

Adverse Reactions: In clinical trials, the use of OPTIPRANOLOL® Ophthalmic Solution has been associated with transient local discomfort.

Other ocular adverse reactions, such as conjunctivitis, eyelid dermatitis, blepharitis, blurred vision, tearing, browache, adnormal vision, photophobia, edema, and uveitis have been reported in small numbers of patients, either in U.S. clinical trials or from post-marketing experience.

Other systemic adverse reactions, such as allergic reaction, headache, asthenia, hypertension, myocardial infarct, atrial fibrillation, angina, palpitation, bradycardia, nausea, rhinitis, dyspnea, epistaxis, bronchitis, coughing, dizziness, anxiety, depression, somnolence, nervousness, arthritis, myalgia, and rash have also been reported in small numbers of patients.

Overdosage: No information is available on overdosage of OPTIPRANOLOL® Ophthalmic Solution in humans. The symptoms which might be expected with an overdose of a systemically administered beta-adrenergic receptor blocking agent are bradycardia, hypotension and acute cardiac failure.

Dosage And Administration: The recommended dose is one drop of OPTIPRANOLOL® Ophthalmic Solution in the affected eye(s) twice a day.

If the patients's IOP is not at a satisfactory level on this regimen, use of more frequent administration or a larger dose of OPTIPRANOLOL® Ophthalmic Solution is not known to be of benefit. Concomitant therapy to lower intraocular pressure can be instituted.

How Supplied: OPTIPRANOLOL® Ophthalmic Solution is supplied in white opaque, plastic ophthalmic bottle dispensers with a controlled drop tip and a yellow plastic screw-top cap as follows

5 mL: NDC 24208-275-07
10 mL: NDC 24208-275-09

Storage: Store at controlled room temperature, 15°–30°C (59°–86°F).

FOR OPHTHALMIC USE ONLY
Rx only
Bausch & Lomb
Pharmaceuticals, Inc.
Tampa, FL 33637

Shown in Product Identification Guide, page 104

RĒV-EYES® ℞

[reev-eyes]
dapiprazole hydrochloride
Ophthalmic Eyedrops, 0.5%—Sterile

Description: For ophthalmic use only.

RĒV-EYES® (dapiprazole hydrochloride) is an alpha-adrenergic blocking agent.

Dapiprazole hydrochloride is 5,6,7,8-tetrahydro-3-[2-(4-*o*.tolyl-1-piperazinyl) ethyl]-*s*-triazolo[4,3-a]pyridine hydrochloride.

Dapiprazole hydrochloride has the empirical formula $C_{19}H_{27}N_5$ HCl and a molecular weight of 361.93.

Dapiprazole hydrochloride is a sterile, white, lyophilized powder soluble in water.

RĒV-EYES® (dapiprazole hydrochloride) Eyedrops is a clear, colorless, slightly viscous solution for topical application. Each mL (when reconstituted as directed) contains 5 mg of dapiprazole hydrochloride as the active ingredient.

The reconstituted solution has a pH of approximately 6.6 and an osmolarity of approximately 415 mOsm.

The inactive ingredients include: mannitol (2%), sodium chloride, hydroxypropyl methylcellulose (0.4%), edetate sodium (0.01%), sodium phosphate dibasic, sodium phosphate monobasic, water for injection, and benzalkonium chloride (0.01%) as a preservative.

RĒV-EYES® Eyedrops, 0.5% is supplied in a kit consisting of one vial of dapiprazole hydrochloride (25 mg), one vial of diluent (5 mL) and one dropper for dispensing.

Clinical Pharmacology: Dapiprazole acts through blocking the alpha-adrenergic receptors in smooth muscle. Dapiprazole produces miosis through an effect on the dilator muscle of the iris.

Dapiprazole does not have any significant activity on ciliary muscle contraction and, therefore does not induce a significant change in the anterior chamber depth or the thickness of the lens.

Dapiprazole has demonstrated safe and rapid reversal of mydriasis produced by phenylephrine and to a lesser degree tropicamide. In patients with decreased accommodative amplitude due to treatment with tropicamide the miotic effect of dapiprazole may partially increase the accommodative amplitude.
Eye color affects the rate of pupillary constriction. In individuals with brown irides, the rate of pupillary constriction may be slightly slower than in individuals with blue or green irides. Eye color does not appear to affect the final pupil size.
Dapiprazole does not significantly alter intraocular pressure in normotensive or in eyes with elevated intraocular pressure.
Indications and Usage: Dapiprazole is indicated in the treatment of iatrogenically induced mydriasis produced by adrenergic (phenylephrine) or parasympatholytic (tropicamide) agents. Dapiprazole is not indicated for the reduction of intraocular pressure or in the treatment of open angle glaucoma.
Contraindications: Miotics are contraindicated where constriction is undesirable; such as acute iritis, and in those subjects showing hypersensitivity to any component of this preparation.
Warning: For Topical Ophthalmic Use Only. NOT FOR INJECTION. Do not touch the dropper up to lids or any surface, as this may contaminate the solution. Dapiprazole should not be used in the same patient more frequently than once a week.
Precautions:
Information to Patients: Miosis may cause difficulty in dark adaptation and may reduce the field of vision. Patients should exercise caution when involved in night driving or other activities in poor illumination.
Carcinogenesis, Mutagenesis, Impairment of Fertility: Dapiprazole has been shown to significantly increase the incidence of liver tumors in rats after continuous dietary administration for 104 weeks. This effect was found only in male rats treated with the highest dose administered in the study, i.e., 300 mg/kg/day, (80,000 times the human dose) and was not observed in male and female rats at doses of 30 and 100 mg/kg/day and female rats at doses of 300 mg/kg/day.
Negative results have been reported on the mutagenicity and impairment of fertility studies with dapiprazole.
Pregnancy: Pregnancy Category B. Reproduction studies have been performed in rats and rabbits at doses up to 128,000 (rat) and 27,000 (rabbit) times the human ophthalmic dose and revealed no evidence of impaired fertility or harm to the fetus due to dapiprazole. There are, however, no adequate and well-controlled studies in pregnant women. Because animal reproduction studies are not always predictive of human response, this drug should be used during pregnancy only if clearly needed.
Nursing Mothers: It is not known whether this drug is excreted in human milk. Because many drugs are excreted in human milk, caution should be exercised when dapiprazole is administered to a nursing woman.
Pediatric Use: Safety and effectiveness in pediatric patients below the age of 4 have not been established.
Adverse Reactions: In controlled studies the most frequent reaction to dapiprazole was conjunctival injection lasting 20 minutes in over 80% of patients. Burning on instillation of dapiprazole was reported in approximately half of all patients. Reactions occurring in 10% to 40% of patients included ptosis, lid erythema, lid edema, chemosis, itching, punctate keratitis, corneal edema, browache, photophobia and headaches. Other reactions reported less frequently included dryness of eyes, tearing and blurring of vision.
Dosage and Administration: Two drops followed 5 minutes later by an additional 2 drops applied topically to the conjunctiva of each eye should be administered after the ophthalmic examination to reverse the diagnostic mydriasis. Dapiprazole should not be used in the same patient more frequently than once per week.

Directions for Preparing Eyedrops:

1. Use aseptic technique.
2. Tear off aluminum seals, remove and discard rubber plugs from both drug and diluent vials.
3. Pour diluent into drug vial.
4. Remove dropper assembly from its sterile wrapping and attach to the drug vial.
5. Shake container for several minutes to ensure mixing.

How Supplied: RĒV-EYES® Eyedrops, 0.5% (NDC 24208-394-07)
Each package contains RĒV-EYES® (dapiprazole hydrochloride) (25 mg), diluent (5 mL) and dropper for dispensing.
Storage and Stability of Eyedrops: Once the eyedrops have been reconstituted they may be stored at room temperature 15°–30°C (59°–86°F) for 21 days. Discard any solution that is not clear and colorless.
Patented U.S. Patent No. 4,252,721
Rx only

Manufactured by
Abbott Laboratories
North Chicago, IL 60064
For
Angelini Pharmaceuticals Inc.
River Edge, NJ 07661
Marketed by
Bausch & Lomb Pharmaceuticals Inc.
Tampa, FL 33637

Shown in Product Identification Guide, page 104

Bausch & Lomb Surgical
555 WEST ARROW HIGHWAY
CLAREMONT, CA 91711

Direct Inquiries to:
Customer Services (800) 338-2020

CATALYST™ SYSTEM

The Catalyst™ is a totally modular microprocessor based precision instrument intended for surgical use in the human eye for anterior segment surgery. A multifunction programmable footswitch gives precise control of low end power, flow, vacuum and memory switching. A touchscreen graphical user interface facilitates set-up and multimode response for 16 surgeon memories. Remote control and automated diagnostics are also included.
System includes phaco, bipolar vitrectomy, remote control and power IV pole. Optional modules include rotary vane advanced fluidics pumps or a fiberoptic module.
Contact your local representative or BAUSCH & LOMB SURGICAL directly at 1(800) 338-2020. For service call 1 (800) 445-7483.

MILLENNIUM™ MICROSURGICAL SYSTEM

The Millennium™ Microsurgical System is a modular designed unit allowing for expanded ophthalmic surgical capability and integration of future technology. It offers anterior and/or posterior segment functionality with unlimited surgeon programming and software upgrades via a CD-ROM. The Millennium, with CONCENTRIX and venturi modules, is the only dual aspiration pump system for ophthalmic surgery, providing both flow and vacuum-based response. Additional features include Dual Linear control, surgeon-controlled parameter and mode adjustment, voice confirmation. Functions include ultrasound, bipolar, vitrectomy, illumination, air/fluid, automated scissors, viscous fluid module, LIGHTNING high speed vitrectomy cutter, cart with automated IV pole.
Contact your local representative or Bausch & Lomb Surgical at 1-800-338-2020.

OCUCOAT™ ℞
(2% HYDROXYPROPYLMETHYLCELLULOSE)

Description: OCUCOAT is a sterile, isotonic, nonpyrogenic viscoelastic solution of highly purified, noninflammatory, 2% hydroxypropylmethylcellulose with a high molecular weight greater than 80,000 daltons. OCUCOAT is supplied in 1 mL syringes. Each mL provides 20 mg/mL of hydroxypropylmethylcellulose dissolved in a physiological balanced salt solution containing 0.49% sodium chloride, 0.075% potassium chloride, 0.048% calcium chloride, 0.03% magnesium chloride, 0.39% sodium acetate, 0.17% sodium citrate and water for injection. The osmolarity of OCUCOAT is 285 ± 32 mOsM, the viscosity is 4000 ± 1500 cst, and the pH is 7.2±0.4.
Characteristics: OCUCOAT is an ophthalmic surgical aid for use in anterior segment surgery.
OCUCOAT:

1. Is a space occupying, tissue protective substance
2. Exhibits excellent flow properties
3. Is completely transparent
4. Is nonantigenic
5. Is easily removed from the anterior chamber
6. Contains no proteins which may cause inflammation or foreign body reactions
7. Requires no refrigeration or restrictive storage conditions
8. Does not interfere with normal wound healing process
9. Clears the trabecular meshwork in 24 hours (98% clearance rate)

Indications: OCUCOAT is indicated for use as an ophthalmic surgical aid in anterior segment surgical procedures, including cataract extraction and intraocular lens implantation. OCUCOAT maintains a deep chamber during anterior segment surgery and thereby allows for more efficient manipulation with less trauma to the corneal endothelium and other ocular tissues. The viscoelasticity of OCUCOAT helps the vitreous face to be pushed back, thus preventing formation of a postoperative flat chamber.
Contraindications: At present, there are no known contraindications to the use of OCUCOAT when used as recommended.
Precautions: Precautions are limited to those normally associated with the ophthalmic surgical procedure being performed.
There may be transient increased intraocular pressure following surgery because of pre-existing glaucoma or due to the surgery itself. For these reasons, the following precautions should be considered:

- OCUCOAT should be removed from the anterior chamber at the end of surgery.
- If the postoperative intraocular pressure increases above expected values, appropriate therapy should be administered.

Adverse Reactions: Clinical testing of OCUCOAT showed it to be extremely well tolerated after injection into the human eye.

Continued on next page

Ocucoat—Cont.

A transient rise in intraocular pressure postoperatively has been reported in some cases. Rarely, postoperative inflammatory reactions (iritis, hypopyon), as well as incidents of corneal edema and corneal decompensation, have been reported with viscoelastic agents. Their relationship to OCUCOAT has not been established.

Clinical Applications: In anterior segment surgery, OCUCOAT should be carefully introduced into the anterior chamber using a 20 gauge or smaller cannula. OCUCOAT may be injected into the chamber prior to or following delivery of the crystalline lens. Injection of OCUCOAT prior to lens delivery will provide additional protection to the corneal endothelium and other ocular tissues. Injection of the material at this point is significant in that a coating of OCUCOAT may protect the corneal endothelium from possible damage arising from surgical instrumentation during the cataract extraction surgery.

OCUCOAT may also be used to coat an intraocular lens as well as tips of surgical instruments prior to implantation surgery. Additional OCUCOAT may be injected during anterior segment surgery to fully maintain the chamber or to replace fluid lost during the surgical procedure. OCUCOAT should be removed from the anterior chamber at the end of surgery. Rather than aspirate OCUCOAT from the eye with the OCUCOAT syringe, it is recommended that OCUCOAT be aspirated using an automated I/A device, or irrigated using an irrigation syringe or a BSS squeeze bottle.

How Supplied: OCUCOAT is a sterile, nonpyrogenic, viscoelastic preparation supplied in a 1 mL single use glass syringe with a Luer tip and a Luer lock cannula. OCUCOAT syringes are aseptically packaged and terminally sterilized. The sterility expiration date is on the outer package.

Store at room temperature; avoid excessive heat (60° C). Protect from light. For intraocular use.

Warning: Manufactured with CFC-12, a substance which harms public health and environment by destroying ozone in the upper atmosphere.

Caution: Federal (USA) law restricts this device to sale by or on the order of a physician. For intraocular use only. Discard unused contents of OCUCOAT syringe after each use. Do not resterilize.

Contact your local representative or Bausch & Lomb Surgical directly at 1 (800) 338-2020 or (909) 624-2020.

Refer to Section 4
for information on
Contact Lenses.

CIBA Vision®
A Novartis Company

11460 JOHNS CREEK PARKWAY
DULUTH, GA 30097-1556

Customer Service (800) 845-6585
FAX (770) 418-4000
www.cibavision.com

ATROPISOL® (atropine sulfate) 1% ℞
Sterile Ophthalmic Solution
How Supplied: 5mL and DROPPERETTE® (12×1mL)

BETIMOL® ℞
(timolol ophthalmic solution) 0.25%, 0.5%
How Supplied: 2.5, 5, 10, and 15mL

CARBASTAT® ℞
(Carbachol Intraocular Solution, USP) 0.01%
How Supplied: 12×1.5mL

DACRIOSE® OTC
Sterile Eye Irrigating Solution
How Supplied: 15mL, 120mL

DEXACIDIN® ℞
(Neomycin and Polymyxin B Sulfates and Dexamethasone, USP)
Sterile Ophthalmic Suspension
How Supplied: 5mL

DEXACINE™ ℞
(Neomycin and Polymyxin B Sulfates and Dexamethasone)
Ophthalmic Ointment
How Supplied: 1/8 oz

EFLONE™ ℞
Fluorometholone Acetate
Sterile Ophthalmic Suspension
How Supplied: 5mL, 10mL

EYE•SCRUB™ OTC
Hypoallergenic Sterile Eyelid Cleanser
How Supplied: Kits (4 fl. oz + 60 pads) and boxes of 30 premoistened pads

FLUOR-OP® (Fluorometholone ℞
Sterile Ophthalmic Suspension, USP) 0.1%
How Supplied: 3, 5, 10, and 15mL

GENTACIDIN® (gentamicin sulfate ℞
sterile ophthalmic solution, USP)
How Supplied: 5mL

GENTAMICIN SULFATE ℞
Ophthalmic Ointment, USP
How Supplied: 3.5g

GENTEAL™ OTC
Lubricant Eye Drops
How Supplied: 15mL, 25mL

GENTEAL™ OTC
Lubricant Eye Gel
How Supplied: 10 mL

GONIOSOL®
(hydroxypropyl methylcellulose) 2.5% Diagnostic
Sterile Ophthalmic Solution
How Supplied: 15mL

HOMATROPINE HYDROBROMIDE ℞
Sterile Ophthalmic Solution, USP 5%
How Supplied: 5mL and DROPPERETTE® (12×1mL)

HYPOTEARS® OTC
Sterile Lubricant Eye Drops
How Supplied: 15mL, 30mL

HYPOTEARS® PF OTC
Lubricant Eye Drops (Preservative Free)
How Supplied: 30 Single-Use Containers (0.02 fl. oz. each)

HYPOTEARS® Ointment OTC
Sterile Eye Lubricant
Preservative Free and Lanolin Free
How Supplied: 3.5g

INFLAMASE® MILD 1/8% ℞
(prednisolone sodium phosphate)
Sterile Ophthalmic Solution
How Supplied: 5mL, 10mL

INFLAMASE® FORTE 1% ℞
(prednisolone sodium phosphate)
Sterile Ophthalmic Solution
How Supplied: 3, 5, 10, and 15mL

IOCARE® Balanced Salt Solution ℞
Sterile Ophthalmic Solution
How Supplied: 15mL

LIVOSTIN™ 0.05% (levocabastine HCl ℞
ophthalmic suspension)
How Supplied: 2.5, 5, and 10mL

MIOCHOL®-E (acetylcholine chloride ℞
intraocular solution) 1:100 with electrolyte diluent
CIBA VISION® Steri-Tags™
How Supplied: 2mL univial,

MIOCHOL®-E System Pak™ ℞
Miochol-E (acetylcholine chloride intraocular solution) 1:100 with electrolyte diluent 2mL univial
CIBA VISION® Steri-Tags™, 3mL B-D® Syringe
0.2 Micron DynaGard™ Filter

OCUPRESS® (carteolol HCl) ℞
Ophthalmic Solution 1% Sterile
How Supplied: 5, 10, and 15 mL

PILOCAR® (pilocarpine HCl) 1/2% ℞
Sterile Ophthalmic Solution
How Supplied: 15mL and Twin Pack (2×15mL)

PILOCAR® (pilocarpine HCl) 1% ℞
Sterile Ophthalmic Solution
How Supplied: 15mL, Twin Pack (2×15mL), DROPPERETTE® (12×1mL)

PILOCAR® (pilocarpine HCl) 2% ℞
Sterile Ophthalmic Solution
How Supplied: 15mL, Twin Pack (2×15mL), DROPPERETTE® (12×1mL)

PILOCAR® (pilocarpine HCl) 3% ℞
Sterile Ophthalmic Solution
How Supplied: 15mL, Twin Pack (2×15mL)

PILOCAR® (pilocarpine HCl) 4% ℞
Sterile Ophthalmic Solution
How Supplied: 15mL, Twin Pack (2×15mL), DROPPERETTE® (12×1mL)

PILOCAR® (pilocarpine HCl) 6% ℞
Sterile Ophthalmic Solution
How Supplied: 15mL, Twin Pack (2×15mL)

TEARISOL® OTC
Sterile Lubricant Eye Drops
How Supplied: 15mL

VASOCIDIN® ℞
(sulfacetamide sodium and prednisolone sodium phosphate sterile
ophthalmic solution, USP) 10%/0.25%
How Supplied: 5mL, 10mL

VASOCINE™ ℞
(sulfacetamide sodium and prednisolone acetate)
Ophthalmic Ointment, USP
How Supplied: 3.5g

VASOCLEAR® OTC
Sterile Lubricant/Redness Reliever Eye Drop
How Supplied: 15mL

VASOCLEAR® A OTC
Sterile Astringent/Lubricant/Redness Reliever Eye Drops
How Supplied: 15mL

VASOCON®-A OTC
Itching/Redness Reliever Eye Drops
(naphazoline HCl 0.05%-antazoline phosphate 0.5%)
Sterile Ophthalmic Solution
How Supplied: 15mL

VASOCON®-Regular ℞
(naphazoline HCl 0.1%
Sterile Ophthalmic Solution, USP)
How Supplied: 15mL

VASOSULF® ℞
(sulfacetamide sodium 15%-phenylephrine hydrochloride 0.125%)
Sterile Ophthalmic Solution
How Supplied: 5mL, 15mL

VITRAVENE™ (formivirsen sodium intravitreal injectable) ℞
How Supplied: 0.25 mL, 6.6 mg/mL

VOLTAREN OPHTHALMIC® ℞
(diclofenac sodium 0.1%)
Sterile Ophthalmic Solution
How Supplied: 2.5mL, 5mL

DROPPERETTES® Applicator—
Sterile Package

ATROPISOL® 1% (atropine sulfate) ℞
Sterile Ophthalmic Solution
How Supplied: 12×1mL DROPPERETTE®

Fluorescein Sodium 2% ℞
Sterile Ophthalmic Solution
How Supplied: 12×1mL DROPPERETTE®

Homatropine HBr ℞
Sterile Ophthalmic Solution, USP 5%
How Supplied: 12×1mL DROPPERETTE®

Phenylephrine HCl 10% (Rfg.) ℞
Sterile Ophthalmic Solution
How Supplied: 12×1mL DROPPERETTE®

PILOCAR® 1% (pilocarpine HCl) ℞
Sterile Ophthalmic Solution
How Supplied: 12×1mL DROPPERETTE®

PILOCAR® 2% (pilocarpine HCl) ℞
Sterile Ophthalmic Solution
How Supplied: 12×1mL DROPPERETTE®

PILOCAR® 4% (pilocarpine HCl) ℞
Sterile Ophthalmic Solution
How Supplied: 12×1mL DROPPERETTE®

SULF-10® (sodium sulfacetamide sterile ophthalmic solution, USP) ℞
How Supplied: 12×1mL DROPPERETTE®

Tetracaine HCl 1/2% ℞
Sterile Ophthalmic Solution
How Supplied: 12×1mL DROPPERETTE®

BETIMOL® ℞

[bət-ĭ-mŏl ″]

(timolol ophthalmic solution) 0.25%, 0.5%

Description: Betimol® (timolol ophthalmic solution), 0.25% and 0.5%, is a non-selective beta-adrenergic antagonist for ophthalmic use. The chemical name of the active ingredient is (S)-1-[(1,1-dimethylethyl)amino]-3-[[4-(4-morpholinyl)-1,2,5-thiadiazol-3-yl]oxy]-2-propanol. Timolol hemihydrate is the levo isomer. Specific rotation is $[\alpha]^{25}_{405nm}$=-16° (C=10% as the hemihydrate form in 1N HCl).
The molecular formula of timolol is $C_{13}H_{24}N_4O_3S$ and its structural formula is:

Timolol (as the hemihydrate) is a white, odorless, crystalline powder which is slightly soluble in water and freely soluble in ethanol. Timolol hemihydrate is stable at room temperature.
Betimol is a clear, colorless, isotonic sterile, microbiologically preserved phosphate buffered aqueous solution. It is supplied in two dosage strengths, 0.25% and 0.5%.
Each mL of Betimol 0.25% contains 2.56 mg of timolol hemihydrate equivalent to 2.5 mg timolol.
Each mL of Betimol 0.5% contains 5.12 mg of timolol hemihydrate equivalent to 5.0 mg timolol.
Inactive ingredients: monosodium and disodium phosphate dihydrate to adjust pH (6.5–7.5) and water for injection, benzalkonium chloride 0.01% added as preservative.
The osmolality of Betimol® is 260 to 320 m0smol/kg.

Clinical Pharmacology: Timolol is a non-selective beta-adrenergic antagonist. It blocks both beta 1- and beta 2- adrenergic receptors. Timolol does not have significant intrinsic sympathomimetic activity, local anesthetic (membrane-stabilizing) or direct myocardial depressant activity.
Timolol, when applied topically in the eye, reduces normal and elevated intraocular pressure (IOP) whether or not accompanied by glaucoma. Elevated intraocular pressure is a major risk factor in the pathogenesis of glaucomatous visual field loss. The higher the level of IOP, the greater the likelihood of glaucomatous visual field loss and optic nerve damage.
The predominant mechanism of ocular hypotensive action of topical beta-adrenergic blocking agents is likely due to a reduction in aqueous humor production.
In general, beta-adrenergic blocking agents reduce cardiac output both in healthy subjects and patients with heart diseases. In patients with severe impairment of myocardial function, beta-adrenergic receptor blocking agents may inhibit sympathetic stimulatory effect necessary to maintain adequate cardiac function. In the bronchi and bronchioles, beta-adrenergic receptor blockade may also increase airway resistance because of unopposed parasympathetic activity.

Pharmacokinetics
When given orally, timolol is well absorbed and undergoes considerable first pass metabolism. Timolol and its metabolites are primarily excreted in the urine. The half-life of timolol in plasma is approximately 4 hours.

Clinical Studies
In two controlled multicenter studies in the U.S., Betimol 0.25% and 0.5% were compared with respective timolol maleate eyedrops. In these studies, the efficacy and safety profile of Betimol was similar to that of timolol maleate.

Indications And Usage: Betimol is indicated in the treatment of elevated intraocular pressure in patients with ocular hypertension or open-angle glaucoma.

Contraindications: Betimol is contraindicated in patients with overt heart failure, cardiogenic shock, sinus bradycardia, second- or third-degree atrioventricular block, bronchial asthma or history of bronchial asthma, or severe chronic obstructive pulmonary disease, or hypersensitivity to any component of this product.

Warnings: As with other topically applied ophthalmic drugs, Betimol is absorbed systemically. The same adverse reactions found with systemic administration of beta-adrenergic blocking agents may occur with topical administration. For example, severe respiratory and cardiac reactions, including death due to bronchospasm in patients with asthma, and rarely, death in association with cardiac failure have been reported following systemic or topical administration of beta-adrenergic blocking agents.
Cardiac Failure: Sympathetic stimulation may be essential for support of the circulation in individuals with diminished myocardial contractility, and its inhibition by beta-adrenergic receptor blockade may precipitate more severe cardiac failure.
In patients without a history of cardiac failure, continued depression of the myocardium with beta-blocking agents over a period of time can, in some cases, lead to cardiac failure. Betimol should be discontinued at the first sign or symptom of cardiac failure.
Obstructive Pulmonary Disease: Patients with chronic obstructive pulmonary disease (e.g. chronic bronchitis, emphysema) of mild or moderate severity, bronchospastic disease, or a history of bronchospastic disease (other than bronchial asthma or a history of bronchial asthma which are contraindications) should in general not receive beta-blocking agents.
Major Surgery: The necessity or desirability of withdrawal of beta-adrenergic blocking agents prior to a major surgery is controversial. Beta-adrenergic receptor blockade impairs the ability of the heart to respond to beta-adrenergically mediated reflex stimuli. This may augment the risk of general anesthesia in surgical procedures. Some patients receiving beta-adrenergic receptor blocking agents have been subject to protracted severe hypotension during anesthesia. Difficulty in restarting and maintaining the heartbeat has also been reported. For these reasons, in patients undergoing elective surgery, gradual withdrawal of beta-adrenergic receptor blocking agents is recommended. If necessary during surgery, the effects of beta-adrenergic blocking agents may be reversed by sufficient doses of beta-adrenergic agonists.
Diabetes Mellitus: Beta-adrenergic blocking agents should be administered with caution in patients subject to spontaneous hypoglycemia or to diabetic patients (especially those with labile diabetes) who are receiving insulin or oral hypoglycemic agents. Beta-adrenergic receptor blocking agents may mask the signs and symptoms of acute hypoglycemia.
Thyrotoxicosis: Beta-adrenergic blocking agents may mask certain clinical signs (e.g. tachycardia) of hyperthyroidism. Patients suspected of developing thyrotoxicosis should be managed carefully to avoid abrupt withdrawal of beta-adrenergic blocking agents which might precipitate a thyroid storm.

Precautions: ***General*** Because of the potential effects of beta-adrenergic blocking agents relative to blood pressure and pulse, these agents should be used with caution in patients with cerebrovascular insufficiency. If signs or symptoms suggesting reduced cerebral blood flow develop following initiation of therapy with Betimol, alternative therapy should be considered.
There have been reports of bacterial keratitis associated with the use of multiple dose containers of topical ophthalmic products. These containers had been inadvertently contaminated by patients who, in most cases, had a concurrent corneal disease or a disruption of the ocular epithelial surface. (See PRECAUTIONS, Information for Patients.)
Muscle Weakness: Beta-adrenergic blockade has been reported to potentiate muscle weakness consistent with certain myasthenic symptoms (e.g. diplopia, ptosis, and generalized weakness). Beta-adrenergic blocking agents have been reported rarely to increase muscle weakness in some patients with myasthenia gravis or myasthenic symptoms.
In angle-closure glaucoma, the goal of the treatment is to reopen the angle. This requires constricting the pupil. Betimol has no effect on the pupil. Therefore, if timolol is used in angle-closure glaucoma, it should always be combined with a miotic and not used alone.
Anaphylaxis: While taking beta-blockers, patients with a history of atopy or a history of severe anaphylactic reactions to a variety of allergens may be more reactive to repeated accidental, diagnostic, or therapeutic challenge with such allergens. Such patients may be unresponsive to the usual doses of epinephrine used to treat anaphylactic reactions.

Continued on next page

Betimol—Cont.

The preservative benzalkonium chloride may be absorbed by soft contact lenses. Patients who wear soft contact lenses should wait 5 minutes after instilling Betimol before they insert their lenses.

Information for Patients

Patients should be instructed to avoid allowing the tip of the dispensing container to contact the eye or surrounding structures.

Patients should also be instructed that ocular solutions can become contaminated by common bacteria known to cause ocular infections. Serious damage to the eye and subsequent loss of vision may result from using contaminated solutions. (See PRECAUTIONS, General.)

Patients requiring concomitant topical ophthalmic medications should be instructed to administer these at least 5 minutes apart.

Patients with bronchial asthma, a history of bronchial asthma, severe chronic obstructive pulmonary disease, sinus bradycardia, second- or third-degree atrioventricular block, or cardiac failure should be advised not to take this product (See CONTRAINDICATIONS.)

Drug Interactions

Beta-adrenergic blocking agents: Patients who are receiving a beta-adrenergic blocking agent orally and Betimol should be observed for a potential additive effect either on the intraocular pressure or on the known systemic effects of beta-blockade.

Patients should not usually receive two topical ophthalmic beta-adrenergic blocking agents concurrently.

Catecholamine-depleting drugs: Close observation of the patient is recommended when a beta-blocker is administered to patients receiving catecholamine-depleting drugs such as reserpine, because of possible additive effects and the production of hypotension and/or marked bradycardia, which may produce vertigo, syncope, or postural hypotension.

Calcium antagonists: Caution should be used in the co-administration of beta-adrenergic blocking agents and oral or intravenous calcium antagonists, because of possible atrioventricular conduction disturbances, left ventricular failure, and hypotension. In patients with impaired cardiac function, co-administration should be avoided.

Digitalis and calcium antagonists: The concomitant use of beta-adrenergic blocking agents with digitalis and calcium antagonists may have additive effects in prolonging atrioventricular conduction time.

Injectable Epinephrine: (See PRECAUTIONS, General, Anaphylaxis.)

Carcinogenesis, Mutagenesis, Impairment of Fertility

Carcinogenicity of timolol (as the maleate) has been studied in mice and rats. In a two-year study orally administrated timolol maleate (300mg/kg/day) (approximately 42,000 times the systemic exposure following the maximum recommended human ophthalmic dose) in male rats caused a significant increase in the incidence of adrenal pheochromocytomas; the lower doses, 25 mg or 100 mg/kg daily did not cause any changes.

In a life span study in mice the overall incidence of neoplasms was significantly increased in female mice at 500 mg/kg/day (approximately 71,000 times the systemic exposure following the maximum recommended human ophthalmic dose). Furthermore, significant increases were observed in the incidences of benign and malignant pulmonary tumors, benign uterine polyps, as well as mammary adenocarcinomas. These changes were not seen at the daily dose level of 5 or 50 mg/kg (approximately 700 or 7,000, respectively, times the systemic exposure following the maximum recommended human ophthalmic dose). For comparison, the maximum recommended human oral dose of timolol maleate is 1 mg/kg/day.

Mutagenic potential of timolol was evaluated *in vivo* in the micronucleus test and cytogenetic assay and *in vitro* in the neoplastic cell transformation assay and Ames test. In the bacterial mutagenicity test (Ames test) high concentrations of timolol maleate (5000 and 10,000 g/plate) statistically significantly increased the number of revertants in Salmonella typhimurium TA100, but not in the other three strains tested. However, no consistent dose-response was observed nor did the number of revertants reach the double of the control value, which is regarded as one of the criteria for a positive result in the Ames test. *In vivo* genotoxicity tests (the mouse micronucleus test and cytogenetic assay) and *in vitro* the neoplastic cell transformation assay were negative up to dose levels of 800 mg/kg and 100 g/mL, respectively.

No adverse effects on male and female fertility were reported in rats at timolol oral doses of up to 150 mg/kg/day (21,000 times the systemic exposure following the maximum recommended human ophthalmic dose).

Pregnancy Teratogenic Effects

Category C: Teratogenicity of timolol (as the maleate) after oral administration was studied in mice and rabbits. No fetal malformations were reported in mice or rabbits at a daily oral dose of 50 mg/kg (7,000 times the systemic exposure following the maximum recommended human ophthalmic dose). Although delayed fetal ossification was observed at this dose in rats, there were no adverse effects on postnatal development of offspring. Doses of 1000 mg/kg/day (142,000 times the systemic exposure following the maximum recommended human ophthalmic dose) were maternotoxic in mice and resulted in an increased number of fetal resorptions. Increased fetal resorptions were also seen in rabbits at doses of 14,000 times the systemic exposure following the maximum recommended human ophthalmic dose in this case without apparent maternotoxicity.

There are no adequate and well-controlled studies in pregnant women. Betimol should be used during pregnancy only if the potential benefit justifies the potential risk to the fetus.

Nursing Mothers

Because of the potential for serious adverse reactions in nursing infants from timolol, a decision should be made whether to discontinue the drug, taking into account the importance of the drug to the mother.

Pediatric Use

Safety and efficacy in pediatric patients have not been established.

Adverse Reactions: The most frequently reported ocular event in clinical trials was burning/stinging on instillation and was comparable between Betimol and timolol maleate (approximately one in eight patients).

The following adverse events were associated with the use of Betimol in frequencies of more than 5% in two controlled, double-masked clinical studies in which 184 patients received 0.25% or 0.5% Betimol:

Ocular Dry eyes, itching, foreign body sensation, discomfort in the eye, eyelid erythema, conjunctival infection, and headache.

Body as a Whole Headache.

The following side effects were reported in frequencies of 1 to 5%:

Ocular Eye pain, epiphora, photophobia, blurred or abnormal vision, corneal fluorescein staining, keratitis, blepharitis and cataract.

Body as a Whole Allergic reaction, asthenia, common cold and pain in extremities.

Cardiovascular Hypertension.

Digestive Nausea.

Metabolic/Nutritional Peripheral edema.

Nervous System/Psychiatry Dizziness and dry mouth.

Respiratory Respiratory infections and sinusitis.

In addition, the following adverse reactions have been reported with ophthalmic use of beta blockers:

Ocular Conjunctivitis, blepharoptosis, decreased corneal sensitivity, visual disturbances including refractive changes, diplopia and retinal vascular disorder.

Body as a Whole Chest pain.

Cardiovascular Arrhythmia, palpitation, bradycardia, hypotension, syncope, heart block, cerebral vascular accident, cerebral ischemia, cardiac failure and cardiac arrest.

Digestive Diarrhea.

Endocrine Masked symptoms of hypoglycemia in insulin dependent diabetics (See WARNINGS).

Nervous System/Psychiatry Depression, impotence, increase in signs and symptoms of myasthenia gravis and paresthesia.

Respiratory Dyspnea, bronchospasm, respiratory failure and nasal congestion.

Skin Alopecia, hypersensitivity including localized and generalized rash, urticaria.

Overdosage: No information is available on overdosage with Betimol. Symptoms that might be expected with an overdose of a beta-adrenergic receptor blocking agent are bronchospasm, hypotension, bradycardia, and acute cardiac failure.

Dosage And Administration: Betimol is available in concentrations of 0.25% and 0.5%. The starting dose is one drop of Betimol, 0.25% or 0.5%, twice daily in the affected eyes(s).

Because in some patients the pressure-lowering response to timolol may require a few weeks to stabilize, evaluation should include a determination of intraocular pressure after approximately 4 weeks of treatment with Betimol.

Dosages higher than one drop of Betimol 0.5% twice a day have not been studied. If the patient's intraocular pressure is still not at a satisfactory level on this regimen, concomitant therapy can be considered.

How Supplied: Betimol (timolol ophthalmic solution) is a clear, colorless solution.

Betimol 0.25% is supplied in a white, opaque, plastic, ophthalmic dispenser bottle with a controlled drop tip as follows:

NDC 58768-898-99 2.5mL
NDC 58768-898-05 5.0mL
NDC 58768-898-10 10mL
NDC 58768-898-15 15mL

Betimol 0.5% is supplied in a white, opaque, plastic, ophthalmic dispenser bottle with a controlled drop tip as follows:

NDC 58768-899-99 2.5mL
NDC 58768-899-05 5.0mL
NDC 58768-899-10 10mL
NDC 58768-899-15 15mL

STORAGE: Store between 15–30°C (59–86°F). Do not freeze. Protect from light.

MADE IN FINLAND
MANUFACTURED BY:
Santen Oy, P.O. Box 33
Fin-33721 Tampere, Finland
CIBA Vision®
A Novartis Company
U.S. Ophthalmics
Atlanta, Georgia 30097
Revised: September 1997 5036-B

Shown in Product Identification Guide, page 105

CARBASTAT® ℞
(CARBACHOL INTRAOCULAR SOLUTION, USP) 0.01%

Description: CARBASTAT® (Carbachol Intraocular Solution, USP) 0.01% is a sterile balanced salt solution of carbachol for intraocular injection. The active ingredient is represented by the structural formula:

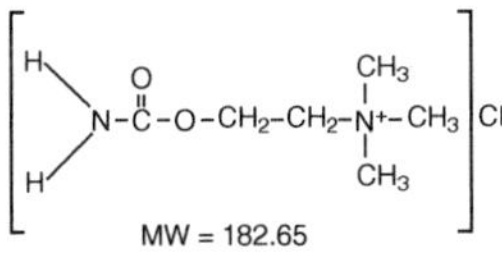

MW = 182.65

Established name: Carbachol
Chemical name: Ethanaminium, 2-[(aminocarbonyl)oxy]-*N,N,N* -trimethyl-, chloride.
Each mL contains: Active: Carbachol 0.01%. Inactive: Sodium chloride 0.64%, potassium chloride 0.075%, calcium chloride dihydrate 0.048%, magnesium chloride hexahydrate 0.03%, sodium acetate trihydrate 0.39%, sodium citrate dihydrate 0.17%, sodium hydroxide and/or hydrochloric acid to adjust pH (5.0–7.5) and water for injection USP.

Clinical Pharmacology: Carbahol is a potent cholinergic (parasympathomimetic) agent which produces constriction of the iris and ciliary body resulting in reduction in intraocular pressure. The exact mechanism by which carbachol lowers intraocular pressure is not precisely known.

Indications and Usage: Intraocular use for obtaining miosis during surgery. In addition, Carbastat® (Carbachol Intraocular Solution USP) reduces the intensity of intraocular pressure elevation in the first 24 hours after cataract surgery.

Contraindications: Should not be used in those persons showing hypersensitivity to any of the components of this preparation.

Warnings: For single-dose intraocular use only. Discard unused portion. Intraocular carbachol 0.01% should be used with caution in patients with acute cardiac failure, bronchial asthma, peptic ulcer, hyperthyroidism, G.I. spasm, urinary tract obstruction and Parkinson's disease.

Precautions: Carcinogenesis: Studies in animals to evaluate the carcinogenic potential have not been conducted.

Pregnancy: Category C. There are no adequate and well controlled studies in pregnant women. Carbastat® should be used during pregnancy only if the potential benefit justifies the potential risk to the fetus.

Nursing Mothers: It is not known if this medication is excreted in breast milk. Exercise caution when administering to a nursing woman.

Pediatric Use: Safety and efficacy in pediatric patients have not been established.

Adverse Reactions: Ocular: Corneal clouding, persistent bullous keratopathy, retinal detachment and postoperative iritis following cataract extraction have been reported.

Systemic: Side effects such as flushing, sweating, epigastric distress, abdominal cramps, tightness in urinary bladder, and headache have been reported with topical or systemic application of carbachol.

Dosage and Administration: Aseptically remove the sterile vial from the blister package by peeling the backing paper and dropping the vial onto a sterile tray. Withdraw the contents into a dry sterile syringe, and replace the needle with an atraumatic cannula prior to intraocular irrigation. No more than one-half milliliter should be gently instilled into the anterior chamber for the production of satisfactory miosis. It may be instilled before or after securing sutures. Miosis is usually maximal within two to five minutes after application.

How Supplied: CARBASTAT (Carbachol Intraocular Solution, USP) 0.01%:
1.5 mL sterile glass vials in cartons of 12 (12 × 1.5 mL)
NDC 58768-735-12

Store at controlled room temperature 15°–30°C (59°–86°F).

CAUTION: Federal law prohibits dispensing without prescription.

Manufactured by OMJ Pharmaceuticals, Inc., San Germán, P.R. 00683

5007-C
Revised: June, 1997

DEXACINE™ ℞

[deks 'a 'cīne]
(Neomycin and Polymyxin B Sulfates and Dexamethasone)
Ophthalmic Ointment

EFLONE™ ℞

[əff-flone]
(fluorometholone acetate)
Sterile Ophthalmic Suspension

Description: EFLONE™ (fluorometholone acetate) is a corticosteroid prepared as a sterile topical ophthalmic suspension. The active ingredient, fluorometholone acetate, is a white to creamy white powder with an empirical formula of $C_{24}H_{31}FO_5$ and a molecular weight of 418.5. Its chemical name is 9-fluoro-11β, 17-dihydrozy-6α -methylpregna-1, 4-diene-3, 20-dione 17-acetate. The chemical structure of Fluorometholone Acetate is presented below:

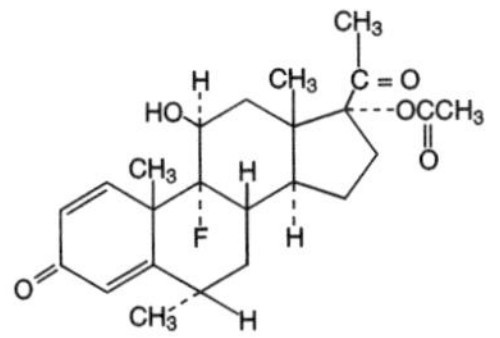

Each mL contains: Active: fluorometholone acetate 1 mg (0.1%). **Preservative:** benzalkonium chloride 0.01%. **Inactive:** sodium chloride, monobasic sodium phosphate, edetate disodium, hydroxyethyl cellulose, tyloxapol, hydrochloric acid and/or sodium hydroxide (to adjust pH), and purified water. DM-00

Clinical Pharmacology: Corticosteroids suppress the inflammatory response to inciting agents of mechanical, chemical or immunological nature. No generally accepted explanation of this steroid property has been advanced. Clinical studies demonstrate that Fluorometholone Acetate is significantly more efficacious than Fluorometholone for the treatment of external ocular inflammation.[1] Corticostgeroids cause a rise in intraocular pressure in susceptible individuals. In a small study, EFLONE Ophthalmic Suspension demonstrated a significantly longer average time to produce a rise in intraocular pressure than did dexamethasone phosphate; however, the ultimate magnitude of the rise was equivalent for both drugs and in a small percentage of individuals a significant rise in intraocular pressure occurred within three days.[2]

Indications and Usage: EFLONE Ophthalmic Suspension is indicated for use in the treatment of steroid responsive inflammatory conditions of the palpebral and bulbar conjunctiva, cornea, and anterior segment of the eye.

Contraindications: Contraindicated in acute superficial herpes simplex keratitis, vaccinia, varicella, and most other viral diseases of cornea and conjunctiva; tuberculosis; fungal diseases; acute purulent untreated infections which, like other diseases caused by microorganisms, may be masked or enhanced by the presence of the steroid; and in those persons who have known hypersensitivity to any component of this preparation.

Warnings: Not for injection. Use in the treatment of herpes simplex infection requires great caution. Prolonged use may result in glaucoma, damage to the optic nerve, defect in visual acuity and visual field, cataract formation and/or may aid in the establishment of secondary ocular infections from pathogens due to suppression of host response. Acute purulent infections of the eye may be masked or exacerbated by presence of steroid medication. In those diseases causing thinning of the cornea or sclera, perforation has been known to occur with chronic use of topical steroids. It is advisable that the intraocular pressure be checked frequently.

Precautions:

General: Fungal infections of the cornea are particularly prone to develop coincidentally with long-term local steroid application. Fungus invasion must be considered in any persistent corneal ulceration where a steriod has been used or is in use.

Information for Patients: Do not touch dropper tip to any surface, as this may contaminate the suspension.

Carcinogenesis, mutagenesis, impairment of fertility: No studies have been conducted in animals or in humans to evaluate the possibility of these effects with fluorometholone.

Pregnancy: Pregnancy Category C. Fluorometholone has been shown to be embryocidal and teratogenic in rabbits when administered at low multiples of the human ocular dose. Fluorometholone was applied ocularly to rabbits daily on days 6–18 of gestation, and dose-related fetal loss and fetal abnormalities including cleft palate, deformed rib cage, anomalous limbs and neural abnormalities such as encephalocele, craniorachischisis, and spina bifida were observed. There are no adequate and well controlled studies of fluorometholone in pregnant women, and it is not known whether fluorometholone can cause fetal harm when administered to a pregnant woman. Fluorometholone should be used during pregnancy only if the potential benefit justifies the potential risk to the fetus.

Nursing Mothers: It is not known whether topical administration of corticosteroids could result in sufficient systemic absorption to produce detectable quantities in human milk. Systemically-administered corticosteroids appear in human milk and could suppress growth, interfere with endogenous corticosteroid production, or cause other untoward effects. Because of the potential for serious adverse reactions in nursing infants from fluorometholone, a decision should be made whether to discontinue nursing or to discontinue the drug.

Pediatric Use: Safety and effectiveness in pediatric patients have not been established.

Adverse Reactions: Glaucoma with optic nerve damage, visual acuity and field defects, cataract formation, secondary ocular infection following suppression of host response, and perforation of the globe may occur.

Dosage and Administration: Shake Well Before Using. One to two drops instilled into the conjunctival sac(s) four times daily. During the initial 24 to 48 hours the dosage may be safely increased to two drops every two hours. If no improvement after two weeks, consult physician. Care should be taken not to discontinue therapy prematurely.

How Supplied: 5mL and 10 mL in plastic dispensers.
5 mL: **NDC** 58768-107-05
10 mL: **NDC** 58768-107-10

Storage: Store upright between 2°–27°C (36°–80°F). Protect From Freezing.

Continued on next page

Eflone—Cont.

If tamper resistant seal on the bottle is broken or missing do not use.

References:

1. Leibowitz, H. M., et. al., Annals of Ophthalmology 1984; 16:1110.
2. Stewart, R. H., et. al., Current Eye Research 1984; 3:835.

Mfd.
by: Alcon Laboratories, Inc.
Fort Worth, TX 76134
Revised: January 1995
CS-700007
341165

EYE•SCRUB™ OTC

Non-irritating, hypoallergenic sterile eyelid cleanser
Lid Cleanser For Daily Eyelid Hygiene

Cleanser Ingredients: Purified Water USP, PEG-200 Glyceryl Tallowate, Disodium Laureth Sulfosuccinate, Cocamidopropylamine Oxide, PEG-78 Glyceryl Cocoate, Benzyl Alcohol and Edetate Disodium.

Ready to use, needs no diluting. For External Use Only. Do Not Use Directly In The Eye.

Manufactured for:
Ciba Vision Ophthalmics®
Atlanta, GA 30155
EYE•SCRUB™ is a trademark of CIBA Vision Ophthalmics Inc. Patented Formula

FLUOR-OP® ℞

(FLUOROMETHOLONE OPHTHALMIC SUSPENSION, USP) 0.1%

Description: FLUOR-OP (fluorometholone ophthalmic suspension, USP) 0.1%, is a topical anti-inflammatory agent for ophthalmic use.

Chemical Name: 9-fluoro-11β,17-dihydroxy-6α-methylpregna-1,4-diene-3,20-dione.

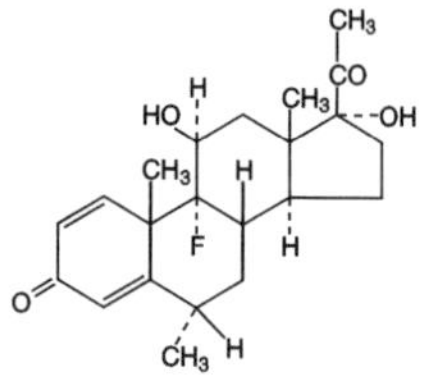

Contains:
Fluorometholone 0.1%
with: polyvinyl alcohol, 1.4%; benzalkonium chloride 0.004%, edetate disodium; sodium chloride; sodium phosphate monobasic, monohydrate; sodium phosphate dibasic, anhydrous; polysorbate 80; sodium hydroxide to adjust the pH and purified water.

Clinical Pharmacology: Corticosteroids inhibit the inflammatory response to a variety of inciting agents and probably delay or slow healing. They inhibit the edema, fibrin deposition, capillary dilation, leukocyte migration, capillary proliferation, fibroblast proliferation, deposition of collagen and scar formation associated with inflammation.

There is no generally accepted explanation for the mechanism of action of ocular corticosteroids. However, corticosteroids are thought to act by the induction of phospholipase A_2 inhibitory proteins, collectively called lipocortins. It is postulated that these proteins control the biosynthesis of potent mediators of inflammation such as prostaglandins and leukotrienes by inhibiting the release of their common precursor, arachidonic acid. Arachidonic and is released from membrane phospholipids by phospholipase A_2.

Corticosteroids are capable of producing a rise in intraocular pressure. In clinical studies on patients' eyes treated with both dexamethasone and fluorometholone 0.1% suspensions, fluorometholone demonstrated a lower propensity to increase intraocular pressure than did dexamethasone.

Indications and Usage: FLUOR-OP is indicated for the treatment of corticosteroid-responsive inflammation of the palpebral and bulbar conjunctiva, cornea and anterior segment of the globe.

Contraindications: FLUOR-OP suspension is contraindicated in most viral diseases of the cornea and conjunctiva, including epithelial herpes simplex keratitis (dendritic keratitis), vaccina, and varicella, and also in mycobacterial infection of the eye and fungal diseases of ocular structures. FLUOR-OP suspension is also contraindicated in individuals with known or suspected hypersensitivity to any of the ingredients of this preparation and to other corticosteroids.

Warnings: Prolonged use of corticosteroids may result in glaucoma with damage to the optic nerve, defects in visual acuity and fields of vision, and in posterior subcapsular cataract formation. Prolonged use may suppress the host immune response and thus increase the hazard of secondary ocular infections.

Various ocular diseases and long-term use of topical corticosteroids have been known to cause corneal and scleral thinning. Use of topical corticosteroids in the presence of thin corneal or scleral tissue may lead to perforation. Acute purulent untreated infections of the eye may be masked or activity enhanced by the presence of corticosteroid medication.

If this product is used for 10 days or longer, intraocular pressure should be routinely monitored even though it may be difficult in children and uncooperative patients. Steroids should be used with caution in the presence of glaucoma. Intraocular pressure should be checked frequently. The use of steroids after cataract surgery may delay healing and increase the incidence of bleb formation.

Use of ocular steroids may prolong the course and may exacerbate the severity of many viral infections of the eye (including herpes simplex). Employment of a corticosteroid medication in the treatment of patients with a history of herpes simplex requires great caution; frequent slit lamp microscopy is recommended.

Corticosteroids are not effective in mustard gas keratitis and Sjögren's keratoconjuntivitis.

Precautions: General: The initial prescription and renewal of the medication order beyond 20 milliliters of FLUOR-OP suspension should be made by a physician only after examination of the patients and with the aid of magnification, such as slit lamp biomicroscopy and, where appropriate, fluorescein staining. If signs and symptoms fail to improve after two days, the patients should be re-evaluated.

As fungal infections of the cornea are particularly prone to develop coincidentally with long-term local corticosteroid applications, fungal invasion should be suspected in any persistent corneal ulceration where a corticosteroid has been used or is in use. Fungal cultures should be taken when appropriate.

If this product is used for 10 days or longer, intraocular pressure should be monitored (see WARNINGS).

Information to the Patients: If inflammation or pain persists longer than 48 hours or becomes aggravated, the patient should be advised to discontinue use of the medication and consult a physician.

This product is sterile when packaged. To prevent contamination, care should be taken to avoid touching the bottle tip to eyelids or to any other surface. The use of this bottle by more than one person may spread infection. Keep bottle tightly closed when not in use. Keep out of reach of children.

Carcinogenesis, mutagenesis, impairment of fertility: No studies have been conducted in animals or in humans to evaluate the possibility of these effects with fluorometholone.

Pregnancy: Teratogenic effects. Pregnancy Category C: Fluorometholone has been shown to be embryocidal and teratogenic in rabbits when administered at low multiples of the human ocular dose. Fluorometholone was applied ocularly to rabbits daily on days 6–18 of gestation, and dose related fetal loss and fetal abnormalities including cleft palate, deformed rib cage, anomalous limbs and neural abnormalities such as encephalocele, craniorachischisis, and spina bifida were observed. There are no adequate and well-controlled studies of fluorometholone in pregnant women, and it is not known whether fluorometholone can cause fetal harm when administered to a pregnant women. Fluorometholone should be used during pregnancy only if the potential benefit justifies the potential risk to the fetus.

Nursing Mothers: It is not known whether topical ophthalmic administration of corticosteroids could result in sufficient systemic absorption to produce detectable quantities in human milk. Systemically administered corticosteroids appear in human milk and could suppress growth, interfere with endogenous corticosteroid production, or cause other untoward effects. Because of the potential for serious adverse reactions in nursing infants from fluorometholone, a decision should be made whether to discontinue nursing or to discontinue the drug, taking into account the importance of the drug to the mother.

Pediatric Use: Safety and effectiveness in children below the age of two years have not been established.

Adverse Reactions: Adverse reactions include, in decreasing order of frequency, elevation of intraocular pressure (IOP) with possible development of glaucoma and infrequent optic nerve damage, posterior subcapsular cataract formation, and delayed wound healing.

Although systemic effects are extremely uncommon, there have been rare occurrences of systemic hypercorticoidism after use of topical steroids.

Corticosteroid-containing preparations have also been reported to cause acute uveitis and perforation of the globe. Keratitis, conjunctivitis, corneal ulcers, mydriasis, conjunctival hyperemia, loss of accommodation and ptosis have occasionally been reported following use of corticosteroids.

The development of secondary ocular infection (bacterial, fungal and viral) has occurred. Fungal and viral infections of the cornea are particularly prone to develop coincidentally with long-term applications of steroids. The possibility of fungal invasion should be considered in any persistent corneal ulceration where steroid treatment has been used (see WARNINGS).

Dosage and Administration: Instill one drop into the conjunctival sac two to four times daily. During the initial 24 to 48 hours, the dosage may be increased to one application every four hours. Care should be taken not to discontinue therapy prematurely.

If signs and symptoms fail to improve after two days, the patient should be re-evaluated (see PRECAUTIONS).

The dosing of FLUOR-OP suspension may be reduced, but care should be taken not to discontinue therapy prematurely. In chronic conditions, withdrawal of treatment should be carried out by gradually decreasing the frequency of applications.

How Supplied: FLUOR-OP (fluorometholone ophthalmic suspension, USP) 0.1% is supplied in plastic dropper bottles in the following sizes:

3 mL NDC 58768-358-99
5 mL NDC 58768-358-05
10 mL NDC 58768-358-10
15 mL NDC 58768-358-15

Store at controlled room temperature 15°–30°C (59°–86°F). **Protect from freezing. Shake well before using. Keep bottle tightly closed when not in use.**
Caution: Federal (U.S.) law prohibits dispensing without prescription.
Mfd. by OMJ Pharmaceuticals, Inc.,
San Germán, P.R., 00683 for:

6069-A
Revised: May, 1995

GENTACIDIN® ℞
(Gentamicin Sulfate)
Ophthalmic Solution, USP, 0.3%
GENTAMICIN SULFATE
Ophthalmic Ointment, USP, 0.3%

GENTEAL™ OTC
LUBRICANT EYE DROPS
PATENTED* NON-IRRITATING PRESERVATIVE

GenTeal differs from ordinary multidose tears because it is preserved in the bottle by a unique disappearing preservative, sodium perborate. Upon contact with the eye, sodium perborate turns into pure water and oxygen, thereby minimizing the irritation that may be caused by traditional preservatives.
FDA Approved Uses: For the temporary relief of discomfort due to minor irritations of the eye from exposure to wind, sun, or other irritants. For use as a protectant against further irritation or to relieve dryness of the eye.
Description: GenTeal is a sterile lubricant eye drop containing hydroxypropyl methylcellulose; with boric acid, sodium chloride, potassium chloride, phosphonic acid, and purified water; sodium perborate added as a preservative.
Directions: Instill 1 or 2 drops in the affected eye(s) as needed.
Warnings: If you experience eye pain, changes in vision, continued redness or irritation of the eye, or if the condition worsens or persists for more than 72 hours, discontinue use and consult a doctor. To avoid contamination, do not touch tip of container to any surface. Do not use this product if you are allergic to any of its ingredients.
Keep this and all drugs out of the reach of children.
Always replace cap after using.
How Supplied: GenTeal is supplied in a dropper-tipped plastic squeeze bottle containing 15mL or 25mL. Use only if tamper-evident seal marked **CIBA Vision** Ophthalmics® is intact at time of purchase. Store at controlled room temperature.
Made in Canada. ©1995

*Patent Pending
Part No. CS400020

Shown in Product Identification Guide, page 105

GENTEAL™ OTC
[gĕn tēēl]
Lubricant Eye Gel
(Hydroxypropyl Methylcellulose)

GenTeal™ Lubricant Eye Gel: The First Long-Lasting Eye Lubricant In Gel Form
GenTeal™ Lubricant Eye Gel:
Multidose Convenience WITHOUT Irritation

GenTeal™ Lubricant Eye Gel differs from ordinary multidose tears because it is preserved in the tube by a unique preservative, sodium perborate. Upon contact with the eye, sodium perborate turns into pure water and oxygen, thereby minimizing the irritation that may be caused by traditional preservatives. So all you feel is soothing relief.
GenTeal™ Lubricant Eye Gel is a clear gel that liquifies upon contact with the eye, spreading rapidly without leaving streaks or causing blurred vision like ointments. And unlike ointments, GenTeal™ Lubricant Eye Gel contains no irritating lanolin or mineral oil. Once in the eye, GenTeal™ Lubricant Eye Gel forms a long-lasting protective film. In fact, only three to four applications per day can provide comfort all day and night.

FDA Approved Uses/Indications: For the temporary relief of discomfort due to minor irritations of the eye from exposure to wind, sun, or other irritants. For use as a protectant against further irritation or to relieve dryness of the eye.

Directions: Instill 1 or 2 drops in the affected eye(s) as needed. The frequency of administration depends on requirements. On average, one drop is administered 3–4 times daily. If required, GenTeal™ Lubricant Eye Gel may be administered more frequently.
Hold the tube vertically. This results in the formation of a small drop which readily becomes detached from the tube opening. This drop is instilled into the conjunctival sac.
Close tube immediately after use.

INCORRECT

CORRECT

Description: GenTeal™ Lubricant Eye Gel contains hydroxypropyl methylcellulose 0.3%; with carbopol 980, phosphonic acid, purified water and sorbitol; sodium perborate (0.028%) added as a preservative.

Warnings: If you experience eye pain, changes in vision, continued redness or irritation of the eye, or if the condition worsens or persists for more than 72 hours, discontinue use and consult a doctor. To avoid contamination, do not touch tip of container to any surface. Do not use this product if you are allergic to any of its ingredients.
Contraindicated in known hypersensitivity to any component of the gel.
If gel changes color or becomes cloudy, do not use.
Keep this and all drugs out of the reach of children.
Always replace cap after using.
Store at 8° – 25°C (46° – 77°F).
How supplied: GenTeal™ Lubricant Eye Gel is supplied in a dropper tipped plastic squeeze tube containing 10 mL. Use only if tamper-evident pull tab is intact at the time of purchase.

Shown in Product Identification Guide, page 105

HYPOTEARS® OTC
LUBRICANT EYE DROPS
HYPOTEARS® PF, Lubricant Eye Drops
HYPOTEARS® OINTMENT Bedtime Eye Lubricant

Shown in Product Identification Guide, page 105

INFLAMASE® MILD 1/8% ℞
[in 'fla-mās]
(prednisolone sodium phosphate)
Ophthalmic Solution
INFLAMASE® FORTE 1%
(prednisolone sodium phosphate)
Ophthalmic Solution

LIVOSTIN™ ℞
0.05% (levocabastine hydrochloride ophthalmic suspension)

Description: LIVOSTIN™ 0.05% (levocabastine hydrochloride ophthalmic suspension) is a selective histamine H_1-receptor antagonist for topical ophthalmic use. Each mL contains 0.54 mg levocabastine hydrochloride equivalent to 0.5 mg levocabastine; 0.15 mg benzalkonium chloride; propylene glycol; polysorbate 80; dibasic sodium phosphate, anhydrous; monobasic sodium phosphate, monohydrate; disodium edetate; hydroxypropyl methylcellulose; and purified water. It has a pH of 6.0 to 8.0.
The chemical name for levocabastine hydrochloride is (–)-*trans*-1-[*cis*-4-Cyano-4-(p-fluorophenyl)cyclohexyl]-3-methyl-4-phenyl-isonipecotic acid monohydrochloride, and is represented by the following chemical structure:

Clinical Pharmacology: Levocabastine is a potent, selective histamine H_1-antagonist.
Antigen challenge studies performed two and four hours after initial drug instillation indicated activity was maintained for at least two hours.
In an environmental study, LIVOSTIN™ 0.05% (levocabastine hydrochloride ophthalmic suspension) instilled four times daily was shown to be significantly more effective than its vehicle in reducing ocular itching associated with seasonal allergic conjunctivitis.
After instillation in the eye, levocabastine is systemically absorbed. However, the amount of systemically absorbed levocabastine after therapeutic ocular doses is low (mean plasma concentrations in the range of 1–2 ng/mL).
Indications and Usage: LIVOSTIN™ 0.05% (levocabastine hydrochloride ophthalmic suspension) is indicated for the temporary relief of the signs and symptoms of seasonal allergic conjunctivitis.
Contraindications: This product is contraindicated in persons with known or suspected hypersensitivity to any of its components. It should not be used while soft contact lenses are being worn.
Warning: For topical use only. Not for injection.
Precautions:
Information for Patients: SHAKE WELL BEFORE USING. To prevent contaminating the dropper tip and suspension, care should be taken not to touch the eyelids or surrounding areas with the dropper tip of the bottle. Keep bottle tightly closed when not in use. Do not use if the suspension has discolored. Store at controlled room temperature. Protect from freezing.

Continued on next page

Livostin—Cont.

Carcinogenesis, Mutugenesis, Impairment of Fertility: Levocabastine was not carcinogenic in male or female rats or in male mice when administered in the diet for up to 24 months. In female mice, levocabastine doses of 5,000 and 21,500 times the maximum recommended ocular human use level resulted in an increased incidence of pituitary gland adenoma and mammary gland adenocarcinoma possibly produced by increased prolactin levels. The clinical relevance of this finding is unknown with regard to the interspecies differences in prolactin physiology and the very low plasma concentrations of levocabastine following ocular administration.

Mutagenic potential was not demonstrated for levocabastine when tested in Ames' Salmonella reversion test or in *Escherichia coli, Drosophila melanogaster*, a mouse Dominant Lethal Assay or in rat Micronucleus test.

In reproduction studies in rats, levocabastine showed no effects on fertility at oral doses of 20 mg/kg/day (8,300 times the maximum recommended human ocular dose).

PREGNANCY: Teratogenic Effects: Pregnancy Category C. Levocabastine has been shown to be teratogenic (polydactyly) in rats when given in doses 16,500 times the maximum recommended human ocular dose. Teratogenicity (polydactyly, hydrocephaly, brachygnathia), embryotoxicity, and maternal toxicity were observed in rats at 66,000 times the maximum recommended ocular human dose. There are no adequate and well-controlled studies in pregnant women. Levocabastine should be used during pregnancy only if the potential benefit justifies the potential risk to the fetus.

Nursing Mothers: Based on determinations of levocabastine in breast milk after ophthalmic administration of the drug to one nursing woman, it was calculated that the daily dose of levocabastine in the infant was about 0.5 µg.

Pediatric Use: Safety and effectiveness in pediatric patients below the age of 12 have not been established.

Adverse Reactions: The most frequent adverse experiences reported with the use of LIVOSTIN™ 0.05% (levocabastine hydrochloride ophthalmic suspension) were mild, transient stinging and burning (29%) and headache (5%).

Other adverse experiences reported in approximately 1–3% of patients treated with LIVOSTIN™ were visual disturbances, dry mouth, fatigue, pharyngitis, eye pain/dryness, somnolence, red eyes, lacrimation/discharge, cough, nausea, rash/erythema, eyelid edema, and dyspnea.

Dosage and Administration: SHAKE WELL BEFORE USING. The usual dose is one drop instilled in affected eyes four times per day.

How Supplied: LIVOSTIN™ 0.05% (levocabastine hydrochloride ophthalmic suspension), 2.5 mL, 5 mL, and 10 mL is provided in white, polyethylene dropper tip squeeze bottles.

Keep tightly closed when not in use.

Do not use if the suspension has discolored.

Store at controlled room temperature 15° to 30°C (59° to 86°F).

Protect from freezing.

NDC 58768-610-10 (10.0 mL)

NDC 58768-610-05 (5.0 mL)

NDC 58768-610-99 (2.5 mL)

Federal law prohibits dispensing without prescription.

Levocabastine hydrochloride is an original product of Janssen Pharmaceutica Inc.

Mfd. by OMJ Pharmaceuticals, Inc.,
San Germán, P.R., 00683 for:

5035-B

Revised: June 1996

Shown in Product Identification Guide, page 105

MIOCHOL®-E ℞

(acetylcholine chloride intraocular solution) 1:100 with Electrolyte Diluent

Description: MIOCHOL®-E (acetylcholine chloride intraocular solution) is a parasympathomimetic preparation for intraocular use packaged in a vial of two compartments; the lower chamber containing acetylcholine chloride 20 mg and mannitol 56 mg; the upper chamber containing 2 mL of a modified diluent of sodium acetate trihydrate, potassium chloride, magnesium chloride hexahydrate, calcium chloride dihydrate and sterile water for injection.

The reconstituted liquid will be a sterile isotonic solution (275–330 milliosmoles/Kg) containing 20 mg acetylcholine chloride (1:100 solution) and 2.8% mannitol. The pH range is 5.0–8.2. Mannitol is used in the process of lyophilizing acetylcholine chloride, and is not considered an active ingredient.

The chemical name for acetylcholine chloride, $C_7H_{16}ClNO_2$, is Ethanaminium, 2-(acetyloxy)-*N,N,N*-trimethyl-, chloride and is represented by the following chemical structure:

$$CH_3\overset{O}{\overset{\|}{C}}O(CH_2)_2N^+(CH_3)_3\ Cl^-$$

Clinical Pharmacology: Acetylcholine is a naturally occurring neurohormone which mediates nerve impulse transmission at all cholinergic sites involving somatic and autonomic nerves. After release from the nerve ending, acetylcholine is rapidly inactivated by the enzyme acetylcholinesterase by hydrolysis to acetic acid and choline.

Direct application of acetylcholine to the iris will cause rapid miosis of short duration. Topical ocular instillation of acetylcholine to the intact eye causes no discernible response as cholinesterase destroys the molecule more rapidly than it can penetrate the cornea.

Indications and Usage: To obtain miosis of the iris in seconds after delivery of the lens in cataract surgery, in penetrating keratoplasty, iridectomy and other anterior segment surgery where rapid miosis may be required.

Contraindications: None known.

Warnings: DO NOT GAS STERILIZE. If blister or peelable backing is damaged or broken, sterility of the enclosed bottle cannot be assured. Open under aseptic conditions only.

Precautions: *General* In the reconstitution of the solution, as described under Directions for Using Univial, if the center rubber plug seal in the univial does not go down or is down, do not use the vial.

If miosis is to be obtained quickly with MIOCHOL-E, anatomical hindrances to miosis, such as anterior or posterior synechiae, must be released, prior to administration of MIOCHOL-E. During cataract surgery, use MIOCHOL-E only after delivery of the lens.

Aqueous solutions of acetylcholine chloride are unstable. Prepare solution immediately before use. Do not use solution which is not clear and colorless. Discard any solution that has not been used.

Drug Interactions: Although clinical studies with acetylcholine chloride and animal studies with acetylcholine or carbachol revealed no interference, and there is no known pharmacological basis for an interaction, there have been reports that acetylcholine chloride and carbachol have been ineffective when used in patients treated with topical nonsteroidal anti-inflammatory agents.

Pediatric Use: Safety and effectiveness in pediatric patients have not been established.

Adverse Reactions: Infrequent cases of corneal edema, corneal clouding, and corneal decompensation have been reported with the use of intraocular acetylcholine.

Adverse reactions have been reported rarely which are indicative of systemic absorption. These include bradycardia, hypotension, flushing, breathing difficulties and sweating.

Overdosage: Atropine sulfate (0.5 to 1 mg) should be given intramuscularly or intravenously and should be readily available to counteract possible overdosage. Epinephrine (0.1 to 1 mg subcutaneously) is also of value in overcoming severe cardiovascular or bronchoconstrictor responses.

Dosage And Administration: With a new needle of sturdy gauge, 18–20, draw all the solution into a dry, sterile syringe. Replace needle with a suitable atraumatic cannulae for intraocular irrigation.

The MIOCHOL-E solution is instilled into the anterior chamber before or after securing one or more sutures. Instillation should be gentle and parallel to the iris face and tangential to pupil border.

If there are no mechanical hindrances, the pupil starts to constrict in seconds and the peripheral iris is drawn away from the angle of the anterior chamber. Any anatomical hindrance to miosis must be released to permit the desired effect of the drug. In most cases, 0.5 to 2 mL produces satisfactory miosis.

In cataract surgery, use MIOCHOL-E only after delivery of the lens.

Aqueous solutions of acetylcholine chloride are unstable. Prepare solution immediately before use. Do not use solution which is not clear and colorless. Discard any solution that has not been used.

DIRECTIONS FOR USING THE UNIVIAL: STERILE UNLESS PACKAGE OPEN OR BROKEN

1. Inspect univial while inside unopened blister. Diluent must be in upper chamber.
2. Peel open blister.
3. Aseptically transfer univial to sterile field. Maintain sterility of outer container during preparation of solution.
4. Immediately before use, give plunger-stopper a quarter turn and press to force diluent and center plug into lower chamber.
5. Shake gently to dissolve drug.
6. Discard univial and any unused solution.

How Supplied: MIOCHOL-E with CIBA Vision® Steri-Tags™: **NDC** 58768-773-52

One MIOCHOL-E 2 mL sterile univial

One pack CIBA Vision® Steri-Tags sterile labels

MIOCHOL-E System Pak™: **NDC** 58768-773-53

One MIOCHOL-E 2 mL sterile univial

One pack CIBA Vision® Steri-Tags sterile labels

One B-D® 3 mL sterile syringe

One Dynagard™ 0.2 micron sterile filter

Store at 4°–25°C (39°–77°F).

KEEP FROM FREEZING.

℞ Only

Mfd. by OMJ Pharmaceuticals, Inc.,
San Germán, P.R., 00683

6110-C

Revised: April 1998

INSTRUCTIONS FOR USING THE SYRINGE TIP FILTER

Injection Procedure:

1. Pre-fill syringe with MIOCHOL®-E.
2. Aseptically open Syringe Filter pouch.
3. Aseptically attach filter onto luer of syringe with twisting motion to assure secure fit.
4. Aseptically attach sterile needle or cannula to male luer of filter.

5. After use discard appropriately.

Precautions

- Do not exceed 50 psi pressure on the inlet side to avoid resultant decrease in flow rates.
- Change filter when pressure buildup makes syringe operation difficult.
- Aspiration through the filter is not recommended.
  However, if utilized, discard needle and syringe filter to prevent recontamination of fluids during injection.

Contraindications

- Chemically resistant to aqueous solutions, dilute acids, bases, and aliphatic and aromatic hydrocarbons.
  Not recommended for use with aldehydes, esters, ketones, alcohols, halogenated hydrocarbons or their derivatives.

OCUPRESS® ℞

[ăk-yu-pres]

(carteolol HCl ophthalmic solution)
1% STERILE

Description: Ocupress® (carteolol hydrochloride) Ophthalmic Solution, 1%, is a nonselective beta-adrenoceptor blocking agent for ophthalmic use.

The chemical name for carteolol hydrochloride is (±)-5-[3-[(1,1-dimethylethyl) amino]-2 hydroxypropoxy]-3, 4-dihydro-2(1H)-quinolinone monohydrochloride. The structural formula is as follows:

$OCH_2CHCH_2NHC(CH_3)_3$ (with OH) • HCl

$C_{16}H_{24}N_2O_3 \cdot HCl$ Mol. Wt. 328.84

Each mL contains 10 mg carteolol HCl and the inactive ingredients—Benzalkonium chloride 0.05 mg (0.005%) as a preservative; sodium chloride; sodium phosphate, dibasic; sodium phosphate, monobasic; and water for injection, USP. The product has a pH of 6.2 to 7.2

Clinical Pharmacology: Carteolol HCl is a nonselective beta-adrenergic blocking agent with associated intrinsic sympathomimetic activity and without significant membrane-stabilizing activity.

Ocupress (carteolol HCl) reduces normal and elevated intraocular pressure (IOP) whether or not accompanied by glaucoma. The exact mechanism of the ocular hypotensive effect of beta-blockers has not been definitely demonstrated.

In general, beta-adrenergic blockers reduce cardiac output in patients in good and poor cardiovascular health. In patients with severe impairment of myocardial function, beta-blockers may inhibit the sympathetic stimulation necessary to maintain adequate cardiac function. Beta-adrenergic blockers may also increase airway resistance in the bronchi and bronchioles due to unopposed parasympathetic activity.

Given topically twice daily in controlled domestic clinical trials ranging from 1.5 to 3 months, Ocupress produced a median percent reduction of IOP 22% to 25%. No significant effects were noted on corneal sensitivity, tear secretion, or pupil size.

Indications and Usage: Ocupress Ophthalmic Solution, 1%, has been shown to be effective in lowering intraocular pressure and may be used in patients with chronic open-angle glaucoma and intraocular hypertension. It may be used alone or in combination with other intraocular pressure lowering medications.

Contraindications: Ocupress Ophthalmic Solution is contraindicated in those individuals with bronchial asthma or with a history of bronchial asthma, or severe chronic obstructive pulmonary disease (see WARNINGS); sinus bradycardia; second- and third-degree atrioventricular block; overt cardiac failure (see WARNINGS); cardiogenic shock; or hypersensitivity to any component of this product.

Warnings: Ocupress Ophthalmic Solution has not been detected in plasma following ocular instillation. However, as with other topically applied ophthalmic preparations, Ocupress may be absorbed systemically. The same adverse reactions found with systemic administration of beta-adrenergic blocking agents may occur with topical administration. For example, severe respiratory reactions and cardiac reactions, including death due to bronchospasm in patients with asthma, and rarely death in association with cardiac failure, have been reported with topical application of beta-adrenergic blocking agents (see CONTRAINDICATIONS).

Cardiac Failure: Sympathetic stimulation may be essential for support of the circulation in individuals with diminished myocardial contractility, and its inhibition by beta-adrenergic receptor blockade may precipitate more severe failure.

In Patients Without a History of Cardiac Failure: Continued depression of the myocardium with beta-blocking agents over a period of time can, in some cases, lead to cardiac failure. At the first sign or symptom of cardiac failure, Ocupress should be discontinued.

Non-allergic Bronchospasm: In patients with non-allergic bronchospasm or with a history of non-allergic bronchospasm (e.g., chronic bronchitis, emphysema), Ocupress should be administered with caution since it may block bronchodilation produced by endogenous and exogenous catecholamine stimulation of $beta_2$ receptors.

Major Surgery: The necessity or desirability of withdrawal of beta-adrenergic blocking agents prior to major surgery is controversial. Beta-adrenergic receptor blockade impairs the ability of the heart to respond to beta-adrenergically mediated reflex stimuli. This may augment the risk of general anesthesia in surgical procedures. Some patients receiving beta-adrenergic receptor blocking agents have been subject to protracted severe hypotension during anesthesia. For these reasons, in patients undergoing elective surgery, gradual withdrawal of beta-adrenergic receptor blocking agents may be appropriate.

If necessary during surgery, the effects of beta-adrenergic blocking agents may be reversed by sufficient doses of such agonists as isoproterenol, dopamine, dobutamine or levarterenol (see OVERDOSAGE).

Diabetes Mellitus: Beta-adrenergic blocking agents should be administered with caution in patients subject to spontaneous hypoglycemia or to diabetic patients (especially those with labile diabetes) who are receiving insulin or oral hypoglycemic agents. Beta-adrenergic receptor blocking agents may mask the signs and symptoms of acute hypoglycemia.

Thyrotoxicosis: Beta-adrenergic blocking agents may mask certain clinical signs (e.g., tachycardia) of hyperthyroidism. Patients suspected of developing thyrotoxicosis should be managed carefully to avoid abrupt withdrawal of beta-adrenergic blocking agents which might precipitate a thyroid storm.

Precautions:

General: Ocupress Ophthalmic Solution should be used with caution in patients with known hypersensitivity to other beta-adrenoceptor blocking agents.

Use with caution in patients with known diminished pulmonary function.

In patients with angle-closure glaucoma, the immediate objective of treatment is to reopen the angle. This requires constricting the pupil with a miotic. Ocupress has little or no effect on the pupil. When Ocupress is used to reduce elevated intraocular pressure in angle-closure glaucoma, it should be used with a miotic and not alone.

Information for the Patient: For topical use only. To prevent contaminating the dropper tip and solution, care should be taken not to touch the eyelids or surrounding areas with the dropper tip of the bottle. Keep bottle tightly closed when not in use. Protect from light.

Risk from Anaphylactic Reaction: While taking beta-blockers, patients with a history of atopy or a history of severe anaphylactic reaction to a variety of allergens may be more reactive to repeated accidental, diagnostic, or therapeutic challenge with such allergens. Such patients may be unresponsive to the usual doses of epinephrine used to treat anaphylactic reactions.

Muscle Weakness: Beta-adrenergic blockade has been reported to potentiate muscle weakness consistent with certain myasthenic symptoms (e.g., diplopia, ptosis and generalized weakness).

Drug Interactions: Ocupress should be used with caution in patients who are receiving a beta-adrenergic blocking agent orally, because of the potential for additive effects on systemic beta-blockade.

Close observation of the patient is recommended when a beta-blocker is administered to patients receiving catecholamine-depleting drugs such as reserpine, because of possible additive effects and the production of hypotension and/or marked bradycardia, which may produce vertigo, syncope, or postural hypotension.

Carcinogenesis, Mutagenesis, Impairment of Fertility: Carteolol hydrochloride did not produce carcinogenic effects at doses up to 40 mg/kg/day in two-year oral rat and mouse studies. Tests of mutagenicity, including the Ames Test, recombinant (rec)-assay, *in vivo* cytogenetics and dominant lethal assay demonstrated no evidence for mutagenic potential. Fertility of male and female rats and male and female mice was unaffected by administration of carteolol hydrochloride dosages up to 150 mg/kg/day.

Pregnancy: Teratogenic Effects: Pregnancy Category C: Carteolol hydrochloride increased resorptions and decreased fetal weights in rabbits and rats at maternally toxic doses approximately 1052 and 5264 times the maximum recommended human oral dose (10 mg/70 kg/day), respectively. A dose-related increase in wavy ribs was noted in the developing rat fetus when pregnant females received daily doses of approximately 212 times the maximum recommended human oral dose. No such effects were noted in pregnant mice subjected to up to 1052 times the maximum recommended human oral dose. There are no adequate and well-controlled studies in pregnant women. Ocupress (carteolol hydrochloride) should be used during pregnancy only if the potential benefit justifies the potential risk to the fetus.

Nursing Mothers: It is not known whether this drug is excreted in human milk, although in animal studies carteolol has been shown to be excreted in breast milk. Caution should be exercised when Ocupress is administered to nursing mothers.

Pediatric Use: Safety and effectiveness in pediatric patients have not been established.

Adverse Reactions: The following adverse reactions have been reported in clinical trials with Ocupress Ophthalmic Solution:

Continued on next page

Ocupress—Cont.

Ocular: Transient eye irritation, burning, tearing, conjunctival hyperemia and edema occurred in about 1 of 4 patients. Ocular symptoms including blurred and cloudy vision, photophobia, decreased night vision, and ptosis and ocular signs including blepharoconjunctivitis, abnormal corneal staining, and corneal sensitivity occurred occassionally.
Systemic: As is characteristic of nonselective adrenergic blocking agents, Ocupress may cause bradycardia and decreased blood pressure (see WARNINGS). The following systemic events have occasionally been reported with the use of Ocupress: cardiac arrhythmia, heart palpitation, dyspnea, asthenia, headache, dizziness, insomnia, sinusitis, and taste perversion.
The following additional adverse reactions have been reported with ophthalmic use of $beta_1$ and $beta_2$ (nonselective) adrenergic receptor blocking agents:
Body As a Whole: Headache
Cardiovascular: Arrhythmia, syncope, heart block, cerebral vascular accident, cerebral ischemia, congestive heart failure, palpitation (see WARNINGS).
Digestive: Nausea
Psychiatric: Depression
Skin: Hypersensitivity, including localized and generalized rash
Respiratory: Bronchospasm (predominantly in patients with pre-existing bronchospastic disease), respiratory failure (see WARNINGS)
Endocrine: Masked symptoms of hypoglycemia in insulin-dependent diabetics (see WARNINGS)
Special Senses: Signs and symptoms of keratitis, blepharoptosis, visual disturbances including refractive changes (due to withdrawal of miotic therapy in some cases), diplopia, ptosis.
Other reactions associated with the oral use of nonselective adrenergic receptor blocking agents should be considered potential effects with ophthalmic use of these agents.
Overdosage: No specific information on emergency treatment of overdosage in humans is available. Should accidental ocular overdosage occur, flush eye(s) with water or normal saline. The most common effects expected with overdosage of a beta-adrenergic blocking agent are bradycardia, bronchospasm, congestive heart failure and hypotension.
In case of ingestion, treatment with Ocupress should be discontinued and gastric lavage considered. The patient should be closely observed and vital signs carefully monitored. The prolonged effects of carteolol must be considered when determining the duration of corrective therapy. On the basis of the pharmacologic profile, the following additional measures should be considered as appropriate:
Symptomatic Sinus Bradycardia or Heart Block: Administer atropine. If there is no response to vagal blockade, administer isoproterenol cautiously.
Bronchospasm: Administer a $beta_2$-stimulating agent such as isoproterenol and/or a theophylline derivative.
Congestive Heart Failure: Administer diuretics and digitalis glycosides as necessary.
Hypotension: Administer vasopressors such as intravenous dopamine, epinephrine or norepinephrine bitartrate.
Dosage and Administration: The usual dose is one drop of Ocupress Ophthalmic Solution, 1%, in the affected eye(s) twice a day.
If the patient's IOP is not a satisfactory level on this regimen, concomitant therapy with pilocarpine and other miotics, and/or epinephrine or dipivefrin, and/or systemically administered carbonic anhydrase inhibitors, such as acetazolamide, can be instituted.
How Supplied: Ocupress Ophthalmic Solution, 1%, is supplied as a sterile ophthalmic solution in plastic dispenser bottles of 5 mL (NDC 58768-001-01), 10 mL (NDC 58768-001-02) and 15 mL (NDC 58768 001 04).
Store at 15° to 25°C (59° to 77°F) (room temperature) and protect from light.
Rx Only
Licensed under U.S. Patent Nos. 3910924 and 4309432.
Made in Canada by:
CIBA Vision Sterile Mfg.,
Mississauga, Ontario L5N 2X5
For: **CIBA Vision®**
A Novartis Company
Duluth, Georgia 30097

I6138-A

Shown in Product Identification Guide, page 105

PILOCAR® ℞
[*pī 'lō-car "*]
(pilocarpine hydrochloride)
Ophthalmic Solution

VASOCINE™ ℞
[*vas 'o 'cīne*]
(sulfacetamide sodium and prednisolone acetate)
Ophthalmic Ointment, USP

VASOCIDIN® ℞
(sulfacetamide sodium-prednisolone sodium phosphate)
Ophthalmic Solution, USP

VASOCON®–A OTC
[*vas "o-kon*]
Itching/Redness Reliever Eye Drops

For temporary relief of minor allergic symptoms of the eye, including itching and redness due to pollen and animal hair.
Description: Active Ingredients—antazoline phosphate (0.5%), naphazoline hydrochloride (0.05%).
Inactive Ingredients—polyethylene glycol 8000, sodium chloride, polyvinyl alcohol, purified water, benzalkonium chloride (0.01%), and edetate disodium (0.03%). (Sodium hydroxide and/or hydrochloric acid to adjust pH. The solution has a pH of 5.5–6.3 and a tonicity of 280–350 mOsm/Kg.)
Directions: Instill 1 or 2 drops in the affected eye(s) as needed up to 4 times daily.

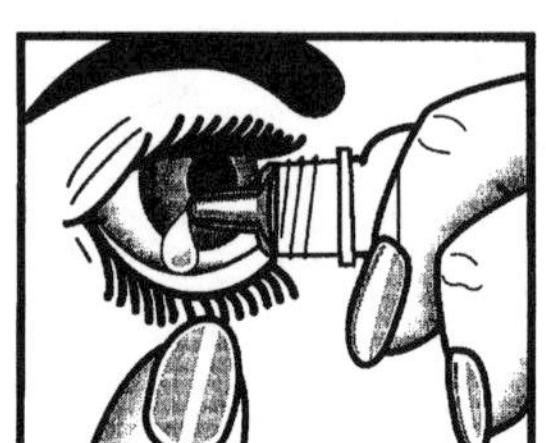

Warnings: To avoid contamination, do not touch tip of container to any surface. Replace cap after using.
If solution changes color or becomes cloudy, do not use.
If you experience eye pain, changes in vision, continued redness or irritation of the eye, or if the condition worsens or persists for more than 72 hours, discontinue use and consult a physician. Transient burning and stinging has been reported with some patients upon instillation. Overuse of this product may produce increased redness of the eye.
If you are sensitive to any ingredient in this product, do not use. Do not use this product if you have heart disease, high blood pressure, or narrow angle glaucoma unless directed by a physician.
Accidental oral ingestion in infants and children may lead to coma and marked reduction in body temperature. Before using in children under 6 years of age, consult your physician.
Keep this and all drugs out of the reach of children. In case of accidental ingestion, seek professional assistance or contact a Poison Control Center immediately.
Remove contact lenses before using.
Store at room temperature (59°–77°F) (15°–25°C).
Protect from light.
Use before the expiration date marked on the carton or bottle.
USE ONLY IF IMPRINTED TAMPER EVIDENT SEAL IS INTACT AT THE TIME OF PURCHASE.
NDC 58768-881-15

Shown in Product Identification Guide, page 105

VASOSULF® ℞
[*vas "o-sulf*]
(sulfacetamide sodium–phenylephrine hydrochloride)
Ophthalmic Solution

VITRAVENE™ ℞
Fomivirsen sodium intravitreal injectable

Description: Vitravene™ (fomivirsen sodium intravitreal injectable) is a sterile, aqueous, preservative-free, bicarbonate-buffered solution for intravitreal injection.
Fomivirsen sodium is represented by the following structural formula:
[See chemical structure at top of next page]
Fomivirsen sodium is a phosphorothioate oligonucleotide, twenty-one nucleotides in length, with the following sequence: 5'-GCG TTT GCT CTT CTT CTT GCG-3'
The chemical name for fomivirsen sodium is as follows:
2'-Deoxyguanosylyl-(3'→5' *O,O*-phosphorothioyl)-2'-deoxycytidylyl-(3'→5' *O,O*-phosphorothioyl)-2'-deoxyguanosylyl-(3'→5' *O,O*-phosphorothioyl)-thymidylyl-(3'→5' *O,O*-phosphorothioyl)-thymidylyl- (3'→5' *O,O*-phosphorothioyl)-thymidylyl-(3'→5' *O,O*-phosphorothioyl)-2'-deoxyguanosylyl- (3'→5' *O,O*-phosphorothioyl) -2'-deoxycytidylyl- (3'→5' *O,O*-phosphorothioyl)-thymidylyl-(3'→5' *O,O*-phosphorothioyl) -2'-deoxycytidylyl -(3'→5' *O,O*-phosphorothioyl)-thymidylyl-(3'→5' *O,O*-phosphorothioyl) -thymidylyl-(3'→5' *O,O*-phosphorothioyl) -2'-deoxycytidylyl -(3'→5' *O,O*-phosphorothioyl)-thymidylyl-(3'→5' *O,O*-phosphorothioyl) -thymidylyl- (3'→5' *O,O*-phosphorothioyl) -2'-deoxycytidylyl- (3'→5' *O,O*-phosphorothioyl)-thymidylyl-(3'→5' *O,O*-phosphorothioyl) -thymidylyl- (3'→5' *O,O*-phosphorothioyl)-2'-deoxyguanosylyl-(3'→5' *O,O* -phosphorothioyl) -2'-deoxycytidylyl-(3'→5' *O,O*-phosphorothioyl)-2'-deoxyguanosine, 20-sodium salt.
Fomivirsen sodium is a white to off-white, hygroscopic, amorphous powder with a molecular formula of $C_{204} H_{243} N_{63} O_{114} P_{20} S_{20} Na_{20}$ and a molecular weight of 7,122.
Each mL of Vitravene™ contains:
ACTIVE: Fomivirsen sodium 6.6 mg

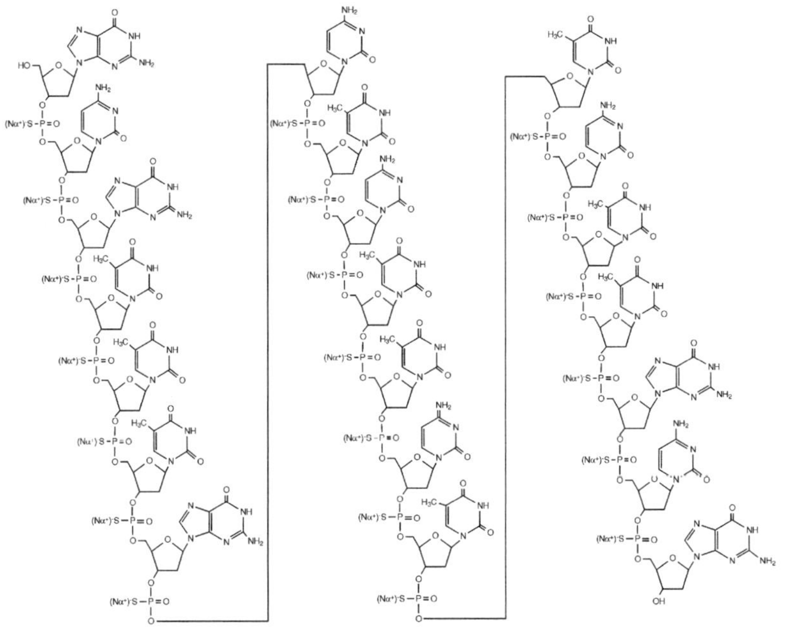

INACTIVES: Sodium chloride, sodium bicarbonate, sodium carbonate and water for injection. Sodium hydroxide and/or hydrochloric acid may be added to adjust pH. Vitravene™ is formulated to have an osmolality of 290 mOsm/kg, and a pH of 8.7.

Clinical Pharmacology

Virology

Mechanism of Action

Fomivirsen is a phosphorothioate oligonucleotide that inhibits human cytomegalovirus (HCMV) replication through an antisense mechanism. The nucleotide sequence of fomivirsen is complementary to a sequence in mRNA transcripts of the major immediate early region 2 (IE2) of HCMV. This region of mRNA encodes several proteins responsible for regulation of viral gene expression that are essential for production of infectious CMV. Binding of fomivirsen to the target mRNA, results in inhibition of IE2 protein synthesis, subsequently inhibiting virus replication.

Resistance

Through persistent selection pressure ***in vitro*** it was possible to isolate a clone of HCMV that was 10-fold less sensitive to inhibition of replication than the parent strain. The molecular basis for the resistance has not been elucidated. It is possible that resistant strains may occur in clinical use.

Cross-resistance

The antisense mechanism of action and molecular target of fomivirsen are different from that of inhibitors of HCMV replication, which function by inhibiting the viral DNA polymerase. Fomivirsen was equally potent against 21 independent clinical HCMV isolates, including several that were resistant to ganciclovir, foscarnet and/or cidofovir. Isolates, which are resistant to fomivirsen, may be sensitive to ganciclovir, foscarnet and/or cidofovir.

Pharmacokinetics

The assessment of ocular pharmacokinetic parameters in patients has been limited and is still ongoing.

ANIMAL STUDIES

Ocular Kinetics: Fomivirsen is cleared from the vitreous in rabbits over the course of 7 to 10 days, by a combination of tissue distribution and metabolism. In the eye, fomivirsen concentrations were greatest in the retina and iris. Fomivirsen was detectable in retina within hours after injection, and concentrations increased over 3 to 5 days.

Metabolism and Elimination: Metabolism is the primary route of elimination from the eye. Metabolites of fomivirsen are detected in the retina and vitreous in animals. Fomivirsen sodium is metabolized by exonucleases in a process that sequentially removes residues from the terminal ends of the oligonucleotide yielding shortened oligonucleotides and mononucleotide metabolites. Data with related compounds indicate that mononucleotide metabolites are further catabolized similar to endogenous nucleotides and are excreted as low molecular weight metabolites. In rabbits, a small amount of fomivirsen-derived radioactivity was eliminated in urine (16%) or feces (3%) as low molecular weight metabolites. Expired air has been shown to be a major route of excretion for CO_2 generated by catabolism of nucleotides after administration of phosphorothioate oligonucleotides.

Systemic Exposure: Systemic exposure to fomivirsen following single or repeated intravitreal injection in monkeys was below limits of quantitation (70 ηg/mL in plasma and 350 ηg/g in tissue). In monkeys treated every other week for up to 3 months with fomivirsen there were isolated instances when fomivirsen's metabolites were observed in liver, kidney, and plasma at a concentration near the level of detection (14 ηg/mL in plasma and 70 ηg/g in tissue).

Protein Binding: Analysis of vitreous samples from treated rabbits and monkeys indicates that approximately 40% of fomivirsen is bound to proteins.

Clinical Studies

Clinical ocular pharmacokinetics studies have not yet been completed.

Limited, open label, controlled clinical studies evaluating the safety and efficacy of Vitravene™ have been conducted in patients with newly diagnosed CMV retinitis and in patients who have failed previous therapies. Based on the assessment of fundus photographs, the median time to CMV retinitis progression was approximately 80 days in patients receiving a dose of 330 µg. Many of these patients were also receiving protease inhibitor treatment. In the subgroup of newly diagnosed patients who received delayed treatment, most had CMV retinitis progression within two weeks. Head to head comparisons with other medications available to treat CMV retinitis has not been completed.

Indications and Usage: Vitravene™ is indicated for the local treatment of cytomegalovirus (CMV) retinitis in patients with acquired immunodeficiency syndrome (AIDS), who are intolerant of or have a contraindication to other treatment(s) for CMV retinitis or who were insufficiently responsive to previous treatment(s) for CMV retinitis.

The diagnosis and evaluation of CMV retinitis is ophthalmologic and should be made by comprehensive retinal examination including indirect ophthalmoscopy. Other conditions that should be considered in the differential diagnosis of CMV retinitis include ocular infections caused by syphilis, candidiasis, toxoplasmosis, histoplasmosis, herpes simplex virus and varicella-zoster virus as well as retinal scars, and cotton wool spots, any of which may produce a retinal appearance similar to CMV. For this reason, it is essential that a physician familiar with the retinal presentation of these conditions establish the diagnosis of CMV retinitis.

Contraindications: Vitravene™ is contraindicated in those persons who have known hypersensitivity to any component of this preparation.

Warnings: Vitravene™ is for intravitreal injection use only.

CMV retinitis may be associated with CMV disease elsewhere in the body. Vitravene™ provides localized therapy limited to the treated eye. The use of Vitravene™ does not provide treatment for systemic CMV disease. Patients should be monitored for extraocular CMV disease or disease in the contralateral eye.

Vitravene™ is not recommended for use in patients who have recently (2–4 weeks) been treated with either intravenous or intravitreal cidofovir because of the risk of exaggerated ocular inflammation.

Precautions

General

FOR OPHTHALMIC USE ONLY.

Ocular inflammation (uveitis) including iritis and vitritis has been reported to occur in approximately 1 in 4 patients. Inflammatory reactions are more common during induction dosing. Topical corticosteroids have been useful in the medical management of inflammatory changes, and with both medical management and time, patients may be able to continue to receive intravitreal injections of Vitravene™ after the inflammation has resolved.

Increased intraocular pressure has been commonly reported. The increase is usually a transient event and in most cases the pressure returns to the normal range without any treatment or with temporary use of topical medications. Intraocular pressure should be monitored at each visit and elevations of intraocular pressure, if sustained, should be managed with medications to lower intraocular pressure.

Information for patients

Vitravene™ is not a cure for CMV retinitis, and some immunocompromised patients may continue to experience progression of retinitis during and following treatment. Patients receiving Vitravene™ should be advised to have regular ophthalmologic follow-up examinations. Patients may also experience other manifestations of CMV disease despite Vitravene™ therapy.

Vitravene™ treats only the eye(s) in which it has been injected. CMV may exist as a systemic disease, in addition to CMV retinitis. Therefore, patients should be monitored for ex-

Continued on next page

Vitravene—Cont.

traocular CMV infections (e.g., pneumonitis, colitis) and retinitis in the opposite eye, if only one infected eye is being treated.
HIV-infected patients should continue taking antiretroviral therapy as otherwise indicated.

Drug Interactions
The interaction in humans between fomivirsen sodium and other drugs has not been studied. Results from *in vitro* tests demonstrated no inhibition of anti-HCMV activity of fomivirsen by AZT or ddC.

Carcinogenesis, Mutagenesis, Impairment of Fertility
No studies have been conducted to evaluate the carcinogenic potential of fomivirsen sodium.
Fomivirsen sodium was not mutagenic in Salmonella/Microsome (Ames) and mouse lymphoma tests or clastogenic in the *in vivo* mouse micronucleus assay. However, equivocal results were observed in the chromosome aberration tests with Chinese hamster ovary cells. No studies have been conducted to evaluate the potential of fomivirsen sodium to affect fertility.

Pregnancy
Teratogenic Effects
Pregnancy Category C. Animal reproductive studies have not been conducted with fomivirsen sodium. It is also not known whether fomivirsen sodium can cause fetal harm when administered to a pregnant woman or can affect reproduction capacity.
There are no adequate and well-controlled studies in pregnant women. Vitravene™ should be used during pregnancy only if the potential benefit justifies the potential risk to the fetus.

Nursing Mothers
It is not known whether fomivirsen sodium is excreted in human milk. Because many drugs are excreted in human milk and because of the potential for serious adverse reactions in nursing infants from Vitravene™, a decision should be made whether to discontinue nursing or to discontinue the drug, taking into account the importance of the drug to the mother.

Pediatric use
Safety and effectiveness in pediatric patients have not been established.

Geriatric use
Clinical studies of Vitravene™ did not include sufficient numbers of subjects aged 65 and over to determine whether they respond differently than younger subjects.

Adverse Reactions: The most frequently observed adverse experiences have been cases of ocular inflammation (uveitis) including iritis and vitritis. Ocular inflammation has been reported to occur in approximately 1 in 4 patients. Inflammatory reactions are more common during induction dosing. Delaying additional treatment with Vitravene™ and the use of topical corticosteroids have been useful in the medical management of inflammatory changes (SEE PRECAUTIONS, General).
Adverse experiences reported in approximately 5 to 20% of patients have included:

Ocular: abnormal vision, anterior chamber inflammation, blurred vision, cataract, conjunctival hemorrhage, decreased visual acuity, desaturation of color vision, eye pain, floaters, increased intraocular pressure, photophobia, retinal detachment, retinal edema, retinal hemorrhage, retinal pigment changes, uveitis, vitritis.

Systemic: abdominal pain, anemia, asthenia, diarrhea, fever, headache, infection, nausea, pneumonia, rash, sepsis, sinusitis, systemic CMV, vomiting.

Adverse experiences reported in approximately 2 to 5% of patients have included:

Ocular: application site reaction, conjunctival hyperemia, conjunctivitis, corneal edema, decreased peripheral vision, eye irritation, hypotony, keratic precipitates, optic neuritis, photopsia, retinal vascular disease, visual field defect, vitreous hemorrhage, vitreous opacity.

Systemic: abnormal liver function, abnormal thinking, allergic reactions, anorexia, back pain, bronchitis, cachexia, catheter infection, chest pain, decreased weight, dehydration, depression, dizziness, dyspnea, flu syndrome, increased cough, increased GGTP, kidney failure, lymphoma like reaction, neuropathy, neutropenia, oral monilia, pain, pancreatitis, sweating, thrombocytopenia.

Overdosage: In clinical trials with Vitravene™, one patient with advanced CMVR unresponsive to other antivitral treatments was accidentally dosed once bilaterally with 990 µg per eye. Anterior chamber paracentesis was performed bilaterally and vision was retained.

Dosage and Administration: Treatment with Vitravene™ involves an induction and a maintenance phase. The recommended dose of Vitravene™ is 330 µg (0.05 mL). The induction dose of Vitravene™ should be one injection every other week for two doses. Subsequent maintenance doses should be administered once every four weeks after induction.
For unacceptable inflammation in the face of controlled CMVR, it is worthwhile interrupting therapy until the level of inflammation decreases and therapy can resume.
For patients whose disease progresses on Vitravene™ during maintenance, an attempt at reinduction at the same dose may result in resumed disease control.

Instructions for Intravitreal Injection
Vitravene™ is administered by intravitreal injection (0.05 mL/eye) into the affected eye following application of standard topical and/or local anesthetics and antimicrobials using a 30 gauge needle on a low-volume (e.g., tuberculin) syringe. The following steps should be used:

- Remove plastic cap from vial containing Vitravene™.
- Disinfect rubber stopper with 70% ethyl alcohol.
- Attach a 5 micron filter needle to the injection syringe for solution withdrawal (to further guard against the introduction of stopper particulate).
- Withdraw approximately 0.15 mL through the filter needle.
- Remove filter needle and attach a 30 gauge needle to syringe containing Vitravene™.
- Eject excess volume and air from syringe.
- Stabilize globe with cotton tip applicator and insert needle fully through an area 3.5 to 4 mm posterior to the limbus (avoiding the horizontal meridian) aiming toward the center of the globe, keeping fingers off the plunger until the needle has been completed inserted. Deliver the injection volume (0.05 mL) by injecting slowly. Roll cotton tip applicator over injection site as needle is withdrawn to reduce loss of eye fluid.

Instructions for Post-Injection Monitoring
Monitor light perception and optic nerve head perfusion: if not completely perfused by 7–10 minutes, perform anterior chamber paracentesis with a 30 gauge needle on a plungerless tuberculin syringe at the slit lamp.

How Supplied: Vitravene™ (fomivirsen sodium intravitreal injectable) is supplied in preservative-free, single-use vials containing 0.25 mL, 6.6 mg/mL. The product is intended for intravitreal injection only.
NDC 58768-902-35
Store between 2–25° C (35–77° F). Protect from excessive heat and light.
Rx only
Manufactured by:
Abbott Laboratories
McPherson, KS 67460
Distributed by:
CIBA Vision®
A Novartis Company
Duluth, GA 30097
This product has been discovered and developed by Isis Pharmaceuticals, Inc., Carlsbad, CA 92008
September 1998 I6127-A

Shown in Product Identification Guide, page 105

VOLTAREN OPHTHALMIC® ℞
(diclofenac sodium ophthalmic solution) 0.1%
Sterile Ophthalmic Solution

Prescribing Information:
Description: Voltaren Ophthalmic (diclofenac sodium ophthalmic solution) 0.1% solution is a sterile, topical, nonsteroidal, anti-inflammatory product for ophthalmic use. Diclofenac sodium is designated chemically as 2-[(2,6-dichlorophenyl)amino] benzeneacetic acid, monosodium salt, with an empirical formula of $C_{14}H_{10}Cl_2NO_2Na$. The structural formula of diclofenac sodium is:

Voltaren Ophthalmic is available as a sterile solution which contains diclofenac sodium 0.1% (1 mg/mL).
Inactive Ingredients: polyoxyl 35 castor oil, boric acid, tromethamine, sorbic acid (2 mg/mL), edetate disodium (1 mg/mL), and purified water.
Diclofenac sodium is a faintly yellow-white to light-beige, slightly hygroscopic crystalline powder. It is freely soluble in methanol, sparingly soluble in water, very slightly soluble in acetonitrile, and insoluble in chloroform and in 0.1 N hydrochloric acid. Its molecular weight is 318.14. Voltaren Ophthalmic 0.1% is an iso-osmotic solution with an osmolality of about 300 mOsmol/1000 g, buffered at approximately pH 7.2. Voltaren Ophthalmic solution has a faint characteristic odor of castor oil.

Clinical Pharmacology:
Pharmacodynamics
Diclofenac sodium is one of a series of phenylacetic acids that has demonstrated anti-inflammatory and analgesic properties in pharmacological studies. It is thought to inhibit the enzyme cyclooxygenase, which is essential in the biosynthesis of prostaglandins.

Animal Studies
Prostaglandins have been shown in many animal models to be mediators of certain kinds of intraocular inflammation. In studies performed in animal eyes, prostaglandins have been shown to produce disruption of the blood-aqueous humor barrier, vasodilation, increased vascular permeability, leukocytosis, and increased intraocular pressure.

Pharmacokinetics
Results from a bioavailability study established that plasma levels of diclofenac following ocular instillation of two drops of Voltaren Ophthalmic to each eye were below the limit of

quantification (10 ng/mL) over a 4-hour period. This study suggests that limited, if any, systemic absorption occurs with Voltaren Ophthalmic.

Clinical Trials

Postoperative Anti-Inflammatory Effects:

In two double-masked, controlled, efficacy studies of postoperative inflammation, a total of 206 cataract patients were treated with Voltaren Ophthalmic and 103 patients were treated with vehicle placebo. Voltaren Ophthalmic was favored over vehicle placebo over a 2-week period for the clinical assessments of inflammation as measured by anterior chamber cells and flare.

In double-masked, controlled studies of corneal refractive surgery (radial keratotomy (RK) and laser photorefractive keratectomy (PRK)) patients were treated with Voltaren Ophthalmic and/or vehicle placebo. The efficacy of Voltaren Ophthalmic given before and shortly after surgery was favored over vehicle placebo during the 6-hour period following surgery for the clinical assessments of pain and photophobia. Patients were permitted to use a hydrogel soft contact lens with Voltaren Ophthalmic for up to three days after PRK.

Indications and Usage: Voltaren Ophthalmic is indicated for the treatment of postoperative inflammation in patients who have undergone cataract extraction and for the temporary relief of pain and photophobia in patients undergoing corneal refractive surgery.

Contraindications: Voltaren Ophthalmic is contraindicated in patients who are hypersensitive to any component of the medication.

Warnings: The refractive stability of patients undergoing corneal refractive procedures and treated with Voltaren has not been established. Patients should be monitored for a year following use in this setting.

With some nonsteroidal anti-inflammatory drugs, there exists the potential for increased bleeding time due to interference with thrombocyte aggregation. There have been reports that ocularly applied nonsteroidal anti-inflammatory drugs may cause increased bleeding of ocular tissues (including hyphemas) in conjunction with ocular surgery.

There is the potential for cross-sensitivity to acetylsalicylic acid, phenylacetic acid derivatives, and other nonsteroidal anti-inflammatory agents. Therefore, caution should be used when treating individuals who have previously exhibited sensitivities to these drugs.

Precautions:

General

It is recommended that Voltaren Ophthalmic, like other NSAIDs, be used with caution in surgical patients with known bleeding tendencies or who are receiving other medications which may prolong bleeding time.

Voltaren may slow or delay healing.

Results from clinical studies indicate that Voltaren Ophthalmic has no significant effect upon ocular pressure; however, elevations in intraocular pressure may occur following cataract surgery.

Information for Patients

Except for the use of a bandage hydrogel soft contact lens during the first 3 days following refractive surgery, Voltaren Ophthalmic should not be used by patients currently wearing soft contact lenses due to adverse events that have occurred in other circumstances.

Carcinogenesis, Mutagenesis, Impairment of Fertility

Long-term carcinogenicity studies in rats given Voltaren in oral doses up to 2 mg/kg/day (approximately the human oral dose) revealed no significant increases in tumor incidence. There was a slight increase in benign rat mammary fibroadenomas in mid-dose females (high-dose females had excessive mortality) but the increase was not significant for this common rat tumor. A 2-year carcinogenicity study conducted in mice employing oral Voltaren up to 2 mg/kg/day did not reveal any oncogenic potential. Voltaren did not show mutagenic potential in various mutagenicity studies including the Ames test. Voltaren administered to male and female rats at 4 mg/kg/day did not affect fertility.

Pregnancy:

Teratogenic Effects

Pregnancy Category C. Reproduction studies performed in mice at oral doses up to 5,000 times (20 mg/kg/day) and in rats and rabbits at oral doses up to 2,500 times (10 mg/kg/day) the human topical dose have revealed no evidence of teratogenicity due to Voltaren despite the induction of maternal toxicity and fetal toxicity. In rats, maternally toxic doses were associated with dystocia, prolonged gestation, reduced fetal weights and growth, and reduced fetal survival. Voltaren has been shown to cross the placental barrier in mice and rats.

There are, however, no adequate and well-controlled studies in pregnant women. Because animal reproduction studies are not always predictive of human response, this drug should be used during pregnancy only if clearly needed.

Non-Teratogenic Effects

Because of the known effects of prostaglandin biosynthesis-inhibiting drugs on the fetal cardiovascular system (closure of ductus arteriosus), the use of Voltaren Ophthalmic during late pregnancy should be avoided.

Pediatric Use

Safety and effectiveness in pediatric patients have not been established.

Adverse Reactions: Ocular: Transient burning and stinging were reported in approximately 15% of patients across studies with the use of Voltaren Ophthalmic. In cataract surgery studies, keratitis was reported in up to 28% of patients receiving Voltaren Ophthalmic, although in many of these cases keratitis was initially noted prior to the initiation of treatment. Elevated intraocular pressure following cataract surgery was reported in approximately 15% of patients undergoing cataract surgery. Lacrimation complaints were reported in approximately 30% of case studies undergoing incisional refractive surgery.

The following adverse reactions were reported in approximately 5% or less of the patients: abnormal vision, acute elevated IOP, blurred vision, conjunctivitis, corneal deposits, corneal edema, corneal opacity, corneal lesions, discharge, eyelid swelling, injection, iritis, irritation, itching, lacrimation disorder and ocular allergy.

Systemic: The following adverse reactions were reported in 3% or less of the patients: abdominal pain, asthenia, chills, dizziness, facial edema, fever, headache, insomnia, nausea, pain, rhinitis, viral infection, and vomiting.

Overdosage: Overdosage will not ordinarily cause acute problems. If Voltaren Ophthalmic is accidentally ingested, fluids should be taken to dilute the medication.

Dosage and Administration: Cataract Surgery: One drop of Voltaren Ophthalmic should be applied to the affected eye, 4 times daily beginning 24 hours after cataract surgery and continuing throughout the first 2 weeks of the postoperative period.

Corneal Refractive Surgery: One or two drops of Voltaren Ophthalmic should be applied to the operative eye within the hour prior to corneal refractive surgery. Within 15 minutes after surgery, one or two drops should be applied to the operative eye and continued 4 times daily for up to 3 days.

How Supplied: Voltaren Ophthalmic 0.1% (1 mg/mL) Sterile Solution is supplied in dropper-tip, plastic, squeeze bottles in the following sizes:

Bottles of 2.5 mL	NDC 58768-100-02
Bottles of 5 mL	NDC 58768-100-05

Store between 59°–86°F (15°–30°C). Protect from light.

Dispense in original, unopened container only.

Rx Only

CS 665635B Printed in Canada (Rev. 7/98)

Made in Canada

Manufactured for:

CIBA Vision®

A Novartis Company

Duluth, Georgia 30097

Progress in Sight™

Shown in Product Identification Guide, page 105

ZADITOR™ ℞

[zăd-ə-tōr]

ketotifen fumarate ophthalmic solution, 0.025%

Description: ZADITOR™ is a sterile ophthalmic solution containing ketotifen for topical administration to the eyes. Ketotifen fumarate is a finely crystalline powder with an empirical formula of $C_{23}H_{23}NO_5S$ and a molecular weight of 425.50.

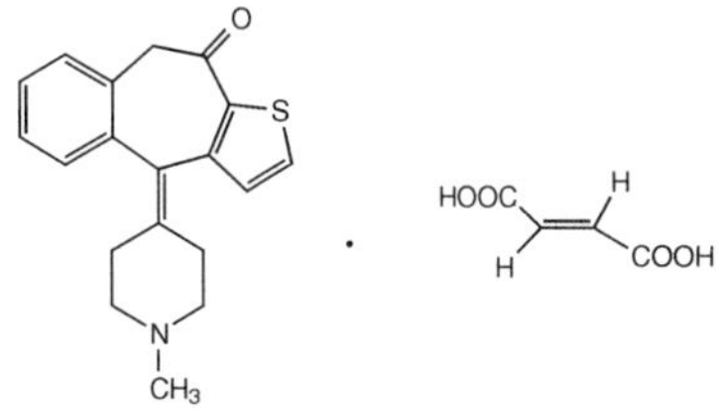

Established Name: Ketotifen Fumarate Ophthalmic Solution

Chemical Name: 4-(1-Methyl-4-piperidylidene)-4*H*-benzo[4,5]cyclohepta[1,2-*b*]thiophen-10(9*H*)-one hydrogen fumarate

Each mL of ZADITOR™ contains: **Active:** 0.345 mg ketotifen fumarate equivalent to 0.25 mg ketotifen. **Inactives:** glycerol, sodium hydroxide/hydrochloric acid (to adjust pH) and purified water. **Preservative:** benzalkonium chloride 0.01%. It has a pH of 4.4 to 5.8 and an osmolality of 210-300 mOsm/kg.

Clinical Pharmacology: Ketotifen is a relatively selective, non-competitive histamine antagonist (H1-receptor) and mast cell stabilizer. Ketotifen inhibits the release of mediators from cells involved in hypersensitivity reactions. Decreased chemotaxis and activation of eosinophils has also been demonstrated.

In human conjunctival allergen challenge studies, ZADITOR™ was significantly more effective than placebo in preventing ocular itching associated with allergic conjunctivitis. The action of ketotifen occurs rapidly with an effect seen within minutes after administration.

Indications And Usage: ZADITOR™ (ketotifen fumarate ophthalmic solution) is indicated for the temporary prevention of itching of the eye due to allergic conjunctivitis.

Contraindications: ZADITOR™ is contraindicated in persons with a known hypersensitivity to any component of this product.

Warnings: For topical ophthalmic use only. Not for injection or oral use.

Precautions:

Information for Patients: To prevent contaminating the dropper tip and solution, care should be taken not to touch the eyelids or surrounding areas with the dropper tip of the bottle. Keep the bottle tightly closed when not in use. Patients should be advised not to wear a contact lens if their eye is red. ZADITOR™ should not be used to treated contact lens related irritation. The preservative in ZADITOR™, benzalkonium chloride, may be absorbed by soft contact lenses. Patients who

Continued on next page

Zaditor—Cont.

wear soft contact lenses and whose eyes are not red, should be instructed to wait at least ten minutes after instilling ZADITOR™ before they insert their contact lenses.

Carcinogenesis, Mutagenesis, Impairment of Fertility:

Ketotifen fumarate was determined to be non-mutagenic in a battery of *in vitro* and *in vivo* mutagenicity assays including: Ames test, *in vitro* chromosomal aberration test with V79 Chinese hamster cells, *in vivo* micronucleus assay in mouse, and mouse dominant lethal test.

Treatment of male rats with oral doses of ketotifen ≥ 10 mg/kg/day orally [6,667 times the maximum recommended human ocular dose of 0.0015 mg/kg/day on a mg/kg basis (MRHOD)] for 70 days prior to mating resulted in mortality and a decrease in fertility. Treatment with ketotifen did not impair fertility in female rats receiving up to 50 mg/kg/day of ketotifen orally (33,333 times the MRHOD) for 15 days prior to mating.

Pregnancy: Pregnancy Category C

Oral treatment of pregnant rabbits during organogenesis with 45 mg/kg/day of ketotifen (30,000 the MRHOD) resulted in an increased incidence of retarded ossification of the sternebrae. However, no effects were observed in rabbits treated with up to 15 mg/kg/day (10,000 times the MRHOD). Similar treatment of rats during organogenesis with 100 mg/kg/day of ketotifen (66,667 times the MRHOD) did not reveal any biologically relevant effects.

Oral treatment of pregnant rats (up to 100 mg/kg/day or 66,667 times the MRHOD) and rabbits (up to 45 mg/kg/day or 30,000 times the MRHOD) during organogenesis did not result in any biologically relevant embryofetal toxicity. In the offspring of the rats that received ketotifen orally from day 15 of pregnancy to day 21 post partum at 50 mg/kg/day (33,333 times the MRHOD), a maternally toxic treatment protocol, the incidence of postnatal mortality was slightly increased, and body weight gain during the first four days post partum was slightly decreased.

Nursing Mothers:

Ketotifen fumarate has been identified in breast milk in rats following oral administration. It is not known whether topical ocular administration could result in sufficient systemic absorption to produce detectable quantities in breast milk. Nevertheless, caution should be exercised when ketotifen fumarate is administered to a nursing mother.

Pediatric Use: Safety and effectiveness in pediatric patients below the age of 3 years have not been established.

Adverse Reactions: In controlled clinical studies, conjunctival injection, headaches, and rhinitis were reported at an incidence of 10 to 25%. The occurrence of these side effects was generally mild. Some of these events were similar to the underlying ocular disease being studied.

The following ocular and non-ocular adverse reactions were reported at an incidence of less than 5%:

Ocular: Allergic reactions, burning or stinging, conjunctivitis, discharge, dry eye, eye pain, eyelid disorder, itching, keratitis, lacrimation disorder, mydriasis, photophobia, and rash.

Non-Ocular: Flu syndrome, pharyngitis.

Overdosage: Oral ingestion of the contents of a 5 mL bottle would be equivalent to 1.725 mg of ketotifen fumarate. Clinical results have shown no serious signs or symptoms after the ingestion of up to 20 mg of ketotifen fumarate.

Dosage And Administration: The recommended dose is one drop in the affected eye(s) every 8 to 12 hours.

How Supplied: ZADITOR™ is supplied as 5 mL solution in white 7.5 mL LDPE plastic bottles with controlled plastic dropper tips and white plastic caps.

NDC 58768-102-05

Storage

Store at 4°–25°C(39°–77°F).

Rx Only

Made in Canada by CIBA Vision Sterile Mfg. for

CIBA Vision®, A Novartis Company
Duluth, GA 30097

Shown in Product Identification Guide, page 105

Lederle Laboratories

Division American Cyanamid Company
PEARL RIVER, NY 10965

DIAMOX® ℞

[*di 'ah-moks*]

Acetazolamide Tablets USP and DIAMOX®
Sterile Acetazolamide Sodium USP Intravenous

Description: DIAMOX acetazolamide, an inhibitor of the enzyme carbonic anhydrase is a white to faintly yellowish white crystalline, odorless powder, weakly acidic, very slightly soluble in water and slightly soluble in alcohol. The chemical name for DIAMOX is *N*-(5-Sulfamoyl-1,3,4-thiadiazol-2yl)-acetamide. Its molecular weight is 222.24. Its chemical formula is $C_4H_6N_4O_3S_2$.

DIAMOX is available as oral tablets containing 125 mg and 250 mg of acetazolamide respectively and the following inactive ingredients: Corn Starch, Dibasic Calcium Phosphate, Magnesium Stearate, Povidone, and Sodium Starch Glycolate.

DIAMOX is also available for intravenous use, and is supplied as a sterile powder requiring reconstitution. Each vial contains an amount of acetazolamide sodium equivalent to 500 mg of acetazolamide. The bulk solution is adjusted to pH 9.2 using sodium hydroxide and, if necessary, hydrochloric acid prior to lyophilization.

Clinical Pharmacology: DIAMOX acetazolamide is a potent carbonic anhydrase inhibitor, effective in the control of fluid secretion (eg, some types of glaucoma), in the treatment of certain convulsive disorders (eg, epilepsy) and in the promotion of diuresis in instances of abnormal fluid retention (eg, cardiac edema).

DIAMOX is not a mercurial diuretic. Rather, it is a nonbacteriostatic sulfonamide possessing a chemical structure and pharmacological activity distinctly different from the bacteriostatic sulfonamides.

DIAMOX is an enzyme inhibitor that acts specifically on carbonic anhydrase, the enzyme that catalyzes the reversible reaction involving the hydration of carbon dioxide and the dehydration of carbonic acid. In the eye, this inhibitory action of acetazolamide decreases the secretion of aqueous humor and results in a drop in intraocular pressure, a reaction considered desirable in cases of glaucoma and even in certain nonglaucomatous conditions. Evidence seems to indicate that DIAMOX has utility as an adjuvant in the treatment of certain dysfunctions of the central nervous system (eg, epilepsy). Inhibition of carbonic anhydrase in this area appears to retard abnormal, paroxysmal, excessive discharge from central nervous system neurons. The diuretic effect of DIAMOX is due to its action in the kidney on the reversible reaction involving hydration of carbon dioxide and dehydration of carbonic acid. The result is renal loss of HCO_3 ion, which carries out sodium, water, and potassium. Alkalinization of the urine and promotion of diuresis are thus effected. Alteration in ammonia metabolism occurs due to increased reabsorption of ammonia by the renal tubules as a result of urinary alkalinization.

Placebo-controlled clinical trials have shown that prophylactic administration of DIAMOX at a dose of 250 mg every eight to 12 hours (or a 500 mg controlled-release capsule once daily) before and during rapid ascent to altitude results in fewer and/or less severe symptoms (such as headache, nausea, shortness of breath, dizziness, drowsiness, and fatigue) of acute mountain sickness (AMS). Pulmonary function (eg, minute ventilation, expired vital capacity, and peak flow) is greater in the DIAMOX treated group, both in subjects with AMS and asymptomatic subjects. The DIAMOX treated climbers also had less difficulty in sleeping.

Indications and Usage: For adjunctive treatment of: edema due to congestive heart failure; drug-induced edema; centrencephalic epilepsies (petit mal, unlocalized seizures); chronic simple (open-angle) glaucoma, secondary glaucoma, and preoperatively in acute angle-closure glaucoma where delay of surgery is desired in order to lower intraocular pressure. DIAMOX is also indicated for the prevention or amelioration of symptoms associated with acute mountain sickness in climbers attempting rapid ascent and in those who are very susceptible to acute mountain sickness despite gradual ascent.

Contraindications: DIAMOX acetazolamide therapy is contraindicated in situations in which sodium and/or potassium blood serum levels are depressed, in cases of marked kidney and liver disease or dysfunction, in suprarenal gland failure, and in hyperchloremic acidosis. It is contraindicated in patients with cirrhosis because of the risk of development of hepatic encephalopathy.

Long-term administration of DIAMOX is contraindicated in patients with chronic noncongestive angle-closure glaucoma since it may permit organic closure of the angle to occur while the worsening glaucoma is masked by lowered intraocular pressure.

Warnings: Fatalities have occurred, although rarely, due to severe reactions to sulfonamides including Stevens-Johnson syndrome, toxic epidermal necrolysis, fulminant hepatic necrosis, agranulocytosis, aplastic anemia, and other blood dyscrasias. Sensitizations may recur when a sulfonamide is readministered irrespective of the route of administration. If signs of hypersensitivity or other serious reactions occur, discontinue use of this drug.

Caution is advised for patients receiving concomitant high-dose aspirin and DIAMOX acetazolamide, as anorexia, tachypnea, lethargy, coma and death have been reported.

Precautions:

General

Increasing the dose does not increase the diuresis and may increase the incidence of drowsiness and/or paresthesia. Increasing the dose often results in a decrease in diuresis. Under certain circumstances, however, very large doses have been given in conjunction with other diuretics in order to secure diuresis in complete refractory failure.

Information for Patients

Adverse reactions common to all sulfonamide derivatives may occur: anaphylaxis, fever, rash (including erythema multiforme, Stevens-Johnson syndrome, toxic epidermal necrolysis), crystalluria, renal calculus, bone marrow depression, thrombocytopenic purpura, hemolytic anemia, leukopenia, pancytopenia, and agranulocytosis. Precaution is advised for early detection of such reactions, and the drug should be discontinued and appropriate therapy instituted.

In patients with pulmonary obstruction or emphysema where alveolar ventilation may be impaired, DIAMOX acetazolamide which may precipitate or aggravate acidosis, should be used with caution.

Gradual ascent is desirable to try to avoid acute mountain sickness. If rapid ascent is undertaken and DIAMOX is used, it should be noted that such use does not obviate the need for prompt descent if severe forms of high altitude sickness occur, ie, high altitude pulmonary edema (HAPE) or high altitude cerebral edema.

Caution is advised for patients receiving concomitant high-dose aspirin and DIAMOX acetazolamide, as anorexia, tachypnea, lethargy, coma and death have been reported (see **Warnings**).

Laboratory Tests

To monitor for hematologic reactions common to all sulfonamides, it is recommended that a baseline CBC and platelet count be obtained on patients prior to initiating DIAMOX therapy and at regular intervals during therapy. If significant changes occur, early discontinuance and institution of appropriate therapy are important. Periodic monitoring of serum electrolytes is recommended.

Carcinogenesis, Mutagenesis, Impairment of Fertility

Long-term studies in animals to evaluate the carcinogenic potential of DIAMOX acetazolamide have not been conducted. In a bacterial mutagenicity assay, DIAMOX was not mutagenic when evaluated with and without metabolic activation.

The drug had no effect on fertility when administered in the diet to male and female rats at a daily intake of up to 4 times the recommended human dose of 1000 mg in a 50 kg individual.

Pregnancy: Pregnancy Category C

Acetazolamide, administered orally or parenterally, has been shown to be teratogenic (defects of the limbs) in mice, rats, hamsters, and rabbits. There are no adequate and well-controlled studies in pregnant women. Acetazolamide should be used in pregnancy only if the potential benefit justifies the potential risk to the fetus.

Nursing Mothers

Because of the potential for serious adverse reaction in nursing infants from DIAMOX, a decision should be made whether to discontinue nursing or to discontinue the drug, taking into account the importance of the drug to the mother.

Pediatric Use

The safety and effectiveness of DIAMOX in pediatric patients have not been established.

Adverse Reactions: Adverse reactions, occurring most often early in therapy, include paresthesias, particularly a "tingling" feeling in the extremities, hearing dysfunction or tinnitus, loss of appetite, taste alteration and gastrointestinal disturbances such as nausea, vomiting and diarrhea; polyuria, and occasional instances of drowsiness and confusion. Metabolic acidosis and electrolyte imbalance may occur.

Transient myopia has been reported. This condition invariably subsides upon diminution or discontinuance of the medication.

Other occasional adverse reactions include urticaria, melena, hematuria, glycosuria, hepatic insufficiency, flaccid paralysis, photosensitivity and convulsions. Also see **Precautions, Information for Patients** for possible reactions common to sulfonamide derivatives. Fatalities have occurred although rarely, due to severe reactions to sulfonamides including Stevens-Johnson syndrome, toxic epidermal necrolysis, fulminant hepatic necrosis, agranulocytosis, aplastic anemia and other blood dyscrasias (see **Warnings**).

Overdosage: No data are available regarding DIAMOX overdosage in humans as no cases of acute poisoning with this drug have been reported. Animal data suggest that DIAMOX is remarkably nontoxic. No specific antidote is known. Treatment should be symptomatic and supportive.

Electrolyte imbalance, development of an acidotic state, and central nervous effects might be expected to occur. Serum electrolyte levels (particularly potassium) and blood pH levels should be monitored.

Supportive measures are required to restore electrolyte and pH balance. The acidotic state can usually be corrected by the administration of bicarbonate.

Despite its high intraerythrocytic distribution and plasma protein binding properties, DIAMOX may be dialyzable. This may be particularly important in the management of DIAMOX overdosage when complicated by the presence of renal failure.

Dosage and Administration: Preparation and Storage of Parenteral Solution

Each 500 mg vial containing DIAMOX sterile acetazolamide sodium parenteral should be reconstituted with at least 5 mL of Sterile Water for Injection prior to use. Reconstituted solutions retain their physical and chemical properties for 3 days under refrigeration at 2° to 8°C (36° to 46°F), or 12 hours at room temperature 15° to 30°C (59° to 86°F). CONTAINS NO PRESERVATIVE. The direct intravenous route of administration is preferred. Intramuscular administration is not recommended.

Glaucoma: DIAMOX should be used as an adjunct to the usual therapy. The dosage employed in the treatment of *chronic simple (open-angle) glaucoma* ranges from 250 mg to 1 g of DIAMOX per 24 hours, usually in divided doses for amounts over 250 mg. It has usually been found that a dosage in excess of 1 g per 24 hours does not produce an increased effect. In all cases, the dosage should be adjusted with careful individual attention both to symptomatology and ocular tension. Continuous supervision by a physician is advisable.

In treatment of secondary glaucoma and in the preoperative treatment of some cases of *acute congestive (closed-angle) glaucoma,* the preferred dosage is 250 mg every four hours, although some cases have responded to 250 mg twice daily on short-term therapy. In some acute cases, it may be more satisfactory to administer an initial dose of 500 mg followed by 125 or 250 mg every four hours depending on the individual case. Intravenous therapy may be used for rapid relief of ocular tension in acute cases. A complementary effect has been noted when DIAMOX has been used in conjunction with miotics or mydriatics as the case demanded.

Epilepsy: It is not clearly known whether the beneficial effects observed in epilepsy are due to direct inhibition of carbonic anhydrase in the central nervous system or whether they are due to the slight degree of acidosis produced by the divided dosage. The best results to date have been seen in petit mal in pediatric patients. Good results, however, have been seen in patients, both pediatric patients and adult, in other types of seizures such as grand mal, mixed seizure patterns, myoclonic jerk patterns, etc. The suggested total daily dose is 8 to 30 mg per kg in divided doses. Although some patients respond to a low dose, the optimum range appears to be from 375 to 1000 mg daily. However, some investigators feel that daily doses in excess of 1 g do not produce any better results than a 1 g dose. When DIAMOX is given in combination with other anticonvulsants, it is suggested that the starting dose should be 250 mg once daily in addition to the existing medications. This can be increased to levels as indicated above.

The change from other medications to DIAMOX should be gradual and in accordance with usual practice in epilepsy therapy.

Congestive Heart Failure: For diuresis in congestive heart failure, the starting dose is usually 250 to 375 mg once daily in the morning (5 mg/kg). If, after an initial response, the patient fails to continue to lose edema fluid, do not increase the dose but allow for kidney recovery by skipping medication for a day. DIAMOX acetazolamide yields best diuretic results when given on alternate days, or for two days alternating with a day of rest.

Failures in therapy may be due to overdosage or too frequent dosage. The use of DIAMOX does not eliminate the need for other therapy such as digitalis, bed rest, and salt restriction.

Drug-Induced Edema: Recommended dosage is 250 to 375 mg of DIAMOX once a day for one or two days, alternating with a day of rest.

Acute Mountain Sickness: Dosage is 500 mg to 1000 mg daily, in divided doses using tablets or sustained-release capsules as appropriate. In circumstances of rapid ascent, such as in rescue or military operations, the higher dose level of 1000 mg is recommended. It is preferable to initiate dosing 24 to 48 hours before ascent and to continue for 48 hours while at high altitude, or longer as necessary to control symptoms.

Note: The dosage recommendations for glaucoma and epilepsy differ considerably from those for congestive heart failure, since the first two conditions are not dependent upon carbonic anhydrase inhibition in the kidney which requires intermittent dosage if it is to recover from the inhibitory effect of the therapeutic agent.

Parenteral drug products should be inspected visually for particulate matter and discoloration prior to administration, whenever solution and container permit.

How Supplied:

DIAMOX® acetazolamide Tablets

125 mg–Round, flat-faced, beveled, white tablets engraved with DIAMOX and 125 on one side and scored in half on the other side. Engraved with LL on the right of the score and D1 on the left, are supplied as follows:

NDC 0005-4398-23—Bottle of 100

250 mg—Round, convex, white tablets engraved with DIAMOX and 250 on one side and scored in quarters on the other side. Engraved with LL in the upper right quadrant and D2 in the lower left quadrant, are supplied as follows:

NDC 0005-4469-23—Bottle of 100
NDC 0005-4469-34—Bottle of 1000
NDC 0005-4469-60—Unit Dose 10 × 10s

Store at controlled room temperature 15°–30°C (59°–86°F).

Manufactured by:
LEDERLE PHARMACEUTICAL DIVISION
American Cyanamid Company
Pearl River, NY 10965

DIAMOX® Sterile acetazolamide sodium, Intravenous

Sterile intravenous (lyophilized) powder.
NDC 0005-4466-96—500 mg Vial

Store at controlled room temperature 15°–30°C (59°–86° F).

Manufactured by:
LEDERLE PARENTERALS, INC.
Carolina, Puerto Rico 00987

Shown in Product Identification Guide, page 105

Continued on next page

DIAMOX® SEQUELS® ℞
Acetazolamide
Sustained-Release Capsules

Description: DIAMOX acetazolamide is an inhibitor of the enzyme carbonic anhydrase. DIAMOX is a white to faintly yellowish white crystalline, odorless powder, weakly acidic, very slightly soluble in water and slightly soluble in alcohol. The chemical name for DIAMOX is *N*-(5-Sulfamoyl-1,3,4-thiadiazol-2-yl) acetamide. Its molecular weight is 222.24. Its chemical formula is $C_4H_6N_4O_3S_2$.
DIAMOX SEQUELS are sustained-release capsules, for oral administration, each containing 500 mg of acetazolamide and the following inactive ingredients: Ethyl Vanillin, FD&C Blue No. 1, FD&C Yellow No. 6, Gelatin, Glycerin, Microcrystalline Cellulose, Methylparaben, Propylene Glycol, Propylparaben, Silicon Dioxide, and Sodium Lauryl Sulfate.

Clinical Pharmacology: DIAMOX is a potent carbonic anhydrase inhibitor, effective in the control of fluid secretion (eg, some types of glaucoma), in the treatment of certain convulsive disorders (eg, epilepsy) and in the promotion of diuresis in instances of abnormal fluid retention (eg, cardiac edema).
DIAMOX is not a mercurial diuretic. Rather, it is a nonbacteriostatic sulfonamide possessing a chemical structure and pharmacological activity distinctly different from the bacteriostatic sulfonamides.
DIAMOX is an enzyme inhibitor that acts specifically on carbonic anhydrase, the enzyme which catalyzes the reversible reaction involving the hydration of carbon dioxide and the dehydration of carbonic acid. In the eye, this inhibitory action of acetazolamide decreases the secretion of aqueous humor and results in a drop in intraocular pressure, a reaction considered desirable in cases of glaucoma and even in certain nonglaucomatous conditions. Evidence seems to indicate that DIAMOX has utility as an adjuvant in the treatment of certain dysfunctions of the central nervous system (eg, epilepsy). Inhibition of carbonic anhydrase in this area appears to retard abnormal, paroxysmal, excessive discharge from central nervous system neurons. The diuretic effect of DIAMOX acetazolamide is due to its action in the kidney on the reversible reaction involving hydration of carbon dioxide and dehydration of carbonic acid. The result is renal loss of HCO_3 ion, which carries out sodium, water, and potassium. Alkalinization of the urine and promotion of diuresis are thus effected. Alteration in ammonia metabolism occurs due to increased reabsorption of ammonia by the renal tubules as a result of urinary alkalinization.
DIAMOX acetazolamide SEQUELS sustained-release capsules provide prolonged action to inhibit aqueous humor secretion for 18 to 24 hours after each dose, whereas tablets act for only eight to 12 hours. The prolonged continuous effect of SEQUELS permits a reduction in dosage frequency.
Plasma concentrations of acetazolamide peak between three to six hours after administration of DIAMOX SEQUELS, compared to one to four hours with tablets. Food does not affect the bioavailability of DIAMOX SEQUELS.
Placebo-controlled clinical trials have shown that prophylactic administration of DIAMOX at a dose of 250 mg every eight to 12 hours (or a 500 mg controlled-release capsule once daily) before and during rapid ascent to altitude results in fewer and/or less severe symptoms (such as headache, nausea, shortness of breath, dizziness, drowsiness, and fatigue) of acute mountain sickness (AMS). Pulmonary function (eg, minute ventilation, expired vital capacity, and peak flow) is greater in the DIAMOX treated group, both in subjects with AMS and asymptomatic subjects. The DIAMOX treated climbers also had less difficulty in sleeping.

Indications and Usage: For adjunctive treatment of: chronic simple (open-angle) glaucoma, secondary glaucoma, and preoperatively in acute angle-closure glaucoma where delay of surgery is desired in order to lower intraocular pressure. DIAMOX is also indicated for the prevention or amelioration of symptoms associated with acute mountain sickness in climbers attempting rapid ascent and in those who are very susceptible to acute mountain sickness despite gradual ascent.

Contraindications: Acetazolamide therapy is contraindicated in situations in which sodium and/or potassium blood serum levels are depressed, in cases of marked kidney and liver disease or dysfunction, in suprarenal gland failure, and in hyperchloremic acidosis. It is contraindicated in patients with cirrhosis because of the risk of development of hepatic encephalopathy.
Long-term administration of DIAMOX acetazolamide is contraindicated in patients with chronic noncongestive angle-closure glaucoma since it may permit organic closure of the angle to occur while the worsening glaucoma is masked by lowered intraocular pressure.

Warnings: Fatalities have occurred, although rarely, due to severe reactions to sulfonamides including Stevens-Johnson syndrome, toxic epidermal necrolysis, fulminant hepatic necrosis, agranulocytosis, aplastic anemia, and other blood dyscrasias. Sensitizations may recur when a sulfonamide is readministered irrespective of the route of administration. If signs of hypersensitivity or other serious reactions occur, discontinue use of this drug.
Caution is advised for patients receiving concomitant high-dose aspirin and DIAMOX acetazolamide, as anorexia, tachypnea, lethargy, coma and death have been reported.

Precautions:

General

Increasing the dose does not increase the diuresis and may increase the incidence of drowsiness and/or paresthesia. Increasing the dose often results in a decrease in diuresis. Under certain circumstances, however, very large doses have been given in conjunction with other diuretics in order to secure diuresis in complete refractory failure.

Information for Patient

Adverse reactions common to all sulfonamide derivatives may occur: anaphylaxis, fever, rash (including erythema multiforme, Stevens-Johnson syndrome, toxic epidermal necrolysis), crystalluria, renal calculus, bone marrow depression, thrombocytopenic purpura, hemolytic anemia, leukopenia, pancytopenia and agranulocytosis. Precaution is advised for early detection of such reactions and the drug should be discontinued and appropriate therapy instituted.
In patients with pulmonary obstruction or emphysema where alveolar ventilation may be impaired, DIAMOX acetazolamide which may aggravate acidosis, should be used with caution.
Gradual ascent is desirable to try to avoid acute mountain sickness. If rapid ascent is undertaken and DIAMOX is used, it should be noted that such use does not obviate the need for prompt descent if severe forms of high altitude sickness occur, ie, high altitude pulmonary edema (HAPE) or high altitude cerebral edema.
Caution is advised for patients receiving concomitant high-dose aspirin and DIAMOX acetazolamide, as anorexia, tachypnea, lethargy, coma and death have been reported (see **Warnings**).

Laboratory Tests

To monitor for hematologic reactions common to all sulfonamides, it is recommended that a baseline CBC and platelet count be obtained on patients prior to initiating DIAMOX therapy and at regular intervals during therapy. If significant changes occur, early discontinuance and institution of appropriate therapy are important. Periodic monitoring of serum electrolytes is recommended.

Carcinogenesis, Mutagenesis, Impairment of Fertility

Long-term studies in animals to evaluate the carcinogenic potential of DIAMOX acetazolamide have not been conducted. In a bacterial mutagenicity assay, DIAMOX was not mutagenic when evaluated with and without metabolic activation. The drug had no effect on fertility when administered in the diet to male and female rats at a daily intake of up to 4 times the maximum recommended human dose of 1000 mg in a 50 kg individual.

Pregnancy Category C

Acetazolamide, administered orally or parenterally, has been shown to be teratogenic (defects of the limbs) in mice, rats, hamsters and rabbits. There are no adequate and well-controlled studies in pregnant women. Acetazolamide should be used in pregnancy only if the potential benefit justifies the potential risk to the fetus.

Nursing Mothers

Because of the potential for serious adverse reactions in nursing infants from DIAMOX, a decision should be made whether to discontinue nursing or to discontinue the drug taking into account the importance of the drug to the mother.

Pediatric Use

The safety and effectiveness of DIAMOX in pediatric patients have not been established.

Adverse Reactions: Adverse reactions, occurring most often early in therapy, include paresthesias, particularly a "tingling" feeling in the extremities, hearing dysfunction or tinnitus, loss of appetite, taste alteration and gastrointestinal disturbances such as nausea, vomiting and diarrhea; polyuria, and occasional instances of drowsiness and confusion. Metabolic acidosis and electrolyte imbalance may occur.
Transient myopia has been reported. This condition invariably subsides upon diminution or discontinuance of the medication.
Other occasional adverse reactions include urticaria, melena, hematuria, glycosuria, hepatic insufficiency, flaccid paralysis, photosensitivity and convulsions. Also see **Precautions: Information for Patients** for possible reactions common to sulfonamide derivatives. Fatalities have occurred although rarely, due to severe reactions to sulfonamides including Stevens-Johnson syndrome, toxic epidermal necrolysis, fulminant hepatic necrosis, agranulocytosis, aplastic anemia and other blood dyscrasias (see **Warnings**).

Overdosage: No data are available regarding DIAMOX overdosage in humans as no cases of acute poisoning with this drug have been reported. Animal data suggest that DIAMOX is remarkably nontoxic. No specific antidote is known. Treatment should be symptomatic and supportive.
Electrolyte imbalance, development of an acidotic state, and central nervous effects might be expected to occur. Serum electrolyte levels (particularly potassium) and blood pH levels should be monitored.
Supportive measures are required to restore electrolyte and pH balance. The acidotic state can usually be corrected by the administration of bicarbonate.
Despite its high intraerythrocytic distribution and plasma protein binding properties, DIAMOX may be dialyzable. This may be particu-

larly important in the management of DIAMOX overdosage when complicated by the presence of renal failure.

Dosage and Administration:

Glaucoma

The recommended dosage is 1 capsule (500 mg) two times a day. Usually 1 capsule is administered in the morning and 1 capsule in the evening. It may be necessary to adjust the dose, but it has usually been found that dosage in excess of 2 capsules (1 g) does not produce an increased effect. The dosage should be adjusted with careful individual attention both to symptomatology and intraocular tension. In all cases, continuous supervision by a physician is advisable.

In those unusual instances where adequate control is not obtained by the twice-a-day administration of DIAMOX acetazolamide SEQUELS sustained-release capsules, the desired control may be established by means of DIAMOX (tablets or parenteral). Use tablets or parenteral in accordance with the more frequent dosage schedules recommended for these dosage forms, such as 250 mg every four hours, or an initial dose of 500 mg followed by 250 mg or 125 mg every four hours, depending on the case in question.

Acute Mountain Sickness

Dosage is 500 mg to 1000 mg daily, in divided doses using tablets or sustained-release capsules as appropriate. In circumstances of rapid ascent, such as in rescue or military operations, the higher dose level of 1000 mg is recommended. It is preferable to initiate dosing 24 to 48 hours before ascent and to continue for 48 hours while at high altitude, or longer as necessary to control symptoms.

How Supplied: DIAMOX® acetazolamide SEQUELS®, 500 mg orange capsules printed with DIAMOX over D3 are supplied as follows:

NDC 0005-0753-23—Bottle of 100

Store at controlled room temperature 15°–30°C (59°–86°F).

Manufactured by:
LEDERLE PHARMACEUTICAL DIVISION
American Cyanamid Company
Pearl River, NY 10965

Shown in Product Identification Guide, page 105

NEPTAZANE® ℞

[*nĕp-ta 'zāne*]

Methazolamide Tablets, USP

Description: NEPTAZANE (methazolamide), a sulfonamide derivative, is a white crystalline powder, weakly acidic, slightly soluble in water, alcohol and acetone. The chemical name for methazolamide is: *N*-[5-(aminosulfonyl)-3-methyl-1,3,4-thiadiazol-2 (3*H*)-ylidene]-acetamide. Its molecular weight is 236.26. Its chemical formula is $C_5H_8N_4O_3S_2$.

NEPTAZANE is available for oral administration as 25 mg and 50 mg tablets containing the following inactive ingredients: Acacia, Alginic Acid, Corn Starch, Dibasic Calcium Phosphate, Gelatin, and Magnesium Stearate.

Clinical Pharmacology: NEPTAZANE is a potent inhibitor of carbonic anhydrase.

NEPTAZANE is well absorbed from the gastrointestinal tract. Peak plasma concentrations are observed 1 to 2 hours after dosing. In a multiple-dose, pharmacokinetic study, administration of NEPTAZANE 25 mg BID, 50 mg BID, and 100 mg BID demonstrated a linear relationship between plasma methazolamide levels and NEPTAZANE dose. Peak plasma concentrations (C_{max}) for the 25 mg, 50 mg, and 100 mg BID regimens were 2.5 mcg/mL, 5.1 mcg/mL, and 10.7 mcg/mL, respectively. The areas under the plasma concentration-time curves (AUC) were 1130 mcg.min/mL, 2571 mcg.min/mL, and 5418 mcg.min/mL for the 25 mg, 50 mg and 100 mg dosage regimens, respectively.

NEPTAZANE is distributed throughout the body including the plasma, cerebrospinal fluid, aqueous humor of the eye, red blood cells,bile and extra-cellular fluid. The mean apparent volume of distribution (V_{area}/F) ranges from 17 to 23 L. Approximately 55% is bound to plasma proteins. The steady-state NEPTAZANE red blood cell: plasma ratio varies with dose and was found to be 27:1, 16:1, and 10:1 following the administration of NEPTAZANE 25 mg BID, 50 mg BID and 100 mg BID, respectively.

The mean steady-state plasma elimination half-life for NEPTAZANE is approximately 14 hours. At steady-state approximately 25% of the dose is recovered unchanged in the urine over the dosing interval. Renal clearance accounts for 20–25% of the total clearance of drug. After repeated BID-TID dosing, NEPTAZANE accumulates to steady state concentrations in 7 days.

Methazolamide's inhibitory action on carbonic anhydrase decreases the secretion of aqueous humor and results in a decrease in intraocular pressure. The onset of the decrease in intraocular pressure generally occurs within two to four hours, has a peak effect in six to eight hours, and a total duration of ten to eighteen hours.

NEPTAZANE is a sulfonamide derivative; however, it does not have any clinically significant antimicrobial properties. Although NEPTAZANE achieves a high concentration in the cerebrospinal fluid, it is not considered an effective anticonvulsant.

NEPTAZANE has a weak and transient diuretic effect, therefore use results in an increase in urinary volume, with excretion of sodium, potassium, and chloride. The drug should not be used as a diuretic. Inhibition of renal bicarbonate reabsorption produces an alkaline urine. Plasma bicarbonate decreases, and a relative, transient metabolic acidosis may occur due to a disequilibrium in carbon dioxide transport in the red cell. Urinary citrate excretion is decreased by approximately 40% after doses of 100 mg every 8 hours. Uric acid output has been shown to decrease 36% in the first 24 hour period.

Indications and Usage: NEPTAZANE is indicated in the treatment of ocular conditions where lowering intraocular pressure is likely to be of therapeutic benefit, such as chronic open-angle glaucoma, secondary glaucoma, and preoperatively in acute angle-closure glaucoma where lowering the intraocular pressure is desired before surgery.

Contraindications: NEPTAZANE therapy is contraindicated in situations in which sodium and/or potassium serum levels are depressed, in cases of marked kidney or liver disease or dysfunction, in adrenal gland failure, and in hyperchloremic acidosis. In patients with cirrhosis, use may precipitate the development of hepatic encephalopathy.

Long-term administration of NEPTAZANE is contraindicated in patients with angle-closure glaucoma, since organic closure of the angle may occur in spite of lowered intraocular pressure.

Warnings: Fatalities have occurred, although rarely, due to severe reactions to sulfonamides including Stevens-Johnson syndrome, toxic epidermal necrolysis, fulminant hepatic necrosis, agranulocytosis, aplastic anemia, and other blood dyscrasias. Hypersensitivity reactions may recur when a sulfonamide is readministered, irrespective of the route of administration.

If hypersensitivity or other serious reactions occur, the use of this drug should be discontinued.

Caution is advised for patients receiving high-dose aspirin and NEPTAZANE concomitantly, as anorexia, tachypnea, lethargy, coma, and death have been reported with concomitant use of high-dose aspirin and carbonic anhydrase inhibitors.

Precautions:

General

Potassium excretion is increased initially upon administration of NEPTAZANE and in patients with cirrhosis or hepatic insufficiency could precipitate a hepatic coma.

In patients with pulmonary obstruction or emphysema, where alveolar ventilation may be impaired NEPTAZANE should be used with caution because it may precipitate or aggravate acidosis.

Information for Patients

Adverse reactions common to all sulfonamide derivatives may occur: anaphylaxis, fever, rash (including erythema multiforme, Stevens-Johnson syndrome, toxic epidermal necrolysis), crystalluria, renal calculus, bone marrow depression, thrombocytopenic purpura, hemolytic anemia, leukopenia, pancytopenia, and agranulocytosis. Precaution is advised for early detection of such reactions and the drug should be discontinued and appropriate therapy instituted.

Caution is advised for patients receiving high-dose aspirin and NEPTAZANE concomitantly.

Laboratory Tests

To monitor for hematologic reactions common to all sulfonamides, it is recommended that a baseline CBC and platelet count be obtained on patients prior to initiating NEPTAZANE therapy and at regular intervals during therapy. If significant changes occur, early discontinuance and institution of appropriate therapy are important. Periodic monitoring of serum electrolytes is also recommended.

Drug Interactions

NEPTAZANE should be used with caution in patients on steroid therapy because of the potential for developing hypokalemia.

Caution is advised for patients receiving high-dose aspirin and NEPTAZANE concomitantly, as anorexia, tachypnea, lethargy, coma, and death have been reported with concomitant use of high-dose aspirin and carbonic anhydrase inhibitors (see **Warnings**).

Carcinogenesis, Mutagenesis, Impairment of Fertility

Long-term studies in animals to evaluate NEPTAZANE's carcinogenic potential and its effect on fertility have not been conducted. NEPTAZANE was not mutagenic in the Ames bacterial test.

Pregnancy

Teratogenic Effects. Pregnancy Category C.

NEPTAZANE has been shown to be teratogenic (skeletal anomalies) in rats when given in doses approximately 40 times the human dose. There are no adequate and well-controlled studies in pregnant women. NEPTAZANE should be used during pregnancy only if the potential benefit justifies the potential risk to the fetus.

Nursing Mothers

It is not known whether this drug is excreted in human milk. Because many drugs are excreted in human milk and because of the potential for serious adverse reactions in nursing infants from NEPTAZANE, a decision should be made whether to discontinue nursing or to discontinue the drug, taking into account the importance of the drug to the mother.

Pediatric Use

The safety and effectiveness of NEPTAZANE in pediatric patients have not been established.

Adverse Reactions: Adverse reactions, occurring most often early in therapy, include paresthesias, particularly a "tingling" feeling in the extremities; hearing dysfunction or tinnitus; fatigue; malaise; loss of appetite; taste

Continued on next page

Neptazane—Cont.

alteration; gastrointestinal disturbances such as nausea, vomiting and diarrhea; polyuria; and occasional instances of drowsiness and confusion.
Metabolic acidosis and electrolyte imbalance may occur.
Transient myopia has been reported. This condition invariably subsides upon diminution or discontinuance of the medication.
Other occasional adverse reactions include urticaria, melena, hematuria, glycosuria, hepatic insufficiency, flaccid paralysis, photosensitivity, convulsions, and rarely, crystalluria and renal calculi. Also see **Precautions: Information for Patients** for possible reactions common to sulfonamide derivatives. Fatalities have occurred, although rarely, due to severe reactions to sulfonamides including Stevens-Johnson syndrome, toxic epidermal necrolysis, fulminant hepatic necrosis, agranulocytosis, aplastic anemia, and other blood dyscrasias (see **Warnings).**
Overdosage: No data are available regarding NEPTAZANE overdosage in humans as no cases of acute poisoning with this drug have been reported. Animal data suggest that even a high dose of NEPTAZANE is nontoxic. No specific antidote is known. Treatment should be symptomatic and supportive.
Electrolyte imbalance, development of an acidotic state, and central nervous system effects might be expected to occur. Serum electrolyte levels (particularly potassium) and blood pH levels should be monitored.
Supportive measures may be required to restore electrolyte and pH balance.
Dosage and Administration: The effective therapeutic dose administered varies from 50 mg to 100 mg 2–3 times daily. The drug may be used concomitantly with miotic and osmotic agents.
How Supplied: NEPTAZANE® (methazolamide) Tablets, USP, 25 mg, are square white tablets with engraved N2 on one side and embossed large N on the other side, supplied as follows:
NDC 0005-4565-23—Bottle of 100
NEPTAZANE® (methazolamide) Tablets, USP, 50 mg, are round white scored tablets engraved with LL on one side and N above and 1 below the score on the other side, supplied as follows:
NDC 0005-4570-23—Bottle of 100
NEPTAZANE (methazolamide) is not available for parenteral use.
Store at controlled room temperature 15°–30°C (59°–86°F).
Manufactured by:
LEDERLE PHARMACEUTICAL DIVISION
American Cyanamid Company
Pearl River, NY 10965

Shown in Product Identification Guide, page 105

Refer to Section 8
for information on
Pharmaceutical Products.

Medical Ophthalmics, Inc.

**40146 U.S. HWY. 19 N.
TARPON SPRINGS, FL 34689**

Direct Inquiries to:
(800)358-7797

Product

Proparacaine 0.5% ℞
Proparacaine HCl 0.5% sterile ophthalmic solution.
15 mL NDC #53012-207-15

Napha-Forte 0.1% ℞
Naphazoline HCl sterile ophthalmic solution.
15 mL NDC #53012-230-15

Bacitracin Ointment ℞
Bacitracin sterile ophthalmic ointment.
3.5 gm NDC #53012-255-35

Polytracin Ointment ℞
Bacitracin, Polymyxin b sterile ophthalmic ointment.
3.5 gm NDC #53012-215-35

Erythromycin Ointment ℞
Erythromycin 0.5% sterile ophthalmic ointment.
3.5 gm NDC #53012-244-35

Gentamicin Sulfate 0.3% ℞
Gentamicin 0.3% sterile ophthalmic solution.
5 mL NDC #53012-216-05

Gentamicin Sulfate Ointment ℞
Gentamicin Sulfate 0.3% sterile ophthalmic ointment.
3.5 gm NDC #53012-217-35

Polymycin ℞
Neomycin, Polymyxin b, Gramicidin sterile ophthalmic solution.
10 mL NDC #53012-218-10

Polymycin Ointment ℞
Neomycin, Polymyxin b, Bacitracin sterile ophthalmic ointment.
3.5 gm NDC #53012-219-35

Sulfacetamide 10% ℞
Sulfacetamide Sodium 10% sterile ophthalmic solution.
15 mL NDC #53012-210-15

Sulfacetamide Ointment ℞
Sulfacetamide Sodium 10% sterile ophthalmic ointment.
3.5 gm NDC #53012-212-35

Neodexasone ℞
Dexamethasone Phosphate, Neomycin sterile ophthalmic solution.
5 mL NDC #53012-246-05

Neopolydex ℞
Dexamethasone, Neomycin, Polymyxin b sterile ophthalmic suspension.
5 mL NDC #53012-220-05

Neopolydex Ointment ℞
Dexamethasone, Neomycin, Polymyxin b sterile ophthalmic ointment.
3.5 gm NDC #53012-221-35

Cortimycin ℞
Hydrocortisone, Neomycin, Polymyxin b sterile ophthalmic suspension.
7.5 mL NDC #53012-225-75

Cortimycin Ointment ℞
Hydrocortisone, Neomycin, Bacitracin, Polymyxin b sterile ophthalmic ointment.
3.5 gm NDC #53012-224-35

Sulfamide ℞
Prednisolone acetate 0.5%, Sulfacetamide Sodium 10%, sterile ophthalmic suspension.
5 mL NDC #53012-222-05

Sulfamide Ointment ℞
Prednisolone acetate 0.5%, Sulfacetamide Sodium 10% sterile ophthalmic ointment.
3.5 gm NDC #53012-223-35

Dexamethasone 0.1% ℞
Dexamethasone Phosphate sterile ophthalmic solution.
5 mL NDC #53012-229-05

Pred-Phosphate 1/8% ℞
Prednisolone Phosphate sterile ophthalmic solution.
5 mL NDC #53012-227-05

Pred-Phosphate 1% ℞
Prednisolone Phosphate sterile ophthalmic solution.
5 mL NDC #53012-228-05

Fluorox ℞
Fluorescein Sodium, Benoxinate, sterile ophthalmic solution.
5 mL NDC #53012-265-05

Fluorocaine ℞
Fluorescein Sodium 0.25%, Proparacaine 0.5%, HCl sterile ophthalmic solution.
5 mL NDC #53012-209-05

Lacri-Tears
Hydroxypropyl methylcellulose, Dextran sterile ophthalmic solution.
15 mL NDC #53012-231-15

Lacri-Gel
(Preservative Free)
Petrolatum, mineral oil, Lanolin sterile ophthalmic ointment.
3.5 gm NDC #53012-235-35

Pilocarpine 1% ℞
Pilocarpine HCl sterile ophthalmic solution.
15 mL NDC #53012-236-15

Pilocarpine 2% ℞
Pilocarpine HCl sterile ophthalmic solution.
15 mL NDC #53012-237-15

Pilocarpine 4% ℞
Pilocarpine HCl sterile ophthalmic solution.
15 mL NDC #53012-239-15

Lubefree Petrolatum, Mineral Oil Lubricant
Sterile Ophthalmic Ointment
3.5 gm NDC #53012-234-35

NACL 5%
Sodium Chloride sterile ophthalmic solution.
15 mL NDC #53012-233-15

NACL Ointment
Sodium Chloride sterile ophthalmic ointment.
3.5 gm NDC #53012-232-35

Eye Wash
Isotonic buffered irrigation solution. sterile ophthalmic solution.
4 fl. oz.

Atropine 1% ℞
Atropine Sulfate sterile ophthalmic solution.
5 mL NDC #53012-206-05

Cyclopentolate 1% ℞
Cyclopentolate HCl sterile ophthalmic solution.
2 mL NDC #53012-202-02
15 mL NDC #53012-202-15

Homatropine 5% ℞
Homatropine sterile ophthalmic solution.
5 mL NDC #53012-205-05

Phenylephrine 2.5% ℞
Phenylephrine HCl sterile ophthalmic solution.
15 mL NDC #53012-201-15

Tropicamide 0.5% ℞
Tropicamide sterile ophthalmic solution.
15 mL NDC #53012-203-15

Tropicamide 1% ℞
Tropicamide sterile ophthalmic solution.
15 mL NDC #53012-204-15

MaxiVision® **OTC**
Multivitamin, multimineral, multinutrient, colloidal minerals. Liquid suspension.
33.5 oz Clear plastic bottle.

MaxiVision® Whole Body Formula **OTC**
Multivitamin, multimineral, multinutrient, plant derived chelated minerals, antioxidants. Powdered capsules.
120 caps brown plastic bottle.

MaxiVision® Ocular Formula **OTC**
Multivitamin, multimineral, multinutrient, antioxidant. Powdered capsules.
60 caps brown plastic bottle.

Merck & Co., Inc.
WEST POINT, PA 19486

CHIBROXIN® ℞
(Norfloxacin), U.S.P.
Sterile Ophthalmic Solution

Description
CHIBROXIN* (Norfloxacin) Ophthalmic Solution is a synthetic broad-spectrum antibacterial agent supplied as a sterile isotonic solution for topical ophthalmic use. Norfloxacin, a fluoroquinolone, is 1-ethyl-6-fluoro-1,4-dihydro-4-oxo-7-(1-piperazinyl) -3- quinoline-carboxylic acid. Its empirical formula is $C_{16}H_{18}FN_3O_3$ and the structural formula is:

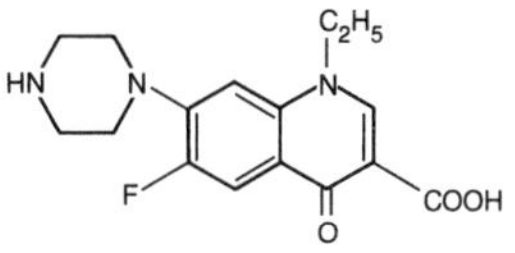

Norfloxacin is a white to pale yellow crystalline powder with a molecular weight of 319.34 and a melting point of about 221°C. It is freely soluble in glacial acetic acid and very slightly soluble in ethanol, methanol and water.
CHIBROXIN Ophthalmic Solution 0.3% is supplied as a sterile isotonic solution. Each mL contains 3 mg norfloxacin. Inactive ingredients: disodium edetate, sodium acetate, sodium chloride, hydrochloric acid (to adjust pH) and water for injection. Benzalkonium chloride 0.0025% is added as preservative. The pH of CHIBROXIN is approximately 5.2 and the osmolarity is approximately 285 mOsmol/liter.
Norfloxacin, a fluoroquinolone, differs from quinolones by having a fluorine atom at the 6 position and a piperazine moiety at the 7 position.

*Registered trademark of MERCK & CO., INC.

Clinical Pharmacology
Microbiology
Norfloxacin has *in vitro* activity against a broad spectrum of gram-positive and gram-negative aerobic bacteria. The fluorine atom at the 6 position provides increased potency against gram-negative organisms and the piperazine moiety at the 7 position is responsible for anti-pseudomonal activity.
Norfloxacin inhibits bacterial deoxyribonucleic acid synthesis and is bactericidal. At the molecular level three specific events are attributed to CHIBROXIN in *E. coli* cells:

1) inhibition of the ATP-dependent DNA supercoiling reaction catalyzed by DNA gyrase;
2) inhibition of the relaxation of supercoiled DNA;
3) promotion of double-stranded DNA breakage.

There is generally no cross-resistance between norfloxacin and other classes of antibacterial agents. Therefore, norfloxacin generally demonstrates activity against indicated organisms resistant to some other antimicrobial agents. When such cross-resistance does occur, it is probably due to decreased entry of the drugs into the bacterial cells. Antagonism has been demonstrated *in vitro* between norfloxacin and nitrofurantoin.
Norfloxacin has been shown to be active against most strains of the following organisms both *in vitro* and clinically in ophthalmic infections (see INDICATIONS AND USAGE):
Gram-positive bacteria including:
Staphylococcus aureus
Staphylococcus epidermidis
Staphylococcus warnerii
Streptococcus pneumoniae
Gram-negative bacteria including:
Acinetobacter calcoaceticus
Aeromonas hydrophila
Haemophilus influenzae
Proteus mirabilis
Pseudomonas aeruginosa
Serratia marcescens
Norfloxacin has been shown to be active *in vitro* against most strains of the following organisms; however, *the clinical significance of these data in ophthalmic infections is unknown.*
Gram-positive bacteria:
Bacillus cereus
Enterococcus faecalis (formerly *Streptococcus faecalis*)
Staphylococcus saprophyticus
Gram-negative bacteria:
Citrobacter diversus
Citrobacter freundii
Edwardsiella tarda
Enterobacter aerogenes
Enterobacter cloacae
Escherichia coli
Hafnia alvei
Haemophilus aegyptius (Koch-Weeks bacillus)
Klebsiella oxytoca
Klebsiella pneumoniae
Klebsiella rhinoscleromatis
Morganella morganii
Neisseria gonorrhoeae
Proteus vulgaris
Providencia alcalifaciens
Providencia rettgeri
Providencia stuartii
Salmonella typhi
Vibrio cholerae
Vibrio parahemolyticus
Yersinia enterocolitica
Other:
Ureaplasma urealyticum
Norfloxacin is not active against obligate anaerobes.
Clinical Studies
Clinical studies were conducted comparing CHIBROXIN Ophthalmic Solution (n=152) with ophthalmic solutions of tobramycin, gentamicin, and chloramphenicol (n=158) in patients with conjunctivitis and positive bacterial cultures. After seven days of therapy with CHIBROXIN Ophthalmic Solution, 72 percent of patients were clinically cured. Of those cured, 85 percent had all their pathogens eradicated. Eradication was also achieved in 62 percent (23/37) of patients whose clinical outcome was not completely cured by day seven. These results were similar among all treatment groups.
Another clinical study compared CHIBROXIN Ophthalmic Solution with placebo in patients with conjunctivitis and positive bacterial cultures. Placebo in this study was the liquid vehicle for CHIBROXIN Ophthalmic Solution and contained the preservative. After five days of therapy, 64 percent (36/56) of patients on CHIBROXIN Ophthalmic Solution were clinically cured compared to 50 percent (23/46) of patients receiving placebo. Of those cured, 78 percent had all their pathogens eradicated. Eradication was also achieved in 50 percent (10/20) of patients whose clinical outcome was not completely cured. The response to CHIBROXIN Ophthalmic Solution was statistically significantly better than the response to placebo.

Indications and Usage
CHIBROXIN Ophthalmic Solution is indicated for the treatment of conjunctivitis when caused by susceptible strains of the following bacteria:
*Acinetobacter calcoaceticus**
*Aeromonas hydrophila**
Haemophilus influenzae
*Proteus mirabilis**
*Pseudomonas aeruginosa**
*Serratia marcescens**
Staphylococcus aureus
Staphylococcus epidermidis
*Staphylococcus warnerii**
Streptococcus pneumoniae
Appropriate monitoring of bacterial response to topical antibiotic therapy should accompany the use of CHIBROXIN Ophthalmic Solution.

*Efficacy for this organism was studied in fewer than 10 infections.

Contraindications
CHIBROXIN Ophthalmic Solution is contraindicated in patients with a history of hypersensitivity to norfloxacin, or the other members of the quinolone group of antibacterial agents or any other component of this medication.

Warnings
NOT FOR INJECTION INTO THE EYE.
Serious and occasionally fatal hypersensitivity (anaphylactoid or anaphylactic) reactions, some following the first dose, have been reported in patients receiving systemic quinolone therapy. Some reactions were accompanied by cardiovascular collapse, loss of consciousness, tingling, pharyngeal or facial edema, dyspnea, urticaria, and itching. Only a few patients had a history of hypersensitivity reactions. Serious anaphylactoid or anaphylactic reactions require immediate emergency treatment with epinephrine. Oxygen, intravenous steroids and airway management, including intubation, should be administered as indicated.

Precautions
General
As with other antibiotic preparations, prolonged use may result in overgrowth of nonsusceptible organisms, including fungi. If superinfection occurs, appropriate measures should be initiated. Whenever clinical judgment dictates, the patient should be examined with the aid of magnification, such as slit lamp biomicroscopy and, where appropriate, fluorescein staining.
There have been reports of bacterial ketatitis associated with the use of multiple dose containers of topical ophthalmic products. These containers have been inadvertently contaminated by patients who, in most cases, had a concurrent corneal disease or a disruption of the ocular epithelial surface. (See PRECAUTIONS, *Information for Patients.*)
Information For Patients
Patients should be instructed to avoid allowing the tip of the dispensing container to contact the eye or surrounding structures.
Patients should also be instructed that ocular preparations, if handled improperly or if the tip of the dispensing container contacts the eye or surrounding structures, can become contaminated by common bacteria known to cause ocular infections. Serious damage to the eye and subsequent loss of vision may result from using contaminated preparations (see PRECAUTIONS, *General*). If redness, irritation, swelling, or pain persists or becomes aggravated, the patient should be advised to consult a physician.
Patients should also be advised that if they have ocular surgery or develop an intercurrent ocular condition (e.g., trauma or infection),

Continued on next page

Information on the Merck & Co., Inc., products listed on these pages is from the full prescribing information in use August 31, 1999.

Chibroxin—Cont.

they should immediately seek their physician's advice concerning the continued use of the present multidose container.

Patients should be advised that norfloxacin may be associated with hypersensitivity reactions, even following a single dose, and to discontinue the drug at the first sign of a skin rash or other allergic reaction.

Patients being treated for bacterial conjunctivitis generally should not wear contact lenses. However, if the physician considers the use of contact lenses appropriate, patients should be advised that CHIBROXIN Ophthalmic Solution contains benzalkonium chloride which may be absorbed by soft contact lenses. Contact lenses should be removed prior to administration of the solution. Lenses may be reinserted 15 minutes following CHIBROXIN Ophthalmic Solution administration.

Drug Interactions

Specific drug interaction studies have not been conducted with norfloxacin ophthalmic solution. However, the systemic administration of some quinolones has been shown to elevate plasma concentrations of theophylline, interfere with the metabolism of caffeine, and enhance the effects of the oral anticoagulant warfarin and its derivatives. Elevated serum levels of cyclosporine have been reported with concomitant use of cyclosporine with norfloxacin. Therefore, cyclosporine serum levels should be monitored and appropriate cyclosporine dosage adjustments made when these drugs are used concomitantly.

Carcinogenesis, Mutagenesis, Impairment of Fertility

No increase in neoplastic changes was observed with norfloxacin as compared to controls in a study in rats, lasting up to 96 weeks at doses eight to nine times the usual human oral dose*.

Norfloxacin was tested for mutagenic activity in a number of *in vivo* and *in vitro* tests. Norfloxacin had no mutagenic effect in the dominant lethal test in mice and did not cause chromosomal aberrations in hamsters or rats at doses 30 to 60 times and usual oral dose*. Norfloxacin had no mutagenic activity *in vitro* in the Ames microbial mutagen test, Chinese hamster fibroblasts and V-79 mammalian cell assay. Although norfloxacin was weakly positive in the Rec-assay for DNA repair, all other mutagenic assays were negative including a more sensitive test (V-79).

Norfloxacin did not adversely affect the fertility of male and female mice at oral doses up to 33 times the usual human oral dose*.

Pregnancy

Pregnancy Category C: Norfloxacin has been shown to produce embryonic loss in monkeys when given in doses 10 times the maximum human oral dose* (400 mg b.i.d.), with peak plasma levels that are two to three times those obtained in humans. There has been no evidence of a teratogenic effect in any of the animal species tested (rat, rabbit, mouse, monkey) at 6 to 50 times the human oral dose. There are no adequate and well-controlled studies in pregnant women. CHIBROXIN Ophthalmic Solution should be used during pregnancy only if the potential benefit justifies the potential risk to the fetus.

Nursing Mothers

It is not known whether norfloxacin is excreted in human milk following ocular administration. Because many drugs are excreted in human milk, and because of the potential for serious adverse reactions in nursing infants from norfloxacin, a decision should be made to discontinue nursing or to discontinue the drug, taking into account the importance of the drug to the mother (see ANIMAL PHARMACOLOGY).

Pediatric Use

Safety and effectiveness in infants below the age of one year have not been established.

Although quinolones including norfloxacin have been shown to cause arthropathy in immature animals after oral administration, topical ocular administration of other quinolones to immature animals has not shown any arthropathy and there is no evidence that the ophthalmic dosage form of those quinolones has any effects on the weight-bearing joints.

Geriatric Use

No overall differences in safety or effectiveness have been observed between elderly and young patients.

---

*All factors are based on a standard patient weight of 50 kg. The usual oral dose of norfloxacin is 800 mg daily. One drop of CHIBROXIN Ophthalmic Solution 0.3% contains about 1/6,666 of this dose (0.12 mg).

Adverse Reactions

In clinical trials, the most frequently reported drug-related adverse reaction was local burning or discomfort. Other drug-related adverse reactions were conjunctival hyperemia, chemosis, photophobia and a bitter taste following instillation.

Dosage and Administration

The recommended dose in adults and pediatric patients (one year and older) is one or two drops of CHIBROXIN Ophthalmic Solution applied topically to the affected eye(s) four times daily for up to seven days. Depending on the severity of the infection, the dosage for the first day of therapy may be one or two drops every two hours during the waking hours.

How Supplied

CHIBROXIN Ophthalmic Solution is a clear, colorless to light yellow solution.

No. 3526—CHIBROXIN Ophthalmic Solution 0.3% is supplied in a white, opaque, plastic OCUMETER* ophthalmic dispenser with a controlled drop tip as follows:

NDC 0006-3526-03, 5 mL.

Storage

Store CHIBROXIN Ophthalmic Solution at room temperature, 15°–30°C (59°–86°F). Protect from light.

Animal Pharmacology

The oral administration of single doses of norfloxacin, six times the recommended human oral dose**, caused lameness in immature dogs. Histologic examination of the weight-bearing joints of these dogs revealed permanent lesions of the cartilage. Related drugs also produced erosions of the cartilage in weight-bearing joints and other signs of arthropathy in immature animals of various species.

---

*Registered trademark of MERCK & CO., INC.

**All factors are based on a standard patient weight of 50 kg. The usual oral dose of norfloxacin is 800 mg daily. One drop of CHIBROXIN Ophthalmic Solution 0.3% contains about 1/6,666 of this dose (0.12 mg).

Additional Cautionary Information

Norfloxacin is available as an oral dosage form in addition to the ophthalmic dosage form. The following adverse effects, while they have not been reported with the ophthalmic dosage form, have been reported with the oral dosage form. However, it should be noted that the usual dosage of oral norfloxacin (800 mg/day) contains 6,666 times the amount in one drop of CHIBROXIN Ophthalmic Solution 0.3% (0.12 mg).

Convulsions have been reported in patients receiving oral norfloxacin. Convulsions, increased intracranial pressure, and toxic psychoses have been reported with other drugs in this class. Orally administered quinolones may also cause central nervous system (CNS) stimulation which may lead to tremors, restlessness, lightheadedness, confusion and hallucinations. If these reactions occur in patients receiving norfloxacin, the drug should be discontinued and appropriate measures instituted.

The effects of norfloxacin on brain function or on the electrical activity of the brain have not been tested. Therefore, as with all quinolones, norfloxacin should be used with caution in patients with known or suspected CNS disorders, such as severe cerebral arteriosclerosis, epilepsy, and other factors which predispose to seizures.

The following adverse effects have been reported with Tablets NOROXIN* (Norfloxacin). *Hypersensitivity Reactions:* Hypersensitivity reactions including anaphylactoid reactions, angioedema, dyspnea, vasculitis, urticaria, arthritis, arthralgia, myalgia; *Gastrointestinal:* Pseudomembranous colitis, hepatitis, jaundice, including cholestatic jaundice, pancreatitis; *Hematologic:* Neutropenia, leukopenia, thrombocytopenia, hemolytic anemia, sometimes associated with glucose-6-phosphate dehydrogenase deficiency; *Musculoskeletal:* Tendinitis, peripheral neuropathy, tendon rupture; and possible exacerbation of myasthenia gravis; *Nervous System/Psychiatric:* CNS effects characterized as generalized seizures and myoclonus; peripheral neuropathy, Guillain-Barre syndrome, ataxia, paresthesia, psychic disturbances including psychotic reactions and confusion, depression; *Renal:* Interstitial nephritis, renal failure; *Skin:* Toxic epidermal necrolysis, Stevens-Johnson syndrome and erythema multiforme, exfoliative dermatitis, rash, photosensitivity; *Special Senses:* Transient hearing loss, tinnitus, diplopia.

Abnormal laboratory values observed with oral norfloxacin included elevation of ALT (SGPT) and AST (SGOT), alkaline phosphatase, BUN, serum creatinine, and LDH.

Please consult the package circular for Tablets NOROXIN (Norfloxacin) for additional information concerning these and other adverse effects and other cautionary information.

---

*Registered trademark of MERCK & CO., INC.

9011206 Issued August 1998

Shown in Product Identification Guide, page 105

COSOPT® ℞

(dorzolamide hydrochloride-timolol maleate ophthalmic solution)
Sterile Ophthalmic Solution

Description

COSOPT* (dorzolamide hydrochloride-timolol maleate ophthalmic solution) is the combination of a topical carbonic anhydrase inhibitor and a topical beta-adrenergic receptor blocking agent.

Dorzolamide hydrochloride is described chemically as: (4*S*-*trans*)-4-(ethylamino)-5,6-dihydro-6-methyl-4*H*-thieno[2,3-*b*]thiopyran-2-sulfonamide 7,7-dioxide monohydrochloride. Dorzolamide hydrochloride is optically active. The specific rotation is:

$$[\alpha]^{25°C}_{405\ nm} \ (C=1,\ water) = \sim -17°.$$

Its empirical formula is $C_{10}H_{16}N_2O_4S_3 \cdot HCl$ and its structural formula is:

[See chemical structure at top of next page]

Dorzolamide hydrochloride has a molecular weight of 360.91. It is a white to off-white, crystalline powder, which is soluble in water and slightly soluble in methanol and ethanol.

Timolol maleate is described chemically as: (-)-1-(*tert*-butylamino)-3-[(4-morpholino-1,2,5-thiadiazol-3-yl)oxy]-2-propanol maleate (1:1) (salt). Timolol maleate possesses an asymmetric carbon atom in its structure and is provided as the levo-isomer. The nominal optical rotation of timolol maleate is:

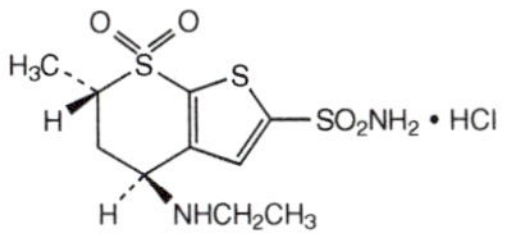

$$[\alpha]^{25°C}_{405\,nm} \text{ in 1N HCl (C=5)} = -12.2°.$$

Its molecular formula is $C_{13}H_{24}N_4O_3S \bullet C_4H_4O_4$ and its structural formula is:

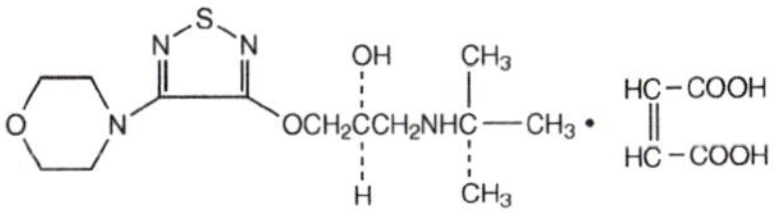

Timolol maleate has a molecular weight of 432.50. It is a white, odorless, crystalline powder which is soluble in water, methanol, and alcohol. Timolol maleate is stable at room temperature.

COSOPT is supplied as a sterile, isotonic, buffered, slightly viscous, aqueous solution. The pH of the solution is approximately 5.65, and the osmolarity is 242-323 mOsM. Each mL of COSOPT contains 20 mg dorzolamide (22.26 mg of dorzolamide hydrochloride) and 5 mg timolol (6.83 mg timolol maleate). Inactive ingredients are sodium citrate, hydroxyethyl cellulose, sodium hydroxide, mannitol, and water for injection. Benzalkonium chloride 0.0075% is added as a preservative.

*Trademark of MERCK & CO., Inc.

Clinical Pharmacology

Mechanism of Action

COSOPT is comprised of two components: dorzolamide hydrochloride and timolol maleate. Each of these two components decreases elevated intraocular pressure, whether or not associated with glaucoma, by reducing aqueous humor secretion. Elevated intraocular pressure is a major risk factor in the pathogenesis of optic nerve damage and glaucomatous visual field loss. The higher the level of intraocular pressure, the greater the likelihood of glaucomatous field loss and optic nerve damage.

Dorzolamide hydrochloride is an inhibitor of human carbonic anhydrase II. Inhibition of carbonic anhydrase in the ciliary processes of the eye decreases aqueous humor secretion, presumably by slowing the formation of bicarbonate ions with subsequent reduction in sodium and fluid transport. Timolol maleate is a $beta_1$ and $beta_2$ (non-selective) adrenergic receptor blocking agent that does not have significant intrinsic sympathomimetic, direct myocardial depressant, or local anesthetic (membrane-stabilizing) activity. The combined effect of these two agents administered as COSOPT b.i.d. results in additional intraocular pressure reduction compared to either component administered alone, but the reduction is not as much as when dorzolamide t.i.d. and timolol b.i.d. are administered concomitantly (see *Clinical Studies*).

Pharmacokinetics/Pharmacodynamics

Dorzolamide Hydrochloride

When topically applied, dorzolamide reaches the systemic circulation. To assess the potential for systemic carbonic anhydrase inhibition following topical administration, drug and metabolite concentrations in RBCs and plasma and carbonic anhydrase inhibition in RBCs were measured. Dorzolamide accumulates in RBCs during chronic dosing as a result of binding to CA-II. The parent drug forms a single N-desethyl metabolite, which inhibits CA-II less potently than the parent drug but also inhibits CA-I. The metabolite also accumulates in RBCs where it binds primarily to CA-I. Plasma concentrations of dorzolamide and metabolite are generally below the assay limit of quantitation (15nM). Dorzolamide binds moderately to plasma proteins (approximately 33%).

Dorzolamide is primarily excreted unchanged in the urine; the metabolite also is excreted in urine. After dosing is stopped, dorzolamide washes out of RBCs nonlinearly, resulting in a rapid decline of drug concentration initially, followed by a slower elimination phase with a half-life of about four months.

To simulate the systemic exposure after long-term topical ocular administration, dorzolamide was given orally to eight healthy subjects for up to 20 weeks. The oral dose of 2 mg b.i.d. closely approximates the amount of drug delivered by topical ocular administration of dorzolamide 2% t.i.d. Steady state was reached within 8 weeks. The inhibition of CA-II and total carbonic anhydrase activities was below the degree of inhibition anticipated to be necessary for a pharmacological effect on renal function and respiration in healthy individuals.

Timolol Maleate

In a study of plasma drug concentrations in six subjects, the systemic exposure to timolol was determined following twice daily topical administration of timolol maleate ophthalmic solution 0.5%. The mean peak plasma concentration following morning dosing was 0.46 ng/mL.

Clinical Studies

Clinical studies of 3 to 15 months duration were conducted to compare the IOP-lowering effect over the course of the day of COSOPT b.i.d. (dosed morning and bedtime) to individually- and concomitantly-administered 0.5% timolol (b.i.d.) and 2.0% dorzolamide (b.i.d. and t.i.d.). The IOP-lowering effect of COSOPT b.i.d. was greater (1-3 mmHg) than that of monotherapy with either 2.0% dorzolamide t.i.d. or 0.5% timolol b.i.d. The IOP-lowering effect of COSOPT b.i.d. was approximately 1 mmHg less than that of concomitant therapy with 2.0% dorzolamide t.i.d. and 0.5% timolol b.i.d.

Open-label extensions of two studies were conducted for up to 12 months. During this period, the IOP-lowering effect of COSOPT b.i.d. was consistent during the 12 month follow-up period.

Indications and Usage

COSOPT is indicated for the reduction of elevated intraocular pressure in patients with open-angle glaucoma or ocular hypertension who are insufficiently responsive to beta-blockers (failed to achieve target IOP determined after multiple measurements over time). The IOP-lowering of COSOPT b.i.d. was slightly less than that seen with the concomitant administration of 0.5% timolol b.i.d. and 2.0% dorzolamide t.i.d. (see CLINICAL PHARMACOLOGY, *Clinical Studies*).

Contraindications

COSOPT is contraindicated in patients with (1) bronchial asthma; (2) a history of bronchial asthma; (3) severe chronic obstructive pulmonary disease (see WARNINGS); (4) sinus bradycardia; (5) second or third degree atrioventricular block; (6) overt cardiac failure (see WARNINGS); (7) cardiogenic shock; or (8) hypersensitivity to any component of this product.

Warnings

Systemic Exposure

COSOPT contains dorzolamide, a sulfonamide, and timolol maleate, a beta-adrenergic blocking agent; and although administered topically, is absorbed systemically. Therefore, the same types of adverse reactions that are attributable to sulfonamides and/or systemic administration of beta-adrenergic blocking agents may occur with topical administration. For example, severe respiratory reactions and cardiac reactions, including death due to bronchospasm in patients with asthma, and rarely death in association with cardiac failure, have been reported following systemic or ophthalmic administration of timolol maleate (see CONTRAINDICATIONS). Fatalities have occurred, although rarely, due to severe reactions to sulfonamides including Stevens-Johnson syndrome, toxic epidermal necrolysis, fulminant hepatic necrosis, agranulocytosis, aplastic anemia, and other blood dyscrasias. Sensitization may recur when a sulfonamide is readministered irrespective of the route of administration. If signs of serious reactions or hypersensitivity occur, discontinue the use of this preparation.

Cardiac Failure

Sympathetic stimulation may be essential for support of the circulation in individuals with diminished myocardial contractility, and its inhibition by beta-adrenergic receptor blockade may precipitate more severe failure.

In Patients Without a History of Cardiac Failure continued depression of the myocardium with beta-blocking agents over a period of time can, in some cases, lead to cardiac failure. At the first sign or symptom of cardiac failure, COSOPT should be discontinued.

Obstructive Pulmonary Disease

Patients with chronic obstructive pulmonary disease (e.g., chronic bronchitis, emphysema) of mild or moderate severity, bronchospastic disease, or a history of bronchospastic disease (other than bronchial asthma or a history of bronchial asthma, in which COSOPT is contraindicated [see CONTRAINDICATIONS]) should, in general, not receive beta-blocking agents, including COSOPT.

Major Surgery

The necessity or desirability of withdrawal of beta-adrenergic blocking agents prior to major surgery is controversial. Beta-adrenergic receptor blockade impairs the ability of the heart to respond to beta-adrenergically mediated reflex stimuli. This may augment the risk of general anesthesia in surgical procedures. Some patients receiving beta-adrenergic receptor blocking agents have experienced protracted severe hypotension during anesthesia. Difficulty in restarting and maintaining the heartbeat has also been reported. For these reasons, in patients undergoing elective surgery, some authorities recommend gradual withdrawal of beta-adrenergic receptor blocking agents.

If necessary during surgery, the effects of beta-adrenergic blocking agents may be reversed by sufficient doses of adrenergic agonists.

Diabetes Mellitus

Beta-adrenergic blocking agents should be administered with caution in patients subject to spontaneous hypoglycemia or to diabetic patients (especially those with labile diabetes) who are receiving insulin or oral hypoglycemic agents. Beta-adrenergic receptor blocking agents may mask the signs and symptoms of acute hypoglycemia.

Thyrotoxicosis

Beta-adrenergic blocking agents may mask certain clinical signs (e.g., tachycardia) of hyperthyroidism. Patients suspected of developing thyrotoxicosis should be managed carefully

Continued on next page

Information on the Merck & Co., Inc., products listed on these pages is from the full prescribing information in use August 31, 1999.

Cosopt—Cont.

to avoid abrupt withdrawal of beta-adrenergic blocking agents that might precipitate a thyroid storm.

Precautions

General

Dorzolamide has not been studied in patients with severe renal impairment (CrCl <30 mL/min). Because dorzolamide and its metabolite are excreted prodominantly by the kidney, COSOPT is not recommended in such patients. Dorzolamide has not been studied in patients with hepatic impairment and should therefore be used with caution in such patients.

While taking beta-blockers, patients with a history of atopy or a history of severe anaphylactic reactions to a variety of allergens may be more reactive to repeated accidental, diagnostic, or therapeutic challenge with such allergens. Such patients may be unresponsive to the usual doses of epinephrine used to treat anaphylactic reactions.

In clinical studies, local ocular adverse effects, primarily conjunctivitis and lid reactions, were reported with chronic administration of COSOPT. Many of these reactions had the clinical appearance and course of an allergic-type reaction that resolved upon discontinuation of drug therapy. If such reactions are observed, COSOPT should be discontinued and the patient evaluated before considering restarting the drug. (See ADVERSE REACTIONS.)

The management of patients with acute angle-closure glaucoma requires therapeutic interventions in addition to ocular hypotensive agents. COSOPT has not been studied in patients with acute angle-closure glaucoma.

Choroidal detachment after filtration procedures has been reported with the administration of aqueous suppressant therapy (e.g., timolol).

Beta-adrenergic blockade has been reported to potentiate muscle weakness consistent with certain myasthenic symptoms (e.g., diplopia, ptosis, and generalized weakness). Timolol has been reported rarely to increase muscle weakness in some patients with myasthenia gravis or myasthenic symptoms.

There have been reports of bacterial keratitis associated with the use of multiple dose containers of topical ophthalmic products. These containers had been inadvertently contaminated by patients who, in most cases, had a concurrent corneal disease or a disruption of the ocular epithelial surface. (See PRECAUTIONS, *Information for Patients*.)

Information for Patients

Patients with bronchial asthma, a history of bronchial asthma, severe chronic obstructive pulmonary disease, sinus bradycardia, second or third degree atrioventricular block, or cardiac failure should be advised not to take this product. (See CONTRAINDICATIONS.)

COSOPT contains dorzolamide (which is a sulfonamide) and although administered topically is absorbed systemically. Therefore the same types of adverse reactions that are attributable to sulfonamides may occur with topical administration. Patients should be advised that if serious or unusual reactions or signs of hypersensitivity occur, they should discontinue the use of the product (see WARNINGS).

Patients should be advised that if they develop any ocular reactions, particularly conjunctivitis and lid reactions, they should discontinue use and seek their physician's advice.

Patients should be instructed to avoid allowing the tip of the dispensing container to contact the eye or surrounding structures.

Patients should also be instructed that ocular solutions, if handled improperly or if the tip of the dispensing container contacts the eye or surrounding structures, can become contaminated by common bacteria known to cause ocular infections. Serious damage to the eye and subsequent loss of vision may result from using contaminated solutions. (See PRECAUTIONS, *General*.)

Patients also should be advised that if they have ocular surgery or develop an intercurrent ocular condition (e.g., trauma or infection), they should immediately seek their physician's advice concerning the continued use of the present multidose container.

If more than one topical ophthalmic drug is being used, the drugs should be administered at least ten minutes apart.

Patients should be advised that COSOPT contains benzalkonium chloride which may be absorbed by soft contact lenses. Contact lenses should be removed prior to administration of the solution. Lenses may be reinserted 15 minutes following administration of COSOPT.

Drug Interactions

Carbonic anhydrase inhibitors: There is a potential for an additive effect on the known systemic effects of carbonic anhydrase inhibition in patients receiving an oral carbonic anhydrase inhibitor and COSOPT. The concomitant administration of COSOPT and oral carbonic anhydrase inhibitors is not recommended.

Acid-base disturbances: Although acid-base and electrolyte disturbances were not reported in the clinical trials with dorzolamide hydrochloride ophthalmic solution, these disturbances have been reported with oral carbonic anhydrase inhibitors and have, in some instances, resulted in drug interactions (e.g., toxicity associated with high-dose salicylate therapy). Therefore, the potential for such drug interactions should be considered in patients receiving COSOPT.

Beta-adrenergic blocking agents: Patients who are receiving a beta-adrenergic blocking agent orally and COSOPT should be observed for potential additive effects of beta-blockade, both systemic and on intraocular pressure. The concomitant use of two topical beta-adrenergic blocking agents is not recommended.

Calcium antagonists: Caution should be used in the coadministration of beta-adrenergic blocking agents, such as COSOPT, and oral or intravenous calcium antagonists because of possible atrioventricular conduction disturbances, left ventricular failure, and hypotension. In patients with impaired cardiac function, coadministration should be avoided.

Catecholamine-depleting drugs: Close observation of the patient is recommended when a beta-blocker is administered to patients receiving catecholamine-depleting drugs such as reserpine, because of possible additive effects and the production of hypotension and/or marked bradycardia, which may result in vertigo, syncope, or postural hypotension.

Digitalis and calcium antagonists: The concomitant use of beta-adrenergic blocking agents with digitalis and calcium antagonists may have additive effects in prolonging atrioventricular conduction time.

Quinidine: Potentiated systemic beta-blockade (e.g., decreased heart rate) has been reported during combined treatment with quinidine and timolol, possibly because quinidine inhibits the metabolism of timolol via the P-450 enzyme, CYP2D6.

Injectable Epinephrine: (See PRECAUTIONS, *General, Anaphylaxis*.)

Carcinogenesis, Mutagenesis, Impairment of Fertility

In a two-year study of dorzolamide hydrochloride administered orally to male and female Sprague-Dawley rats, urinary bladder papillomas were seen in male rats in the highest dosage group of 20 mg/kg/day (250 times the recommended human ophthalmic dose). Papillomas were not seen in rats given oral doses equivalent to approximately 12 times the recommended human ophthalmic dose. No treatment-related tumors were seen in a 21-month study in female and male mice given oral doses up to 75 mg/kg/day (~900 times the recommended human ophthalmic dose).

The increased incidence of urinary bladder papillomas seen in the high-dose male rats is a class-effect of carbonic anhydrase inhibitors in rats. Rats are particularly prone to developing papillomas in response to foreign bodies, compounds causing crystalluria, and diverse sodium salts.

No changes in bladder urothelium were seen in dogs given oral dorzolamide hydrochloride for one year at 2 mg/kg/day (25 times the recommended human ophthalmic dose) or monkeys dosed topically to the eye at 0.4 mg/kg/day (~5 times the recommended human ophthalmic dose) for one year.

In a two-year study of timolol maleate administered orally to rats, there was a statistically significant increase in the incidence of adrenal pheochromocytomas in male rats administered 300 mg/kg/day (approximately 42,000 times the systemic exposure following the maximum recommended human ophthalmic dose). Similar differences were not observed in rats administered oral doses equivalent to approximately 14,000 times the maximum recommended human ophthalmic dose.

In a lifetime oral study of timolol maleate in mice, there were statistically significant increases in the incidence of benign and malignant pulmonary tumors, benign uterine polyps and mammary adenocarcinomas in female mice at 500 mg/kg/day, (approximately 71,000 times the systemic exposure following the maximum recommended human ophthalmic dose), but not at 5 or 50 mg/kg/day (approximately 700 or 7,000, respectively, times the systemic exposure following the maximum recommended human ophthalmic dose). In a subsequent study in female mice, in which postmortem examinations were limited to the uterus and the lungs, a statistically significant increase in the incidence of pulmonary tumors was again observed at 500 mg/kg/day.

The increased occurrence of mammary adenocarcinomas was associated with elevations in serum prolactin which occurred in female mice administered oral timolol at 500 mg/kg/day, but not at doses of 5 or 50 mg/kg/day. An increased incidence of mammary adenocarcinomas in rodents has been associated with administration of several other therapeutic agents that elevate serum prolactin, but no correlation between serum prolactin levels and mammary tumors has been established in humans. Furthermore, in adult human female subjects who received oral dosages of up to 60 mg of timolol maleate (the maximum recommended human oral dosage), there were no clinically meaningful changes in serum prolactin.

The following tests for mutagenic potential were negative for dorzolamide: (1) *in vivo* (mouse) cytogenetic assay; (2) *in vitro* chromosomal aberration assay; (3) alkaline elution assay; (4) V-79 assay; and (5) Ames test.

Timolol maleate was devoid of mutagenic potential when tested *in vivo* (mouse) in the micronucleus test and cytogenetic assay (doses up to 800 mg/kg) and *in vitro* in a neoplastic cell transformation assay (up to 100 µg/mL). In Ames tests the highest concentrations of timolol employed, 5,000 or 10,000 µg/plate, were associated with statistically significant elevations of revertants observed with tester strain TA100 (in seven replicate assays), but not in the remaining three strains. In the assays with tester strain TA100, no consistent dose response relationship was observed, and the ratio of test to control revertants did not reach 2. A ratio of 2 is usually considered the criterion for a positive Ames test.

Reproduction and fertility studies in rats with either timolol maleate or dorzolamide hydrochloride demonstrated no adverse effect on male or female fertility at doses up to approximately 100 times the systemic exposure following the maximum recommended human ophthalmic dose.

Pregnancy

Teratogenic Effects. Pregnancy Category C. Developmental toxicity studies with dorzolamide hydrochloride in rabbits at oral doses of ≥2.5 mg/kg/day (31 times the recommended human ophthalmic dose) revealed malformations of the vertebral bodies. These malformations occurred at doses that caused metabolic acidosis with decreased body weight gain in dams and decreased fetal weights. No treatment-related malformations were seen at 1.0 mg/kg/day (13 times the recommended human ophthalmic dose).

Teratogenicity studies with timolol in mice, rats, and rabbits at oral doses up to 50 mg/kg/day (7,000 times the systemic exposure following the maximum recommended human ophthalmic dose) demonstrated no evidence of fetal malformations. Although delayed fetal ossification was observed at this dose in rats, there were no adverse effects on postnatal development of offspring. Doses of 1000 mg/kg/day (142,000 times the systemic exposure following the maximum recommended human ophthalmic dose) were maternotoxic in mice and resulted in an increased number of fetal resorptions. Increased fetal resorptions were also seen in rabbits at doses of 14,000 times the systemic exposure following the maximum recommended human ophthalmic dose, in this case without apparent maternotoxicity.

There are no adequate and well-controlled studies in pregnant women. COSOPT should be used during pregnancy only if the potential benefit justifies the potential risk to the fetus.

Nursing Mothers

It is not known whether dorzolamide is excreted in human milk. Timolol maleate has been detected in human milk following oral and ophthalmic drug administration. Because of the potential for serious adverse reactions from COSOPT in nursing infants, a decision should be made whether to discontinue nursing or to discontinue the drug, taking into account the importance of the drug to the mother.

Pediatric Use

Safety and effectiveness in pediatric patients have not been established.

Adverse Reactions

COSOPT was evaluated for safety in 1035 patients with elevated intraocular pressure treated for open-angle-glaucoma or ocular hypertension. Approximately 5% of all patients discontinued therapy with COSOPT because of adverse reactions. The most frequently reported adverse events were taste perversion (bitter, sour, or unusual taste) or ocular burning and/or stinging in up to 30% of patients. Conjunctival hyperemia, blurred vision, superficial punctate keratitis or eye itching were reported between 5-15% of patients. The following adverse events were reported in 1-5% of patients: abdominal pain, back pain, blepharitis, bronchitis, cloudy vision, conjunctival discharge, conjunctival edema, conjunctival follicles, conjunctival injection, conjunctivitis, corneal erosion, corneal staining, cortical lens opacity, cough, dizziness, dryness of eyes, dyspepsia, eye debris, eye discharge, eye pain, eye tearing, eyelid edema, eyelid erythema, eyelid exudate/scales, eyelid pain or discomfort, foreign body sensation, glaucomatous cupping, headache, hypertension, influenza, lens nucleus coloration, lens opacity, nausea, nuclear lens opacity, pharyngitis, post-subcapsular cataract, sinusitis, upper respiratory infection, urinary tract infection, visual field defect, vitreous detachment.

The following adverse events have occurred either at low incidence (<1%) during clinical trials or have been reported during the use of COSOPT in clinical practice where these events were reported voluntarily from a population of unknown size and frequency of occurrence cannot be determined precisely. They have been chosen for inclusion based on factors such as seriousness, frequency of reporting, possible causal connection to COSOPT, or a combination of these factors: bradycardia, cardiac failure, chest pain, cerebral vascular accident, depression, diarrhea, dry mouth, dyspnea, hypotension, iridocyclitis, myocardial infarction, nasal congestion, skin rashes, paresthesia, photophobia, urolithiasis and vomiting.

Other adverse reactions that have been reported with the individual components are listed below:

Dorzolamide — Allergic/Hypersensitivity: Signs and symptoms of systemic allergic reactions including angioedema, bronchospasm, pruritus, urticaria; *Body as a Whole:* Asthenia/fatigue; *Skin/Mucous Membranes:* Contact dermatitis, throat irritation; *Special Senses:* Signs and symptoms of ocular allergic reaction, and transient myopia.

Timolol (ocular administration) — Body as a Whole: Asthenia/fatigue; *Cardiovascular:* Arrhythmia, syncope, heart block, cerebral ischemia, worsening of angina pectoris, palpitation, cardiac arrest, pulmonary edema, edema, claudication, Raynaud's phenomenon, and cold hands and feet; *Digestive:* Anorexia; *Immunologic:* Systemic lupus erythematosus; *Nervous System/Psychiatric:* Increase in signs and symptoms of myasthenia gravis, somnolence, insomnia, nightmares, behavioral changes and psychic disturbances including confusion, hallucinations, anxiety, disorientation, nervousness, and memory loss; *Skin:* Alopecia, psoriasiform rash or exacerbation of psoriasis; *Hypersensitivity:* Signs and symptoms of systemic allergic reactions, including angioedema, urticaria, and localized and generalized rash; *Respiratory:* Bronchospasm (predominantly in patients with pre-existing bronchospastic disease), respiratory failure; *Endocrine:* Masked symptoms of hypoglycemia in diabetic patients (see WARNINGS); *Special Senses:* Ptosis; decreased corneal sensitivity; cystoid macular edema; visual disturbances including refractive changes and diplopia; pseudopemphigoid; choroidal detachment following filtration surgery (see PRECAUTIONS, *General*); and tinnitus; *Urogenital:* Retroperitoneal fibrosis, decreased libido, impotence, and Peyronie's disease.

The following additional adverse effects have been reported in clinical experience with ORAL timolol maleate or other ORAL beta-blocking agents and may be considered potential effects of ophthalmic timolol maleate: *Allergic:* Erythematous rash, fever combined with aching and sore throat, laryngospasm with respiratory distress; *Body as a Whole:* Extremity pain, decreased exercise tolerance, weight loss; *Cardiovascular:* Worsening of arterial insufficiency, vasodilatation; *Digestive:* Gastrointestinal pain, hepatomegaly, mesenteric arterial thrombosis, ischemic colitis; *Hematologic:* Nonthrombocytopenic purpura; thrombocytopenic purpura, agranulocytosis; *Endocrine:* Hyperglycemia, hypoglycemia; *Skin:* Pruritus, skin irritation, increased pigmentation, sweating; *Musculoskeletal:* Arthralgia; *Nervous System/Psychiatric:* Vertigo, local weakness, diminished concentration, reversible mental depression progressing to catatonia, an acute reversible syndrome characterized by disorientation for time and place, emotional lability, slightly clouded sensorium, and decreased performance on neuropsychometrics; *Respiratory:* Rales, bronchial obstruction; *Urogenital:* Urination difficulties.

Overdosage

There are no human data available on overdosage with COSOPT.

Symptoms consistent with systemic administration of beta-blockers or carbonic anhydrase inhibitors may occur, including electrolyte imbalance, development of an acidotic state, dizziness, headache, shortness of breath, bradycardia, bronchospasm, cardiac arrest and possible central nervous system effects. Serum electrolyte levels (particularly potassium) and blood pH levels should be monitored (see also ADVERSE REACTIONS).

A study of patients with renal failure showed that timolol did not dialyze readily.

Dosage and Administration

The dose is one drop of COSOPT in the affected eye(s) two times daily.

If more than one topical ophthalmic drug is being used, the drugs should be administered at least ten minutes apart (see also PRECAUTIONS, *Drug Interactions*).

How Supplied

COSOPT Ophthalmic Solution is a clear, colorless to nearly colorless, slightly viscous solution.

No. 3628 — COSOPT Ophthalmic Solution is supplied in an OCUMETER®*, a white, opaque, plastic ophthalmic dispenser with a controlled drop tip as follows:

NDC 0006-3628-03, 5 mL

NDC 0006-3628-10, 10 mL.

Storage

Store COSOPT between 15 and 25°C (59–77°F). Protect from light.

9098901 Issued October 1998

Shown in Product Identification Guide, page 105

DARANIDE® ℞

(Dichlorphenamide), U.S.P.

Tablets

Description

DARANIDE* (Dichlorphenamide) is an oral carbonic anhydrase inhibitor. Dichlorphenamide, a dichlorinated benzenedisulfonamide, is known chemically as 4,5-dichloro-1,3-benzenedisulfonamide. Its empirical formula is $C_6H_6Cl_2N_2O_4S_2$ and its structural formula is:

SO_2NH_2 / Cl / SO_2NH_2 / Cl

Dichlorphenamide is a white or practically white, crystalline compound with a molecular weight of 305.16. It is very slightly soluble in water but soluble in dilute solutions of sodium carbonate and sodium hydroxide. Dilute alkaline solutions of dichlorphenamide are stable at room temperature.

DARANIDE is supplied as tablets, for oral administration, each containing 50 mg dichlor-

Continued on next page

Information on the Merck & Co., Inc., products listed on these pages is from the full prescribing information in use August 31, 1999.

Daranide—Cont.

phenamide. Inactive ingredients are D&C Yellow 10, lactose, magnesium stearate, and starch.

---

*Registered trademark of MERCK & CO., INC.

Clinical Pharmacology

Carbonic anhydrase inhibitors reduce intraocular pressure by partially suppressing the secretion of aqueous humor (inflow), although the mechanism by which they do this is not fully understood. Evidence suggests that HCO_3^- ions are produced in the ciliary body by hydration of carbon dioxide under the influence of carbonic anhydrase and diffuse into the posterior chamber with Na+ ions. The aqueous fluid contains more Na+ and HCO_3^- ions than does plasma and consequently is hypertonic. Water is attracted to the posterior chamber by osmosis. Systemic administration of a carbonic anhydrase inhibitor has been shown to inactivate carbonic anhydrase in the ciliary body of the rabbit's eye and to reduce the high concentration of HCO_3^- ions in ocular fluids. As is the case with all carbonic anhydrase inhibitors, DARANIDE in high doses causes some decrease in renal blood flow and glomerular filtration rate.

In man, DARANIDE begins to act within an hour and maximal effect is observed in two to four hours. The lowered intraocular tension may be maintained for approximately 6 to 12 hours.

Indications and Usage

For adjunctive treatment of: chronic simple (open-angle) glaucoma, secondary glaucoma, and preoperatively in acute angle-closure glaucoma where delay of surgery is desired in order to lower intraocular pressure.

Contraindications

DARANIDE is contraindicated in hepatic insufficiency, renal failure, adrenocortical insufficiency, hyperchloremic acidosis, or in conditions in which serum levels of sodium or potassium are depressed. DARANIDE should not be used in patients with severe pulmonary obstruction who are unable to increase their alveolar ventilation since their acidosis may be increased.

DARANIDE is contraindicated in patients who are hypersensitive to this product.

Precautions

General

Potassium excretion is increased by DARANIDE and hypokalemia may develop with brisk diuresis, when severe cirrhosis is present, or during concomitant use of steroids or ACTH.

Interference with adequate oral electrolyte intake will also contribute to hypokalemia. Hypokalemia can sensitize or exaggerate the response of the heart to the toxic effects of digitalis (e.g., increased ventricular irritability). Hypokalemia may be avoided or treated by use of potassium supplements such as foods with a high potassium content. DARANIDE should be used with caution in patients with respiratory acidosis.

Drug Interactions

Caution is advised in patients receiving concomitant high-dose aspirin and carbonic anhydrase inhibitors, as anorexia, tachypnea, lethargy and coma have been rarely reported due to a possible drug interaction.

Carcinogenesis, Mutagenesis, Impairment of Fertility

Long-term studies in animals have not been performed to evaluate the effects upon fertility or carcinogenic potential of DARANIDE.

Pregnancy

Pregnancy Category C. Dichlorphenamide has been shown to be teratogenic in the rat (skeletal anomalies) when given in doses 100 times the human dose. There are no adequate and well-controlled studies in pregnant women. DARANIDE should not be used in women of childbearing age or in pregnancy, especially during the first trimester, unless the potential benefits outweigh the potential risks.

Nursing Mothers

It is not known whether dichlorphenamide is excreted in human milk. Because many drugs are excreted in human milk, caution should be exercised when dichlorphenamide is administered to a nursing woman.

Pediatric Use

Safety and effectiveness in pediatric patients have not been established.

Adverse Reactions

Certain side effects characteristic of carbonic anhydrase inhibitors may occur with DARANIDE, particularly with increasing doses. The most common effects include gastrointestinal disturbances (anorexia, nausea, and vomiting), drowsiness and paresthesias.

Included in the listing which follows are some adverse reactions which have not been reported with DARANIDE. However, pharmacological similarities among the carbonic anhydrase inhibitors make it advisable to consider the following reactions when dichlorphenamide is administered. *Central Nervous System/Psychiatric:* ataxia, tremor, tinnitus, headache, weakness, nervousness, globus hystericus, lassitude, depression, confusion, disorientation, dizziness; *Gastrointestinal:* constipation, hepatic insufficiency; *Metabolic:* loss of weight, metabolic acidosis, electrolyte imbalance (hypokalemia, hyperchloremia), hyperuricemia; *Hypersensitivity:* skin eruptions, pruritus, fever; *Hematologic:* leukopenia, agranulocytosis, thrombocytopenia; *Genitourinary:* urinary frequency, renal colic, renal calculi, phosphaturia.

Overdosage

The oral LD_{50} of DARANIDE is 1710 and 2600 mg/kg in the mouse and rat respectively.

Symptoms of overdosage or toxicity may include drowsiness, anorexia, nausea, vomiting, dizziness, paresthesias, ataxia, tremor and tinnitus.

In the event of overdosage, induce emesis or perform gastric lavage. The electrolyte disturbance most likely to be encountered from overdosage is hyperchloremic acidosis that may respond to bicarbonate administration. Potassium supplementation may be required. The patient should be carefully observed and given supportive treatment.

Dosage and Administration

DARANIDE is usually given in conjunction with topical ocular hypotensive agents. In acute angle-closure glaucoma, it may be used together with miotics and osmotic agents in an attempt to reduce intraocular tension rapidly. If this is not quickly relieved, surgery may be mandatory.

Dosage must be adjusted carefully to meet the requirements of the individual patient. A priming dose of 100 to 200 mg of DARANIDE (2 to 4 tablets) is suggested for adults, followed by 100 mg (2 tablets) every 12 hours until the desired response has been obtained. The recommended maintenance dosage for adults is 25 to 50 mg (1/2 to 1 tablet) once to three times daily.

How Supplied

No. 3256—Tablets DARANIDE, 50 mg each, are yellow, round, scored, compressed tablets, coded MSD 49 on one side and DARANIDE on the other. They are supplied as follows:

NDC 0006-0049-68 bottles of 100.

7870319 Issued October 1996

Shown in Product Identification Guide, page 105

DECADRON® Phosphate ℞

(Dexamethasone Sodium Phosphate), U.S.P.
0.05% Dexamethasone Phosphate Equivalent
Sterile Ophthalmic Ointment

Description

Dexamethasone sodium phosphate is 9-fluoro-11β, 17-dihydroxy-16α-methyl-21-(phosphonooxy)pregna-1,4-diene-3,20-dione disodium salt. Its empirical formula is $C_{22}H_{28}FNa_2O_8P$ and its structural formula is:

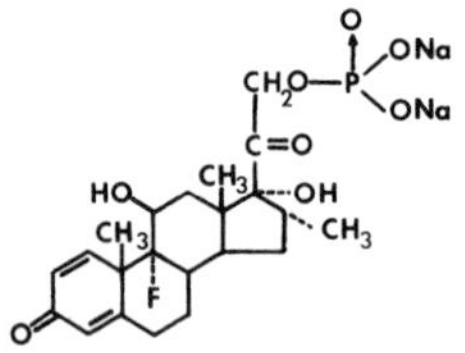

Glucocorticoids are adrenocortical steroids, both naturally occurring and synthetic. Dexamethasone is a synthetic analog of naturally occurring glucocorticoids (hydrocortisone and cortisone). Dexamethasone sodium phosphate is a water soluble, inorganic ester of dexamethasone. Its molecular weight is 516.41.

Sterile Ophthalmic Ointment DECADRON* Phosphate (Dexamethasone Sodium Phosphate) is a topical steroid ointment containing dexamethasone sodium phosphate equivalent to 0.5 mg (0.05%) dexamethasone phosphate in each gram. Inactive ingredients: white petrolatum and mineral oil.

Dexamethasone sodium phosphate is an inorganic ester of dexamethasone.

---

*Registered trademark of MERCK & CO., INC.

Clinical Pharmacology

Dexamethasone sodium phosphate suppresses the inflammatory response to a variety of agents and it probably delays or slows healing. No generally accepted explanation of these steroid properties have been advanced.

Indications and Usage

For the treatment of the following conditions: Steroid responsive inflammatory conditions of the palpebral and bulbar conjunctiva, cornea, and anterior segment of the globe, such as allergic conjunctivitis, acne rosacea, superficial punctate keratitis, herpes zoster keratitis, iritis, cyclitis, selected infective conjunctivitis when the inherent hazard of steroid use is accepted to obtain an advisable diminution in edema and inflammation; corneal injury from chemical or thermal burns, or penetration of foreign bodies.

Contraindications

Epithelial herpes simplex keratitis (dendritic keratitis).

Acute infectious stages of vaccinia, varicella, and many other viral diseases of the cornea and conjunctiva.

Mycobacterial infection of the eye.

Fungal diseases of ocular structures.

Hypersensitivity to a component of the medication.

Warnings

Prolonged use may result in ocular hypertension and/or glaucoma, with damage to the optic nerve, defects in visual acuity and fields of vision, and posterior subcapsular cataract formation. Prolonged use may suppress the host response and thus increase the hazard of secondary ocular infections. In those diseases causing thinning of the cornea or sclera, perforations have been known to occur with the use of topical corticosteroids. In acute purulent conditions of the eye, corticosteroids may mask infection or enhance existing infection. If these products are used for 10 days or longer, intraocular pressure should be routinely monitored even though it may be difficult in children and uncooperative patients.

Employment of corticosteroid medication in the treatment of herpes simplex other than epithelial herpes simplex keratitis, in which it is contraindicated, requires great caution; periodic slit-lamp microscopy is essential.

Precautions

General

The possibility of persistent fungal infections of the cornea should be considered after prolonged corticosteroid dosing.

There have been reports of bacterial keratitis associated with the use of multiple dose containers of topical ophthalmic products. These containers had been inadvertently contaminated by patients who, in most cases, had a concurrent corneal disease or a disruption of the ocular epithelial surface. (See PRECAUTIONS, *Information for Patients.*)

Information for Patients

Patients should be instructed to avoid allowing the tip of the dispensing container to contact the eye or surrounding structures.

Patients should also be instructed that ocular preparations, if handled improperly, can become contaminated by common bacteria known to cause ocular infections. Serious damage to the eye and subsequent loss of vision may result from using contaminated preparations. (See PRECAUTIONS, *General.*)

Patients should also be advised that if they develop an intercurrent ocular condition (e.g., trauma, ocular surgery or infection), they should immediately seek their physician's advice concerning the continued use of the present multidose container.

Carcinogenesis, Mutagenesis, Impairment of Fertility

Long-term animal studies have not been performed to evaluate the carcinogenic potential or the effect on fertility of Ophthalmic Ointment DECADRON Phosphate.

Pregnancy

Pregnancy Category C. Dexamethasone has been shown to be teratogenic in mice and rabbits following topical ophthalmic application in multiples of the therapeutic dose.

In the mouse, corticosteroids produce fetal resorptions and a specific abnormality, cleft palate. In the rabbit, corticosteroids have produced fetal resorptions and multiple abnormalities involving the head, ears, limbs, palate, etc.

There are no adequate or well-controlled studies in pregnant women. Ophthalmic Ointment DECADRON Phosphate should be used during pregnancy only if the potential benefit to the mother justifies the potential risk to the embryo or fetus. Infants born of mothers who have received substantial doses of corticosteroids during pregnancy should be observed carefully for signs of hypoadrenalism.

Nursing Mothers

Topically applied steroids are absorbed systemically. Therefore, because of the potential for serious adverse reactions in nursing infants from dexamethasone sodium phosphate, a decision should be made whether to discontinue nursing or discontinue the drug, taking into account the importance of the drug to the mother.

Pediatric Use

Safety and effectiveness in children have not been established.

Adverse Reactions

Glaucoma with optic nerve damage, visual acuity and field defects, posterior subcapsular cataract formation, secondary ocular infection from pathogens including herpes simplex, perforation of the globe.

Rarely, filtering blebs have been reported when topical steroids have been used following cataract surgery.

Rarely, stinging or burning may occur.

Dosage and Administration

The duration of treatment will vary with the type of lesion and may extend from a few days to several weeks, according to therapeutic response. Relapses, more common in chronic active lesions than in self-limited conditions, usually respond to retreatment.

Apply a thin coating of ointment three or four times a day. When a favorable response is observed, reduce the number of daily applications to two, and later to one a day as a maintenance dose if this is sufficient to control symptoms.

Ophthalmic Ointment DECADRON Phosphate is particularly convenient when an eye pad is used. It may also be the preparation of choice for patients in whom therapeutic benefit depends on prolonged contact of the active ingredients with ocular tissues.

How Supplied

No. 7615—0.05% Sterile Ophthalmic Ointment DECADRON Phosphate is a clear unctuous ointment and is supplied as follows:

NDC 0006-7615-04 in 3.5 g tubes
(6505-00-961-5508 0.05% 3.5 g).
7612331 Issued October 1993

Shown in Product Identification Guide, page 105

DECADRON® Phosphate ℞
(Dexamethasone Sodium Phosphate), U.S.P.
0.1% Dexamethasone Phosphate Equivalent
Sterile Ophthalmic Solution

Description

Dexamethasone sodium phosphate is 9-fluoro-11β, 17-dihydroxy-16α-methyl-21-(phosphonooxy)pregna-1,4-diene-3,20-dione disodium salt. Its empirical formula is $C_{22}H_{28}FNa_2O_8P$ and its structural formula is:

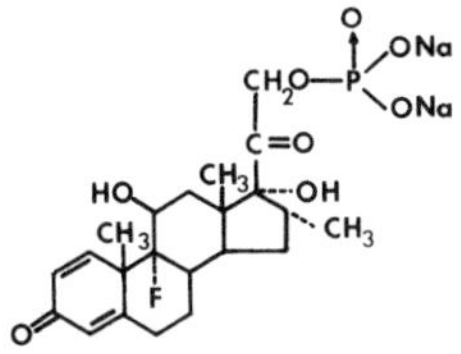

Glucocorticoids are adrenocortical steroids, both naturally occurring and synthetic. Dexamethasone is a synthetic analog of naturally occurring glucocorticoids (hydrocortisone and cortisone). Dexamethasone sodium phosphate is a water soluble, inorganic ester of dexamethasone. It is approximately three thousand times more soluble in water at 25°C than hydrocortisone. Its molecular weight is 516.41.

Ophthalmic Solution DECADRON* Phosphate (Dexamethasone Sodium Phosphate) in the 5 mL OCUMETER* ophthalmic dispenser is a topical steroid solution containing dexamethasone sodium phosphate equivalent to 1 mg (0.1%) dexamethasone phosphate in each milliliter of buffered solution. Inactive ingredients: creatinine, sodium citrate, sodium borate, polysorbate 80, disodium edetate, hydrochloric acid to adjust pH, and water for injection. Sodium bisulfite 0.1%, phenylethanol 0.25% and benzalkonium chloride 0.02% added as preservatives.

*Registered trademark of MERCK & CO., INC.

Clinical Pharmacology

Dexamethasone sodium phosphate suppresses the inflammatory response to a variety of agents and it probably delays or slows healing. No generally accepted explanation of these steroid properties has been advanced.

Indications and Usage

For the treatment of the following conditions:

Ophthalmic:

Steroid responsive inflammatory conditions of the palpebral and bulbar conjunctiva, cornea, and anterior segment of the globe, such as allergic conjunctivitis, acne rosacea, superficial punctate keratitis, herpes zoster keratitis, iritis, cyclitis, selected infective conjunctivitis when the inherent hazard of steroid use is accepted to obtain an advisable diminution in edema and inflammation; corneal injury from chemical or thermal burns, or penetration of foreign bodies.

Otic:

Steroid responsive inflammatory conditions of the external auditory meatus, such as allergic otitis externa, selected purulent and nonpurulent infective otitis externa when the hazard of steroid use is accepted to obtain an advisable diminution in edema and inflammation.

Contraindications

Epithelial herpes simplex keratitis (dendritic keratitis).

Acute infectious stages of vaccinia, varicella, and many other viral diseases of the cornea and conjunctiva.

Mycobacterial infection of the eye.

Fungal diseases of ocular or auricular structures.

Hypersensitivity to any component of this product, including sulfites (see WARNINGS).

Perforation of a drum membrane.

Warnings

Prolonged use may result in ocular hypertension and/or glaucoma, with damage to the optic nerve, defects in visual acuity and fields of vision, and posterior subcapsular cataract formation. Prolonged use may suppress the host response and thus increase the hazard of secondary ocular infections. In those diseases causing thinning of the cornea or sclera, perforations have been known to occur with the use of topical corticosteroids. In acute purulent conditions of the eye or ear, corticosteroids may mask infection or enhance existing infection. If these products are used for 10 days or longer, intraocular pressure should be routinely monitored even though it may be difficult in children and uncooperative patients.

Employment of corticosteroid medication in the treatment of herpes simplex other than epithelial herpes simplex keratitis, in which it is contraindicated, requires great caution; periodic slit-lamp microscopy is essential.

Ophthalmic Solution DECADRON Phosphate contains sodium bisulfite, a sulfite that may cause allergic-type reactions including anaphylactic symptoms and life-threatening or less severe asthmatic episodes in certain susceptible people. The overall prevalence of sulfite sensitivity in the general population is unknown and probably low. Sulfite sensitivity is seen more frequently in asthmatic than in nonasthmatic people.

Precautions

General

The possibility of persistent fungal infections of the cornea should be considered after prolonged corticosteroid dosing.

There have been reports of bacterial keratitis associated with the use of multiple dose containers of topical ophthalmic products. These containers had been inadvertently contaminated by patients who, in most cases, had a concurrent corneal disease or a disruption of the ocular epithelial surface. (See PRECAUTIONS, *Information for Patients.*)

Continued on next page

Information on the Merck & Co., Inc., products listed on these pages is from the full prescribing information in use August 31, 1999.

Decadron Phosphate Sol.—Cont.

Information for Patients
Patients should be instructed to avoid allowing the tip of the dispensing container to contact the eye or surrounding structures.
Patients should also be instructed that ocular solutions, if handled improperly, can become contaminated by common bacteria known to cause ocular infections. Serious damage to the eye and subsequent loss of vision may result from using contaminated solutions. (See PRECAUTIONS, *General.*)
Patients should also be advised that if they develop an intercurrent ocular condition (e.g., trauma, ocular surgery or infection), they should immediately seek their physician's advice concerning the continued use of the present multidose container.
One of the preservatives in Ophthalmic Solution DECADRON Phosphate, benzalkonium chloride, may be absorbed by soft contact lenses. Patients wearing soft contact lenses should be instructed to wait at least 15 minutes after instilling Ophthalmic Solution DECADRON Phosphate before they insert their lenses.
Carcinogenesis, Mutagenesis, Impairment of Fertility
Long-term animal studies have not been performed to evaluate the carcinogenic potential or the effect on fertility of Ophthalmic Solution DECADRON Phosphate.
Pregnancy
Pregnancy Category C. Dexamethasone has been shown to be teratogenic in mice and rabbits following topical ophthalmic application in multiples of the therapeutic dose.
In the mouse, corticosteroids produce fetal resorptions and a specific abnormality, cleft palate. In the rabbit, corticosteroids have produced fetal resorptions and multiple abnormalities involving the head, ears, limbs, palate, etc.
There are no adequate or well-controlled studies in pregnant women. Ophthalmic Solution DECADRON Phosphate should be used during pregnancy only if the potential benefit to the mother justifies the potential risk to the embryo or fetus. Infants born of mothers who have received substantial doses of corticosteroids during pregnancy should be observed carefully for signs of hypoadrenalism.
Nursing Mothers
Topically applied steroids are absorbed systemically. Therefore, because of the potential for serious adverse reactions in nursing infants from dexamethasone sodium phosphate, a decision should be made whether to discontinue nursing or discontinue the drug, taking into account the importance of the drug to the mother.
Pediatric Use
Safety and effectiveness in pediatric patients have not been established.

Adverse Reactions
Glaucoma with optic nerve damage, visual acuity and field defects, posterior subcapsular cataract formation, secondary ocular infection from pathogens including herpes simplex, perforation of the globe.
Rarely, filtering blebs have been reported when topical steroids have been used following cataract surgery.
Rarely, stinging or burning may occur.

Dosage and Administration
The duration of treatment will vary with the type of lesion and may extend from a few days to several weeks, according to therapeutic response. Relapses, more common in chronic active lesions than in self-limited conditions, usually respond to retreatment.
Eye —Instill one or two drops of solution into the conjunctival sac every hour during the day and every two hours during the night as initial therapy. When a favorable response is observed, reduce dosage to one drop every four hours. Later, further reduction in dosage to one drop three or four times daily may suffice to control symptoms.
Ear —Clean the aural canal thoroughly and sponge dry. Instill the solution directly into the aural canal. A suggested initial dosage is three or four drops two or three times a day. When a favorable response is obtained, reduce dosage gradually and eventually discontinue.
If preferred, the aural canal may be packed with a gauze wick saturated with solution. Keep the wick moist with the preparation and remove from the ear after 12 to 24 hours. Treatment may be repeated as often as necessary at the discretion of the physician.

How Supplied
Sterile Ophthalmic Solution DECADRON Phosphate is a clear, colorless to pale yellow solution.
No. 7643—Ophthalmic Solution DECADRON Phosphate is supplied as follows:
NDC 0006-7643-03 in 5 mL white, opaque, plastic OCUMETER ophthalmic dispenser with a controlled drop tip.
(6505-00-007-4536 0.1% 5 mL).

7261522 Issued September 1996

Shown in Product Identification Guide, page 106

HUMORSOL® ℞

(Demecarium Bromide)
Sterile Ophthalmic Solution
For Topical Application into the Conjunctival Sac Only

Description
Ophthalmic Solution HUMORSOL* (Demecarium Bromide) is a sterile solution supplied in two dosage strengths: 0.125 percent and 0.25 percent. The inactive ingredients are sodium chloride and water for injection; benzalkonium chloride 1:5000 is added as preservative. Demecarium bromide is a quaternary ammonium compound with a molecular weight of 716.60. Its chemical name is 3,3′-[1,10-decanediylbis [(methylimino)carbonyloxy]] bis [*N,N,N* -trimethylbenzenaminium] dibromide. Its empirical formula is $C_{32}H_{52}Br_2N_4O_4$ and its structural formula is:

*Registered trademark of MERCK & CO., INC.

Clinical Pharmacology
HUMORSOL is a cholinesterase inhibitor with sustained activity. It acts mainly on true (erythrocyte) cholinesterase. Application of HUMORSOL to the eye produces intense miosis and ciliary muscle contraction due to inhibition of cholinesterase, allowing acetylcholine to accumulate at sites of cholinergic transmission. These effects are accompanied by increased capillary permeability of the ciliary body and iris, increased permeability of the blood-aqueous barrier, and vasodilation. Myopia may be induced or, if present, may be augmented by the increased refractive power of the lens that results from the accommodative effect of the drug. HUMORSOL indirectly produces some of the muscarinic and nicotinic effects of acetylcholine as quantities of the latter accumulate.

Indications and Usage
Open-angle glaucoma (HUMORSOL should be used in glaucoma only when shorter-acting miotics have proved inadequate).
Conditions obstructing aqueous outflow, such as synechial formation, that are amenable to miotic therapy
Following iridectomy
Accommodative esotropia (accommodative convergent strabismus)

Contraindications
Hypersensitivity to any component of this product.
Because of the toxicity of cholinesterase inhibitors in general, HUMORSOL is contraindicated in women who are or who may become pregnant. If this drug is used during pregnancy, or if the patient becomes pregnant while taking this drug, the patient should be apprised of the potential hazard to the fetus.
Because miotics may aggravate inflammation, HUMORSOL should not be used in active uveal inflammation and/or glaucoma associated with iridocyclitis.

Warnings
In patients receiving cholinesterase inhibitors such as HUMORSOL, succinylcholine should be administered with extreme caution before and during general anesthesia.
Because of possible adverse additive effects, HUMORSOL should be administered only with extreme caution to patients with myasthenia gravis who are receiving systemic anticholinesterase therapy; conversely, extreme caution should be exercised in the use of an anticholinesterase drug for the treatment of myasthenia gravis patients who are already undergoing topical therapy with cholinesterase inhibitors.

Precautions
General
Gonioscopy is recommended prior to medication with HUMORSOL.
HUMORSOL should be used with caution in patients with chronic angle-closure (narrow-angle) glaucoma or in patients with narrow angles, because of the possibility of producing pupillary block and increasing angle blockage.
When an intraocular inflammatory process is present, the intensity and persistence of miosis and ciliary muscle contraction that result from anticholinesterase therapy require abstention from, or cautious use of, HUMORSOL.
Systemic effects are infrequent when HUMORSOL is instilled carefully. Compression of the lacrimal duct for several seconds immediately following instillation minimizes drainage into the nasal chamber with its extensive absorption surface. Wash the hands immediately after instillation.
Discontinue HUMORSOL if salivation, urinary incontinence, diarrhea, profuse sweating, muscle weakness, respiratory difficulties, shock, or cardiac irregularities occur.
Persons receiving cholinesterase inhibitors who are exposed to organophosphate-type insecticides and pesticides (gardeners, organophosphate plant or warehouse workers, farmers, residents of communities which are undergoing insecticide spraying or dusting, etc.) should be warned of the added systemic effects possible from absorption through the respiratory tract or skin. Wearing of respiratory masks, frequent washing, and clothing changes may be advisable.
Anticholinesterase drugs should be used with extreme caution, if at all, in patients with marked vagotonia, bronchial asthma, spastic gastrointestinal disturbances, peptic ulcer, pronounced bradycardia and hypotension, recent myocardial infarction, epilepsy, parkinsonism, and other disorders that may respond adversely to vagotonic effects.
After long-term use of HUMORSOL, dilation of blood vessels and resulting greater permeability increase the possibility of hyphema during ophthalmic surgery. Therefore, this drug should be discontinued before surgery.

Despite observance of all precautions and the use of only the recommended dose, there is some evidence that repeated administration may cause depression of the concentration of cholinesterase in the serum and erythrocytes, with resultant systemic effects.

There have been reports of bacterial keratitis associated with the use of multiple dose containers of topical ophthalmic products. These containers had been inadvertently contaminated by patients who, in most cases, had a concurrent corneal disease or a disruption of the ocular epithelial surface. (See PRECAUTIONS, *Information for Patients.*)

Information for Patients

Patients should be instructed to avoid allowing the tip of the dispensing container to contact the eye or surrounding structures.

Patients should also be instructed that ocular solutions, if handled improperly, can become contaminated by common bacteria known to cause ocular infections. Serious damage to the eye and subsequent loss of vision may result from using contaminated solutions. (See PRECAUTIONS, *General.*)

Patients should also be advised that if they develop an intercurrent ocular condition (e.g., trauma, ocular surgery or infection), they should immediately seek their physician's advice concerning the continued use of the present multidose container.

The preservative in HUMORSOL, benzalkonium chloride, may be absorbed by soft contact lenses. Patients wearing soft contact lenses should be instructed to wait at least 15 minutes after instilling HUMORSOL before they insert their lenses.

Drug Interactions

See WARNINGS regarding possible drug interactions of HUMORSOL with succinylcholine or with other anticholinesterase agents.

Carcinogenesis, Mutagenesis, Impairment of Fertility

Long-term studies in animals have not been performed to evaluate the effects of HUMORSOL on fertility or carcinogenic potential.

Pregnancy

Pregnancy Category X: See CONTRAINDICATIONS.

Nursing Mothers

It is not known whether this drug is excreted in human milk. Because of the potential for serious adverse reactions in nursing infants from HUMORSOL, a decision should be made whether to discontinue nursing or to discontinue the drug, taking into account the importance of the drug to the mother.

Pediatric Use

The occurrence of iris cysts is more frequent in pediatric patients. (See ADVERSE REACTIONS and DOSAGE AND ADMINISTRATION.)

Extreme caution should be exercised in pediatric patients receiving HUMORSOL who may require general anesthesia (see WARNINGS).

Since HUMORSOL is a potent cholinesterase inhibitor it should be kept out of the reach of children.

Adverse Reactions

Stinging, burning, lacrimation, lid muscle twitching, conjunctival and ciliary redness, brow ache, headache, and induced myopia with visual blurring may occur.

Activation of latent iritis or uveitis may occur.

As with all miotic therapy, retinal detachment has been reported occasionally.

Iris cysts may form, enlarge, and obscure vision. Occurrence is more frequent in children. The iris cyst usually shrinks upon discontinuance of the miotic. Rarely, the cyst may rupture or break free into the aqueous. Frequent examination for this occurrence is advised.

Lens opacities have been reported in patients on miotic therapy. Routine slit-lamp examinations, including the lens, should accompany prolonged use.

Paradoxical increase in intraocular pressure may follow anticholinesterase instillation. This may be alleviated by pupil-dilating medication.

Prolonged use may cause conjunctival thickening and obstruction of nasolacrimal canals.

Systemic effects, which occur rarely, are suggestive of increased cholinergic activity. Such effects may include nausea, vomiting, abdominal cramps, diarrhea, urinary incontinence, salivation, sweating, difficulty in breathing, bradycardia, or cardiac irregularities. Medical management of systemic effects may be indicated (see TREATMENT OF ADVERSE EFFECTS).

Treatment of Adverse Effects

If HUMORSOL is taken systemically by accident, or if systemic effects occur after topical application in the eye or from accidental skin contact, administer atropine sulfate parenterally (intravenously if necessary) in a dose (for adults) of 0.4 to 0.6 mg or more. The recommended dosage of atropine in infants and children up to 12 years of age is 0.01 mg/kg repeated every two hours as needed until the desired effect is obtained, or adverse effects of atropine preclude further usage. The maximum single dose should not exceed 0.4 mg.

The use of much larger doses of atropine in treating anticholinesterase intoxication in adults has been reported in the literature. Initially 2 to 6 mg may be given followed by 2 mg every hour or more often, as long as muscarinic effects continue. The greater possibility of atropinization with large doses, particularly in sensitive individuals, should be borne in mind.

Pralidoxime* chloride has been reported to be useful in treating systemic effects due to cholinesterase inhibitors. However, its use is recommended in addition to and not as a substitute for atropine.

A short-acting barbiturate is indicated if convulsions occur that are not entirely relieved by atropine. Barbiturate dosage should be carefully adjusted to avoid central respiratory depression. Marked weakness or paralysis of muscles of respiration should be treated promptly by artificial respiration and maintenance of a clear airway.

The oral LD_{50} of HUMORSOL is 2.96 mg/kg in the mouse.

*PROTOPAM® Chloride (Pralidoxime Chloride), Ayerst Laboratories

Dosage and Administration

HUMORSOL *is intended solely for topical use in the conjunctival sac.*

As HUMORSOL is an extremely potent drug, the physician should thoroughly familiarize himself with its use and the technic of instillation.

The required dose is applied in the conjunctival sac, with the patient supine, care being taken not to touch the cornea with the tip of the OCUMETER* ophthalmic dispenser. *The patient or person administering the medication should apply continuous gentle pressure on the lacrimal duct with the index finger for several seconds immediately following instillation of the drops. This is to prevent drainage overflow of solution into the nasal and pharyngeal spaces, which might cause systemic absorption. Wash the hands immediately after administration.*

HUMORSOL *should not be used more often than directed. Caution is necessary to avoid overdosage.*

Initial titration and dosage adjustments with HUMORSOL must be individualized to obtain maximal therapeutic effect. The patient must be closely observed during the initial period. If the response is not adequate within the first 24 hours, other measures should be considered.

Keep frequency of use to a minimum in all patients, but especially in children, to reduce the chance of iris cyst development (see ADVERSE REACTIONS).

Glaucoma

For initial therapy with HUMORSOL (0.125 percent or 0.25 percent) place 1 drop (children) or 1 or 2 drops (adults) in the glaucomatous eye. A decrease in intraocular pressure should occur within a few hours. During this period, keep the patient under supervision and make tonometric examinations at least hourly for 3 or 4 hours to be sure that no immediate rise in pressure occurs (see ADVERSE REACTIONS).

Duration of effect varies with the individual. The usual dosage can vary from as much as 1 or 2 drops twice a day to as little as 1 or 2 drops twice a week. The 0.125 percent strength used twice a day usually results in smooth control of the physiologic diurnal variation in intraocular pressure. This is probably the preferred dosage for most wide (open) angle glaucoma patients.

Strabismus

Essentially equal visual acuity of both eyes is a prerequisite to the successful treatment of esotropia with HUMORSOL. For initial evaluation it may be used as a diagnostic aid to determine if an accommodative factor exists. This is especially useful preoperatively in young children and in patients with normal hypermetropic refractive errors. One drop is given daily for 2 weeks, then 1 drop every 2 days for 2 to 3 weeks. If the eyes become straighter, an accommodative factor is demonstrated. This technic may supplement or complement standard testing with atropine and trial with glasses for the accommodative factor.

In esotropia uncomplicated by amblyopia or anisometropia, HUMORSOL may be instilled in both eyes, *not more than 1 drop at a time every day for 2 to 3 weeks,* as too severe a degree of miosis may interfere with vision. Then reduce the dosage to 1 drop every other day for 3 to 4 weeks and reevaluate the patient's status.

HUMORSOL may be continued in a dosage of 1 drop every 2 days to 1 drop twice a week. (The latter dosage may be maintained for several months.) Evaluate the patient's condition every 4 to 12 weeks. If improvement continues, change the schedule to 1 drop once a week and eventually to a trial without medication. However, if after 4 months, control of the condition still requires 1 drop every 2 days, therapy with HUMORSOL should be stopped.

*Registered trademark of MERCK & CO., INC.

How Supplied

Sterile Ophthalmic Solution HUMORSOL is a clear, colorless, aqueous solution and is supplied in a 5 mL white, opaque, plastic OCUMETER ophthalmic dispenser with a controlled-drop tip:

No. 3255—0.125 percent solution.
NDC 0006-3255-03.

No. 3267—0.25 percent solution.
NDC 0006-3267-03.

Storage

Protect from freezing and excessive heat.

7414315 Issued September 1996

Continued on next page

Information on the Merck & Co., Inc., products listed on these pages is from the full prescribing information in use August 31, 1999.

Humorsol—Cont.

Shown in Product Identification Guide, page 106

LACRISERT® Sterile Ophthalmic Insert ℞ (Hydroxypropyl Cellulose Ophthalmic Insert), U.S.P.

Description

LACRISERT* (hydroxypropyl cellulose ophthalmic insert) is a sterile, translucent, rod-shaped, water soluble, ophthalmic insert made of hydroxypropyl cellulose, for administration into the inferior cul-de-sac of the eye.

The chemical name for hydroxypropyl cellulose is cellulose, 2-hydroxypropyl ether. It is an ether of cellulose in which hydroxypropyl groups (-$CH_2CHOHCH_3$) are attached to the hydroxyls present in the anhydroglucose rings of cellulose by ether linkages. A representative structure of the monomer is: The molecular weight is typically 1×10^6.

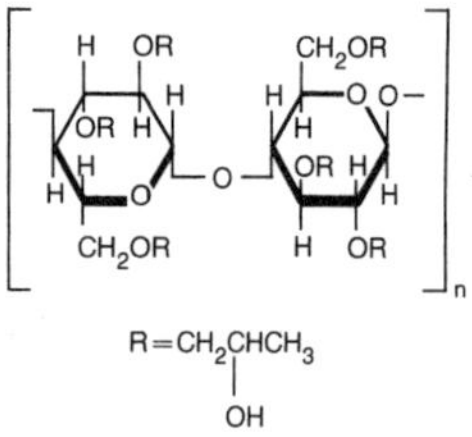

R = $CH_2CH(OH)CH_3$

Hydroxypropyl cellulose is an off-white, odorless, tasteless powder. It is soluble in water below 38°C, and in many polar organic solvents such as ethanol, propylene glycol, dioxane, methanol, isopropyl alcohol (95%), dimethyl sulfoxide, and dimethyl formamide.

Each LACRISERT is 5 mg of hydroxypropyl cellulose. LACRISERT contains no preservatives or other ingredients. It is about 1.27 mm in diameter by about 3.5 mm long.

LACRISERT is supplied in packages of 60 units, together with illustrated instructions and a special applicator for removing LACRISERT from the unit dose blister and inserting it into the eye. A spare applicator is included in each package.

---

*Registered trademark of MERCK & CO., INC.

Clinical Pharmacology

Pharmacodynamics

LACRISERT acts to stabilize and thicken the precorneal tear film and prolong the tear film breakup time which is usually accelerated in patients with dry eye states. LACRISERT also acts to lubricate and protect the eye.

LACRISERT usually reduces the signs and symptoms resulting from moderate to severe dry eye syndromes, such as conjunctival hyperemia, corneal and conjunctival staining with rose bengal, exudation, itching, burning, foreign body sensation, smarting, photophobia, dryness and blurred or cloudy vision. Progressive visual deterioration which occurs in some patients may be retarded, halted, or sometimes reversed.

In a multicenter crossover study the 5 mg LACRISERT administered once a day during the waking hours was compared to artificial tears used four or more times daily. There was a prolongation of tear film breakup time and a decrease in foreign body sensation associated with dry eye syndrome in patients during treatment with inserts as compared to artificial tears; these findings were statistically significantly different between the treatment groups. Improvement, as measured by amelioration of symptoms, by slit lamp examination and by rose bengal staining of the cornea and conjunctiva, was greater in most patients with moderate to severe symptoms during treatment with LACRISERT. Patient comfort was usually better with LACRISERT than with artificial tears solution, and most patients preferred LACRISERT.

In most patients treated with LACRISERT for over one year, improvement was observed as evidenced by amelioration of symptoms generally associated with keratoconjunctivitis sicca such as burning, tearing, foreign body sensation, itching, photophobia and blurred or cloudy vision.

During studies in healthy volunteers, a thickened precorneal tear film was usually observed through the slit-lamp while LACRISERT was present in the conjunctival sac.

Pharmacokinetics and Metabolism

Hydroxypropyl cellulose is a physiologically inert substance. In a study of rats fed hydroxypropyl cellulose or unmodified cellulose at levels up to 5% of their diet, it was found that the two were biologically equivalent in that neither was metabolized.

Studies conducted in rats fed ^{14}C -labeled hydroxypropyl cellulose demonstrated that when orally administered, hydroxypropyl cellulose is not absorbed from the gastrointestinal tract and is quantitatively excreted in the feces.

Dissolution studies in rabbits showed that hydroxypropyl cellulose inserts became softer within 1 hour after they were placed in the conjunctival sac. Most of the inserts dissolved completely in 14 to 18 hours; with a single exception, all had disappeared by 24 hours after insertion. Similar dissolution of the inserts was observed during prolonged administration (up to 54 weeks).

Indications and Usage

LACRISERT is indicated in patients with moderate to severe dry eye syndromes, including keratoconjunctivitis sicca. LACRISERT is indicated especially in patients who remain symptomatic after an adequate trial of therapy with artifical tear solutions.

LACRISERT is also indicated for patients with:

Exposure keratitis
Decreased corneal sensitivity
Recurrent corneal erosions

Contraindications

LACRISERT is contraindicated in patients who are hypersensitive to hydroxypropyl cellulose.

Warnings

Instructions for inserting and removing LACRISERT should be carefully followed.

Precautions

General

If improperly placed, LACRISERT may result in corneal abrasion (see DOSAGE AND ADMINISTRATION).

Information for Patients

Patients should be advised to follow the instructions for using LACRISERT which accompany the package.

Because this product may produce transient blurring of vision, patients should be instructed to exercise caution when operating hazardous machinery or driving a motor vehicle.

Drug Interactions

Application of hydroxypropyl cellulose ophthalmic inserts to the eyes of unanesthetized rabbits immediately prior to or two hours before instilling pilocarpine, proparacaine HCl (0.5%), or phenylephrine (5%) did not markedly alter the magnitude and/or duration of the miotic, local corneal anesthetic, or mydriatic activity, respectively, of these agents.

Under various treatment schedules, the anti-inflammatory effect of ocularly instilled dexamethasone (0.1%) in unanesthetized rabbits with primary uveitis was not affected by the presence of hydroxypropyl cellulose inserts.

Carcinogenesis, Mutagenesis, Impairment of Fertility

Feeding of hydroxypropyl cellulose to rats at levels up to 5% of their diet produced no gross or histopathologic changes or other deleterious effects.

Pediatric Use

Safety and effectiveness in pediatric patients have not been established.

Adverse Reactions

The following adverse reactions have been reported in patients treated with LACRISERT, but were in most instances mild and transient:

Transient blurring of vision
(See PRECAUTIONS)
Ocular discomfort or irritation
Matting or stickiness of eyelashes
Photophobia
Hypersensitivity
Edema of the eyelids
Hyperemia

Dosage and Administration

One LACRISERT ophthalmic insert in each eye once daily is usually sufficient to relieve the symptoms associated with moderate to severe dry eye syndromes. Individual patients may require more flexibility in the use of LACRISERT; some patients may require twice daily use for optimal results.

Clinical experience with LACRISERT indicates that in some patients several weeks may be required before satisfactory improvement of symptoms is achieved.

LACRISERT is inserted into the inferior cul-de-sac of the eye beneath the base of the tarsus, not in apposition to the cornea, nor beneath the eyelid at the level of the tarsal plate. If not properly positioned, it will be expelled into the interpalpebral fissure, and may cause symptoms of a foreign body. Illustrated instructions are included in each package. While in the licensed practitioner's office, the patient should read the instructions, then practice insertion and removal of LACRISERT until proficiency is achieved.

NOTE: Occasionally LACRISERT is inadvertently expelled from the eye, especially in patients with shallow conjunctival fornices. The patient should be cautioned against rubbing the eye(s) containing LACRISERT, especially upon awakening, so as not to dislodge or expel the insert. If required, another LACRISERT ophthalmic insert may be inserted. If experience indicates that transient blurred vision develops in an individual patient, the patient may want to remove LACRISERT a few hours after insertion to avoid this. Another LACRISERT ophthalmic insert may be inserted if needed.

If LACRISERT causes worsening of symptoms, the patient should be instructed to inspect the conjunctival sac to make certain LACRISERT is in the proper location, deep in the inferior cul-de-sac of the eye beneath the base of the tarsus. If these symptoms persist, LACRISERT should be removed and the patient should contact the practitioner.

How Supplied

No. 3380—LACRISERT, a sterile, translucent, rod-shaped, water soluble, ophthalmic insert made of hydroxypropyl cellulose, 5 mg, is supplied as follows:

NDC 0006-3380-60 in packages containing 60 unit doses, two reusable applicators and a storage container

(6505-01-153-4360, 5 mg 60's).

Storage

Store below 30°C (86°F).

7415111 Issued October 1997

Shown in Product Identification Guide, page 106

NEODECADRON® ℞

(Neomycin Sulfate-Dexamethasone Sodium Phosphate)
Sterile Ophthalmic Ointment

Description

Sterile Ophthalmic Ointment NEODECADRON* (Neomycin Sulfate-Dexamethasone Sodium Phosphate) is a topical corticosteroid-antibiotic ointment for ophthalmic use.

Dexamethasone sodium phosphate is 9-fluoro-11β, 17-dihydroxy- 16α-methyl-21-(phosphonooxy)pregna-1, 4-diene-3, 20-dione disodium salt. Its empirical formula is $C_{22}H_{28}FNa_2O_8P$ and its structural formula is:

Dexamethasone is a synthetic analog of naturally occurring glucocorticoids (hydrocortisone and cortisone).

Dexamethasone sodium phosphate is a water soluble, inorganic ester of dexamethasone. Its molecular weight is 516.41.

Neomycin sulfate, an antibiotic of the aminoglycoside group, is a mixture of the sulfate salts of neomycin, produced by the growth of *Streptomyces fradiae* Waksman (Fam. Streptomycetaceae). Neomycin is a complex typically containing 8-13% neomycin C, less than 0.2% neomycin A, and the rest, neomycin B. The empirical formula for both neomycin B and neomycin C is $C_{23}H_{46}N_6O_{13}$, and the molecular weight for each is 614.65. Neomycin A (also referred to as neamine) has an empirical formula of $C_{12}H_{26}N_4O_6$ and a molecular weight of 322.36. The structural formulae for neomycin sulfate are:

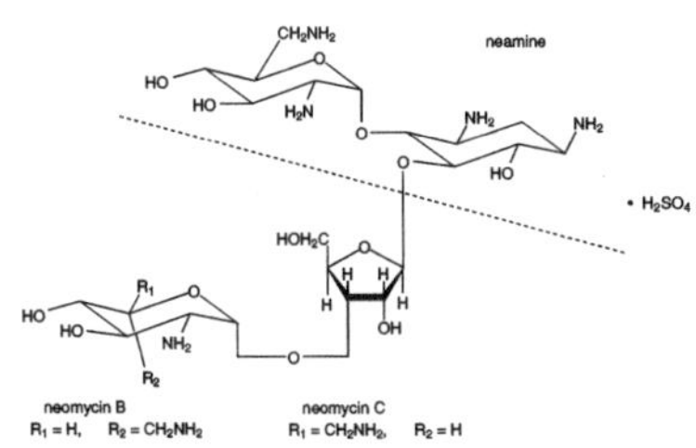

Ophthalmic Ointment NEODECADRON contains in each gram: dexamethasone sodium phosphate equivalent to 0.5 mg (0.05%) dexamethasone phosphate and neomycin sulfate equivalent to 3.5 mg neomycin base. Inactive ingredients: white petrolatum and mineral oil.

---

*Registered trademark of MERCK & CO., Inc.

Clinical Pharmacology

Corticosteroids suppress the inflammatory response to a variety of agents, and they probably delay or slow healing. Since corticosteroids may inhibit the body's defense mechanism against infection, a concomitant antimicrobial drug may be used when this inhibition is considered to be clinically significant in a particular case.

When a decision to administer both a corticosteroid and an antimicrobial is made, the administration of such drugs in combination has the advantage of greater patient compliance and convenience, with the added assurance that the appropriate dosage of both drugs is administered, plus assured compatibility of ingredient when both types of drug are in the same formulation and, particularly, that the correct volume of drug is delivered and retained.

The relative potency of corticosteroids depends on the molecular structure, concentration, and release from the vehicle.

Microbiology

The anti-infective component in Ophthalmic Ointment NEODECADRON is included to provide action against specific organisms susceptible to it. Neomycin sulfate is active *in vitro* against susceptible strains of the following microorganisms: *Staphylococcus aureus, Escherichia coli, Haemophilus influenzae, Klebsiella / Enterobacter* species, and *Neisseria* species. The product does not provide adequate coverage against: *Pseudomonas aeruginosa, Seratia marcescens,* Streptococci, including *Streptococcus pneumoniae*. (See INDICATIONS AND USAGE.)

Indications and Usage

For steroid-responsive inflammatory ocular conditions for which a corticosteroid is indicated and where bacterial infection or a risk of bacterial ocular infection exists.

Ocular steroids are indicated in inflammatory conditions of the palpebral and bulbar conjunctiva, cornea, and anterior segment of the globe where the inherent risk of steroid use in certain infective conjuctivitides is accepted to obtain a diminution in edema and inflammation. They are also indicated in chronic anterior uveitis and corneal injury from chemical, radiation, or thermal burns, or penetration of foreign bodies.

The use of a combination drug with an anti-infective component is indicated where the risk of infection is high or where there is an expectation that potentially dangerous numbers of bacteria will be present in the eye.

The particular anti-infective drug in this product is active against the following common bacterial eye pathogens:

Staphylococcus aureus
Escherichia coli
Haemophilus influenzae
Klebsiella / Enterobacter species
Neisseria species

The product does not provide adequate coverage against:

Pseudomonas aeruginosa
Serratia marcescens
Streptococci, including *Streptococcus pneumaniae*

Contraindications

NEODECADRON is contraindicated in most viral diseases of the cornea and conjunctiva including epithelial herpes simplex keratitis (dendritic keratitis), vaccinia, and varicella, and also in mycobacterial infection of the eye and fungal diseases of ocular structures. NEODECADRON is also contraindicated in individuals with known or suspected hypersensitivity to any of the ingredients of this preparation and to other corticosteroids (see WARNINGS). Hypersensitivity to the antibiotic component occurs at a higher rate than for other components.

Warnings

NOT FOR INJECTION INTO THE EYE

Prolonged use of corticosteroids may result in ocular hypertension and/or glaucoma with damage to the optic nerve, defects in visual acuity and fields of vision, and in posterior subcapsular cataract formation.

Prolonged use of corticosteroids may suppress the host response and thus increase the hazard of secondary ocular infections. In those diseases causing thinning of the cornea or sclera, perforations have been known to occur with the use of topical corticosteroids. In acute purulent conditions of the eye, corticosteroids may mask infection or enhance existing infection.

If this product is used for 10 days or longer, intraocular pressure should be routinely monitored even though it may be difficult in children and uncooperative patients. Corticosteroids should be used with caution in the presence of ocular hypertension and/or glaucoma. Intraocular pressure should be checked frequently.

The use of corticosteroids after cataract surgery may delay healing and increase the incidence of filtering blebs.

Use of ocular corticosteroids may prolong the course and may exacerbate the severity of many viral infections of the eye (including herpes simplex). Employment of a corticosteroid medication in the treatment of patients with a history of herpes simplex requires great caution; periodic slit lamp microscopy is essential. (See CONTRAINDICATIONS.)

Neomycin sulfate may occasionally cause cutaneous sensitization. If any reaction indicating such sensitivity is observed, discontinue use.

Precautions

General

The initial prescription and renewal of the medication order beyond 8 grams should be made by a physician only after examination of the patient with the aid of magnification, such as slit lamp biomicroscopy and, where appropriate, fluorescein staining. If signs and symptoms fail to improve after two days, the patient should be re-evaluated.

The possibility of fungal infections of the cornea should be considered after prolonged corticosteroid dosing. Fungal cultures should be taken when appropriate.

If this product is used for 10 days or longer, intraocular pressure should be monitored (see WARNINGS).

There have been reports of bacterial keratitis associated with the use of multiple dose containers of topical ophthalmic products. These containers had been inadvertently contaminated by patients who, in most cases, had a concurrent corneal disease or a disruption of the ocular epithelial surface. (See PRECAUTIONS, *Information for Patients.*)

Information for Patients

Patients should also be instructed to avoid allowing the tip of the dispensing container to contact the eye, eyelid, fingers, or any other surface. The use of this product by more than one person may spread infection. Keep tightly closed when not in use.

Patients should also be instructed that ocular preparations, if handled improperly, can become contaminated by common bacteria known to cause ocular infections. Serious damage to the eye and subsequent loss of vision may result from using contaminated preparations. (See PRECAUTIONS, *General.)*

If redness, irritation, swelling or pain persists or becomes aggravated, the patient should be advised to consult a physician. Patients should also be advised that if they have ocular surgery or develop an intercurrent ocular condition (e.g., trauma or infection), they should immediately seek their physician's advice.

Keep out of the reach of children.

Continued on next page

Information on the Merck & Co., Inc., products listed on these pages is from the full prescribing information in use August 31, 1999.

Neodecadron Ointment—Cont.

Carcinogenesis, Mutagenesis, Impairment of Fertility
Long term animal studies have not been performed to evaluate the carcinogenic potential or the effect on fertility of Ophthalmic Ointment NEODECADRON. Treatment of human lymphocytes *in-vitro* with neomycin increased the frequency of chromosome aberrations at the highest concentration (80μg/mL) tested; however, the effects of neomycin on carcinogenesis and mutagenesis in humans are unknown.
Pregnancy
Teratogenic effects
Pregnancy Category C
Corrticosteroids have been found to be teratogenic in animal studies. Ocular administration of 0.1% dexamethasone resulted in 15.6% and 32.3% incidence of fetal anomalies in two groups of pregnant rabbits. Fetal growth retardation and increased mortality rates have been observed in rats with chronic dexamethasone therapy. There are no adequate and well-controlled studies in pregnant women. Ophthalmic Ointment NEODECADRON should be used during pregnancy only if the potential benefit justifies the potential risk to the fetus. Infants born of mothers who have received substantial doses of corticosteroids during pregnancy should be observed carefully for signs of hypoadrenalism.
Nursing Mothers
It is not known whether topical administration of corticosteroids could result in sufficient systemic absorption to produce detectable quantities in human milk. Systemically-administered corticosteroids appear in human milk and could suppress growth, interfere with endogenous corticosteroid production, or cause other untoward effects. Because of the potential for serious adverse reactions in nursing infants from Ophthalmic Ointment NEODECADRON, a decision should be made whether to discontinue nursing or to discontinue the drug, taking into account the importance of the drug to the mother.
Pediatric Use
Safety and effectiveness in pediatric patients have not been established.

Adverse Reactions
Adverse reactions have occurred with corticosteroid/anti-infective combination drugs which can be attributed to the corticosteroid component, the anti-infective component, or the combination. Exact incidence figures are not available since no denominator of treated patients is available.
Reactions occurring most often from the presence of the anti-infective ingredient are allergic sensitizations. The reactions due to the corticosteroid component in decreasing order of frequency are: elevation of intraocular pressure (IOP) with possible development of glaucoma, and infrequent optic nerve damage, posterior subcapsular cataract formation; and delayed wound healing.
Secondary Infection: The development of secondary infection has occurred after use of combinations containing corticosteriods and antimicrobials. Fungal and viral infections of the cornea are particularly prone to develop coincidentally with long-term applications of a corticosteroid. The possibility of fungal invasion must be considered in any persistent corneal ulceration where corticosteroid treatment has been used.

Dosage and Administration
NOT FOR INJECTION INTO THE EYE
The duration of treatment will vary with the type of lesion and may extend from a few days to several weeks, according to therapeutic response.
Apply a thin coating of Ophthalmic Ointment NEODECADRON three or four times a day. When a favorable response is observed, reduce the number of daily applications to two, and later to one a day as maintenance dose if this is sufficient to control symptoms.
Not more than 8 grams should be prescribed initially and the prescription should not be refilled without further evaluation as outlined in PRECAUTIONS above.

How Supplied
No. 7617—Sterile Ophthalmic Ointment NEODECADRON is a clear, unctuous ointment, and is supplied as follows:
NDC 0006-7617-04 in 3.5 g tubes
(6505-00-982-0291 0.05% 3.5 g)
Storage
Store at controlled room temperature, 15°–30°C (59°–86°F).
7612628 Issued December 1995

Shown in Product Identification Guide, page 106

NEODECADRON® ℞
(Neomycin Sulfate-Dexamethasone Sodium Phosphate)
Sterile Ophthalmic Solution

Description
Ophthalmic Solution NEODECADRON* (Neomycin Sulfate-Dexamethasone Sodium Phosphate) is a topical corticosteroid-antibiotic solution for ophthalmic use.
Dexamethasone sodium phosphate is 9-fluoro-11β, 17-dihydroxy-16α-methyl-21-(phosphonooxy)pregna-1, 4-diene-3, 20-dione disodium salt. Its empirical formula is $C_{22}H_{28}FNa_2O_8P$ and its structural formula is:

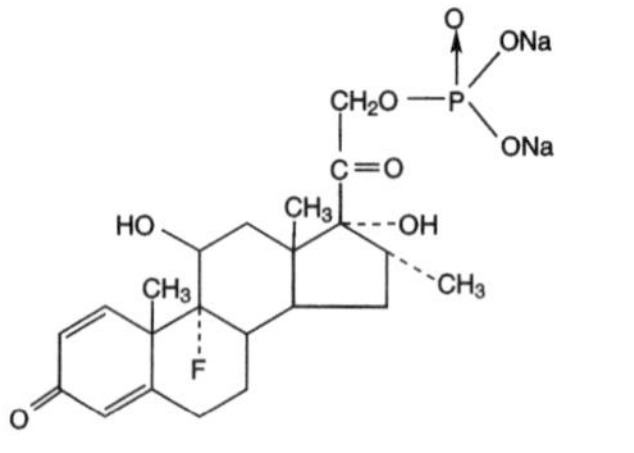

Dexamethasone is a synthetic analog of naturally occurring glucocorticoids (hydrocortisone and cortisone).
Dexamethasone sodium phosphate is a water soluble, inorganic ester of dexamethasone. Its molecular weight is 516.41.
Neomycin sulfate, an antibiotic of the aminoglycoside group, is a mixture of the sulfate salts of neomycin, produced by the growth of *Streptomyces fradiae* Waksman (Fam. Streptomycetaceae). Neomycin is a complex typically containing 8–13% neomycin C, less than 0.2% neomycin A, and the rest, neomycin B. The empirical formula for both neomycin B and neomycin C is $C_{23}H_{46}N_6O_{13}$, and the molecular weight for each is 614.65. Neomycin A (also referred to as neamine) has an empirical formula of $C_{12}H_{26}N_4O_6$ and a molecular weight of 322.36. The structural formulae for neomycin sulfate are:
[See chemical structure at top of next column]
Each milliliter of buffered Ophthalmic Solution NEODECADRON in the OCUMETER* ophthalmic dispenser contains: dexamethasone sodium phosphate equivalent to 1 mg (0.1%) dexamethasone phosphate, and neomycin sulfate equivalent to 3.5 mg neomycin base. Inactive ingredients: creatinine, sodium citrate, sodium borate, polysorbate 80, disodium edetate, hydrochloric acid to adjust pH to

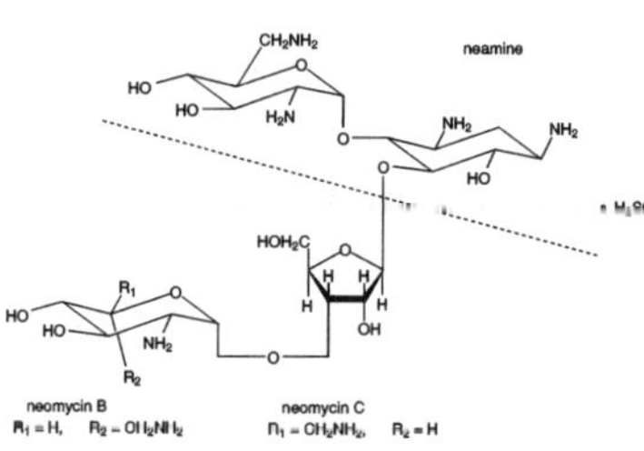

6.6–7.2, and water for injection. Benzalkonium chloride 0.02% and sodium bisulfite 0.1% added as preservatives.

*Registered trademark of MERCK & CO., Inc.

Clinical Pharmacology
Corticosteroids suppress the inflammatory response to a variety of agents, and they probably delay or slow healing. Since corticosteroids may inhibit the body's defense mechanism against infection, a concomitant antimicrobial drug may be used when this inhibition is considered to be clinically significant in a particular case.
When a decision to administer both a corticosteroid and an antimicrobial is made, the administration of such drugs in combination has the advantage of greater patient compliance and convenience, with the added assurance that the appropriate dosage of both drugs is administered, plus assured compatibility of ingredients when both types of drug are in the same formulation and, particularly, that the correct volume of drug is delivered and retained.
The relative potency of corticosteroids depends on the molecular structure, concentration, and release from the vehicle.
Microbiology
The anti-infective component in Ophthalmic Solution NEODECADRON is included to provide action against specific organisms susceptible to it. Neomycin sulfate is active *in vitro* against susceptible strains of the following microorganisms: *Staphylococcus aureus, Escherichia coli, Haemophilus influenzae, Klebsiella / Enterobacter* species, and *Neisseria* species. The product does not provide adequate coverage against: *Pseudomonas aeruginosa, Serratia marcescens,* and streptococci, including *Streptococcus pneumoniae*. (See INDICATIONS AND USAGE.)

Indications and Usage
For steroid-responsive inflammatory ocular conditions for which a corticosteroid is indicated and where bacterial infection or a risk of bacterial ocular infection exists.
Ocular steroids are indicated in inflammatory conditions of the palpebral and bulbar conjunctiva, cornea, and anterior segment of the globe where the inherent risk of steroid use in certain infective conjunctivitides is accepted to obtain a diminution in edema and inflammation. They are also indicated in chronic anterior uveitis and corneal injury from chemical, radiation, or thermal burns, or penetration of foreign bodies.
The use of a combination drug with an anti-infective component is indicated where the risk of infection is high or where there is an expectation that potentially dangerous numbers of bacteria will be present in the eye.
The particular anti-infective drug in this product is active against the following common bacterial eye pathogens:
Staphylococcus aureus
Escherichia coli
Haemophilus influenzae
Klebsiella / Enterobacter species
Neisseria species

The product does not provide adequate coverage against:
Pseudomonas aeruginosa
Serratia marcescens
Streptococci, including *Streptococcus pneumoniae*

Contraindications

NEODECADRON is contraindicated in most viral diseases of the cornea and conjunctiva including epithelial herpes simplex keratitis (dendritic keratitis), vaccinia, varicella, and also in mycobacterial infection of the eye and fungal diseases of ocular structures. NEODECADRON is also contraindicated in individuals with known or suspected hypersensitivity to any of the ingredients of this preparation, including sulfites, and to other corticosteroids (see WARNINGS). (Hypersensitivity to the antibiotic component occurs at a higher rate than for other components.)

Warnings

NOT FOR INJECTION INTO THE EYE

Prolonged use of corticosteroids may result in ocular hypertension and/or glaucoma with damage to the optic nerve, defects in visual acuity and fields of vision, and in posterior subcapsular cataract formation.

Prolonged use of corticosteroids may suppress the host response and thus increase the hazard of secondary ocular infections. In those diseases causing thinning of the cornea or sclera, perforations have been known to occur with the use of topical corticosteroids. In acute purulent conditions of the eye, corticosteroids may mask infection or enhance existing infection.

If this product is used for 10 days or longer, intraocular pressure should be routinely monitored even though it may be difficult in children and uncooperative patients. Corticosteroids should be used with caution in the presence of ocular hypertension and/or glaucoma. Intraocular pressure should be checked frequently.

The use of corticosteroids after cataract surgery may delay healing and increase the incidence of filtering blebs.

Use of ocular corticosteroids may prolong the course and may exacerbate the severity of many viral infections of the eye (including herpes simplex). Employment of a corticosteroid medication in the treatment of patients with a history of herpes simplex requires great caution; periodic slit lamp microscopy is essential. (See CONTRAINDICATIONS.)

Neomycin sulfate may occasionally cause cutaneous sensitization. If any reaction indicating such sensitivity is observed, discontinue use.

Ophthalmic Solution NEODECADRON contains sodium bisulfite, a sulfite that may cause allergic-type reactions including anaphylactic symptoms and life-threatening or less severe asthmatic episodes in certain susceptible people. The overall prevalence of sulfite sensitivity in the general population is unknown and probably low. Sulfite sensitivity is seen more frequently in asthmatic than in nonasthmatic people.

Precautions

General

The initial prescription and renewal of the medication order beyond 20 milliliters should be made by a physician only after examination of the patient with the aid of magnification, such as slit lamp biomicroscopy and, where appropriate, fluorescein staining. If signs and symptoms fail to improve after two days, the patient should be re-evaluated.

The possibility of fungal infections of the cornea should be considered after prolonged corticosteroid dosing. Fungal cultures should be taken when appropriate.

If this product is used for 10 days or longer, intraocular pressure should be monitored (see WARNINGS).

There have been reports of bacterial keratitis associated with the use of multiple dose containers of topical ophthalmic products. These containers had been inadvertently contaminated by patients who, in most cases, had a concurrent corneal disease or a disruption of the ocular epithelial surface. (See PRECAUTIONS, *Information for Patients.*)

Information for Patients

Patients should be instructed to avoid allowing the tip of the dispensing container to contact the eye, eyelid, fingers, or any other surface. The use of this product by more than one person may spread infection. Keep tightly closed when not in use.

Patients should also be instructed that ocular preparations, if handled improperly, can become contaminated by common bacteria known to cause ocular infections. Serious damage to the eye and subsequent loss of vision may result from using contaminated preparations (see PRECAUTIONS, *General*).

If redness, irritation, swelling or pain persists or becomes aggravated, the patient should be advised to consult a physician. Patients should also be advised that if they have ocular surgery or develop an intercurrent ocular condition (e.g., trauma or infection), they should immediately seek their physician's advice.

One of the preservatives in Ophthalmic Solution NEODECADRON, benzalkonium chloride, may be absorbed by soft contact lenses. Patients wearing soft contact lenses should be instructed to wait at least 15 minutes after instilling Ophthalmic Solution NEODECADRON before they insert their lenses.

Keep out of the reach of children.

Carcinogenesis, Mutagenesis, Impairment of Fertility

Long term animal studies have not been performed to evaluate the carcinogenic potential or the effect on fertility of Ophthalmic Solution NEODECADRON. Treatment of human lymphocytes *in-vitro* with neomycin increased the frequency of chromosome aberrations at the highest concentration (80 μg/mL) tested; however, the effects of neomycin or carcinogenesis and mutagenesis in humans are unknown.

Pregnancy

Teratogenic effects

Pregnancy Category C.

Corticosteroids have been found to be teratogenic in animal studies. Ocular administration of 0.1% dexamethasone resulted in 15.6% and 32.3% incidence of fetal anomalies in two groups of pregnant rabbits. Fetal growth retardation and increased mortality rates have been observed in rats with chronic dexamethasone therapy. There are no adequate and well-controlled studies in pregnant women. Ophthalmic Solution NEODECADRON should be used during pregnancy only if the potential benefit justifies the potential risk to the fetus. Infants born of mothers who have received substantial doses of corticosteroids during pregnancy should be observed carefully for signs of hypoadrenalism.

Nursing Mothers

It is not known whether topical administration of corticosteroids could result in sufficient systemic absorption to produce detectable quantities in human milk. Systemically-administered corticosteroids appear in human milk and could suppress growth, interfere with endogenous corticosteroid production, or cause other untoward effects. Because of the potential for serious adverse reactions in nursing infants from Ophthalmic Solution NEODECADRON, a decision should be made whether to discontinue nursing or to discontinue the drug, taking into account the importance of the drug to the mother.

Pediatric Use

Safety and effectiveness in pediatric patients have not been established.

Adverse Reactions

Adverse reactions have occurred with corticosteroid/anti-infective combination drugs which can be attributed to the corticosteroid component, the anti-infective component, the combination, or any other component of the product. Exact incidence figures are not available since no denominator of treated patients is available.

Reactions occurring most often from the presence of the anti-infective ingredient are allergic sensitizations. The reactions due to the corticosteroid component in decreasing order of frequency are: elevation of intraocular pressure (IOP) with possible development of glaucoma, and infrequent optic nerve damage; posterior subcapsular cataract formation; and delayed wound healing.

Secondary Infection: The development of secondary infection has occurred after use of combinations containing corticosteroids and antimicrobials. Fungal and viral infections of the cornea are particularly prone to develop coincidentally with long-term applications of a corticosteroid. The possibility of fungal invasion must be considered in any persistent corneal ulceration where corticosteroid treatment has been used.

Dosage and Administration

The duration of treatment will vary with the type of lesion and may extend from a few days to several weeks, according to therapeutic response.

Instill one or two drops of Ophthalmic Solution NEODECADRON into the conjunctival sac every hour during the day and every two hours during the night as initial therapy. When a favorable response is observed, reduce dosage to one drop every four hours. Later, further reduction in dosage to one drop three or four times daily may suffice to control symptoms.

Not more than 20 milliliters should be prescribed initially and the prescription should not be refilled without further evaluation as outlined in PRECAUTIONS above.

How Supplied

Sterile Ophthalmic Solution NEODECADRON is a clear, colorless to pale yellow solution.

No. 7639—Ophthalmic Solution NEODECADRON is supplied as follows:

NDC 0006-7639-03 in 5 mL white opaque, plastic OCUMETER ophthalmic dispenser with a controlled drop tip.

(6505-01-039-4352 0.1% 5 mL).

Storage

Store at controlled room temperature, 15°–30°C (59°–86°F). Protect from light.

7261326 Issued December 1995

Shown in Product Identification Guide, page 106

TIMOPTIC® ℞
0.25% and 0.5%
(Timolol Maleate Ophthalmic Solution), U.S.P.
Sterile Ophthalmic Solution

Description

TIMOPTIC* (timolol maleate ophthalmic solution) is a non-selective beta-adrenergic receptor blocking agent. Its chemical name is (-)-1-(*tert*-butylamino)-3-[(4-morpholino-1,2,5-thiadiazol-3-yl)oxy]-2-propanol maleate (1:1)

Continued on next page

Information on the Merck & Co., Inc., products listed on these pages is from the full prescribing information in use August 31, 1999.

Timoptic—Cont.

(salt). Timolol maleate possesses an asymmetric carbon atom in its structure and is provided as the levo-isomer. The nominal optical rotation of timolol maleate is:

$$[\alpha]^{25°}_{405\ nm} \text{ in } 0.1N\ HCl\ (C = 5\%) = -12.2°.$$

Its molecular formula is $C_{13}H_{24}N_4O_3S \cdot C_4H_4O_4$ and its structural formula is:

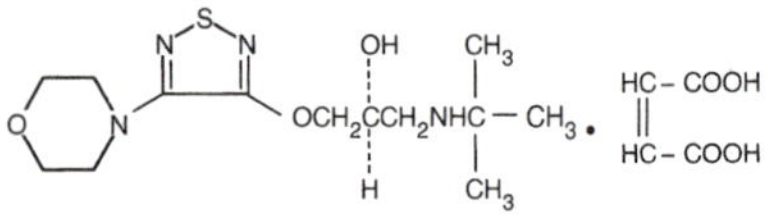

Timolol maleate has a molecular weight of 432.50. It is a white, odorless, crystalline powder which is soluble in water, methanol, and alcohol. TIMOPTIC is stable at room temperature.

TIMOPTIC Ophthalmic Solution is supplied as a sterile, isotonic, buffered, aqueous solution of timolol maleate in two dosage strengths: Each mL of TIMOPTIC 0.25% contains 2.5 mg of timolol (3.4 mg of timolol maleate). Each mL of TIMOPTIC 0.5% contains 5.0 mg of timolol (6.8 mg of timolol maleate). Inactive ingredients: monobasic and dibasic sodium phosphate, sodium hydroxide to adjust pH, and water for injection. Benzalkonium chloride 0.01% is added as preservative.

---

*Registered trademark of MERCK & CO., INC.

Clinical Pharmacology

Mechanism of Action

Timolol maleate is a $beta_1$ and $beta_2$ (non-selective) adrenergic receptor blocking agent that does not have significant intrinsic sympathomimetic, direct myocardial depressant, or local anesthetic (membrane-stabilizing) activity.

Beta-adrenergic receptor blockade reduces cardiac output in both healthy subjects and patients with heart disease. In patients with severe impairment of myocardial function, beta-adrenergic receptor blockade may inhibit the stimulatory effect of the sympathetic nervous system necessary to maintain adequate cardiac function.

Beta-adrenergic receptor blockade in the bronchi and bronchioles results in increased airway resistance from unopposed parasympathetic activity. Such an effect in patients with asthma or other bronchospastic conditions is potentially dangerous.

TIMOPTIC Ophthalmic Solution, when applied topically on the eye, has the action of reducing elevated as well as normal intraocular pressure, whether or not accompanied by glaucoma. Elevated intraocular pressure is a major risk factor in the pathogenesis of glaucomatous visual field loss. The higher the level of intraocular pressure, the greater the likelihood of glaucomatous visual field loss and optic nerve damage.

The onset of reduction in intraocular pressure following administration of TIMOPTIC can usually be detected within one-half hour after a single dose. The maximum effect usually occurs in one to two hours and significant lowering of intraocular pressure can be maintained for periods as long as 24 hours with a single dose. Repeated observations over a period of one year indicate that the intraocular pressure-lowering effect of TIMOPTIC is well maintained.

The precise mechanism of the ocular hypotensive action of TIMOPTIC is not clearly established at this time. Tonography and fluorophotometry studies in man suggest that its predominant action may be related to reduced aqueous formation. However, in some studies a slight increase in outflow facility was also observed.

Pharmacokinetics

In a study of plasma drug concentration in six subjects, the systemic exposure to timolol was determined following twice daily administration of TIMOPTIC 0.5%. The mean peak plasma concentration following morning dosing was 0.46 ng/mL and following afternoon dosing was 0.35 ng/mL.

Clinical Studies

In controlled multiclinic studies in patients with untreated intraocular pressures of 22 mmHg or greater, TIMOPTIC 0.25 percent or 0.5 percent administered twice a day produced a greater reduction in intraocular pressure than 1, 2, 3, or 4 percent pilocarpine solution administered four times a day or 0.5, 1, or 2 percent epinephrine hydrochloride solution administered twice a day.

In these studies, TIMOPTIC was generally well tolerated and produced fewer and less severe side effects than either pilocarpine or epinephrine. A slight reduction of resting heart rate in some patients receiving TIMOPTIC (mean reduction 2.9 beats/minute standard deviation 10.2) was observed.

Indications and Usage

Timoptic Ophthalmic Solution is indicated in the treatment of elevated intraocular pressure in patients with ocular hypertension or open-angle glaucoma.

Contraindications

TIMOPTIC is contraindicated in patients with (1) bronchial asthma; (2) a history of bronchial asthma; (3) severe chronic obstructive pulmonary disease (see **WARNINGS**); (4) sinus bradycardia; (5) second or third degree atrioventricular block; (6) overt cardiac failure (see **WARNINGS**); (7) cardiogenic shock; or (8) hypersensitivity to any component of this product.

Warnings

As with many topically applied ophthalmic drugs, this drug is absorbed systemically.

The same adverse reactions found with systemic administration of beta-adrenergic blocking agents may occur with topical administration. For example, severe respiratory reactions and cardiac reactions, including death due to bronchospasm in patients with asthma, and rarely death in association with cardiac failure, have been reported following systemic or ophthalmic administration of timolol maleate (see CONTRAINDICATIONS).

Cardiac Failure

Sympathetic stimulation may be essential for support of the circulation in individuals with diminished myocardial contractility, and its inhibition by beta-adrenergic receptor blockade may precipitate more severe failure.

In Patients Without a History of Cardiac Failure continued depression of the myocardium with beta-blocking agents over a period of time can, in some cases, lead to cardiac failure. At the first sign or symptom of cardiac failure TIMOPTIC should be discontinued.

Obstructive Pulmonary Disease

Patients with chronic obstructive pulmonary disease (e.g., chronic bronchitis, emphysema) of mild or moderate severity, bronchospastic disease, or a history of bronchospastic disease (other than bronchial asthma or a history of bronchial asthma, in which TIMOPTIC is contraindicated [see **CONTRAINDICATIONS**]) should, in general, not receive beta-blockers, including TIMOPTIC.

Major Surgery

The necessity or desirability of withdrawal of beta-adrenergic blocking agents prior to major surgery is controversial. Beta-adrenergic receptor blockade impairs the ability of the heart to respond to beta-adrenergically mediated reflex stimuli. This may augment the risk of general anesthesia in surgical procedures. Some patients receiving beta-adrenergic receptor blocking agents have experienced protracted severe hypotension during anesthesia. Difficulty in restarting and maintaining the heartbeat has also been reported. For these reasons, in patients undergoing elective surgery, some authorities recommend gradual withdrawal of beta-adrenergic receptor blocking agents.

If necessary during surgery, the effects of beta-adrenergic blocking agents may be reversed by sufficient doses of adrenergic agonists.

Diabetes Mellitus

Beta-adrenergic blocking agents should be administered with caution in patients subject to spontaneous hypoglycemia or to diabetic patients (especially those with labile diabetes) who are receiving insulin or oral hypoglycemic agents. Beta-adrenergic receptor blocking agents may mask the signs and symptoms of acute hypoglycemia.

Thyrotoxicosis

Beta-adrenergic blocking agents may mask certain clinical signs (e.g., tachycardia) of hyperthyroidism. Patients suspected of developing thyrotoxicosis should be managed carefully to avoid abrupt withdrawal of beta-adrenergic blocking agents that might precipitate a thyroid storm.

Precautions

General

Because of potential effects of beta-adrenergic blocking agents on blood pressure and pulse, these agents should be used with caution in patients with cerebrovascular insufficiency. If signs or symptoms suggesting reduced cerebral blood flow develop following initiation of therapy with TIMOPTIC, alternative therapy should be considered.

There have been reports of bacterial keratitis associated with the use of multiple dose containers of topical ophthalmic products. These containers had been inadvertently contaminated by patients who, in most cases, had a concurrent corneal disease or a disruption of the ocular epithelial surface. (See **PRECAUTIONS**, *Information for Patients.*)

Choroidal detachment after filtration procedures has been reported with the administration of aqueous suppressant therapy (e.g. timolol).

Angle-closure glaucoma: In patients with angle-closure glaucoma, the immediate objective of treatment is to reopen the angle. This requires constricting the pupil. Timolol maleate has little or no effect on the pupil. TIMOPTIC should not be used alone in the treatment of angle-closure glaucoma.

Anaphylaxis: While taking beta-blockers, patients with a history of atopy or a history of severe anaphylactic reactions to a variety of allergens may be more reactive to repeated accidental, diagnostic, or therapeutic challenge with such allergens. Such patients may be unresponsive to the usual doses of epinephrine used to treat anaphylactic reactions.

Muscle Weakness: Beta-adrenergic blockade has been reported to potentiate muscle weakness consistent with certain myasthenic symptoms (e.g., diplopia, ptosis, and generalized weakness). Timolol has been reported rarely to increase muscle weakness in some patients with myasthenia gravis or myasthenic symptoms.

Information for Patients

Patients should be instructed to avoid allowing the tip of the dispensing container to contact the eye or surrounding structures.

Patients should also be instructed that ocular solutions, if handled improperly, can become contaminated by common bacteria known to cause ocular infections. Serious damage to the eye and subsequent loss of vision may result from using contaminated solutions. (See **PRECAUTIONS**, *General.*)

Patients should also be advised that if they have ocular surgery or develop an intercurrent ocular condition (e.g., trauma or infection), they should immediately seek their physician's advice concerning the continued use of the present multidose container.

Patients with bronchial asthma, a history of bronchial asthma, severe chronic obstructive pulmonary disease, sinus bradycardia, second or third degree atrioventricular block, or cardiac failure should be advised not to take this product. (See **CONTRAINDICATIONS**.)

Patients should be advised that TIMOPTIC contains benzalkonium chloride which may be absorbed by soft contact lenses. Contact lenses should be removed prior to administration of the solution. Lenses may be reinserted 15 minutes following TIMOPTIC administration.

Drug Interactions

Although TIMOPTIC used alone has little or no effect on pupil size, mydriasis resulting from concomitant therapy with TIMOPTIC and epinephrine has been reported occasionally.

Beta-adrenergic blocking agents: Patients who are receiving a beta-adrenergic blocking agent orally and TIMOPTIC should be observed for potential additive effects of beta-blockade, both systemic and on intraocular pressure. The concomitant use of two topical beta-adrenergic blocking agents is not recommended.

Calcium antagonists: Caution should be used in the coadministration of beta-adrenergic blocking agents, such as TIMOPTIC, and oral or intravenous calcium antagonists because of possible atrioventricular conduction disturbances, left ventricular failure, and hypotension. In patients with impaired cardiac function, coadministration should be avoided.

Catecholamine-depleting drugs: Close observation of the patient is recommended when a beta blocker is administered to patients receiving catecholamine-depleting drugs such as reserpine, because of possible additive effects and the production of hypotension and/or marked bradycardia, which may result in vertigo, syncope, or postural hypotension.

Digitalis and calcium antagonists: The concomitant use of beta-adrenergic blocking agents with digitalis and calcium antagonists may have additive effects in prolonging atrioventricular conduction time.

Quinidine: Potentiated systemic beta-blockade (e.g., decreased heart rate) has been reported during combined treatment with quinidine and timolol, possibly because quinidine inhibits the metabolism of timolol via the P-450 enzyme, CYP2D6.

Injectable Epinephrine: (See **PRECAUTIONS**, *General, Anaphylaxis*)

Carcinogenesis, Mutagenesis, Impairment of Fertility

In a two-year oral study of timolol maleate administered orally to rats, there was a statistically significant increase in the incidence of adrenal pheochromocytomas in male rats administered 300 mg/kg/day (approximately 42,000 times the systemic exposure following the maximum recommended human ophthalmic dose). Similar difference were not observed in rats administered oral doses equivalent to approximately 14,000 times the maximum recommended human ophthalmic dose.

In a lifetime oral study in mice, there were statistically significant increases in the incidence of benign and malignant pulmonary tumors, benign uterine polyps and mammary adenocarcinomas in female mice at 500 mg/kg/day, (approximately 71,000 times the systemic exposure following the maximum recommended human ophthalmic dose), but not at 5 or 50 mg/kg/day (approximately 700 or 7,000, respectively, times the systemic exposure following the maximum recommended human ophthalmic dose). In a subsequent study in female mice, in which post-mortem examinations were limited to the uterus and the lungs, a statistically significant increase in the incidence of pulmonary tumors was again observed at 500 mg/kg/day.

The increased occurrence of mammary adenocarcinomas was associated with elevations in serum prolactin which occurred in female mice administered oral timolol at 500 mg/kg/day, but not at doses of 5 or 50 mg/kg/day. An increased incidence of mammary adenocarcinomas in rodents has been associated with administration of several other therapeutic agents that elevate serum prolactin, but no correlation between serum prolactin levels and mammary tumors has been established in humans. Furthermore, in adult human female subjects who received oral dosages of up to 60 mg of timolol maleate (the maximum recommended human oral dosage), there were no clinically meaningful changes in serum prolactin.

Timolol maleate was devoid of mutagenic potential when tested *in vivo* (mouse) in the micronucleus test and cytogenetic assay (doses up to 800 mg/kg) and *in vitro* in a neoplastic cell transformation assay (up to 100 µg/mL). In Ames tests the highest concentrations of timolol employed, 5000 or 10,000 µg/plate, were associated with statistically significant elevations of revertants observed with tester strain TA100 (in seven replicate assays), but not in the remaining three strains. In the assays with tester strain TA100, no consistent dose response relationship was observed, and the ratio of test to control revertants did not reach 2. A ratio of 2 is usually considered the criterion for a positive Ames test.

Reproduction and fertility studies in rats demonstrated no adverse effect on male or female fertility at doses up to 21,000 times the systemic exposure following the maximum recommended human ophthalmic dose.

Pregnancy-Teratogenic effects:

Pregnancy Category C. Teratogenicity studies with timolol in mice, rats, and rabbits at oral doses up to 50 mg/kg/day (7,000 times the systemic exposure following the maximum recommended human ophthalmic dose) demonstrated no evidence of fetal malformations. Although delayed fetal ossification was observed at this dose in rats, there were no adverse effects on postnatal development of offspring. Doses of 1000 mg/kg/day (142,000 times the systemic exposure following the maximum recommended human ophthalmic dose) were maternotoxic in mice and resulted in an increased number of fetal resorptions. Increased fetal resorptions were also seen in rabbits at doses of 14,000 times the systemic exposure following the maximum recommended human ophthalmic dose, in this case without apparent maternotoxicity.

There are no adequate and well-controlled studies in pregnant women. TIMOPTIC should be used during pregnancy only if the potential benefit justifies the potential risk to the fetus.

Nursing Mothers

Timolol maleate has been detected in human milk following oral and ophthalmic drug administration. Because of the potential for serious adverse reactions from TIMOPTIC in nursing infants, a decision should be made whether to discontinue nursing or to discontinue the drug, taking into account the importance of the drug to the mother.

Pediatric Use

Safety and effectiveness in pediatric patients have not been established.

Adverse Reactions

The most frequently reported adverse experiences have been burning and stinging upon instillation (approximately one in eight patients).

The following additional adverse experiences have been reported less frequently with ocular administration of this or other timolol maleate formulations:

BODY AS A WHOLE

Headache, asthenia/fatigue, and chest pain.

CARDIOVASCULAR

Bradycardia, arrhythmia, hypotension, hypertension, syncope, heart block, cerebral vascular accident, cerebral ischemia, cardiac failure, worsening of angina pectoris, palpitation, cardiac arrest, pulmonary edema, edema, claudication, Raynaud's phenomenon, and cold hands and feet.

DIGESTIVE

Nausea, diarrhea, dyspepsia, anorexia, and dry mouth.

IMMUNOLOGIC

Systemic lupus erythematosus.

NERVOUS SYSTEM/PSYCHIATRIC

Dizziness, increase in signs and symptoms of myasthenia gravis, paresthesia, somnolence, insomnia, nightmares, behavioral changes and psychic disturbances including depression, confusion, hallucinations, anxiety, disorientation, nervousness, and memory loss.

SKIN

Alopecia and psoriasiform rash or exacerbation of psoriasis.

HYPERSENSITIVITY

Signs and symptoms of allergic reactions, including angioedema, urticaria, and localized and generalized rash.

RESPIRATORY

Bronchospasm (predominantly in patients with pre-existing bronchospastic disease), respiratory failure, dyspnea, nasal congestion, cough and upper respiratory infections.

ENDOCRINE

Masked symptoms of hypoglycemia in diabetic patients (see **WARNINGS**).

SPECIAL SENSES

Signs and symptoms of ocular irritation including conjunctivitis, blepharitis, keratitis, ocular pain, discharge (e.g., crusting), foreign body sensation, itching and tearing, and dry eyes; ptosis; decreased corneal sensitivity; cystoid macular edema; visual disturbances including refractive changes and diplopia; pseudopemphigoid; and choroidal detachment following filtration surgery (see **PRECAUTIONS**, *General*), and tinnitus.

UROGENITAL

Retroperitoneal fibrosis, decreased libido, impotence, and Peyronie's disease.

The following additional adverse effects have been reported in clinical experience with ORAL timolol maleate or other ORAL beta-blocking agents and may be considered potential effects of ophthalmic timolol maleate: *Allergic:* Erythematous rash, fever combined with aching and sore throat, laryngospasm with respiratory distress; *Body as a Whole:* Extremity pain, decreased exercise tolerance, weight loss; *Cardiovascular:* Worsening of arterial insufficiency, vasodilatation; *Digestive:* Gastrointestinal pain, hepatomegaly, vomiting, mesenteric arterial thrombosis, ischemic colitis; *Hematologic:* Nonthrombocytopenic purpura; thrombocytopenic purpura, agranulocytosis; *Endocrine:* Hyperglycemia, hypoglycemia; *Skin:* Pruritus, skin irritation, increased pigmentation, sweating; *Musculoskeletal:* Arthralgia; *Nervous System/Psychiatric:* Vertigo, local weakness, diminished concentration, reversible mental depression progressing to catatonia, and acute reversible syndrome characterized by disorien-

Continued on next page

Information on the Merck & Co., Inc., products listed on these pages is from the full prescribing information in use August 31, 1999.

Timoptic—Cont.

tation for time and place, emotional lability, slightly clouded sensorium, and decreased performance on neuropsychometrics; *Respiratory:* Rales, bronchial obstruction; *Urogenital:* Urination difficulties.

Overdosage

There have been reports of inadvertent overdosage with TIMOPTIC Ophthalmic Solution resulting in systemic effects similar to those seen with systemic beta-adrenergic blocking agents such as dizziness, headache, shortness of breath, bradycardia, bronchospasm, and cardiac arrest (see also ADVERSE REACTIONS).

Overdosage has been reported with Tablets BLOCADREN* (timolol maleate). A 30 year old female ingested 650 mg of BLOCADREN (maximum recommended oral daily dose is 60 mg) and experienced second and third degree heart block. She recovered without treatment but approximately two months later developed irregular heartbeat, hypertension, dizziness, tinnitus, faintness, increased pulse rate, and borderline first degree heart block.

Significant lethality was observed in female rats and female mice after a single dose of 900 and 1190 mg/kg (5310 and 3570 mg/m^2) of timolol, respectively.

An *in vitro* hemodialysis study, using ^{14}C timolol added to human plasma or whole blood, showed that timolol was readily dialyzed from these fluids; however, a study of patients with renal failure showed that timolol did not dialyze readily.

---

*Registered trademark of MERCK & CO., INC.

Dosage and Administration

TIMOPTIC Ophthalmic Solution is available in concentrations of 0.25 and 0.5 percent. The usual starting dose is one drop of 0.25 percent TIMOPTIC in the affected eye(s) twice a day. If the clinical response is not adequate, the dosage may be changed to one drop of 0.5 percent solution in the affected eye(s) twice a day.

Since in some patients the pressure-lowering response to TIMOPTIC may require a few weeks to stabilize, evaluation should include a determination of intraocular pressure after approximately 4 weeks of treatment with TIMOPTIC.

If the intraocular pressure is maintained at satisfactory levels, the dosage schedule may be changed to one drop once a day in the affected eye(s). Because of diurnal variations in intraocular pressure, satisfactory response to the once-a-day dose is best determined by measuring the intraocular pressure at different times during the day.

Dosages above one drop of 0.5 percent TIMOPTIC twice a day generally have not been shown to produce further reduction in intraocular pressure. If the patient's intraocular pressure is still not at a satisfactory level on this regimen, concomitant therapy with other agent(s) for lowering intraocular pressure can be instituted. The concomitant use of two topical beta-adrenergic blocking agents is not recommended. (See PRECAUTIONS, *Drug Interactions, Beta-adrenergic blocking agents.*)

How Supplied

Sterile Ophthalmic Solution TIMOPTIC is a clear, colorless to light yellow solution.

No. 3366—TIMOPTIC Ophthalmic Solution, 0.25% timolol equivalent, is supplied in a white, opaque, plastic OCUMETER* ophthalmic dispenser with a controlled drop tip as follows:

NDC 0006-3366-32, 2.5 mL
NDC 0006-3366-03, 5 mL
(6505-01-069-6518, 0.25% 5 mL)
NDC 0006-3366-10, 10 mL
(6505-01-093-5458, 0.25% 10 mL)
NDC 0006-3366-12, 15 mL.

No. 3367—TIMOPTIC Ophthalmic Solution, 0.5% timolol equivalent, is supplied in a white, opaque, plastic OCUMETER ophthalmic dispenser with a controlled drop tip as follows:

NDC 0006-3367-32, 2.5 mL
NDC 0006-3367-03, 5 mL
(6505-01-069-6519, 0.5% 5 mL)
NDC 0006-3367-10, 10 mL
(6505-01-092-0422, 0.5% 10 mL)
NDC 0006-3367-12, 15 mL.

---

*Registered trademark of MERCK & CO., INC.

Storage

Store at room temperature, 15–30°C (59–86°F). Protect from freezing. Protect from light.

9010840 Issued August 1997

Shown in Product Identification Guide, page 106

TIMOPTIC® ℞

0.25% and 0.5%
(Timolol Maleate Ophthalmic Solution)
in OCUDOSE® (Dispenser), U.S.P.
Preservative-Free Sterile Ophthalmic Solution
in a Sterile Ophthalmic Unit Dose Dispenser

Description

Timolol maleate is a non-selective beta-adrenergic receptor blocking agent. Its chemical name is (-)-1-(*tert*-butylamino)-3-[(4-morpholino-1,2,5-thiadiazol-3-yl)oxy]-2-propanol maleate (1:1) (salt). Timolol maleate possesses an asymmetric carbon atom in its structure and is provided as the levo-isomer. The nominal optical rotation of timolol maleate is

$$[\alpha]^{25°}_{405\ nm} \text{ in 0.1N HCl (C = 5\%)} = -12.2°.$$

Its molecular formula is $C_{13}H_{24}N_4O_3S{\cdot}C_4H_4O_4$ and its structural formula is:

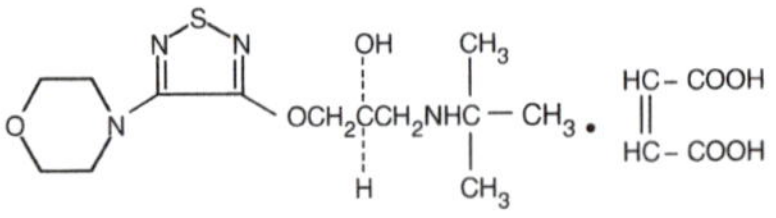

Timolol maleate has a molecular weight of 432.50. It is a white, odorless, crystalline powder which is soluble in water, methanol, and alcohol. Timolol maleate is stable at room temperature.

Timolol maleate ophthalmic solution is supplied in two formulations: Ophthalmic Solution TIMOPTIC* (timolol maleate ophthalmic solution), which contains the preservative benzalkonium chloride; and Ophthalmic Solution TIMOPTIC* (timolol maleate ophthalmic solution), the preservative-free formulation.

Preservative-free Ophthalmic Solution TIMOPTIC is supplied in OCUDOSE*, a unit dose container, as a sterile, isotonic, buffered, aqueous solution of timolol maleate in two dosage strengths: Each mL of Preservative-free TIMOPTIC in OCUDOSE 0.25% contains 2.5 mg of timolol (3.4 mg of timolol maleate). Each mL of Preservative-free TIMOPTIC in OCUDOSE 0.5% contains 5.0 mg of timolol (6.8 mg of timolol maleate). Inactive ingredients: monobasic and dibasic sodium phosphate, sodium hydroxide to adjust pH, and water for injection.

---

*Registered trademark of MERCK & CO., INC.

Clinical Pharmacology

Mechanism of Action

Timolol maleate is a $beta_1$ and $beta_2$ (non-selective) adrenergic receptor blocking agent that does not have significant intrinsic sympathomimetic, direct myocardial depressant, or local anesthetic (membrane-stabilizing) activity.

Beta-adrenergic receptor blockade reduces cardiac output in both healthy subjects and patients with heart disease. In patients with severe impairment of myocardial function beta-adrenergic receptor blockade may inhibit the stimulatory effect of the sympathetic nervous system necessary to maintain adequate cardiac function.

Beta-adrenergic receptor blockade in the bronchi and bronchioles results in increased airway resistance from unopposed parasympathetic activity. Such an effect in patients with asthma or other bronchospastic conditions is potentially dangerous.

TIMOPTIC (timolol maleate ophthalmic solution), when applied topically on the eye, has the action of reducing elevated as well as normal intraocular pressure, whether or not accompanied by glaucoma. Elevated intraocular pressure is a major risk factor in the pathogenesis of glaucomatous visual field loss. The higher the level of intraocular pressure, the greater the likelihood of glaucomatous visual field loss and optic nerve damage.

The onset of reduction in intraocular pressure following administration of TIMOPTIC (timolol maleate ophthalmic solution) can usually be detected within one-half hour after a single dose. The maximum effect usually occurs in one to two hours and significant lowering of intraocular pressure can be maintained for periods as long as 24 hours with a single dose. Repeated observations over a period of one year indicate that the intraocular pressure-lowering effect of TIMOPTIC (timolol maleate ophthalmic solution) is well maintained.

The precise mechanism of the ocular hypotensive action of TIMOPTIC (timolol maleate ophthalmic solution) is not clearly established at this time. Tonography and fluorophotometry studies in man suggest that its predominant action may be related to reduced aqueous formation. However, in some studies a slight increase in outflow facility was also observed.

Pharmacokinetics

In a study of plasma drug concentration in six subjects, the systemic exposure to timolol was determined following twice daily administration of TIMOPTIC 0.5%. The mean peak plasma concentration following morning dosing was 0.46 ng/mL and following afternoon dosing was 0.35 ng/mL.

Clinical Studies

In controlled multiclinic studies in patients with untreated intraocular pressures of 22 mmHg or greater, TIMOPTIC (timolol maleate ophthalmic solution) 0.25 percent or 0.5 percent administered twice a day produced a greater reduction in intraocular pressure than 1,2,3, or 4 percent pilocarpine solution administered four times a day or 0.5, 1, or 2 percent epinephrine hydrochloride solution administered twice a day.

In these studies, TIMOPTIC (timolol maleate ophthalmic solution) was generally well tolerated and produced fewer and less severe side effects than either pilocarpine or epinephrine. A slight reduction of resting heart rate in some patients receiving TIMOPTIC (timolol maleate ophthalmic solution) (mean reduction 2.9 beats/minute standard deviation 10.2) was observed.

Indications and Usage

Preservative-free TIMOPTIC in OCUDOSE is indicated in the treatment of elevated intraocular pressure in patients with ocular hypertension or open-angle glaucoma.

Preservative-free TIMOPTIC in OCUDOSE may be used when a patient is sensitive to the preservative in TIMOPTIC (timolol maleate ophthalmic solution), benzalkonium chloride, or when use of a preservative-free topical medication is advisable.

Contraindications

Preservative-free TIMOPTIC in OCUDOSE is contraindicated in patients with (1) bronchial asthma; (2) a history of bronchial asthma; (3) severe chronic obstructive pulmonary disease (see **WARNINGS**); (4) sinus bradycardia; (5) second or third degree atrioventricular block; (6) overt cardiac failure (see **WARNINGS**); (7) cardiogenic shock; or (8) hypersensitivity to any component of this product.

Warnings

As with many topically applied ophthalmic drugs, this drug is absorbed systemically.

The same adverse reactions found with systemic administration of beta-adrenergic blocking agents may occur with topical administration. For example, severe respiratory reactions and cardiac reactions, including death due to bronchospasm in patients with asthma, and rarely death in association with cardiac failure, have been reported following systemic or ophthalmic administration of timolol maleate (see CONTRAINDICATIONS).

Cardiac Failure

Sympathetic stimulation may be essential for support of the circulation in individuals with diminished myocardial contractility, and its inhibition by beta-adrenergic receptor blockade may precipitate more severe failure.

In Patients Without a History of Cardiac Failure continued depression of the myocardium with beta-blocking agents over a period of time can, in some cases, lead to cardiac failure. At the first sign or symptom of cardiac failure Preservative-free TIMOPTIC in OCUDOSE should be discontinued.

Obstructive Pulmonary Disease

Patients with chronic obstructive pulmonary disease (e.g., chronic bronchitis, emphysema) of mild or moderate severity, bronchospastic disease, or a history of bronchospastic disease (other than bronchial asthma or a history of bronchial asthma, in which TIMOPTIC in OCUDOSE is contraindicated [see **CONTRAINDICATIONS**]) should, in general, not receive beta-blockers, including Preservative-free TIMOPTIC in OCUDOSE.

Major Surgery

The necessity or desirability of withdrawal of beta-adrenergic blocking agents prior to major surgery is controversial. Beta-adrenergic receptor blockade impairs the ability of the heart to respond to beta-adrenergically mediated reflex stimuli. This may augment the risk of general anesthesia in surgical procedures. Some patients receiving beta-adrenergic receptor blocking agents have experienced protracted severe hypotension during anesthesia. Difficulty in restarting and maintaining the heartbeat has also been reported. For these reasons, in patients undergoing elective surgery, some authorities recommend gradual withdrawal of beta-adrenergic receptor blocking agents.

If necessary during surgery, the effects of beta-adrenergic blocking agents may be reversed by sufficient doses of adrenergic agonists.

Diabetes Mellitus

Beta-adrenergic blocking agents should be administered with caution in patients subject to spontaneous hypoglycemia or to diabetic patients (especially those with labile diabetes) who are receiving insulin or oral hypoglycemic agents. Beta-adrenergic receptor blocking agents may mask the signs and symptoms of acute hypoglycemia.

Thyrotoxicosis

Beta-adrenergic blocking agents may mask certain clinical signs (e.g., tachycardia) of hyperthyroidism. Patients suspected of developing thyrotoxicosis should be managed carefully to avoid abrupt withdrawal of beta-adrenergic blocking agents that might precipitate a thyroid storm.

Precautions

General

Because of potential effects of beta-adrenergic blocking agents on blood pressure and pulse, these agents should be used with caution in patients with cerebrovascular insufficiency. If signs or symptoms suggesting reduced cerebral blood flow develop following initiation of therapy with Preservative-free TIMOPTIC in OCUDOSE, alternative therapy should be considered.

Choroidal detachment after filtration procedures has been reported with the administration of aqueous suppressant therapy (e.g. timolol).

Angle-closure glaucoma: In patients with angle-closure glaucoma, the immediate objective of treatment is to reopen the angle. This requires constricting the pupil. Timolol maleate has little or no effect on the pupil. TIMOPTIC in OCUDOSE should not be used alone in the treatment of angle-closure glaucoma.

Anaphylaxis: While taking beta-blockers, patients with a history of atopy or a history of severe anaphylactic reactions to a variety of allergens may be more reactive to repeated accidental, diagnostic, or therapeutic challenge with such allergens. Such patients may be unresponsive to the usual doses of epinephrine used to treat anaphylactic reactions.

Muscle Weakness: Beta-adrenergic blockade has been reported to potentiate muscle weakness consistent with certain myasthenic symptoms (e.g., diplopia, ptosis, and generalized weakness). Timolol has been reported rarely to increase muscle weakness in some patients with myasthenia gravis or myasthenic symptoms.

Information for Patients

Patients should be instructed about the use of Preservative-free TIMOPTIC in OCUDOSE.

Since sterility cannot be maintained after the individual unit is opened, patients should be instructed to use the product immediately after opening, and to discard the individual unit and any remaining contents immediately after use.

Patients with bronchial asthma, a history of bronchial asthma, severe chronic obstructive pulmonary disease, sinus bradycardia, second or third degree atrioventricular block, or cardiac failure should be advised not to take this product. (See **CONTRAINDICATIONS**.)

Drug Interactions

Although TIMOPTIC (timolol maleate ophthalmic solution) used alone has little or no effect on pupil size, mydriasis resulting from concomitant therapy with TIMOPTIC (timolol maleate ophthalmic solution) and epinephrine has been reported occasionally.

Beta-adrenergic blocking agents: Patients who are receiving a beta-adrenergic blocking agent orally and Preservative-free TIMOPTIC in OCUDOSE should be observed for potential additive effects of beta-blockade, both systemic and on intraocular pressure. The concomitant use of two topical beta-adrenergic blocking agents is not recommended.

Calcium antagonists: Caution should be used in the coadministration of beta-adrenergic blocking agents, such as Preservative-free TIMOPTIC in OCUDOSE, and oral or intravenous calcium antagonists, because of possible atrioventricular conduction disturbances, left ventricular failure, and hypotension. In patients with impaired cardiac function, coadministration should be avoided.

Catecholamine-depleting drugs: Close observation of the patient is recommended when a beta blocker is administered to patients receiving catecholamine-depleting drugs such as reserpine, because of possible additive effects and the production of hypotension and/or marked bradycardia, which may result in vertigo, syncope, or postural hypotension.

Digitalis and calcium antagonists: The concomitant use of beta-adrenergic blocking agents with digitalis and calcium antagonists may have additive effects in prolonging atrioventricular conduction time.

Quinidine: Potentiated systemic beta-blockade (e.g., decreased heart rate) has been reported during combined treatment with quinidine and timolol, possibly because quinidine inhibits the metabolism of timolol via the P-450 enzyme, CYP2D6.

Injectable Epinephrine: (See **PRECAUTIONS**, *General, Anaphylaxis)*

Carcinogenesis, Mutagenesis, Impairment of Fertility

In a two-year oral study of timolol maleate administered orally to rats, there was a statistically significant increase in the incidence of adrenal pheochromocytomas in male rats administered 300 mg/kg/day (approximately 42,000 times the systemic exposure following the maximum recommended human ophthalmic dose). Similar differences were not observed in rats administered oral doses equivalent to approximately 14,000 times the maximum recommended human ophthalmic dose.

In a lifetime oral study in mice, there were statistically significant increases in the incidence of benign and malignant pulmonary tumors, benign uterine polyps and mammary adenocarcinomas in female mice at 500 mg/kg/day (approximately 71,000 times the systemic exposure following the maximum recommended human ophthalmic dose), but not at 5 or 50 mg/kg/day (approximately 700 or 7,000 times, respectively, the systemic exposure following the maximum recommended human ophthalmic dose). In a subsequent study in female mice, in which post-mortem examinations were limited to the uterus and the lungs, a statistically significant increase in the incidence of pulmonary tumors was again observed at 500 mg/kg/day.

The increased occurrence of mammary adenocarcinomas was associated with elevations in serum prolactin which occurred in female mice administered oral timolol at 500 mg/kg/day, but not at doses of 5 or 50 mg/kg/day. An increased incidence of mammary adenocarcinomas in rodents has been associated with administration of several other therapeutic agents that elevate serum prolactin, but no correlation between serum prolactin levels and mammary tumors has been established in humans. Furthermore, in adult human female subjects who received oral dosages of up to 60 mg of timolol maleate (the maximum recommended human oral dosage), there were no clinically meaningful changes in serum prolactin.

Timolol maleate was devoid of mutagenic potential when tested *in vivo* (mouse) in the micronucleus test and cytogenetic assay (doses up to 800 mg/kg) and *in vitro* in a neoplastic cell transformation assay (up to 100 µg/mL). In Ames tests the highest concentrations of timolol employed, 5000 or 10,000 µg/plate, were associated with statistically significant elevations of revertants observed with tester strain TA 100 (in seven replicate assays), but not in the remaining three strains. In the assays with tester strain TA 100, no consistent dose response relationship was observed, and the ratio of test to control revertants did not reach 2. A ratio of 2 is usually considered the criterion for a positive Ames test.

Reproduction and fertility studies in rats demonstrated no adverse effect on male or female

Continued on next page

Information on the Merck & Co., Inc., products listed on these pages is from the full prescribing information in use August 31, 1999.

Timoptic in Ocudose—Cont.

fertility at doses up to 21,000 times the systemic exposure following the maximum recommended human ophthalmic dose.

Pregnancy-Teratogenic effects:

Pregnancy Category C. Teratogenicity studies with timolol in mice, rats and rabbits at oral doses up to 50 mg/kg/day (7,000 times the systemic exposure following the maximum recommended human ophthalmic dose) demonstrated no evidence of fetal malformations. Although delayed fetal ossification was observed at this dose in rats, there were no adverse effects on postnatal development of offspring. Doses of 1000 mg/kg/day (142,000 times the systemic exposure following the maximum recommended human ophthalmic dose) were maternotoxic in mice and resulted in an increased number of fetal resorptions. Increased fetal resorptions were also seen in rabbits at doses of 14,000 times the systemic exposure following the maximum recommended human ophthalmic dose, in this case without apparent maternotoxicity.

There are no adequate and well-controlled studies in pregnant women. Preservative-free TIMOPTIC in OCUDOSE should be used during pregnancy only if the potential benefit justifies the potential risk to the fetus.

Nursing Mothers

Timolol maleate has been detected in human milk following oral and ophthalmic drug administration. Because of the potential for serious adverse reactions from timolol in nursing infants, a decision should be made whether to discontinue nursing or to discontinue the drug, taking into account the importance of the drug to the mother.

Pediatric Use

Safety and effectiveness in pediatric patients have not been established.

Adverse Reactions

The most frequently reported adverse experiences have been burning and stinging upon instillation (approximately one in eight patients).

The following additional adverse experiences have been reported less frequently with ocular administration of this or other timolol maleate formulations:

BODY AS A WHOLE

Headache, asthenia/fatigue, chest pain.

CARDIOVASCULAR

Bradycardia, arrhythmia, hypotension, hypertension, syncope, heart block, cerebral vascular accident, cerebral ischemia, cardiac failure, worsening of angina pectoris, palpitation, cardiac arrest, pulmonary edema, edema, claudication, Raynaud's phenomenon, and cold hands and feet.

DIGESTIVE

Nausea, diarrhea. dyspepsia, anorexia, and dry mouth.

IMMUNOLOGIC

Systemic lupus erythematosus.

NERVOUS SYSTEM/PSYCHIATRIC

Dizziness, increase in signs and symptoms of myasthenia gravis, paresthesia, somnolence, insomnia, nightmares, behavioral changes and psychic disturbances including depression, confusion, hallucinations, anxiety, disorientation, nervousness, and memory loss.

SKIN

Alopecia and psoriasiform rash or exacerbation of psoriasis.

HYPERSENSITIVITY

Signs and symptoms of allergic reactions, including angioedema, urticaria, and localized and generalized rash.

RESPIRATORY

Bronchospasm (predominantly in patients with pre-existing bronchospastic disease), respiratory failure, dyspnea, nasal congestion, cough and upper respiratory infections.

ENDOCRINE

Masked symptoms of hypoglycemia in diabetic patients (see **WARNINGS**).

SPECIAL SENSES

Signs and symptoms of ocular irritation including conjunctivitis, blepharitis, keratitis, ocular pain, discharge (e.g., crusting), foreign body sensation, itching and tearing, and dry eyes; ptosis; decreased corneal sensitivity; cystoid macular edema; visual disturbances including refractive changes and diplopia; pseudopemphigoid; and choroidal detachment following filtration surgery (see **PRECAUTIONS**, *General*), and tinnitus.

UROGENITAL

Retroperitoneal fibrosis, decreased libido, impotence, and Peyronie's disease.

The following additional adverse effects have been reported in clinical experience with ORAL timolol maleate or other ORAL beta blocking agents, and may be considered potential effects of ophthalmic timolol maleate: *Allergic:* Erythematous rash, fever combined with aching and sore throat, laryngospasm with respiratory distress; *Body as a Whole:* Extremity pain, decreased exercise tolerance, weight loss; *Cardiovascular:* Worsening of arterial insufficiency, vasodilatation; *Digestive:* Gastrointestinal pain, hepatomegaly, vomiting, mesenteric arterial thrombosis, ischemic colitis; *Hematologic:* Nonthrombocytopenic purpura; thrombocytopenic purpura; agranulocytosis; *Endocrine:* Hyperglycemia, hypoglycemia; *Skin:* Pruritus, skin irritation, increased pigmentation, sweating; *Musculoskeletal:* Arthralgia; *Nervous System/Psychiatric:* Vertigo, local weakness, diminished concentration, reversible mental depression progressing to catatonia; an acute reversible syndrome characterized by disorientation for time and place, emotional lability, slightly clouded sensorium, and decreased performance on neuropsychometrics; *Respiratory:* Rales, bronchial obstruction; *Urogenital:* Urination difficulties.

Overdosage

There have been reports of inadvertent overdosage with Ophthalmic Solution TIMOPTIC (timolol maleate ophthalmic solution) resulting in systemic effects similar to those seen with systemic beta-adrenergic blocking agents such as dizziness, headache, shortness of breath, bradycardia, bronchospasm, and cardiac arrest (see also **ADVERSE REACTIONS**).

Overdosage has been reported with Tablets BLOCADREN* (timolol maleate). A 30 year old female ingested 650 mg of BLOCADREN (maximum recommended oral daily dose is 60 mg) and experienced second and third degree heart block. She recovered without treatment but approximately two months later developed irregular heartbeat, hypertension, dizziness, tinnitus, faintness, increased pulse rate, and borderline first degree heart block.

Significant lethality was observed in female rats and female mice after a single dose of 900 and 1190 mg/kg (5310 and 3570 mg/m^2) of timolol, respectively.

An *in vitro* hemodialysis study, using ^{14}C timolol added to human plasma or whole blood, showed that timolol was readily dialyzed from these fluids; however, a study of patients with renal failure showed that timolol did not dialyze readily.

* Registered trademark of MERCK & CO., INC.

Dosage and Administration

Preservative-free TIMOPTIC in OCUDOSE is a sterile solution that does not contain a preservative. The solution from one individual unit is to be used immediately after opening for administration to one or both eyes. Since sterility cannot be guaranteed after the individual unit is opened, the remaining contents should be discarded immediately after administration.

Preservative-free TIMOPTIC in OCUDOSE is available in concentrations of 0.25 and 0.5 percent. The usual starting dose is one drop of 0.25 percent Preservative-free TIMOPTIC in OCUDOSE in the affected eye(s) administered twice a day. Apply enough gentle pressure on the individual container to obtain a single drop of solution. If the clinical response is not adequate, the dosage may be changed to one drop of 0.5 percent solution in the affected eye(s) administered twice a day.

Since in some patients the pressure-lowering response to Preservative-free TIMOPTIC in OCUDOSE may require a few weeks to stabilize, evaluation should include a determination of intraocular pressure after approximately 4 weeks of treatment with Preservative-free TIMOPTIC in OCUDOSE.

If the intraocular pressure is maintained at satisfactory levels, the dosage schedule may be changed to one drop once a day in the affected eye(s). Because of diurnal variations in intraocular pressure, satisfactory response to the once-a-day dose is best determined by measuring the intraocular pressure at different times during the day.

Dosages above one drop of 0.5 percent TIMOPTIC (timolol maleate ophthalmic solution) twice a day generally have not been shown to produce further reduction in intraocular pressure. If the patient's intraocular pressure is still not at a satisfactory level on this regimen, concomitant therapy with other agent(s) for lowering intraocular pressure can be instituted taking into consideration that the preparation(s) used concomitantly may contain one or more preservatives. The concomitant use of two topical beta-adrenergic blocking agents is not recommended. (See **PRECAUTIONS,** *Drug Interactions*, *Beta-adrenergic blocking agents.*)

How Supplied

Preservative-free Sterile Ophthalmic Solution TIMOPTIC in OCUDOSE is a clear, colorless to light yellow solution.

No. 3542—Preservative-free TIMOPTIC, 0.25% timolol equivalent, is supplied in OCUDOSE, a clear polyethylene unit dose container. Each individual unit contains 0.3 mL of solution, and is available in a foil laminate overwrapped pouch as follows:

NDC 0006-3542-60; 60 Individual Unit Doses (6505-01-316-8791, 0.25% 60 Individual Unit Doses).

No. 3543—Preservative-free TIMOPTIC, 0.5% timolol equivalent, is supplied in OCUDOSE, a clear polyethylene unit dose container. Each individual unit contains 0.3 mL of solution, and is available in a foil laminate overwrapped pouch as follows:

NDC 0006-3543-60; 60 Individual Unit Doses (6505-01-284-5154, 0.5% 60 Individual Unit Doses).

Storage

Store at room temperature, 15–30°C (59–86°F). Protect from freezing. Protect from light.

Because evaporation can occur through the unprotected polyethylene unit dose container and prolonged exposure to direct light can modify the product, the unit dose container should be kept in the protective foil overwrap and used within one month after the foil package has been opened.

7950515 Issued August 1997

Shown in Product Identification Guide, page 106

TIMOPTIC-XE® ℞
0.25% and 0.5%
(Timolol Maleate Ophthalmic Gel Forming Solution)
Sterile Ophthalmic Gel Forming Solution

Description

TIMOPTIC-XE* (timolol maleate ophthalmic gel forming solution) is a non-selective beta-adrenergic receptor blocking agent. Its chemical name is (-)-1-(*tert*-butyl-amino)-3-[(4-morpholino-1,2,5-thiadiazol-3-yl)oxy]-2-propanol maleate (1:1) (salt). Timolol maleate possesses an asymmetric carbon atom in its structure and is provided as the levo-isomer. The nominal optical rotation of timolol maleate is:

$$[\alpha]^{25^\circ}_{405\ nm} \text{ in 0.1N HCl (C=5\%)} = -12.2^\circ.$$

Its molecular formula is $C_{13}H_{24}N_4O_3S \cdot C_4H_4O_4$ and its structural formula is:

Timolol maleate has a molecular weight of 432.50. It is a white, odorless, crystalline powder which is soluble in water, methanol, and alcohol.

TIMOPTIC-XE Sterile Ophthalmic Gel Forming Solution is supplied as a sterile, isotonic, buffered, aqueous solution of timolol maleate in two dosage strengths. Each mL of TIMOPTIC-XE 0.25% contains 2.5 mg of timolol (3.4 mg of timolol maleate). Each mL of TIMOPTIC-XE 0.5% contains 5.0 mg of timolol (6.8 mg of timolol maleate). Inactive ingredients: GELRITE* gellan gum, tromethamine, mannitol, and water for injection. Preservative: benzododecinium bromide 0.012%.

GELRITE is a purified anionic heteropolysaccharide derived from gellan gum. An aqueous solution of GELRITE, in the presence of a cation, has the ability to gel. Upon contact with the precorneal tear film, TIMOPTIC-XE forms a gel that is subsequently removed by the flow of tears.

* Registered trademark of MERCK & CO., INC.

Clinical Pharmacology

Mechanism of Action

Timolol maleate is a $beta_1$ and $beta_2$ (non-selective) adrenergic receptor blocking agent that does not have significant intrinsic sympathomimetic, direct myocardial depressant, or local anesthetic (membrane-stabilizing) activity.

TIMOPTIC-XE, when applied topically on the eye, has the action of reducing elevated, as well as normal intraocular pressure, whether or not accompanied by glaucoma. Elevated intraocular pressure is a major risk factor in the pathogenesis of glaucomatous visual field loss and optic nerve damage.

The precise mechanism of the ocular hypotensive action of TIMOPTIC-XE is not clearly established at this time. Tonography and fluorophotometry studies of TIMOPTIC* (timolol maleate ophthalmic solution) in man suggest that its predominant action may be related to reduced aqueous formation. However, in some studies, a slight increase in outflow facility was also observed.

Beta-adrenergic receptor blockade reduces cardiac output in both healthy subjects and patients with heart disease. In patients with severe impairment of myocardial function beta-adrenergic receptor blockade may inhibit the stimulatory effect of the sympathetic nervous system necessary to maintain adequate cardiac function.

Beta-adrenergic receptor blockade in the bronchi and bronchioles results in increased airway resistance from unopposed parasympathetic activity. Such an effect in patients with asthma or other bronchospastic conditions is potentially dangerous.

Pharmacokinetics

In a study of plasma drug concentration in six subjects, the systemic exposure to timolol was determined following once daily administration of TIMOPTIC-XE 0.5% in the morning. The mean peak plasma concentration following this morning dose was 0.28 ng/mL.

Clinical Studies

In controlled, double-masked, multicenter clinical studies, comparing TIMOPTIC-XE 0.25% to TIMOPTIC 0.25% and TIMOPTIC-XE 0.5% to TIMOPTIC 0.5%, TIMOPTIC-XE administered once a day was shown to be equally effective in lowering intraocular pressure as the equivalent concentration of TIMOPTIC administered twice a day. The effect of timolol in lowering intraocular pressure was evident for 24 hours with a single dose of TIMOPTIC-XE. Repeated observations over a period of six months indicate that the intraocular pressure-lowering effect of TIMOPTIC-XE was consistent. The results from the largest U.S. and international clinical trials comparing TIMOPTIC-XE 0.5% to TIMOPTIC 0.5% are shown in Figure 1.

Figure 1

Mean IOP and Std Deviation (mm Hg) by Treatment Group

U.S. Study

TIMOPTIC-XE 0.5% q.d. N=191
TIMOPTIC 0.5% b.i.d. N=95

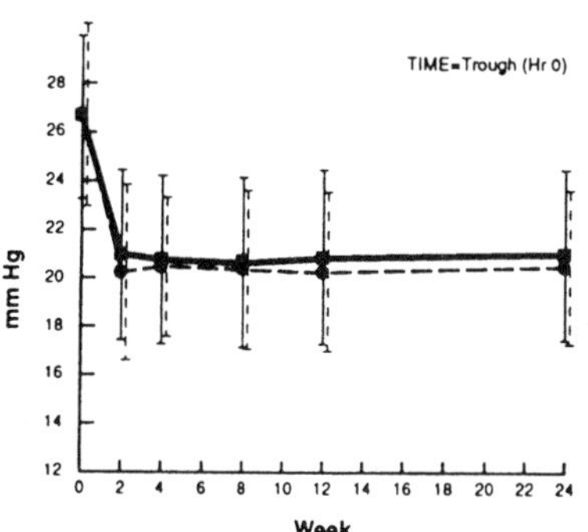

[See figures in next column]

TIMOPTIC-XE administered once daily had a safety profile similar to that of an equivalent concentration of TIMOPTIC administered twice daily. Due to the physical characteristics of the formulation, there was a higher incidence of transient blurred vision in patients administered TIMOPTIC-XE. A slight reduction in resting heart rate was observed in some patients receiving TIMOPTIC-XE 0.5% (mean reduction 24 hours post-dose 0.8 beats/minute, mean reduction 2 hours post-dose 3.8 beats/minute). (See **ADVERSE REACTIONS**.)

TIMOPTIC-XE has not been studied in patients wearing contact lenses.

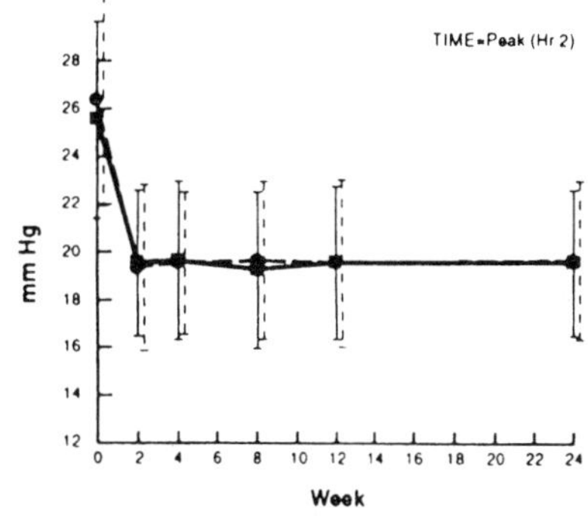

International Study

TIMOPTIC-XE 0.5% q.d. N=226
TIMOPTIC 0.5% b.i.d. N=116

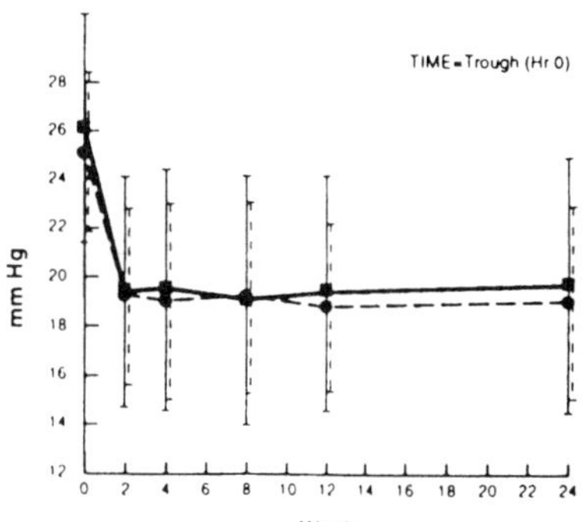

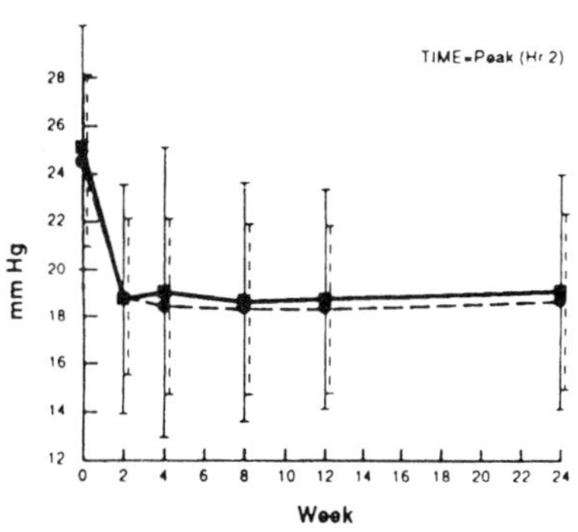

* Registered trademark of MERCK & CO., INC.

Indications and Usage

TIMOPTIC-XE Sterile Ophthalmic Gel Forming Solution is indicated in the treatment of elevated intraocular pressure in patients with ocular hypertension or open-angle glaucoma.

Contraindications

TIMOPTIC-XE is contraindicated in patients with (1) bronchial asthma; (2) a history of bronchial asthma; (3) severe chronic obstructive pulmonary disease (see **WARNINGS**) ; (4) sinus bradycardia; (5) second or third degree atrioventricular block; (6) overt cardiac failure

Continued on next page

Information on the Merck & Co., Inc., products listed on these pages is from the full prescribing information in use August 31, 1999.

Timoptic-XE—Cont.

(see **WARNINGS**) ; (7) cardiogenic shock; or (8) hypersensitivity to any component of this product.

Warnings

As with many topically applied ophthalmic drugs, this drug is absorbed systemically.

The same adverse reactions found with systemic administration of beta-adrenergic blocking agents may occur with topical ophthalmic administration. For example, severe respiratory reactions and cardiac reactions, including death due to bronchospasm in patients with asthma, and rarely death in association with cardiac failure, have been reported following systemic or ophthalmic administration of timolol maleate. (See CONTRAINDICATIONS.)

Cardiac Failure

Sympathetic stimulation may be essential for support of the circulation in individuals with diminished myocardial contractility, and its inhibition by beta-adrenergic receptor blockade may precipitate more severe failure.

In Patients Without a History of Cardiac Failure, continued depression of the myocardium with beta-blocking agents over a period of time can, in some cases, lead to cardiac failure. At the first sign or symptom of cardiac failure, TIMOPTIC-XE should be discontinued.

Obstructive Pulmonary Disease

Patients with chronic obstructive pulmonary disease (e.g., chronic bronchitis, emphysema) of mild or moderate severity, bronchospastic disease, or a history of bronchospastic disease (other than bronchial asthma or a history of bronchial asthma, in which TIMOPTIC-XE is contraindicated [see **CONTRAINDICATIONS**]) should, in general, not receive betablockers, including TIMOPTIC-XE.

Major Surgery

The necessity or desirability of withdrawal of beta-adrenergic blocking agents prior to major surgery is controversial. Beta-adrenergic receptor blockade impairs the ability of the heart to respond to beta-adrenergically mediated reflex stimuli. This may augment the risk of general anesthesia in surgical procedures. Some patients receiving beta-adrenergic receptor blocking agents have experienced protracted, severe hypotension during anesthesia. Difficulty in restarting and maintaining the heartbeat has also been reported. For these reasons, in patients undergoing elective surgery, some authorities recommend gradual withdrawal of beta-adrenergic receptor blocking agents.

If necessary during surgery, the effects of beta-adrenergic blocking agents may be reversed by sufficient doses of adrenergic agonists.

Diabetes Mellitus

Beta-adrenergic blocking agents should be administered with caution in patients subject to spontaneous hypoglycemia or to diabetic patients (especially those with labile diabetes) who are receiving insulin or oral hypoglycemic agents. Beta-adrenergic receptor blocking agents may mask the signs and symptoms of acute hypoglycemia.

Thyrotoxicosis

Beta-adrenergic blocking agents may mask certain clinical signs (e.g., tachycardia) of hyperthyroidism. Patients suspected of developing thyrotoxicosis should be managed carefully to avoid abrupt withdrawal of beta-adrenergic blocking agents that might precipitate a thyroid storm.

Precautions

General

Because of potential effects of beta-adrenergic blocking agents on blood pressure and pulse, these agents should be used with caution in patients with cerebrovascular insufficiency. If signs or symptoms suggesting reduced cerebral blood flow develop following initiation of therapy with TIMOPTIC-XE, alternative therapy should be considered.

There have been reports of bacterial keratitis associated with the use of multiple dose containers of topical ophthalmic products. These containers had been inadvertently contaminated by patients who, in most cases, had a concurrent corneal disease or a disruption of the ocular epithelial surface. (See **PRECAUTIONS,** *Information for Patients.*)

Choroidal detachment after filtration procedures has been reported with the administration of aqueous suppressant therapy (e.g. timolol).

Angle-closure glaucoma: In patients with angle-closure glaucoma, the immediate objective of treatment is to reopen the angle. This may require constricting the pupil. Timolol maleate has little or no effect on the pupil. TIMOPTIC-XE should not be used alone in the treatment of angle-closure glaucoma.

Anaphylaxis: While taking beta-blockers, patients with a history of atopy or a history of severe anaphylactic reactions to a variety of allergens may be more reactive to repeated accidental, diagnostic, or therapeutic challenge with such allergens. Such patients may be unresponsive to the usual doses of epinephrine used to treat anaphylactic reactions.

Muscle Weakness: Beta-adrenergic blockade has been reported to potentiate muscle weakness consistent with certain myasthenic symptoms (e.g., diplopia, ptosis, and generalized weakness). Timolol has been reported rarely to increase muscle weakness in some patients with myasthenia gravis or myasthenic symptoms.

Information for Patients

Patients should be instructed to avoid allowing the tip of the dispensing container to contact the eye or surrounding structures.

Patients should also be instructed that ocular solutions, if handled improperly or if the tip of the dispensing container contacts the eye or surrounding structures, can become contaminated by common bacteria known to cause ocular infections. Serious damage to the eye and subsequent loss of vision may result from using contaminated solutions. (See **PRECAUTIONS,** *General.*)

Patients should also be advised that if they have ocular surgery or develop an intercurrent ocular condition (e.g., trauma or infection), they should immediately seek their physician's advice concerning the continued use of the present multidose container.

Patients should be instructed to invert the closed container and shake once before each use. It is not necessary to shake the container more than once.

Patients requiring concomitant topical ophthalmic medications should be instructed to administer these at least 10 minutes before instilling TIMOPTIC-XE.

Patients with bronchial asthma, a history of bronchial asthma, severe chronic obstructive pulmonary disease, sinus bradycardia, second or third degree atrioventricular block, or cardiac failure should be advised not to take this product. (See **CONTRAINDICATIONS.**)

Transient blurred vision, generally lasting from 30 seconds to 5 minutes, following instillation, and potential visual disturbances may impair the ability to perform hazardous tasks such as operating machinery or driving a motor vehicle.

Drug Interactions

Beta-adrenergic blocking agents: Patients who are receiving a beta-adrenergic blocking agent orally and TIMOPTIC-XE should be observed for potential additive effects of beta-blockade, both systemic and on intraocular pressure. The concomitant use of two topical beta-adrenergic blocking agents is not recommended.

Calcium antagonists: Caution should be used in the coadministration of beta-adrenergic blocking agents, such as TIMOPTIC-XE, and oral or intravenous calcium antagonists because of possible atrioventricular conduction disturbances, left ventricular failure, or hypotension. In patients with impaired cardiac function, coadministration should be avoided.

Catecholamine-depleting drugs: Close observation of the patient is recommended when a beta blocker is administered to patients receiving catecholamine-depleting drugs such as reserpine, because of possible additive effects and the production of hypotension and/or marked bradycardia, which may result in vertigo, syncope, or postural hypotension.

Digitalis and calcium antagonists: The concomitant use of beta-adrenergic blocking agents with digitalis and calcium antagonists may have additive effects in prolonging atrioventricular conduction time.

Quinidine: Potentiated systemic beta-blockade (e.g., decreased heart rate) has been reported during combined treatment with quinidine and timolol, possibly because quinidine inhibits the metabolism of timolol via the P-450 enzyme, CYP2D6.

Injectable Epinephrine: (See **PRECAUTIONS,** *General, Anaphylaxis:*)

Carcinogenesis, Mutagenesis, Impairment of Fertility

In a two-year study of timolol maleate administered orally to rats, there was a statistically significant increase in the incidence of adrenal pheochromocytomas in male rats administered 300 mg/kg/day (approximately 42,000 times the systemic exposure following the maximum recommended human ophthalmic dose). Similar differences were not observed in rats administered oral doses equivalent to approximately 14,000 times the maximum recommended human ophthalmic dose.

In a lifetime oral study in mice, there were statistically significant increases in the incidence of benign and malignant pulmonary tumors, benign uterine polyps, and mammary adenocarcinomas in female mice at 500 mg/kg/day (approximately 71,000 times the systemic exposure following the maximum recommended human ophthalmic dose), but not at 5 or 50 mg/kg/day (approximately 700 or 7,000, respectively, times the systemic exposure following the maximum recommended human ophthalmic dose). In a subsequent study in female mice, in which post-mortem examinations were limited to the uterus and the lungs, a statistically significant increase in the incidence of pulmonary tumors was again observed at 500 mg/kg/day.

The increased occurrence of mammary adenocarcinomas was associated with elevations in serum prolactin, which occurred in female mice administered oral timolol at 500 mg/kg/day, but not at oral doses of 5 or 50 mg/kg/day. An increased incidence of mammary adenocarcinomas in rodents has been associated with administration of several other therapeutic agents that elevate serum prolactin, but no correlation between serum prolactin levels and mammary tumors has been established in humans. Furthermore, in adult human female subjects who received oral dosages of up to 60 mg of timolol maleate (the maximum recommended human oral dosage), there were no clinically meaningful changes in serum prolactin.

Timolol maleate was devoid of mutagenic potential when tested *in vivo* (mouse) in the micronucleus test and cytogenetic assay (doses up to 800 mg) and *in vitro* in a neoplastic cell transformation assay (up to 100 μg/mL). In Ames tests, the highest concentrations of timolol employed, 5,000 or 10,000 μg/plate, were associated with statistically significant elevations of revertants observed with tester strain TA100 (in seven replicate assays), but not in the remaining three strains. In the assays with tester strain TA100, no consistent dose response relationship was observed, and the ratio of test to control revertants did not reach 2. A ratio of 2 is usually considered the criterion for a positive Ames test.

Reproduction and fertility studies in rats demonstrated no adverse effect on male or female fertility at doses up to 21,000 times the systemic exposure following the maximum recommended human ophthalmic dose.

Pregnancy—Teratogenic effects:

Pregnancy Category C. Teratogenicity studies with timolol in mice and rabbits at oral doses up to 50 mg/kg/day (7,000 times the systemic exposure following the maximum recommended human ophthalmic dose) demonstrated no evidence of fetal malformations. Although delayed fetal ossification was observed at this dose in rats, there were no adverse effects on postnatal development of offspring. Doses of 1000 mg/kg/day (142,000 times the systemic exposure following the maximum recommended human ophthalmic dose) were maternotoxic in mice and resulted in an increased number of fetal resorptions. Increased fetal resorptions were also seen in rabbits at doses of 14,000 times the systemic exposure following the maximum recommended human ophthalmic dose, in this case without apparent maternotoxicity.

There are no adequate and well-controlled studies in pregnant women. TIMOPTIC-XE should be used during pregnancy only if the potential benefit justifies the potential risk to the fetus.

Nursing Mothers

Timolol maleate has been detected in human milk following oral and ophthalmic drug administration. Because of the potential for serious adverse reactions from TIMOPTIC-XE in nursing infants, a decision should be made whether to discontinue nursing or to discontinue the drug, taking into account the importance of the drug to the mother.

Pediatric Use

Safety and effectiveness in pediatric patients have not been established.

Geriatric Use

Of the total number of patients in clinical studies of TIMOPTIC-XE, 46% were 65 years of age and over, while 14% were 75 years of age and over. No overall differences in effectiveness or safety were observed between these patients and younger patients, but greater sensitivity of some older individuals to the product cannot be ruled out.

Adverse Reactions

In clinical trials, transient blurred vision upon instillation of the drop was reported in approximately one in three patients (lasting from 30 seconds to 5 minutes). Less than 1% of patients discontinued from the studies due to blurred vision. The frequency of patients reporting burning and stinging upon instillation was comparable between TIMOPTIC-XE and TIMOPTIC (approximately one in eight patients).

Adverse experiences reported in 1–5% of patients were:

Ocular: Pain, conjunctivitis, discharge (e.g. crusting), foreign body sensation, itching and tearing;

Systemic: Headache, dizziness, and upper respiratory infections.

The following additional adverse experiences have been reported with the ocular administration of this or other timolol maleate formulations:

BODY AS A WHOLE

Asthenia/fatigue, and chest pain.

CARDIOVASCULAR

Bradycardia, arrhythmia, hypotension, hypertension, syncope, heart block, cerebral vascular accident, cerebral ischemia, cardiac failure, worsening of angina pectoris, palpitation, cardiac arrest, pulmonary edema, edema, claudication, Raynaud's phenomenon, and cold hands and feet.

DIGESTIVE

Nausea, diarrhea, dyspepsia, anorexia, and dry mouth.

IMMUNOLOGIC

Systemic lupus erythematosus.

NERVOUS SYSTEM/PSYCHIATRIC

Increase in signs and symptoms of myasthenia gravis, paresthesia, somnolence, insomnia, nightmares, behavioral changes and psychic disturbances including depression, confusion, hallucinations, anxiety, disorientation, nervousness, and memory loss.

SKIN

Alopecia and psoriasiform rash or exacerbation of psoriasis.

HYPERSENSITIVITY

Signs and symptoms of allergic reactions, including angioedema, urticaria, and localized and generalized rash.

RESPIRATORY

Bronchospasm (predominantly in patients with preexisting bronchospastic disease), respiratory failure, dyspnea, nasal congestion, and cough.

ENDOCRINE

Masked symptoms of hypoglycemia in diabetic patients (see **WARNINGS**).

SPECIAL SENSES

Signs and symptoms of ocular irritation including blepharitis, keratitis, and dry eyes; ptosis; decreased corneal sensitivity; cystoid macular edema; visual disturbances including refractive changes and diplopia; pseudopemphigoid; choroidal detachment following filtration surgery (see **PRECAUTIONS,** *General*); and tinnitus.

UROGENITAL

Retroperitoneal fibrosis, decreased libido, impotence, and Peyronie's disease.

The following additional adverse effects have been reported in clinical experience with ORAL timolol maleate or other ORAL beta-blocking agents and may be considered potential effects of ophthalmic timolol maleate: *Allergic:* Erythematous rash, fever combined with aching and sore throat, laryngospasm with respiratory distress; *Body as a Whole:* Extremity pain, decreased exercise tolerance, weight loss; *Cardiovascular:* Worsening of arterial insufficiency, vasodilatation; *Digestive:* Gastrointestinal pain, hepatomegaly, vomiting, mesenteric arterial thrombosis, ischemic colitis; *Hematologic:* Nonthrombocytopenic purpura, thrombocytopenic purpura, agranulocytosis; *Endocrine:* Hyperglycemia, hypoglycemia; *Skin:* Pruritus, skin irritation, increased pigmentation, sweating; *Musculoskeletal:* Arthralgia; *Nervous System/Psychiatric:* Vertigo, local weakness, diminished concentration, reversible mental depression progressing to catatonia, an acute reversible syndrome characterized by disorientation for time and place, emotional lability, slightly clouded sensorium, and decreased performance on neuropsychometrics; *Respiratory:* Rales, bronchial obstruction; *Urogenital:* Urination difficulties.

Overdosage

No data are available in regard to human overdosage with or accidental oral ingestion of TIMOPTIC-XE.

There have been reports of inadvertent overdosage with TIMOPTIC Ophthalmic Solution resulting in systemic effects similar to those seen with systemic beta-adrenergic blocking agents such as dizziness, headache, shortness of breath, bradycardia, bronchospasm, and cardiac arrest (see also **ADVERSE REACTIONS**).

Overdosage has been reported with Tablets BLOCADREN* (Timolol Maleate). A 30 year old female ingested 650 mg of BLOCADREN (maximum recommended oral daily dose is 60 mg) and experienced second and third degree heart block. She recovered without treatment but approximately two months later developed irregular heartbeat, hypertension, dizziness, tinnitus, faintness, increased pulse rate, and borderline first degree heart block.

Significant lethality was observed in female rats and female mice after a single oral dose of 900 and 1190 mg/kg (5310 and 3570 mg/m^2) of timolol, respectively.

An *in vitro* hemodialysis study, using ^{14}C timolol added to human plasma or whole blood, showed that timolol was readily dialyzed from these fluids; however, a study of patients with renal failure showed that timolol did not dialyze readily.

---

*Registered trademark of MERCK & CO., Inc.

Dosage and Administration

Patients should be instructed to invert the closed container and shake once before each use. It is not necessary to shake the container more than once. Other topically applied ophthalmic medications should be administered at least 10 minutes before TIMOPTIC-XE. (See **PRECAUTIONS,** *Information for Patients* and accompanying INSTRUCTIONS FOR USE.)

TIMOPTIC-XE Sterile Ophthalmic Gel Forming Solution is available in concentrations of 0.25% and 0.5%. The dose is one drop of TIMOPTIC-XE (either 0.25% or 0.5%) in the affected eye(s) once a day.

Because in some patients the pressure-lowering response to TIMOPTIC-XE may require a few weeks to stabilize, evaluation should include a determination of intraocular pressure after approximately 4 weeks of treatment with TIMOPTIC-XE.

Dosages higher than one drop of 0.5% TIMOPTIC-XE once a day have not been studied. If the patient's intraocular pressure is still not at a satisfactory level on this regimen, concomitant therapy can be considered. The concomitant use of two topical beta-adrenergic blocking agents is not recommended. (See **PRECAUTIONS**, *Drug Interactions, Beta-adrenergic blocking agents.*)

When patients have been switched from therapy with TIMOPTIC administered twice daily to TIMOPTIC-XE administered once daily, the ocular hypotensive effect has remained consistent.

How Supplied

TIMOPTIC-XE Sterile Ophthalmic Gel Forming Solution is a colorless to nearly colorless, slightly opalescent, and slightly viscous solution.

No. 3557—TIMOPTIC-XE Sterile Ophthalmic Gel Forming Solution, 0.25% timolol equivalent, is supplied in OCUMETER*, a white, opaque, plastic, ophthalmic dispenser with a controlled drop tip as follows:

NDC 0006-3557-32, 2.5 mL

(6505-01-388-0967, 0.25% 2.5 mL)

NDC 0006-3557-03, 5 mL

(6505-01-387-9495, 0.25% 5 mL).

No. 3558—TIMOPTIC-XE Sterile Ophthalmic Gel Forming Solution, 0.5% timolol equivalent, is supplied in OCUMETER, a white, opaque, plastic, ophthalmic dispenser with a controlled drop tip as follows:

NDC 0006-3558-32, 2.5 mL

(6505-01-388-0964, 0.5% 2.5 mL)

NDC 0006-3558-03, 5 mL

(6505-01-387-9482, 0.5% 5 mL).

Continued on next page

Information on the Merck & Co., Inc., products listed on these pages is from the full prescribing information in use August 31, 1999.

Timoptic-XE—Cont.

Storage
Store between 15° and 25°C (59° and 77°F). **AVOID FREEZING.** Protect from light.

*Registered trademark of MERCK & CO., INC.
9028708 Issued June 1997

TIMOPTIC-XE®
0.25% AND 0.5%
(Timolol Maleate Ophthalmic Gel Forming Solution)

INSTRUCTIONS FOR USE

Please follow these instructions carefully when using TIMOPTIC-XE*. Use TIMOPTIC-XE as prescribed by your doctor.

1. If you use other topically applied ophthalmic medications, they should be administered at least 10 minutes before TIMOPTIC-XE.
2. Wash hands before each use.
3. Invert the closed bottle and shake ONCE before each use. (It is not necessary to shake the bottle more than once.)

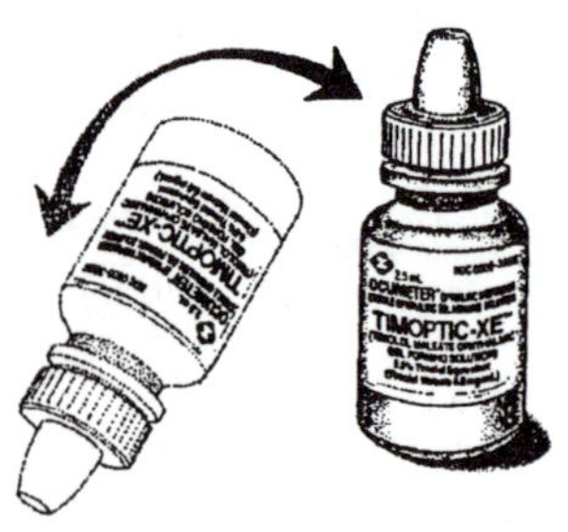

4. Remove the cap from the bottle carefully so that the dispenser tip does not touch anything. Place the cap in a clean, dry area.
5. Hold the bottle between the thumb and index finger. Use the index finger of the other hand to pull down the lower eyelid to form a pocket for the eye drop. Tilt your head back.

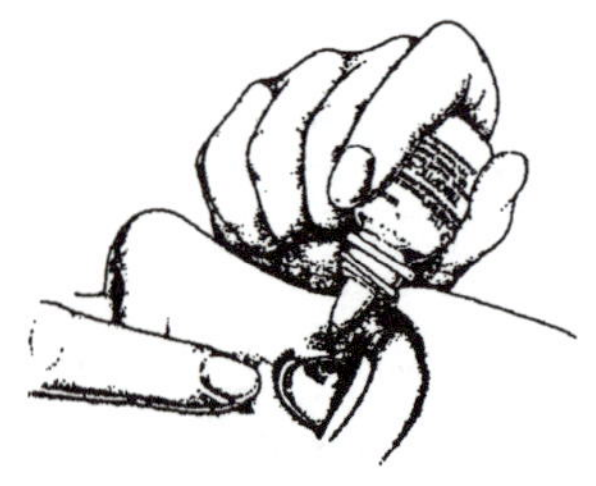

6. Place the dispenser tip close to your eye and gently squeeze the bottle to administer one drop. Remove pressure after a single drop has been released. If instructed, repeat steps 5 and 6 in the other eye.
7. **DO NOT ALLOW THE DISPENSER TIP TO TOUCH THE EYE OR SURROUNDING AREAS.** Ophthalmic medications, if handled improperly, can become contaminated by common bacteria known to cause eye infections. Serious damage to the eye and subsequent loss of vision may result from using contaminated ophthalmic medications. If you think your medication may be contaminated, or you develop an eye infection, contact your doctor immediately concerning continued use of this bottle.
8. Replace the cap. Store the bottle at room temperature in an upright position in a clean area.

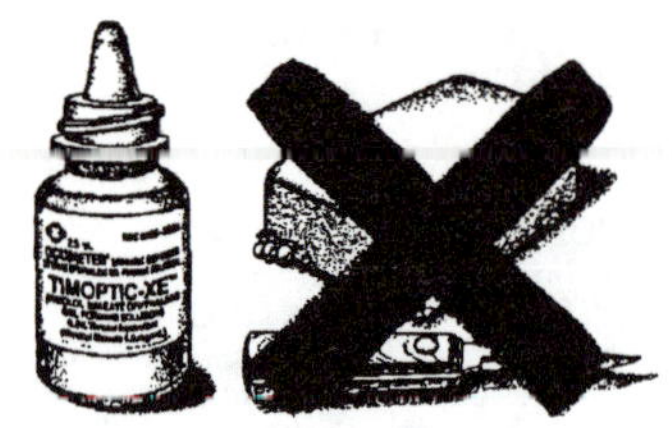

9. The dispenser tip is designed to provide a pre-measured drop; therefore, do NOT enlarge the hold of the dispenser.
10. Do NOT wash the tip of the dispenser with water, soap, or any other cleaner.

WARNING: Keep out of reach of children.
If you have any questions about the use of TIMOPTIC-XE, please consult your doctor.

*Registered trademark of MERCK & CO., Inc.

Issued June 1997
MERCK & CO., Inc.
West Point, PA 19486, USA
Shown in Product Identification Guide, page 106

TRUSOPT® ℞
Sterile Ophthalmic Solution 2%
(dorzolamide hydrochloride ophthalmic solution)

Description

TRUSOPT* (dorzolamide hydrochloride ophthalmic solution) is a carbonic anhydrase inhibitor formulated for topical ophthalmic use. Dorzolamide hydrochloride is described chemically as: (4*S-trans*)-4-(ethylamino)-5,6-dihydro-6-methyl-4*H*-thieno [2,3-*b*]thiopyran-2-sulfonamide 7,7-dioxide monohydrochloride. Dorzolamide hydrochloride is optically active. The specific rotation is

$$\alpha^{25°}_{405} \text{ (C = 1, water)} = \sim -17°.$$

Its empirical formula is $C_{10}H_{16}N_2O_4S_3 \cdot HCl$ and its structural formula is:

[Structural formula: H_3C, H, O, O, S, S, $SO_2NH_2 \cdot HCl$, H, $NHCH_2CH_3$]

Dorzolamide hydrochloride has a molecular weight of 360.9 and a melting point of about 264°C. It is a white to off-white, crystalline powder, which is soluble in water and slightly soluble in methanol and ethanol.

TRUSOPT Sterile Ophthalmic Solution is supplied as a sterile, isotonic, buffered, slightly viscous, aqueous solution of dorzolamide hydrochloride. The pH of the solution is approximately 5.6, and the osmolarity is 260–330 mOsM. Each mL of TRUSOPT 2% contains 20 mg dorzolamide (22.3 mg of dorzolamide hydrochloride). Inactive ingredients are hydroxyethyl cellulose, mannitol, sodium citrate dihydrate, sodium hydroxide (to adjust pH) and water for injection. Benzalkonium chloride 0.0075% is added as a preservative.

*Registered trademark of MERCK & CO., Inc.

Clinical Pharmacology

Mechanism of Action
Carbonic anhydrase (CA) is an enzyme found in many tissues of the body including the eye. It catalyzes the reversible reaction involving the hydration of carbon dioxide and the dehydration of carbonic acid. In humans, carbonic anhydrase exists as a number of isoenzymes, the most active being carbonic anhydrase II (CA-II), found primarily in red blood cells (RBCs), but also in other tissues. Inhibition of carbonic anhydrase in the ciliary processes of the eye decreases aqueous humor secretion, presumably by slowing the formation of bicarbonate ions with subsequent reduction in sodium and fluid transport. The result is a reduction in intraocular pressure (IOP).

TRUSOPT Ophthalmic Solution contains dorzolamide hydrochloride, an inhibitor of human carbonic anhydrase II. Following topical ocular administration, TRUSOPT reduces elevated intraocular pressure. Elevated intraocular pressure is a major risk factor in the pathogenesis of optic nerve damage and glaucomatous visual field loss.

Pharmacokinetics / Pharmacodynamics
When topically applied, dorzolamide reaches the systemic circulation. To assess the potential for systemic carbonic anhydrase inhibition following topical administration, drug and metabolite concentrations in RBCs and plasma and carbonic anhydrase inhibition in RBCs were measured. Dorzolamide accumulates in RBCs during chronic dosing as a result of binding to CA-II. The parent drug forms a single N-desethyl metabolite, which inhibits CA-II less potently than the parent drug but also inhibits CA-I. The metabolite also accumulates in RBCs where it binds primarily to CA-I. Plasma concentrations of dorzolamide and metabolite are generally below the assay limit of quantitation (15nM). Dorzolamide binds moderately to plasma proteins (approximately 33%). Dorzolamide is primarily excreted unchanged in the urine; the metabolite also is excreted in urine. After dosing is stopped, dorzolamide washes out of RBCs nonlinearly, resulting in a rapid decline of drug concentration initially, followed by a slower elimination phase with a half-life of about four months.

To simulate the systemic exposure after long-term topical ocular administration, dorzolamide was given orally to eight healthy subjects for up to 20 weeks. The oral dose of 2 mg b.i.d. closely approximates the amount of drug delivered by topical ocular administration of TRUSOPT 2% t.i.d. Steady state was reached within 8 weeks. The inhibition of CA-II and total carbonic anhydrase activities was below the degree of inhibition anticipated to be necessary for a pharmacological effect on renal function and respiration in healthy individuals.

Clinical Studies
The efficacy of TRUSOPT was demonstrated in clinical studies in the treatment of elevated intraocular pressure in patients with glaucoma or ocular hypertension (baseline IOP ≥23 mmHg). The IOP-lowering effect of TRUSOPT was approximately 3 to 5 mmHg throughout the day and this was consistent in clinical studies of up to one year duration.

The efficacy of TRUSOPT when dosed less frequently than three times a day (alone or in combination with other products) has not been established.

In a one year clinical study, the effect of TRUSOPT 2% t.i.d. on the corneal endothelium was compared to that of betaxolol ophthalmic solution b.i.d. and timolol maleate ophthalmic solution 0.5% b.i.d. There were no statistically significant differences between groups in corneal endothelial cell counts or in corneal thickness measurements. There was a mean loss of approximately 4% in the endothelial cell counts for each group over the one year period.

Indications and Usage
TRUSOPT Ophthalmic Solution is indicated in the treatment of elevated intraocular pressure in patients with ocular hypertension or open-angle glaucoma.

Contraindications
TRUSOPT is contraindicated in patients who are hypersensitive to any component of this product.

Warnings
TRUSOPT is a sulfonamide and although administered topically is absorbed systemically. Therefore, the same types of adverse reactions that are attributable to sulfonamides may occur with topical administration with TRUSOPT. Fatalities have occurred, although rarely, due to severe reactions to sulfonamides including Stevens-Johnson syndrome, toxic epidermal necrolysis, fulminant hepatic necrosis, agranulocytosis, aplastic anemia, and other blood dyscrasias. Sensitization may recur when a sulfonamide is readministered irrespective of the route of administration. If signs of serious reactions or hypersensitivity occur, discontinue the use of this preparation.

Precautions
General
The management of patients with acute angle-closure glaucoma requires therapeutic interventions in addition to ocular hypotensive agents. TRUSOPT has not been studied in patients with acute angle-closure glaucoma.
TRUSOPT has not been studied in patients with severe renal impairment (CrCl < 30 mL/min). Because TRUSOPT and its metabolite are excreted predominantly by the kidney, TRUSOPT is not recommended in such patients.
TRUSOPT has not been studied in patients with hepatic impairment and should therefore be used with caution in such patients.
In clinical studies, local ocular adverse effects, primarily conjunctivitis and lid reactions, were reported with chronic administration of TRUSOPT. Many of these reactions had the clinical appearance and course of an allergic-type reaction that resolved upon discontinuation of drug therapy. If such reactions are observed, TRUSOPT should be discontinued and the patient evaluated before considering restarting the drug. (See **ADVERSE REACTIONS**.)
There is a potential for an additive effect on the known systemic effects of carbonic anhydrase inhibition in patients receiving an oral carbonic anhydrase inhibitor and TRUSOPT. The concomitant administration of TRUSOPT and oral carbonic anhydrase inhibitors is not recommended.
There have been reports of bacterial keratitis associated with the use of multiple dose containers of topical ophthalmic products. These containers had been inadvertently contaminated by patients who, in most cases, had a concurrent corneal disease or a disruption of the ocular epithelial surface.
Information for Patients
TRUSOPT is a sulfonamide and although administered topically is absorbed systemically. Therefore the same types of adverse reactions that are attributable to sulfonamides may occur with topical administration. Patients should be advised that if serious or unusual reactions or signs of hypersensitivity occur, they should discontinue the use of the product (see **WARNINGS**).
Patients should be advised that if they develop any ocular reactions, particularly conjunctivitis and lid reactions, they should discontinue use and seek their physician's advice.
Patients should be instructed to avoid allowing the tip of the dispensing container to contact the eye or surrounding structures.
Patients should also be instructed that ocular solutions, if handled improperly or if the tip of the dispensing container contacts the eye or surrounding structures, can become contaminated by common bacteria known to cause ocular infections. Serious damage to the eye and subsequent loss of vision may result from using contaminated solutions.
Patients also should be advised that if they have ocular surgery or develop an intercurrent ocular condition (e.g., trauma or infection), they should immediately seek their physician's advice concerning the continued use of the present multidose container.
If more than one topical ophthalmic drug is being used, the drugs should be administered at least ten minutes apart.
Patients should be advised that TRUSOPT contains benzalkonium chloride which may be absorbed by soft contact lenses. Contact lenses should be removed prior to administration of the solution. Lenses may be reinserted 15 minutes following TRUSOPT administration.
Drug Interactions
Although acid-base and electrolyte disturbances were not reported in the clinical trials with TRUSOPT, these disturbances have been reported with oral carbonic anhydrase inhibitors and have, in some instances, resulted in drug interactions (e.g., toxicity associated with high-dose salicylate therapy). Therefore, the potential for such drug interactions should be considered in patients receiving TRUSOPT.
Carcinogenesis, Mutagenesis, Impairment of Fertility
In a two-year study of dorzolamide hydrochloride administered orally to male and female Sprague-Dawley rats, urinary bladder papillomas were seen in male rats in the highest dosage group of 20 mg/kg/day (250 times the recommended human ophthalmic dose). Papillomas were not seen in rats given oral doses equivalent to approximately 12 times the recommended human ophthalmic dose. No treatment-related tumors were seen in a 21-month study in female and male mice given oral doses up to 75 mg/kg/day (900 times the recommended human ophthalmic dose).
The increased incidence of urinary bladder papillomas seen in the high-dose male rats is a class-effect of carbonic anhydrase inhibitors in rats. Rats are particularly prone to developing papillomas in response to foreign bodies, compounds causing crystalluria, and diverse sodium salts.
No changes in bladder urothelium were seen in dogs given oral dorzolamide hydrochloride for one year at 2 mg/kg/day (25 times the recommended human ophthalmic dose) or monkeys dosed topically to the eye at 0.4 mg/kg/day (5 times the recommended human ophthalmic dose) for one year.
The following tests for mutagenic potential were negative: (1) *in vivo* (mouse) cytogenetic assay; (2) *in vitro* chromosomal aberration assay; (3) alkaline elution assay; (4) V-79 assay; and (5) Ames test.
In reproduction studies of dorzolamide hydrochloride in rats, there were no adverse effects on the reproductive capacity of males or females at doses up to 188 or 94 times, respectively, the recommended human ophthalmic dose.
Pregnancy
Teratogenic Effects. Pregnancy Category C. Developmental toxicity studies with dorzolamide hydrochloride in rabbits at oral doses of ≥2.5 mg/kg/day (31 times the recommended human ophthalmic dose) revealed malformations of the vertebral bodies. These malformations occurred at doses that caused metabolic acidosis with decreased body weight gain in dams and decreased fetal weights. No treatment-related malformations were seen at 1.0 mg/kg/day (13 times the recommended human ophthalmic dose). There are no adequate and well-controlled studies in pregnant women. TRUSOPT should be used during pregnancy only if the potential benefit justifies the potential risk to the fetus.
Nursing Mothers
In a study of dorzolamide hydrochloride in lactating rats, decreases in body weight gain of 5 to 7% in offspring at an oral dose of 7.5 mg/kg/day (94 times the recommended human ophthalmic dose) were seen during lactation. A slight delay in postnatal development (incisor eruption, vaginal canalization and eye openings), secondary to lower fetal body weight, was noted.
It is not known whether this drug is excreted in human milk. Because many drugs are excreted in human milk and because of the potential for serious adverse reactions in nursing infants from TRUSOPT, a decision should be made whether to discontinue nursing or to discontinue the drug, taking into account the importance of the drug to the mother.
Pediatric Use
Safety and effectiveness in pediatric patients have not been established.

Adverse Reactions
Controlled clinical trials: The most frequent adverse events associated with TRUSOPT were ocular burning, stinging, or discomfort immediately following ocular administration (approximately one-third of patients). Approximately one-quarter of patients noted a bitter taste following administration. Superficial punctate keratitis occurred in 10–15% of patients and signs and symptoms of ocular allergic reaction in approximately 10%. Events occurring in approximately 1–5% of patients were conjunctivitis and lid reactions (see PRECAUTIONS, *General*), blurred vision, eye redness, tearing, dryness, and photophobia. Other ocular events and systemic events were reported infrequently, including headache, nausea, asthenia/fatigue; and, rarely, skin rashes, urolithiasis, and iridocyclitis.
Clinical practice: The following adverse events have occurred either at low incidence (<1%) during clinical trials or have been reported during the use of TRUSOPT in clinical practice where these events were reported voluntarily from a population of unknown size and frequency of occurrence cannot be determined precisely. They have been chosen for inclusion based on factors such as seriousness, frequency of reporting, possible causal connection to TRUSOPT, or a combination of these factors: signs and symptoms of systemic allergic reactions including angioedema, bronchospasm, pruritus, and urticaria; dizziness, paresthesia; ocular pain, transient myopia, eyelid crusting; dyspnea; contact dermatitis and throat irritation.

Overdosage
Electrolyte imbalance, development of an acidotic state, and possible central nervous system effects may occur. Serum electrolyte levels (particularly potassium) and blood pH levels should be monitored.

Dosage and Administration
The dose is one drop of TRUSOPT Ophthalmic Solution in the affected eyes(s) three times daily.
TRUSOPT may be used concomitantly with other topical ophthalmic drug products to lower intraocular pressure. If more than one topical ophthalmic drug is being used, the drugs should be administered at least ten minutes apart.

How Supplied
TRUSOPT Ophthalmic Solution is a slightly opalescent, nearly colorless, slightly viscous solution.

Continued on next page

Information on the Merck & Co., Inc., products listed on these pages is from the full prescribing information in use August 31, 1999.

Trusopt—Cont.

No. 3519—TRUSOPT Ophthalmic Solution 2% is supplied in OCUMETER®*, a white, opaque, plastic ophthalmic dispenser with a controlled drop tip as follows:
NDC 0006-3519-03, 5 mL
(6505-01-439-8632)
NDC 0006-3519-10, 10 mL
(6505-01-416-4328).
Storage
Store TRUSOPT Ophthalmic Solution at 15–30°C (59–86°F). Protect from light.

*Registered trademark of MERCK & CO., Inc.

9010007 Issued February 1999

Shown in Product Identification Guide, page 106

Monarch Pharmaceuticals
355 BEECHAM STREET
BRISTOL, TN 37620

CHLOROMYCETIN® ℞
Ophthalmic Ointment, 1%
[*chlorō mycētin*]
(Chloramphenicol Ophthalmic Ointment, USP)

> **Warning:** Bone marrow hypoplasia including aplastic anemia and death has been reported following local application of chloramphenicol. Chloramphenicol should not be used when less potentially dangerous agents would be expected to provide effective treatment.

Description: Each gram of Chloromycetin Ophthalmic Ointment, 1% contains 10 mg chloramphenicol in a special base of liquid petrolatum and polyethylene. It contains no preservatives. Sterile ointment.
The chemical names for chloramphenicol are:
(1) Acetamide, 2,2-dichloro-*N*-[2-hydroxy-1-(hydroxymethyl) -2-(4-nitrophenyl) ethyl]-, and
(2) D-*threo*-(—)-2,2-Dichloro-*N*-[β-hydroxy-α-(hydroxymethyl) -*p*-nitrophenethyl] acetamide.
Chloramphenicol has the following empirical and structural formulas:

$O_2N-C_6H_4-CH(OH)-CH(NHCOCHCl_2)-CH_2OH$

$C_{11}H_{12}Cl_2N_2O_5$ Mol Wt 323.13

Clinical Pharmacology: Chloramphenicol is a broad-spectrum antibiotic originally isolated from *Streptomyces venezuelae*. It is primarily bacteriostatic and acts by inhibition of protein synthesis by interfering with the transfer of activated amino acids from soluble RNA to ribosomes. It has been noted that chloramphenicol is found in measurable amounts in the aqueous humor following local application to the eye. Development of resistance to chloramphenicol can be regarded as minimal for staphylococci and many other species of bacteria.
Indications and Usage: Chloramphenicol should be used only in those serious infections for which less potentially dangerous drugs are ineffective or contraindicated. Bacteriological studies should be performed to determine the causative organisms and their sensitivity to chloramphenicol (see Boxed Warning).
Chloromycetin Ophthalmic Ointment, 1% (Chloramphenicol Ophthalmic Ointment, USP) is indicated for the treatment of surface ocular infections involving the conjunctiva and/or cornea caused by chloramphenicol-susceptible organisms.
The particular antiinfective drug in this product is active against the following common bacterial eye pathogens:
Staphylococcus aureus
Streptococci, including *Streptococcus pneumoniae*
Escherichia coli
Haemophilus influenzae
Klebsiella/Enterobacter species
Moraxella lacunata
(Morax-Axenfeld bacillus)
Neisseria species
The product does not provide adequate coverage against:
Pseudomonas aeruginosa
Serratia marcescens
Contraindications: This product is contraindicated in persons sensitive to any of its components.
Warnings: See Boxed Warning
Ophthalmic ointments may retard corneal wound healing.
Precautions: The prolonged use of antibiotics may occasionally result in overgrowth of nonsusceptible organisms, including fungi. If new infections appear during medication, the drug should be discontinued and appropriate measures should be taken.
In all serious infections the topical use of chloramphenicol should be supplemented by appropriate systemic medication.
Adverse Reactions: Blood dyscrasias have been reported in association with the use of chloramphenicol (see Warnings).
Allergic or inflammatory reactions due to individual hypersensitivity and occasional burning or stinging may occur with the use of Chloromycetin Ophthalmic Ointment.
Dosage and Administration: A small amount of ointment placed in the lower conjunctival sac every three hours, or more frequently if deemed advisable by the prescribing physician. Administration should be continued day and night for the first 48 hours, after which the interval between applications may be increased. Treatment should be continued for at least 48 hours after the eye appears normal.
How Supplied: NDC 61570-307-01
Chloromycetin Ophthalmic Ointment, 1% (Chloramphenicol Ophthalmic Ointment, USP) is supplied, sterile, in ophthalmic ointment tubes of 3.5 grams.
Chloromycetin, brand of chloramphenicol. Reg US Pat Off
Rx only.
Distributed by: Monarch Pharmaceuticals, Inc., Bristol, TN 37620

CHLOROMYCETIN® OPHTHALMIC ℞
[*chlŏrō ' mycētin*]
(Chloramphenicol for Ophthalmic Solution, USP)

> **Warning:** Bone marrow hypoplasia including aplastic anemia and death has been reported following local application of chloramphenicol. Chloramphenicol should not be used when less potentially dangerous agents would be expected to provide effective treatment

Description: Each vial of Chloromycetin Ophthalmic contains 25 mg of Chloromycetin (chloramphenicol) with boric acid-sodium borate buffer. Sodium hydroxide may have been added for adjustment of pH. A 15 mL bottle of Sterile Distilled Water is included in each package for use as a diluent in the preparation of a solution of Chloromycetin suitable for ophthalmic use. By varying the quantity of diluent used, solutions ranging in strength from 0.16% to 0.5% may be prepared. Both the powder for solution and the diluent contain no preservatives. Sterile powder.
The chemical names for chloramphenicol are
(1) Acetamide, 2,2-dichloro-*N*-[2-hydroxy-1-(hydroxymethyl)-2-(4-nitrophenyl) ethyl]-, and
(2) D-*tbreo*(—)-2,2-Dichloro-*N*-[β-hydroxy-α-(hydroxymethyl)-*p*-nitrophenethyl] acetamide.
Chloramphenicol has the following empirical and structural formulas:

$O_2N-C_6H_4-CH(OH)-CH(NHCOCHCl_2)-CH_2OH$

$C_{11}H_{12}Cl_2N_2O_3$ Mol. Wt. 323.13

Clinical Pharmacology: Chloramphenicol is a broad-spectrum antibiotic originally isolated from *Streptomyces venezuelae*. It is primarily bacteriostatic and acts by inhibition of protein synthesis by interfering with the transfer or activated amino acids from soluble RNA to ribosomes. It has been noted that chloramphenicol is found in measurable amounts in the aqueous humor following local application to the eye. Development of resistance to chloramphenicol can be regarded as minimal for staphylococci and many other species of bacteria.
Indications and Usage: Chloramphenicol should be used only in those serious infections for which less potentially dangerous drugs are ineffective or contraindicated. Bacteriological studies should be performed to determine the causative organisms and their sensitivity to chloramphenicol (see Boxed Warning).
Chloromycetin Ophthalmic (Chloramphenicol for Ophthalmic Solution, USP) is indicated for the treatment of surface ocular infections involving the conjunctiva and/or cornea caused by chloramphenicol-susceptible organisms.
The particular antiinfective drug in this product is active against the following common bacterial eye pathogens:
Staphylococcus aureus
Streptococci, including *Streptococcus pneumoniae*
Escberichia coli
Haemophilus influenzae
Klebsiella/Enterobacter species
Moraxella lacunata
(Morax-Axenfeld bacillus)
Neisseria species
The product does not provide adequate coverage against:
Pseudomonas aeruginosa
Serratia marcescens
Contraindications: This product is contraindicated in persons sensitive to any of its components.
Warnings: See Boxed Warning
Precautions: The prolonged use of antibiotics may occasionally result in overgrowth of nonsusceptible organisms, including fungi. If new infections appear during medication, the drug should be discontinued and appropriate measures should be taken.
In all serious infections the topical use of chloramphenicol should be supplemented by appropriate systemic medication.
Adverse Reactions: Blood dyscrasias have been reported in association with the use of chloramphenicol (see Warnings).
Transient burning or stinging sensations may occur with use of Chloromycetin Ophthalmic Solution.

Dosage and Administration: Two drops applied to the affected eye every three hours, or more frequently if deemed advisable by the prescribing physician. Administration should be continued day and night for the first 48 hours, after which the interval between applications may be increased. Treatment should be continued for at least 48 hours after the eye appears normal.

Directions for dispensing—Prepare solution by adding sterile distilled water to the vial as follows:

Strength of solution desired	Add sterile distilled water
0.5%	5 mL
0.25%	10 mL
0.16%	15 mL

Solutions remain stable at room temperature for ten days.

How Supplied: NDC 61570-321-31 Chloromycetin Ophthalmic (Chloramphenicol for Ophthalmic Solution, USP) is supplied in a package containing dry ingredients in a 15 mL vial and also a vial containing 15 mL of Sterile Distilled Water for use as a diluent in preparing the solution for ophthalmic use. A sterilized dropper-cap assembly for use on the vial of solution is included in the package.

Store below 30°C (86°F).

Chloromycetin, brand of chloramphenicol. Reg US Pat Off

Rx only

Distributed by: Monarch Pharmaceuticals, Inc. Bristol, TN 37620

CORTISPORIN® ℞
Ophthalmic Ointment Sterile

[cŏr 'tĭ-spŏrin]

(neomycin and polymyxin B sulfates, bacitracin zinc, and hydrocortisone ophthalmic ointment, USP)

Description: CORTISPORIN® Ophthalmic Ointment (neomycin and polymyxin B sulfates, bacitracin zinc, and hydrocortisone ophthalmic ointment) is a sterile antimicrobial and anti-inflammatory ointment for ophthalmic use. Each gram contains: neomycin sulfate equivalent to 3.5 mg neomycin base, polymyxin B sulfate equivalent to 10,000 polymyxin B units, bacitracin zinc equivalent to 400 bacitracin units, hydrocortisone 10 mg (1%), and white petrolatum, q.s.

Neomycin sulfate is the sulfate salt of neomycin B and C, which are produced by the growth of *Streptomyces fradiae* Waksman (Fam. Streptomycetaceae). It has a potency equivalent of not less than 600 µg of neomycin standard per mg, calculated on an anhydrous basis. The structural formulae are:

Neomycin B (R_1=H, R_2=CH_2NH_2)
Neomycin C (R_1=CH_2NH_2, R_2=H)

Polymyxin B sulfate is the sulfate salt of polymyxin B_1 and B_2, which are produced by the growth of *Bacillus polymyxa* (Prazmowski) Migula (Fam. Bacillaceae). It has a potency of not less than 6,000 polymyxin B units per mg, calculated on an anhydrous basis. The structural formulae are:

Polymyxin B_1 (R=CH_3)
Polymyxin B_2 (R=H)
DAB=α,γ-diaminobutyric acid

Bacitracin zinc is the zinc salt of bacitracin, a mixture of related cyclic polypeptides (mainly bacitracin A) produced by the growth of an organism of the *licheniformis* group of *Bacillus subtilis* var Tracy. It has a potency of not less than 40 bacitracin units per mg. The structural formula is:

Hydrocortisone, 11β, 17, 21-trihydroxypregn-4-ene-3, 20-dione, is an anti-inflammatory hormone. Its structural formula is:

Clinical Pharmacology: Corticosteroids suppress the inflammatory response to a variety of agents and they probably delay or slow healing. Since corticosteroids may inhibit the body's defense mechanism against infection, concomitant antimicrobial drugs may be used when this inhibition is considered to be clinically significant in a particular case.

When a decision to administer both a corticosteroid and antimicrobials is made, the administration of such drugs in combination has the advantage of greater patient compliance and convenience, with the added assurance that the appropriate dosage of all drugs is administered. When each type of drug is in the same formulation, compatibility of ingredients is assured and the correct volume of drug is delivered and retained.

The relative potency of corticosteroids depends on the molecular structure, concentration, and release from the vehicle.

Microbiology: The anti-infective components in CORTISPORIN Ophthalmic Ointment are included to provide action against specific organisms susceptible to it. Neomycin sulfate and polymyxin B sulfate are active in vitro against susceptible strains of the following microorganisms: *Staphylococcus aureus,* streptococci including *Streptococcus pneumoniae, Escherichia coli, Haemophilus influenzae, Klebsiella / Enterobacter* species, *Neisseria* species, and *Pseudomonas aeruginosa.* The product does not provide adequate coverage against *Serratia marcescens* (see Indications and Usage).

Indications and Usage: CORTISPORIN Ophthalmic Ointment is indicated for steroid-responsive inflammatory ocular conditions for which a corticosteroid is indicated and where bacterial infection or a risk of bacterial infection exists.

Ocular corticosteroids are indicated in inflammatory conditions of the palpebral and bulbar conjunctiva, cornea, and anterior segment of the globe where the inherent risk of corticosteroid use in certain infective conjunctivitides is accepted to obtain a diminution in edema and inflammation. They are also indicated in chronic anterior uveitis and corneal injury from chemical, radiation, or thermal burns, or penetration of foreign bodies.

The use of a combination drug with an anti-infective component is indicated where the risk of infection is high or where there is an expectation that potentially dangerous numbers of bacteria will be present in the eye (see Clinical Pharmacology: Microbiology).

The particular anti-infective drugs in this product are active against the following common bacterial eye pathogens: *Staphylococcus aureus,* streptococci, including *Streptococcus pneumoniae, Escherichia coli, Haemophilus influenzae, Klebsiella / Enterobacter* species, *Neisseria* species, and *Pseudomonas aeruginosa.*

The product does not provide adequate coverage against *Serratia marcescens.*

Contraindications: CORTISPORIN Ophthalmic Ointment is contraindicated in most viral diseases of the cornea and conjunctiva including: epithelial herpes simplex keratitis (dendritic keratitis), vaccinia and varicella, and also in mycobacterial infection of the eye and fungal diseases of ocular structures.

CORTISPORIN Ophthalmic Ointment is also contraindicated in individuals who have shown hypersensitivity to any of its components. Hypersensitivity to the antibiotic component occurs at a higher rate than for other components.

Warnings: NOT FOR INJECTION INTO THE EYE. CORTISPORIN Ophthalmic Ointment should never be directly introduced into the anterior chamber of the eye. Ophthalmic ointments may retard corneal wound healing. Prolonged use of corticosteroids may result in ocular hypertension and/or glaucoma, with damage to the optic nerve, defects in visual acuity and fields of vision, and in posterior subcapsular cataract formation.

Prolonged use may suppress the host response and thus increase the hazard of secondary ocular infections. In those diseases causing thinning of the cornea or sclera, perforations have been known to occur with the use of topical corticosteroids. In acute purulent conditions of the eye, corticosteroids may mask infection or enhance existing infection.

If these products are used for 10 days or longer, intraocular pressure should be routinely monitored even though it may be difficult in uncooperative patients. Corticosteroids should be used with caution in the presence of glaucoma. The use of corticosteroids after cataract surgery may delay healing and increase the incidence of filtering blebs.

Use of the ocular corticosteroids may prolong the course and may exacerbate the severity of many viral infections of the eye (including herpes simplex). Employment of corticosteroid medication in the treatment of herpes simplex requires great caution.

Topical antibiotics, particularly neomycin sulfate, may cause cutaneous sensitization. A precise incidence of hypersensitivity reactions (primarily skin rash) due to topical antibiotics is not known. The manifestations of sensitization to topical antibiotics are usually itching, reddening, and edema of the conjunctiva and

Continued on next page

Cortisporin Ointment—Cont.

eyelid. A sensitization reaction may manifest simply as a failure to heal. During long-term use of topical antibiotic products, periodic examination for such signs is advisable, and the patient should be told to discontinue the product if they are observed. Symptoms usually subside quickly on withdrawing the medication. Applications of products containing these ingredients should be avoided for the patient thereafter (see Precautions: General).

Precautions:

General: The initial prescription and renewal of the medication order beyond 8 grams should be made by a physician only after examination of the patient with the aid of magnification, such as slit lamp biomicroscopy and, where appropriate, fluorescein staining. If signs and symptoms fail to improve after two days, the patient should be re-evaluated.

The possibility of fungal infections of the cornea should be considered after prolonged corticosteroid dosing. Fungal cultures should be taken when appropriate.

If this product is used for 10 days or longer, intraocular pressure should be monitored (see Warnings).

There have been reports of bacterial keratitis associated with the use of topical ophthalmic products in multiple-dose containers which have been inadvertently contaminated by patients, most of whom had a concurrent corneal disease or a disruption of the ocular epithelial surface (see Precautions: Information for Patients).

Allergic cross-reactions may occur which could prevent the use of any or all of the following antibiotics for the treatment of future infections: kanamycin, paromomycin, streptomycin, and possibly gentamicin.

Information for Patients: Patients should be instructed to avoid allowing the tip of the dispensing container to contact the eye, eyelid, fingers, or any other surface. The use of this product by more than one person may spread infection.

Patients should also be instructed that ocular products, if handled improperly, can become contaminated by common bacteria known to cause ocular infections. Serious damage to the eye and subsequent loss of vision may result from using contaminated products (see Precautions: General).

If the condition persists or gets worse, or if a rash or allergic reaction develops, the patient should be advised to stop use and consult a physician. Do not use this product if you are allergic to any of the listed ingredients.

Keep tightly closed when not in use. Keep out of the reach of children.

Carcinogenesis, Mutagenesis, Impairment of Fertility: Long-term studies in animals to evaluate carcinogenic or mutagenic potential have not been conducted with polymyxin B sulfate or bacitracin. Treatment of cultured human lymphocytes in vitro with neomycin increased the frequency of chromosome aberrations at the highest concentrations (80 µg/mL) tested; however, the effects of neomycin on carcinogenesis and mutagenesis in humans are unknown.

Long-term studies in animals (rats, rabbits, mice) showed no evidence of carcinogenicity or mutagenicity attributable to oral administration of corticosteroids. Long-term animal studies have not been performed to evaluate the carcinogenic potential of topical corticosteroids. Studies to determine mutagenicity with hydrocortisone have revealed negative results. Polymyxin B has been reported to impair the motility of equine sperm, but its effects on male or female fertility are unknown. No adverse effects on male or female fertility, litter size, or survival were observed in rabbits given bacitracin zinc 100 gm/ton of diet. Long-term animal studies have not been performed to evaluate the effect on fertility of topical corticosteroids.

Pregnancy: ***Teratogenic Effects:*** Pregnancy Category C. Corticosteroids have been found to be teratogenic in rabbits when applied topically at concentrations of 0.5% on days 6 to 18 of gestation and in mice when applied topically at a concentration of 15% on days 10 to 13 of gestation. There are no adequate and well-controlled studies in pregnant women. CORTISPORIN Ophthalmic Ointment should be used during pregnancy only if the potential benefit justifies the potential risk to the fetus.

Nursing Mothers: It is not known whether topical administration of corticosteroids could result in sufficient systemic absorption to produce detectable quantities in human milk. Systemically administered corticosteroids appear in human milk and could suppress growth, interfere with endogenous corticosteroid production, or cause other untoward effects. Because of the potential for serious adverse reactions in nursing infants from CORTISPORIN Ophthalmic Ointment, a decision should be made whether to discontinue nursing or to discontinue the drug, taking into account the importance of the drug to the mother.

Pediatric Use: Safety and effectiveness in children have not been established.

Adverse Reactions: Adverse reactions have occurred with corticosteroid/anti-infective combination drugs which can be attributed to the corticosteroid component, the anti-infective component, or the combination. The exact incidence is not known.

Reactions occurring most often from the presence of the anti-infective ingredient are allergic sensitization reactions including itching, swelling, and conjunctival erythema (see Warnings). More serious hypersensitivity reactions, including anaphylaxis, have been reported rarely.

The reactions due to the corticosteroid component in decreasing order of frequency are: elevation of intraocular pressure (IOP) with possible development of glaucoma, and infrequent optic nerve damage; posterior subcapsular cataract formation; and delayed wound healing.

Secondary Infection: The development of the secondary infection has occurred after use of combinations containing corticosteroids and antimicrobials. Fungal and viral infections of the cornea are particularly prone to develop coincidentally with long-term applications of a corticosteroid. The possibility of fungal invasion must be considered in any persistent corneal ulceration where corticosteroid treatment has been used.

Local irritation on installation has been reported.

Dosage and Administration: Apply the ointment in the affected eye every 3 or 4 hours, depending on the severity of the condition.

Not more than 8 grams should be prescribed initially and the prescription should not be refilled without further evaluation as outlined in Precautions above.

How Supplied: Tube of 1/8 oz. (3.5 g) with ophthalmic tip (NDC 61570-035-35).

Rx only

Store at 15° to 25°C (59° to 77°F).

Distributed by: Monarch Pharmaceuticals, Inc., Bristol, TN 37620

Manufactured by: Catalytica Pharmaceuticals, Inc., Greenville, NC 27834

CORTISPORIN® ℞
OPHTHALMIC SUSPENSION STERILE
(neomycin and polymyxin B sulfates and hydrocortisone ophthalmic suspension, USP)

Description: CORTISPORIN Ophthalmic Suspension (neomycin and polymyxin B sulfates and hydrocortisone ophthalmic suspension) is a sterile antimicrobial and anti-inflammatory suspension for ophthalmic use. Each mL contains: neomycin sulfate equivalent to 3.5 mg neomycin base, polymyxin B sulfate equivalent to 10,000 polymyxin B units, and hydrocortisone 10 mg (1%). The vehicle contains thimerosal 0.001% (added as a preservative) and the inactive ingredients cetyl alcohol, glyceryl monostearate, mineral oil, polyoxyl 40 stearate, propylene glycol, and Water for Injection. Sulfuric acid may be added to adjust pH.

Neomycin sulfate is the sulfate salt of neomycin B and C, which are produced by the growth of *Streptomyces fradiae* Waksman (Fam. Streptomycetaceae). It has a potency equivalent of not less than 600 µg of neomycin standard per mg, calculated on an anhydrous basis. The structural formulae are:

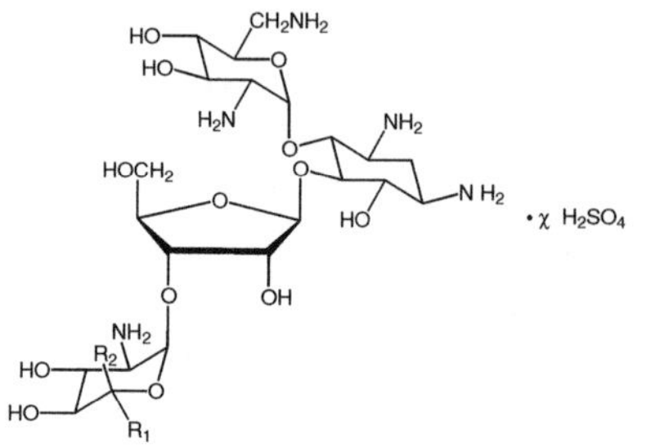

Neomycin B (R_1=H, R_2=CH_2NH_2)
Neomycin C (R_1=CH_2NH_2, R_2=H)

Polymyxin B sulfate is the sulfate salt of polymyxin B_1 and B_2, which are produced by the growth of *Bacillus polymyxa* (Prazmowski) Migula (Fam. Bacillaceae). It has a potency of not less than 6,000 polymyxin B units per mg, calculated on an anhydrous basis. The structural formulae are:

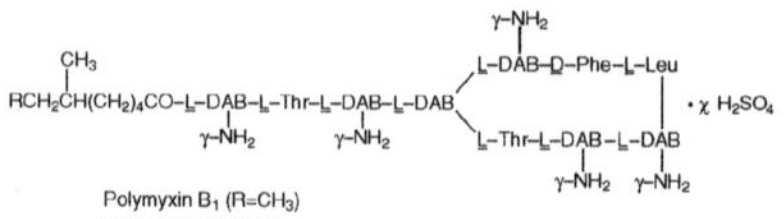

Polymyxin B_1 (R=CH_3)
Polymyxin B_2 (R=H)
DAB=α, γ-diaminobutyric acid

Hydrocortisone, 11β,17,21-trihydroxypregn-4-ene-3,20-dione, is an anti-inflammatory hormone. Its structural formula is:

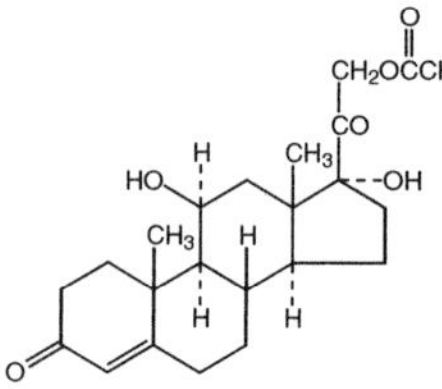

Clinical Pharmacology: Corticosteroids suppress the inflammatory response to a variety of agents, and they probably delay or slow healing. Since corticosteroids may inhibit the body's defense mechanism against infection, concomitant antimicrobial drugs may be used when this inhibition is considered to be clinically significant in a particular case.

When a decision to administer both a corticosteroid and antimicrobials is made, the administration of such drugs in combination has the advantage of greater patient compliance and convenience, with the added assurance that the appropriate dosage of all drugs is administered. When each type of drug is in the same formulation, compatibility of ingredients is assured and the correct volume of drug is delivered and retained.

The relative potency of corticosteroids depends on the molecular structure, concentration, and release from the vehicle.

Microbiology: The anti-infective components in CORTISPORIN Ophthalmic Suspension are included to provide action against specific organisms susceptible to it. Neomycin sulfate and polymyxin B sulfate are active in vitro against susceptible strains of the following microorganisms: *Staphylococcus aureus, Escherichia coli, Haemophilus influenzae, Klebsiella / Enterobacter species, Neisseria species,* and *Pseudomonas aeruginosa*. The product does not provide adequate coverage against Serratia marcescens and streptococci, including Streptococcus pneumoniae (see Indications and Usage).

Indications and Usage: CORTISPORIN Ophthalmic Suspension is indicated for steroid-responsive inflammatory ocular conditions for which a corticosteroid is indicated and where bacterial infection or a risk of bacterial infection exists.

Ocular corticosteroids are indicated in inflammatory conditions of the palpebral and bulbar conjunctiva, cornea, and anterior segment of the globe where the inherent risk of corticosteroid use in certain infective conjunctivitides is accepted to obtain a diminution in edema and inflammation. They are also indicated in chronic anterior uveitis and corneal injury from chemical, radiation, or thermal burns, or penetration of foreign bodies.

The use of a combination drug with an anti-infective component is indicated where the risk of infection is high or where there is an expectation that potentially dangerous numbers of bacteria will be present in the eye (see Clinical Pharmacology: Microbiology).

The particular anti-infective drugs in this product are active against the following common bacterial eye pathogens: *Staphylococcus aureus, Escherichia coli, Haemophilus influenzae, Klebsiella / Enterobacter species, Neisseria species,* and *Pseudomonas aeruginosa.*

The product does not provide adequate coverage against Serratia marcescens and streptococci, including *Streptococcus pneumoniae.*

Contraindications: CORTISPORIN Ophthalmic Suspension is contraindicated in most viral diseases of the cornea and conjunctiva including: epithelial herpes simplex keratitis (dendritic keratitis), vaccinia and varicella, and also in mycobacterial infection of the eye and fungal diseases of ocular structures.

CORTISPORIN Ophthalmic Suspension is also contraindicated in individuals who have shown hypersensitivity to any of its components. Hypersensitivity to the antibiotic component occurs at a higher rate than for other components.

Warnings: NOT FOR INJECTION INTO THE EYE. CORTISPORIN Ophthalmic Suspension should never be directly introduced into the anterior chamber of the eye.

Prolonged use of corticosteroids may result in ocular hypertension and/or glaucoma, with damage to the optic nerve, defects in visual acuity and fields of vision, and in posterior subcapsular cataract formation.

Prolonged use may suppress the host response and thus increase the hazard of secondary ocular infections. In those diseases causing thinning of the cornea or sclera, perforations have been known to occur with the use of topical corticosteroids. In acute purulent conditions of the eye, corticosteroids may mask infection or enhance existing infection.

If these products are used for 10 days or longer, intraocular pressure should be routinely monitored even though it may be difficult in uncooperative patients. Corticosteroids should be used with caution in the presence of glaucoma. The use of corticosteroids after cataract surgery may delay healing and increase the incidence of filtering blebs.

Use of ocular corticosteroids may prolong the course and may exacerbate the severity of many viral infections of the eye (including herpes simplex). Employment of corticosteroid medication in the treatment of herpes simplex requires great caution.

Topical antibiotics, particularly, neomycin sulfate, may cause cutaneous sensitization. A precise incidence of hypersensitivity reactions (primarily skin rash) due to topical antibiotics is not known. The manifestations of sensitization to topical antibiotics are usually itching, reddening, and edema of the conjunctiva and eyelid. A sensitization reaction may manifest simply as a failure to heal. During long-term use of topical antibiotic products, periodic examination for such signs is advisable, and the patient should be told to discontinue the product if they are observed. Symptoms usually subside quickly on withdrawing the medication. Application of products containing these ingredients should be avoided for the patient thereafter (see Precautions: General).

Precautions:

General: The initial prescription and renewal of the medication order beyond 20 milliliters should be made by a physician only after examination of the patient with the aid of magnification, such as slit lamp biomicroscopy and, where appropriate, fluorescein staining. If signs and symptoms fail to improve after 2 days, the patient should be re-evaluated.

The possibility of fungal infections of the cornea should be considered after prolonged corticosteroid dosing. Fungal cultures should be taken when appropriate.

If this product is used for 10 days or longer, intraocular pressure should be monitored (see Warnings).

There have been reports of bacterial keratitis associated with the use of topical ophthalmic products in multiple-dose containers which have been inadvertently contaminated by patients, most of whom had a concurrent corneal disease or a disruption of the ocular epithelial surface (see Precautions: Information for Patients).

Allergic cross-reactions may occur which could prevent the use of any or all of the following antibiotics for the treatment of future infections: kanamycin, paromomycin, streptomycin, and possibly gentamicin.

Information for Patients: Patients should be instructed to avoid allowing the tip of the dispensing container to contact the eye, eyelid, fingers, or any other surface. The use of this product by more than one person may spread infection.

Patients should also be instructed that ocular products, if handled improperly, can become contaminated by common bacteria known to cause ocular infections. Serious damage to the eye and subsequent loss of vision may result from using contaminated products (see Precautions: General).

If the condition persists or gets worse, or if a rash or allergic reaction develops, the patient should be advised to stop use and consult a physician. Do not use this product if you are allergic to any of the listed ingredients.

Keep tightly closed when not in use. Keep out of reach of children.

Carcinogenesis, Mutagenesis, Impairment of Fertility: Long-term studies in animals to evaluate carcinogenic or mutagenic potential have not been conducted with polymyxin B sulfate. Treatment of cultured human lymphocytes in vitro with neomycin increased the frequency of chromosome aberrations at the highest concentrations (80 mg/mL) tested; however, the effects of neomycin on carcinogenesis and mutagenesis in humans are unknown.

Long-term studies in animals (rats, rabbits, mice) showed no evidence of carcinogenicity or mutagenicity attributable to oral administration of corticosteroids. Long-term animal studies have not been performed to evaluate the carcinogenic potential of topical corticosteroids. Studies to determine mutagenicity with hydrocortisone have revealed negative results.

Polymyxin B has been reported to impair the motility of equine sperm, but its effects on male or female fertility are unknown. Long-term animal studies have not been performed to evaluate the effect on fertility of topical corticosteroids.

Pregnancy: ***Teratogenic Effects:*** Pregnancy Category C. Corticosteroids have been found to be teratogenic in rabbits when applied topically at concentrations of 0.5% on days 6 to 18 of gestation and in mice when applied topically at a concentration of 15% on days 10 to 13 of gestation. There are no adequate and well-controlled studies in pregnant women. CORTISPORIN Ophthalmic Suspension should be used during pregnancy only if the potential benefit justifies the potential risk to the fetus.

Nursing Mothers: It is not known whether topical administration of corticosteroids could result in sufficient systemic absorption to produce detectable quantities in human milk. Systemically administered corticosteroids appear in human milk and could suppress growth, interfere with endogenous corticosteroid production, or cause other untoward effects. Because of the potential for serious adverse reactions in nursing infants from CORTISPORIN Ophthalmic Suspension, a decision should be made whether to discontinue nursing or to discontinue the drug, taking into account the importance of the drug to the mother.

Pediatric Use: Safety and effectiveness in pediatric patients have not been established.

Adverse Reactions: Adverse reactions have occurred with corticosteroid/anti-infective combination drugs which can be attributed to the corticosteroid component, the anti-infective component, or the combination. The exact incidence is not known.

Reactions occurring most often from the presence of the anti-infective ingredient are allergic sensitization reactions including itching, swelling, and conjunctival erythema (see Warnings). More serious hypersensitivity reactions, including anaphylaxis, have been reported rarely.

The reactions due to the corticosteroid component in decreasing order of frequency are: elevation of intraocular pressure (IOP) with possible development of glaucoma, and infrequent optic nerve damage; posterior subcapsular cataract formation; and delayed wound healing.

Secondary Infection: The development of secondary infection has occurred after use of combinations containing corticosteroids and antimicrobials. Fungal and viral infections of the cornea are particularly prone to develop coincidentally with long-term applications of a corticosteroid. The possibility of fungal invasion must be considered in any persistent corneal ulceration where corticosteroid treatment has been used.

Local irritation on instillation has also been reported.

Dosage and Administration: One or two drops in the affected eye every 3 or 4 hours,

Continued on next page

Cortisporin Solution—Cont.

depending on the severity of the condition. The suspension may be used more frequently if necessary.

Not more than 20 milliliters should be prescribed initially and the prescription should not be refilled without further evaluation as outlined in Precautions above.

SHAKE WELL BEFORE USING.

How Supplied: Plastic DROP DOSE® dispenser bottle of 7.5 mL (NDC 61570-036-75).

Rx only

Store at 15° to 25°C (59° to 77°F).

Distributed by: Monarch Pharmaceuticals, Inc., Bristol, TN 37620

Manufactured by: Catalytica Pharmaceutical, Inc.

Greenville, NC 27835]

5/97
0932678

Shown in Product Identification Guide, page 106

NEOSPORIN® ℞

[*nē "ō-spor 'ĭn*]

Ophthalmic Ointment Sterile
(neomycin and polymyxin B sulfates and bacitracin zinc ophthalmic ointment, USP)

Description: NEOSPORIN OPHTHALMIC OINTMENT (neomycin and polymyxin B sulfates and bacitracin zinc ophthalmic ointment) is a sterile antimicrobial ointment for ophthalmic use. Each gram contains: neomycin sulfate equivalent to 3.5 mg neomycin base, polymyxin B sulfate equivalent to 10,000 polymyxin B units, bacitracin zinc equivalent to 400 bacitracin units, and white petrolatum, q.s.

Neomycin sulfate is the sulfate salt of neomycin B and C, which are produced by the growth of *Streptomyces fradiae* Waksman (Fam. Streptomycetaceae). It has a potency equivalent of not less than 600 µg of neomycin standard per mg, calculated on an anhydrous basis. The structural formulae are:

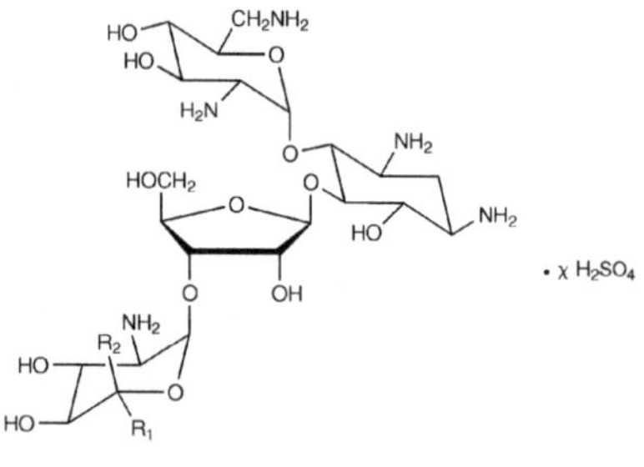

Neomycin B (R_1=H, R_2=CH_2NH_2)
Neomycin C (R_1=CH_2NH_2, R_2=H)

Polymyxin B sulfate is the sulfate salt of polymyxin B_1 and B_2, which are produced by the growth of *Bacillus polymyxa* (Prazmowski) Migula (Fam. Bacillaceae). It has a potency of not less than 6,000 polymyxin B units per mg, calculated on an anhydrous basis. The structural formulae are:

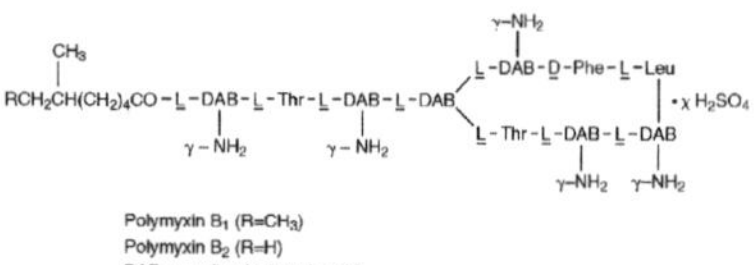

Polymyxin B_1 (R=CH_3)
Polymyxin B_2 (R=H)
DAB=α,γ-diaminobutyric acid

Bacitracin zinc is the zinc salt of bacitracin, a mixture of related cyclic polypeptides (mainly bacitracin A) produced by the growth of an organism of the *licheniformis* group of *Bacillus subtilis* var Tracy. It has a potency of not less than 40 bacitracin units per mg. The structural formula is:

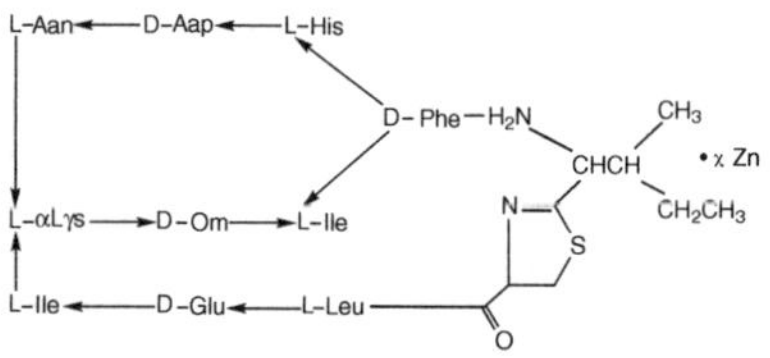

Clinical Pharmacology: A wide range of antibacterial action is provided by the overlapping spectra of neomycin, polymyxin B sulfate, and bacitracin.

Neomycin is bactericidal for many gram-positive and gram-negative organisms. It is an aminoglycoside antibiotic which inhibits protein synthesis by binding with ribosomal RNA and causing misreading of the bacterial genetic code.

Polymyxin B is bactericidal for a variety of gram-negative organisms. It increases the permeability of the bacterial cell membrane by interacting with the phospholipid components of the membrane.

Bacitracin is bactericidal for a variety of gram-positive and gram-negative organisms. It interferes with bacterial cell wall synthesis by inhibition of the regeneration of phospholipid receptors involved in peptidoglycan synthesis.

Microbiology: Neomycin sulfate, polymyxin B sulfate, and bacitracin zinc together are considered active against the following microorganisms: *Staphylococcus aureus*, streptococci including *Streptococcus pneumoniae, Escherichia coli, Haemophilus influenzae, Klebsiella / Enterobacter* species, *Neisseria* species, and *Pseudomonas aeruginosa*. The product does not provide adequate coverage against *Serratia marcescens*.

Indications and Usage: Neosporin Ophthalmic Ointment is indicated for the topical treatment of superficial infections of the external eye and its adnexa caused by susceptible bacteria. Such infections encompass conjunctivitis, keratitis and keratoconjunctivitis, blepharitis and blepharoconjunctivitis.

Contraindications: Neosporin Ophthalmic Ointment is contraindicated in individuals who have shown hypersensitivity to any of its components.

Warnings: NOT FOR INJECTION INTO THE EYE. NEOSPORIN OPHTHALMIC OINTMENT should never be directly introduced into the anterior chamber of the eye. Ophthalmic ointments may retard corneal wound healing.

Topical antibiotics, particularly neomycin sulfate, may cause cutaneous sensitization. A precise incidence of hypersensitivity reactions (primarily skin rash) due to topical antibiotics is not known. The manifestations of sensitization to topical antibiotics are usually itching, reddening, and edema of the conjunctiva and eyelid. A sensitization reaction may manifest simply as a failure to heal. During long-term use of topical antibiotic products, periodic examination for such signs is advisable, and the patient should be told to discontinue the product if they are observed. Symptoms usually subside quickly on withdrawing the medication. Application of products containing these ingredients should be avoided for the patient thereafter (see Precautions: General).

Precautions:

General: As with other antibiotic preparations, prolonged use of Neosporin Ophthalmic Ointment may result in overgrowth of nonsusceptible organisms including fungi. If superinfection occurs, appropriate measures should be initiated.

Bacterial resistance to Neosporin Ophthalmic Ointment may also develop. If purulent discharge, inflammation, or pain become aggravated, the patient should discontinue use of the medication and consult a physician.

There have been reports of bacterial keratitis associated with the use of topical ophthalmic products in multiple-dose containers which have been inadvertently contaminated by patients, most of whom had a concurrent corneal disease or a disruption of the ocular epithelial surface (see Precautions: Information for Patients).

Allergic cross-reactions may occur which could prevent the use of any or all of the following antibiotics for the treatment of future infections: kanamycin, paromomycin, streptomycin, and possibly gentamicin.

Information for Patients: Patients should be instructed to avoid allowing the tip of the dispensing container to contact the eye, eyelid, fingers, or any other surface. The use of this product by more than one person may spread infection.

Patients should also be instructed that ocular products, if handled improperly, can become contaminated by common bacteria known to cause ocular infections. Serious damage to the eye and subsequent loss of vision may result from using contaminated products (see Precautions: General).

If the condition persists or gets worse, or if a rash or allergic reaction develops, the patient should be advised to stop use and consult a physician. Do not use this product if you are allergic to any of the listed ingredients.

Keep tightly closed when not in use. Keep out of reach of children.

Carcinogenesis, Mutagenesis, Impairment of Fertility: Long-term studies in animals to evaluate carcinogenic or mutagenic potential have not been conducted with polymyxin B sulfate or bacitracin. Treatment of cultured human lymphocytes in vitro with neomycin increased the frequency of chromosome aberrations at the highest concentration (80 µg/mL) tested; however, the effects of neomycin on carcinogenesis and mutagenesis in humans are unknown.

Polymyxin B has been reported to impair the motility of equine sperm, but its effects on male or female fertility are unknown. No adverse effects on male or female fertility, litter size or survival were observed in rabbits given bacitracin zinc 100 gm/ton of diet.

Pregnancy: ***Teratogenic Effects:*** Pregnancy Category C. Animal reproduction studies have not been conducted with neomycin sulfate, polymyxin B sulfate, or bacitracin. It is also not known whether NEOSPORIN® Ophthalmic Ointment can cause fetal harm when administered to a pregnant woman or can affect reproduction capacity. NEOSPORIN OPHTHALMIC OINTMENT should be given to a pregnant woman only if clearly needed.

Nursing Mothers: It is not known whether this drug is excreted in human milk. Because many drugs are excreted in human milk, caution should be exercised when NEOSPORIN OPHTHALMIC OINTMENT is administered to a nursing woman.

Pediatric Use: Safety and effectiveness in pediatric patients have not been established.

Adverse Reactions: Adverse reactions have occurred with the anti-infective components of NEOSPORIN OPHTHALMIC OINTMENT. The exact incidence is not known. Reactions occurring most often are allergic sensitization reactions including itching, swelling, and conjunctival erythema (see Warnings). More serious hypersensitivity reactions, including anaphylaxis, have been reported rarely.

Local irritation on instillation has also been reported.

Dosage and Administration: Apply the ointment every 3 or 4 hours for 7 to 10 days, depending on the severity of the infection.
How Supplied: Tube of 1/8 oz (3.5 g) with ophthalmic tip (NDC 61570-046-35).
Rx only.
Store at 15° to 25°C (59° to 77°F).
Distributed by: Monarch Pharmaceuticals, Inc., Bristol, TN 37620

NEOSPORIN® Ophthalmic Solution Sterile ℞

[*nē ″ō-spor ′ĭn*]
(neomycin and polymyxin B sulfates and gramicidin ophthalmic solution, USP)

Description: NEOSPORIN Ophthalmic Solution (neomycin and polymyxin B sulfates and gramicidin ophthalmic solution) is a sterile antimicrobial solution for ophthalmic use. Each mL contains: neomycin sulfate equivalent to 1.75 mg neomycin base, polymyxin B sulfate equivalent to 10,000 polymyxin B units, and gramicidin 0.025 mg. The vehicle contains alcohol 0.5%, thimerosal 0.001% (added as a preservative), and the inactive ingredients propylene glycol, polyoxyethylene polyoxypropylene compound, sodium chloride, and Water for Injection.

Neomycin sulfate is the sulfate salt of neomycin B and C, which are produced by the growth of *Streptomyces fradiae* Waksman (Fam. Streptomycetaceae). It has a potency equivalent of not less than 600 mg of neomycin standard per mg, calculated on an anhydrous basis. The structural formulae are:

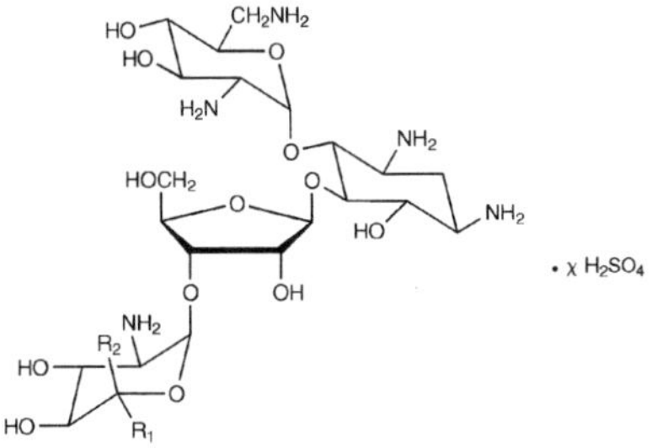

Neomycin B (R_1=H, R_2=CH_2NH_2)
Neomycin C (R_1=CH_2NH_2, R_2=H)

Polymyxin B sulfate is the sulfate salt of polymyxin B_1 and B_2 which are produced by the growth of *Bacillus polymyxa* (Prazmowski) Migula (Fam. Bacillaceae). It has a potency of not less than 6,000 polymyxin B units per mg, calculated on an anhydrous basis. The structural formulae are:

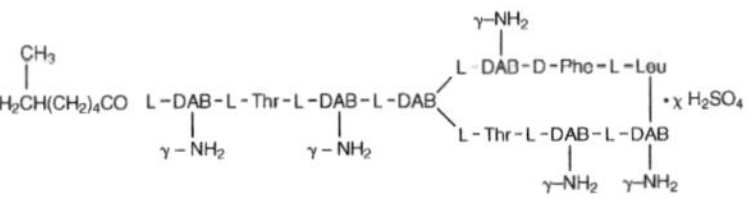

Polymyxin B_1 (R=CH_3)
Polymyxin B_2 (R=H)
DAB=α,γ-diaminobutyric acid

Gramicidin (also called Gramicidin D) is a mixture of three pairs of antibacterial substances (Gramicidin A, B, and C) produced by the growth of *Bacillus brevis* Dubos (Fam. Bacillaceae). It has a potency of not less than 900 µg of standard gramicidin per mg. The structural formulae are:

[See chemical structure at top of next column]

Clinical Pharmacology: A wide range of antibacterial action is provided by the overlapping spectra of neomycin, polymyxin B sulfate, and gramicidin.

Neomycin is bactericidal for many gram-positive and gram-negative organisms. It is an aminoglycoside antibiotic which inhibits pro-

Gramicidin D

HC(=O)-X-Gly-Ala-D-Leu-Ala-D-Val-Val-D-Val-Trp-D-Leu-Y-D-Leu-Trp-D-Leu-Trp-$NHCH_2CH_2OH$

	X	Y
Valine-gramicidin A	Val	Trp
Isoleucine-gramicidin A	Ile	Trp
Valine-gramicidin B	Val	Phe
Isoleucine-gramicidin B	Ile	Phe
Valine-gramicidin C	Val	Tyr
Isoleucine-gramicidin C	Ile	Tyr

tein synthesis by binding with ribosomal RNA and causing misreading of the bacterial genetic code.

Polymyxin B is bactericidal for a variety of gram-negative organisms. It increases the permeability of the bacterial cell membrane by interacting with the phospholipid components of the membrane.

Gramicidin is bactericidal for a variety of gram-positive organisms. It increases the permeability of the bacterial cell membrane to inorganic cations by forming a network of channels through the normal lipid bilayer of the membrane.

Microbiology: Neomycin sulfate, polymyxin B sulfate, and gramicidin together are considered active against the following microorganisms: *Staphylococcus aureus*, streptococci, including *Streptococcus pneumoniae*, *Escherichia coli, Haemophilus influenzae, Klebsiella / Enterobacter* species, *Neisseria species*, and *Pseudomonas aeruginosa*. The product does not provide adequate coverage against *Serratia marcescens*.

Indications and Usage: NEOSPORIN Ophthalmic Solution is indicated for the topical treatment of superficial infections of the external eye and its adnexa caused by susceptible bacteria. Such infections encompass conjunctivitis, keratitis and keratoconjunctivitis, blepharitis and blepharoconjunctivitis.

Contraindications: NEOSPORIN Ophthalmic Solution is contraindicated in individuals who have shown hypersensitivity to any of its components.

Warnings: NOT FOR INJECTION INTO THE EYE. NEOSPORIN Ophthalmic Solution should never be directly introduced into the anterior chamber of the eye or injected subconjunctivally.

Topical antibiotics, particularly neomycin sulfate, may cause cutaneous sensitization. A precise incidence of hypersensitivity reactions (primarily skin rash) due to topical antibiotics is not known. The manifestations of sensitization to topical antibiotics are usually itching, reddening, and edema of the conjunctiva and eyelid. A sensitization reaction may manifest simply as a failure to heal. During long-term use of topical antibiotic products, periodic examination for such signs is advisable, and the patient should be told to discontinue the product if they are observed. Symptoms usually subside quickly on withdrawing the medication. Application of products containing these ingredients should be avoided for the patient thereafter (see Precautions: General).

Precautions:

General: As with other antibiotic preparations, prolonged use of NEOSPORIN Ophthalmic Solution may result in overgrowth of nonsusceptible organisms including fungi. If superinfection occurs, appropriate measures should be initiated.

Bacterial resistance to NEOSPORIN Ophthalmic Solution may also develop. If purulent discharge, inflammation, or pain becomes aggravated, the patient should discontinue use of the medication and consult a physician.

There have been reports of bacterial keratitis associated with the use of topical ophthalmic products in multiple-dose containers which have been inadvertently contaminated by patients, most of whom had a concurrent corneal disease or a disruption of the ocular epithelial surface (see Precautions: Information for Patients).

Allergic cross-reactions may occur which could prevent the use of any or all of the following antibiotics for the treatment of future infections: kanamycin, paromomycin, streptomycin, and possibly gentamicin.

Information for Patients: Patients should be instructed to avoid allowing the tip of the dispensing container to contact the eye, eyelid, fingers, or any other surface. The use of this product by more than one person may spread infection.

Patients should also be instructed that ocular products, if handled improperly, can become contaminated by common bacteria known to cause ocular infections. Serious damage to the eye and subsequent loss of vision may result from using contaminated products (see Precautions: General).

If the condition persists or gets worse, or if a rash or other allergic reaction develops, the patient should be advised to stop use and consult a physician. Do not use this product if you are allergic to any of the listed ingredients.

Keep tightly closed when not in use. Keep out of reach of children.

Carcinogenesis, Mutagenesis, Impairment of Fertility: Long-term studies in animals to evaluate carcinogenic or mutagenic potential have not been conducted with polymyxin B sulfate or gramicidin. Treatment of cultured human lymphocytes in vitro with neomycin increased the frequency of chromosome aberrations at the highest concentration (80 µg/mL) tested. However, the effects of neomycin on carcinogenesis and mutagenesis in humans are unknown.

Polymyxin B has been reported to impair the motility of equine sperm, but its effects on male or female fertility are unknown.

Pregnancy: ***Teratogenic Effects:*** Pregnancy Category C. Animal reproduction studies have not been conducted with neomycin sulfate, polymyxin B sulfate, or gramicidin. It is also not known whether NEOSPORIN Ophthalmic Solution can cause fetal harm when administered to a pregnant woman or can affect reproduction capacity. NEOSPORIN Ophthalmic Solution should be given to a pregnant woman only if clearly needed.

Nursing Mothers: It is not known whether this drug is excreted in human milk. Because many drugs are excreted in human milk, caution should be exercised when NEOSPORIN Ophthalmic Solution is administered to a nursing woman.

Pediatric Use: Safety and effectiveness in pediatric patients have not been established.

Adverse Reactions: Adverse reactions have occurred with the anti-infective components of NEOSPORIN Ophthalmic Solution. The exact incidence is not known. Reactions occurring most often are allergic sensitization reactions including itching, swelling, and conjunctival erythema (see Warnings). More serious hypersensitivity reactions, including anaphylaxis, have been reported rarely.

Local irritation on instillation has also been reported.

Dosage And Administration: Instill one or two drops into the affected eye every 4 hours for 7 to 10 days. In severe infections, dosage may be increased to as much as two drops every hour.

How Supplied: Drop Dose® of 10 mL (plastic dispenser bottle) (NDC 61570-045-10).

Rx only

Store at 15° to 25°C (59° to 77°F) and protect from light.

Distributed by: Monarch Pharmaceuticals, Inc., Bristol, TN 37620

Continued on next page

POLYSPORIN® OPHTHALMIC OINTMENT ℞

[pŏly-spor 'in]

Sterile

(bacitracin zinc and polymyxin B sulfate ophthalmic ointment, USP)

Description: POLYSPORIN Ophthalmic Ointment (bacitracin zinc and polymyxin B sulfate ophthalmic ointment) is a sterile antimicrobial ointment for ophthalmic use. Each gram contains: bacitracin zinc equivalent to 500 bacitracin units, polymyxin B sulfate equivalent to 10,000 polymyxin B units, and white petrolatum, q.s.

Bacitracin zinc is the zinc salt of bacitracin, a mixture of related cyclic polypeptides (mainly bacitracin A) produced by the growth of an organism of the *licheniformis* group of *Bacillus subtilis* var Tracy. It has a potency of not less than 40 bacitracin units per mg. The structural formula for bacitracin A is:

Polymyxin B sulfate is the sulfate salt of polymyxin B_1 and B_2 which are produced by the growth of *Bacillus polymyxa* (Prazmowski) Migula (Fam. Bacillaceae). It has a potency of not less than 6,000 polymyxin B units per mg. calculated on an anhydrous basis. The structural formulae are:

Polymyxin B_1 (R=CH_3)
Polymyxin B_2 (R=H)
DAB=α,γ-diaminobutyric acid

Clinical Pharmacology: A wide range of antibacterial action is provided by the overlapping spectra of bacitracin and polymyxin B sulfate.

Bacitracin is bactericidal for a variety of gram-positive and gram-negative organisms. It interferes with bacterial cell wall synthesis by inhibition of the regeneration of phospholipid receptors involved in peptidoglycan synthesis.

Polymyxin B is bactericidal for a variety of gram-negative organisms. It increases the permeability of the bacterial cell membrane by interacting with the phospholipid components of the membrane.

Microbiology: Bacitracin zinc and polymyxin B sulfate together are considered active against the following microorganisms: *Staphylococcus aureus,* streptococci including *Streptococcus pneumoniae, Escherichia coli, Haemophilus influenzae, Klebsiella/Enterobacter* species, *Neisseria* species and *Pseudomonas aeruginosa.* The product does not provide adequate coverage against *Serratia marcescens.*

Indications and Usage: POLYSPORIN Ophthalmic Ointment is indicated for the topical treatment of superficial infections of the external eye and its adnexa caused by susceptible bacteria. Such infections encompass conjunctivitis, keratitis and keratoconjunctivitis, blepharitis and blepharoconjunctivitis.

Contraindications: POLYSPORIN Ophthalmic Ointment is contraindicated in individuals who have shown hypersensitivity to any of its components.

Warnings: NOT FOR INJECTION INTO THE EYE. POLYSPORIN Ophthalmic Ointment should never by directly introduced into the anterior chamber of the eye. Opthalmic ointments may retard corneal wound healing. Topical antibiotics may cause cutaneous sensitization. A precise incidence of hypersensitivity reactions (primarily skin rash) due to topical antibiotics is not known. The manifestations of sensitization to topical antibiotics are usually itching, reddening, and edema of the conjunctiva and eyelid. A sensitization reaction may manifest simply as a failure to heal. During long-term use of topical antibiotic products, periodic examination for such signs is advisable, and the patient should be told to discontinue the product if they are observed. Symptoms usually subside quickly on withdrawing the medication. Application of products containing these ingredients should be avoided for the patient thereafter (see Precautions: General).

Precautions:

General: As with other antibiotic preparations, prolonged use of POLYSPORIN Ophthalmic Ointment may result in overgrowth of nonsusceptible organisms including fungi. If superinfection occurs, appropriate measures should be initiated.

Bacterial resistance to POLYSPORIN Ophthalmic Ointment may also develop. If purulent discharge, inflammation, or pain become aggravated, the patient should discontinue use of the medication and consult a physician.

There have been reports of bacterial keratitis associated with the use of topical ophthalmic products in multiple-dose containers which have been inadvertently contaminated by patients, most of whom had a concurrent corneal disease or a disruption of the ocular epithelial surface (see Precautions: Information for Patients).

Allergic cross-reactions may occur which could prevent the use of any or all of the following antibiotics for the treatment of future infections: kanamycin, paromomycin, streptomycin, and possibly gentamicin.

Information for Patients: Patients should be instructed to avoid allowing the tip of the dispensing container to contact the eye, eyelid, fingers, or any other surface. The use of this product by more than one person may spread infection.

Patients should also be instructed that ocular products, if handled improperly, can become contaminated by common bacteria known to cause ocular infections. Serious damage to the eye and subsequent loss of vision may result from using contaminated products (see Precautions: General).

If the condition persists or gets worse, or if a rash or other allergic reaction develops, the patient should be advised to stop use and consult a physician. Do not use this product if you are allergic to any of the listed ingredients.

Keep tightly closed when not in use. Keep out of reach of children.

Carcinogenesis, Mutagenesis, Impairment of Fertility: Long-term studies in animals to evaluate carcinogenic or mutagenic potential have not been conducted with polymyxin B sulfate or bacitracin. Polymyxin B has been reported to impair the motility of equine sperm, but its effects on male or female fertility are unknown. No adverse effects on male or female fertility, litter size, or survival were observed in rabbits given bacitracin zinc 100 gm/ton of diet.

Pregnancy: ***Teratogenic Effects:*** Pregnancy Category C Animal reproduction studies have not been conducted with polymyxin B sulfate or bacitracin. It is also not known whether POLYSPORIN Ophthalmic Ointment can cause fetal harm when administered to a pregnant woman or can affect reproduction capacity POLYSPORIN Ophthalmic Ointment should be given to a pregnant woman only if clearly needed.

Nursing Mothers: It is not known whether this drug is excreted in human milk. Because many drugs are excreted in human milk, caution should be exercised when POLYSPORIN Ophthalmic Ointment is administered to a nursing woman.

Pediatric Use: Sales and effectiveness in pediatric patients have not been established.

Adverse Reactions: Adverse reactions have occurred with the anti-infective components of POLYSPORIN Ophthalmic Ointment. The exact incidence is not known. Reactions occurring most often are allergic sensitization reactions including itching, swelling, and conjunctival erythema (see Warnings). More serious hypersensitivity reactions including anaphylaxis, have been reported rarely.

Local irritation on installation has also been reported.

Dosage and Administration: Apply the ointment every 3 or 4 hours for 7 to 10 days, depending on the severity of the infection.

How Supplied: POLYSPORIN Ophthalmic Ointment (bacitracin zinc and polymyxin B sulfate ophthalmic ointment, USP) is available as a tube of 1/8 oz (3.5 g) with ophthalmic tip (NDC 61570-049-35)

Rx Only

Store at 15° to 25° C (59° to 77° F).

Distributed by: Monarch Pharmaceuticals, Inc., Bristol, TN 37620

VIRA-A® ℞

[vī 'ra-ā]

(Vidarabine Ophthalmic Ointment, USP) 3%

Description: VIRA-A is the trade name for vidarabine (also known as adenine arabinoside and Ara-A), an antiviral drug for the topical treatment of epithelial keratitis caused by Herpes simplex virus. The chemical name is 9H-Purin-6-amine, 9-$_b$-D-arabinofuranosyl-, monohydrate. Each gram of the ophthalmic ointment contains 30 mg of vidarabine monohydrate equivalent to 28.11 mg of vidarabine in a sterile, inert, petrolatum base.

The empirical and structural formulas are:

$C_{10}H_{13}H_5O_4 \cdot H_2O$ Mol. Wt. 285.26

Clinical Pharmacology: VIRA-A is rapidly deaminated to arabinosylhypoxanthine (Ara-Hx), the principal metabolite. Ara-Hx also possesses *in vitro* antiviral activity but this activity is less than that of VIRA-A. Because of the low solubility of VIRA-A, trace amounts of both VIRA-A and Ara-Hx can be detected in the aqueous humor only if there is an epithelial defect in the cornea. If the cornea is normal, only trace amounts of Ara-Hx can be recovered from the aqueous humor.

Systemic absorption of VIRA-A should not be expected to occur following ocular administration and swallowing lacrimal secretions. In laboratory animals, VIRA-A is rapidly deaminated in the gastrointestinal tract to Ara-Hx.

In contrast to topical idoxuridine, VIRA-A demonstrated less cellular toxicity in the regenerating corneal epithelium of the rabbit.

In controlled and uncontrolled clinical trials, an average of seven and nine days of continuous VIRA-A Ophthalmic Ointment, 3%, therapy was required to achieve corneal re-epithelialization. In the controlled trials, 70 of 81 subjects (86%) re-epithelialized at the end of three weeks of therapy. In the uncontrolled trials, 101 of 142 subjects (71%) re-epithelialized at the end of three weeks. Seventy-five percent of the subjects in these uncontrolled trials had either not healed previously or had developed hypersensitivity to topical idoxuridine therapy.

Microbiology

Vidarabine is a purine nucleoside obtained from fermentation cultures of *Streptomyces antibioticus*. The antiviral mechanism of action has not been established. Vidarabine appears to interfere with the early steps of viral DNA synthesis.

Vidarabine has been shown to possess antiviral activity against the following viruses *in vitro*:

Herpes simplex types 1 and 2
Vaccinia
Varicella-Zoster

Except for Rhabdovirus and Oncornavirus, vidarabine does not display *in vitro* antiviral activity against other RNA or DNA viruses, including Adenovirus.

Susceptibility Tests—No universal, standardized, quantitative *in vitro* procedures have as yet been developed to estimate the susceptibility of viruses to antiviral agents.

Indications and Usage: VIRA-A Ophthalmic Ointment, 3%, is indicated for the treatment of acute keratoconjunctivitis and recurrent epithelial keratitis due to Herpes simplex virus types 1 and 2. The clinical diagnosis of keratitis caused by Herpes simplex virus is usually established by the presence of typical dendritic or geographic lesions on slit-lamp examination. It is also effective in superficial keratitis caused by Herpes simplex virus which has not responded to topical idoxuridine or when toxic or hypersensitivity reactions due to idoxuridine have occurred. The effectiveness of VIRA-A Ophthalmic Ointment, 3%, against stromal keratitis and uveitis due to Herpes simplex virus has not been established.

Contraindications: VIRA-A Ophthalmic Ointment, 3%, is contraindicated in patients who develop hypersensitivity reactions to it.

Warnings: Normally, corticosteroids alone are contraindicated in Herpes simplex virus infections of the eye. If VIRA-A Ophthalmic Ointment, 3%, is administered concurrently with topical corticosteroid therapy, corticosteroid-induced ocular side effects must be considered. These include corticosteroid-induced glaucoma or cataract formation and progression of a bacterial or viral infection.

VIRA-A is not effective against RNA virus or adenoviral ocular infections. It is also not effective against bacterial, fungal, or chlamydial infections of the cornea or nonviral trophic ulcers.

Although viral resistance to VIRA-A has not been observed, this possibility may exist.

Precautions:

General

The diagnosis of keratoconjunctivitis due to Herpes simplex virus should be established clinically prior to prescribing VIRA-A Ophthalmic Ointment, 3%.

Patients should be forewarned that VIRA-A Ophthalmic Ointment, 3%, like any ophthalmic ointment, may produce a temporary visual haze.

Carcinogenesis

Chronic parenteral (IM) studies of vidarabine have been conducted in mice and rats.

In the mouse study, there was a statistically significant increase in liver tumor incidence among the vidarabine-treated females. In the same study some vidarabine-treated male mice developed kidney neoplasia. No renal tumors were found in the vehicle-treated control mice or the vidarabine-treated female mice.

In the rat study, intestinal, testicular, and thyroid neoplasia occurred with greater frequency among the vidarabine-treated animals than in the vehicle-treated controls. The increases in thyroid adenoma incidence in the high-dose (50 mg/kg) males and the low-dose (30 mg/kg) females were statistically significant.

Hepatic megalocytosis, associated with vidarabine treatment, has been found in short and long-term rodent (rat and mouse) studies. It is not clear whether or not this represents a preneoplastic change.

The recommended frequency and duration of administration should not be exceeded (see Dosage and Administration).

Mutagenesis

Results of *in vitro* experiments indicate that vidarabine can be incorporated into mammalian DNA and can induce mutation in mammalian cells (mouse L5178Y cell line). Thus far, *in vivo* studies have not been as conclusive, but there is some evidence (dominant lethal assay in mice) that vidarabine may be capable of producing mutagenic effects in male germ cells.

It has also been reported that vidarabine causes chromosome breaks and gaps when added to human leukocytes *in vitro*. While the significance of these effects in terms of mutagenicity is not fully understood, there is a well-known correlation between the ability of various agents to produce such effects and their ability to produce heritable genetic damage.

Pregnancy Category C

VIRA-A parenterally is teratogenic in rats and rabbits. Ten percent VIRA-A ointment applied to 10% of the body surface during organogenesis induced fetal abnormalities in rabbits. When 10% VIRA-A ointment was applied to 2% to 3% of the body surface of rabbits, no fetal abnormalities were found. This dose greatly exceeds the total recommended ophthalmic dose in humans. The possibility of embryonic or fetal damage in pregnant women receiving VIRA-A Ophthalmic Ointment, 3%, is remote. The topical ophthalmic dose is small, and the drug relatively insoluble. Its ocular penetration is very low. However, a safe dose for a human embryo or fetus has not been established. There are no adequate and well-controlled studies in pregnant women. VIRA-A should be used during pregnancy only if the potential benefit justifies the potential risk to the fetus.

Nursing Mothers

It is not known whether VIRA-A is secreted in human milk. Because many drugs are excreted in human milk and because of the potential for tumorigenicity shown for VIRA-A in animal studies, a decision should be made whether to discontinue nursing or to discontinue the drug, taking into account the importance of the drug to the mother. However, breast milk excretion is unlikely because VIRA-A is rapidly deaminated in the gastrointestinal tract.

Pediatric Use

The safety and effectiveness in pediatric patients below the age of 2 years have not been established.

Adverse Reactions: Lacrimation, foreign body sensation, conjunctival injection, burning, irritation, superficial punctate keratitis, pain, photophobia, punctal occlusion, and sensitivity have been reported with VIRA-A Ophthalmic Ointment, 3%. The following have also been reported but appear disease-related: uveitis, stromal edema, secondary glaucoma, trophic defects, corneal vascularization, and hyphema.

Overdosage: Acute massive overdosage by oral ingestion of the ophthalmic ointment has not occurred. However, the rapid deamination to arabinosylhypoxanthine should preclude any difficulty. The oral LD50 for vidarabine is greater than 5020 mg/kg in mice and rats. No untoward effects should result from ingestion of the entire contents of the tube.

Overdosage by ocular instillation is unlikely because any excess should be quickly expelled from the conjunctival sac.

Dosage and Administration: Administer approximately one-half inch of VIRA-A Ophthalmic Ointment, 3%, into the lower conjunctival sac five times daily at three-hour intervals.

If there are no signs of improvement after 7 days, or complete re-epithelialization has not occurred by 21 days, other forms of therapy should be considered. Some severe cases may require longer treatment.

Too frequent administration should be avoided.

After re-epithelialization has occurred, treatment for an additional 7 days at a reduced dosage (such as twice daily) is recommended in order to prevent recurrence.

The following topical antibiotics: gentamicin, erythromycin, chloramphenicol; or topical steroids: prednisolone or dexamethasone have been administered concurrently with VIRA-A Ophthalmic Ointment, 3%.

How Supplied: NDC 61570-367-71

VIRA-A Ophthalmic Ointment, 3%, is supplied sterile in ophthalmic ointment tubes of 3.5 g. The base is a 60:40 mixture of solid and liquid petrolatum.

Store at room temperature 15°-30°C (59°F-86°F).

Rx only.

Distributed by: Monarch Pharmaceuticals, Inc.
Bristol, TN 37620
Manufactured by: Parkedale Pharmaceuticals, Inc., Rochester, MI 48307

Rev. 4/98

Shown in Product Identification Guide, page 106

VIROPTIC® Ophthalmic Solution, 1% Sterile ℞
(trifluridine ophthalmic solution)

Description: VIROPTIC is the brand name for trifluridine (also known as trifluorothymidine, F_3T_dR, F_3T), an antiviral drug for topical treatment of epithelial keratitis caused by herpes simplex virus. The chemical name of trifluridine is α,α,α-trifluorothymidine; it has the following structural formula:

M.W. = 296.21 $C_{10}H_{11}F_3N_2O_5$

VIROPTIC sterile ophthalmic solution contains 1% trifluridine in an aqueous solution with acetic acid and sodium acetate (buffers), sodium chloride, and thimerosal 0.001% (added as a preservative). The pH range is 5.5 to 6.0 and osmolality is approximately 283 mOsm.

Clinical Pharmacology: Trifluridine is a fluorinated pyrimidine nucleoside with *in vitro* and *in vivo* activity against herpes simplex virus, types 1 and 2 and vacciniavirus. Some strains of adenovirus are also inhibited *in vitro*.

VIROPTIC is also effective in the treatment of epithelial keratitis that has not responded clinically to the topical administration of idoxuridine or when ocular toxicity or hyper-

Continued on next page

Viroptic—Cont.

sensitivity to idoxuridine has occurred. In a smaller number of patients found to be resistant to topical vidarabine, VIROPTIC was also effective.

Trifluridine interferes with DNA synthesis in cultured mammalian cells. However, its antiviral mechanism of action is not completely known.

In vitro perfusion studies on excised rabbit corneas have shown that trifluridine penetrates the intact cornea as evidenced by recovery of parental drug and its major metabolite, 5-carboxy-2′-deoxyuridine, on the endothelial side of the cornea. Absence of the corneal epithelium enhances the penetration of trifluridine approximately two-fold.

Intraocular penetration of trifluridine occurs after topical instillation of VIROPTIC into human eyes. Decreased corneal integrity or stromal or uveal inflammation may enhance the penetration of trifluridine into the aqueous humor. Unlike the results of ocular penetration of trifluridine *in vitro*, 5-carboxy-2′-deoxyuridine was not found in detectable concentrations within the aqueous humor of the human eye.

Systemic absorption of trifluridine following therapeutic dosing with VIROPTIC appears to be negligible. No detectable concentrations of trifluridine or 5-carboxy-2′-deoxyuridine were found in the sera of adult healthy normal subjects who had VIROPTIC instilled into their eyes seven times daily for 14 consecutive days.

Clinical Studies: During a controlled multicenter clinical trial, 92 of 97 (95%) patients (78 of 81 with dendritic and 14 of 16 with geographic ulcers) responded to therapy with VIROPTIC as evidenced by complete corneal re-epithelialization within the 14-day therapy period. Fifty-six of 75 (75%) patients (49 of 58 with dendritic and 7 of 17 with geographic ulcers) responded to idoxuridine therapy. The mean time to corneal re-epithelialization for dendritic ulcers (6 days) and geographic ulcers (7 days) was similar for both therapies.

In other clinical studies. VIROPTIC was evaluated in the treatment of herpes simplex virus keratitis in patients who were unresponsive or intolerant to the topical administration of idoxuridine or vidarabine. VIROPTIC was effective in 138 of 150 (92%) patients (109 of 114 with dendritic and 29 of 36 with geographic ulcers) as evidenced by corneal re-epithelialization. The mean time to corneal re-epithelialization was 6 days for patients with dendritic ulcers and 12 days for patients with geographic ulcers.

The clinical efficacy of VIROPTIC in the treatment of stromal keratitis and uveitis due to herpes simplex virus or ophthalmic infections caused by vacciniavirus and adenovirus has not been established by well-controlled clinical trials. VIROPTIC has not been shown to be effective in the prophylaxis of herpes simplex virus keratoconjunctivitis and epithelial keratitis by well-controlled clinical trials. VIROPTIC is not effective against bacterial, fungal, or chlamydial infections of the cornea or nonviral trophic lesions.

Indications and Usage: VIROPTIC Ophthalmic Solution, 1% (trifluridine ophthalmic solution) is indicated for the treatment of primay keratoconjunctivitis and recurrent epithelial keratitis due to herpes simplex virus, types 1 and 2.

Contraindications: VIROPTIC Ophthalmic Solution, 1% is contraindicated for patients who develop hypersensitivity reactions or chemical intolerance to trifluridine.

Warnings: The recommended dosage and frequency of administration should not be exceeded (see **Dosage and Administration**).

Precautions:

General: VIROPTIC Ophthalmic Solution, 1% should be prescribed only for patients who have a clinical diagnosis of herpetic keratitis. VIROPTIC may cause mild local irritation of the conjunctiva and cornea when instilled, but these effects are usually transient.

Although documented *in vitro* viral resistance to trifluridine has not been reported following multiple exposures to VIROPTIC, the possibility of the development of viral resistance exists.

Carcinogenesis, Mutagenesis, Impairment of Fertility: ***Mutagenic Potential:*** Trifluridine has been shown to exert mutagenic, DNA-damaging and cell-transforming activities in various standard *in vitro* test systems, and clastogenic activity in *Vicia faba* cells. It did not induce chromosome aberrations in bone marrow cells of male or female rats following a single subcutaneous dose of 100 mg/kg, but was weakly positive in female, but not in male, rats following daily subcutaneous administration at 700 mg/kg/day for 5 days.

Although the significance of these test results is not clear or fully understood, there exists the possibility that mutagenic agents may cause genetic damage in humans.

Oncogenic Potential: Lifetime carcinogenicity bioassays in rats and mice given daily subcutaneous doses of trifluridine have been performed. Rats tested at 1.5, 7.5, and 15 mg/kg/day had increased incidences of adenocarcinomas of the intestinal tract and mammary glands, hemangiosarcomas of the spleen and liver, carcinosarcomas of the prostate gland, and granulosa-thecal cell tumors of the ovary. Mice were tested at 1, 5, and 10 mg/kg/day; those given 10 mg/kg/day trifluridine had significantly increased incidences of adenocarcinomas of the intestinal tract and uterus. Those given 10 mg/kg/day also had a significantly increased incidence of testicular atrophy as compared to vehicle control mice.

Pregnancy: ***Teratogenic Effects:*** Pregnancy Category C. Trifluridine was not teratogenic at doses up to 5 mg/kg/day (23 times the estimated human exposure) when given subcutaneously to rats and rabbits. However, fetal toxicity consisting of delayed ossification of portions of the skeleton occurred at dose levels of 2.5 and 5 mg/kg/day in rats and at 2.5 resorption in rabbits. In both rats and rabbits, 1 mg/kg/day (5 times the estimated human exposure) was a no-effect level. There were no teratogenic or fetotoxic effects after topical application of VIROPTIC Ophthalmic Solution, 1% (approximately 5 times the estimated human exposure) to the eyes of rabbits on the 6th through the 18th days of pregnancy. In a non-standard test, trifluridine solution has been shown to be teratogenic when injected directly into the yolk sac of chicken eggs. There are no adequate and well-controlled studies in pregnant women. VIROPTIC Ophthalmic Solution, 1% should be used during pregnancy only if the potential benefit justifies the potential risk to the fetus.

Nursing Mothers: It is unlikely that trifluridine is excreted in human milk after ophthalmic instillation of VIROPTIC because of the relatively small dosage (≤5 mg/day), its dilution in body fluids and its extremely short half-life (approximately 12 minutes). The drug should not be prescribed for nursing mothers unless the potential benefits outweigh the potential risks.

Pediatric Use: Safety and effectiveness in pediatric patients below six years of age have not been established.

Adverse Reactions: The most frequent adverse reactions reported during controlled clinical trials were mild, transient burning or stinging upon instillation (4.6%) and palpebral edema (2.8%). Other adverse reactions in decreasing order of reported frequency were superficial punctate keratopathy, epithelial keratopathy, hypersensitivity reaction, stromal edema, irritation, keratitis sicca, hyperemia, and increased intraocular pressure.

Overdosage: Overdosage by ocular instillation is unlikely because any excess solution should be quickly expelled from the conjunctival sac.

Acute overdosage by accidental oral ingestion of VIROPTIC has not occurred. However, should such ingestion occur, the 75 mg dosage of trifluridine in a 7.5 mL bottle of VIROPTIC is not likely to produce adverse effects. Single intravenous doses of 1.5 to 30 mg/kg/day in children and adults with neoplastic disease produce reversible bone marrow depression as the only potentially serious toxic effect and only after three to five courses of therapy. The acute oral LD_{50} in the mouse and rat was 4379 mg/kg or higher.

Dosage and Administration: Instill one drop of VIROPTIC Ophthalmic Solution, 1% onto the cornea of the affected eye every 2 hours while awake for a maximum daily dosage of nine drops until the corneal ulcer has completely re-epithelialized. Following re-epithelialization, treatment for an additional 7 days of one drop every 4 hours while awake for a minimum daily dosage of five drops is recommended.

If there are no signs of improvement after 7 days of therapy or complete re-epithelialization has not occurred after 14 days of therapy, other forms of therapy should be considered. Continuous administration of VIROPTIC for periods exceeding 21 days should be avoided because of potential ocular toxicity.

How Supplied: VIROPTIC Ophthalmic Solution, 1% is supplied as a sterile ophthalmic solution in a plastic Drop Dose® dispenser bottle of 7.5 mL (NDC 61570-037-75).

Store under refrigeration 2° to 8°C (36° to 46°F).
Rx Only

Animal Pharmacology and Animal Toxicology: Corneal wound healing studies in rabbits showed that VIROPTIC did not significantly retard closure of epithelial wounds. However, mild toxic changes such as intracellular edema of the basal cell layer, mild thinning of the overlying epithelium and reduced strength of stromal wounds were observed.

Whereas instillation of VIROPTIC into rabbit eyes during a subchronic toxicity study produced some degree of corneal epithelial thinning, a 12-month chronic toxicity study in rabbits in which VIROPTIC was instilled into eyes in intermittent, multiple, full-therapy courses showed no drug-related changes in the cornea.

Distributed by: Monarch Pharmaceuticals®, Inc., Bristol, TN 37620
Manufactured by: Catalytica Pharmaceutical, Inc., Greenville, NC 27835

11/97

Ocumed, Inc.

119 HARRISON AVENUE
ROSELAND, NJ 07068

(UNIT DOSE) PRODUCTS

OCU-TEARS PF™

in Ophtha-Dose™ unit dispenser
Preservative Free, (Polyvinyl Alcohol ocular lubricant), Sterile Ophthalmic Solution.

How Supplied: 60 Ophtha-Dose™ Single Use Container NDC #51944-4485-01
120 Ophtha-Dose™ Single Use Container NDC #51944-4485-02

(MULTI-DOSE) PRODUCTS

EYE-ZINE
(tetrahydrozoline hydrochloride 0.05%)
Sterile eye drops
How Supplied: In 0.5 fl. oz. plastic dropper bottle.

IRI-SOL
(irrigating eye wash)
Sterile isotonic buffered solution
How Supplied: In 0.5 fl. oz., 1 fl. oz. and 4 fl. oz. plastic dispenser bottle.

OCU-CAINE ℞
(proparacaine hydrochloride 0.5%)
Sterile Ophthalmic Solution
How Supplied: In 2 ml and 15 ml plastic dropper bottle.

OCU-CARPINE ℞
(pilocarpine hydrochloride)
(0.5%, 1%, 2%, 3%, 4%. 5% and 6%)
Sterile Ophthalmic Solution
How Supplied: 15 ml Plastic Dropper Bottles.

OCU-LUBE
(white petrolatum base ocular lubricant)
Sterile ophthalmic Ointment
How Supplied: In 3.5 g tube with ophthalmic tip.

OCU-MYCIN ℞
(gentamicin sulfate—equiv. 3.0 mg)
Sterile Ophthalmic Ointment
How Supplied: In 3.5 g tubes with ophthalmic tip.

OCU-MYCIN ℞
(gentamicin sulfate—equiv. 3.0 mg)
Sterile Ophthalmic Solution
How Supplied: In 5 ml and 15 ml plastic dropper bottle.

OCU-PENTOLATE ℞
(cyclopentolate hydrochloride 1%)
Sterile Ophthalmic Solution
How Supplied: In 2 ml, 5 ml and 15 ml plastic dropper bottle.

OCU-PHRIN
(phenylephrine hydrochloride 0.12%)
Sterile Eye Drops
How Supplied: In 0.5 fl. oz. plastic dropper bottle.

OCU-PHRIN ℞
(phenylephrine hydrochloride 2.5% and 10%)
Sterile Ophthalmic Solution
How Supplied: In 5 ml and 15 ml plastic dropper bottle.

OCU-TEARS
(polyvinyl alcohol ocular lubricant)
Sterile Ophthalmic Solution
How Supplied: In 0.5 fl. oz. plastic dropper bottle.

OCU-TROL ℞
(polymyxin B sulfate 10,000 u/g)
(neomycin sulfate—equiv. 3.5 mg/g)
(dexamethasone 0.1%)
Sterile Ophthalmic Ointment
How Supplied: In 3.5 g tube with ophthalmic tip.

OCU-TROL ℞
(polymyxin B sulfate 10,000 u/g)
(neomycin sulfate—equiv. 3.5 mg/g)
dexamethesone 0.1%)
Sterile Ophthalmic Suspension
How Supplied: In 5 ml plastic dropper bottle.

OCU-TROPIC ℞
(tropicamide 0.5% and 1.0%)
Sterile Ophthalmic Solution
How Supplied: In 15 ml plastic dropper bottle.

OCU-TROPINE ℞
(atropine sulfate 1%)
Sterile Ophthalmic Ointment
How Supplied: In 3.5 g tubes with ophthalmic tip.

OCU-TROPINE ℞
(atropine sulfate 1%)
Sterile Ophthalmic Solution
How Supplied: In 15 ml plastic dropper bottle.

OCU-SPOR-B ℞
(polymyxin B sulfate—10,000 u/cc)
(neomycin sulfate—equiv. 3.5 mg/g)
(zinc bacitracin 400 u/g)
Sterile Ophthalmic Ointment
How Supplied: In 3.5 g tubes with ophthalmic tip.

OCU-SPOR-G ℞
(polymyxin B sulfate—10,000 u/cc)
(neomycin sulfate—equiv. 1.75 mg/cc)
(gramicidin 0.025%)
Sterile Ophthalmic Solution
How Supplied: In 10 cc plastic dropper bottle.

Pfizer Consumer Health Care Group

Pfizer Inc
235 EAST 42nd ST.
NEW YORK, NY 10017

Direct Inquiries to:
Consumer Relations Group
(212) 573-5656
FAX (212) 973-7437

OCUHIST®
Eye Allergy Relief
Itching & Redness Reliever Eye Drops
ANTIHISTAMINE & DECONGESTANT

OcuHist is an antihistamine/decongestant eye drop, clinically proven to temporarily relieve itching and redness of the eye.
Indications: For the temporary relief of itching and redness of the eye due to pollen, ragweed, grass, animal hair and dander.
Directions: Adults and children 6 years of age or older: Place 1 or 2 drops in the affected eye(s) up to four times a day. Some users may experience a brief tingling sensation.
Active Ingredients: pheniramine maleate 0.3%, naphazoline hydrochloride 0.025%.
Inactive Ingredients: boric acid and sodium borate buffer system preserved with benzalkonium chloride (0.01%) and edetate disodium (0.1%), sodium hydroxide and/or hydrochloric acid (to adjust pH) and purified water. The solution has a pH of 5.5–6.5 and a tonicity of 245—305 mOsm/Kg.
Warnings: If you experience eye pain, changes in vision, continued redness or irritation of the eye, or if the condition worsens or persists for more than 72 hours, discontinue use and consult a physician.
Do not use this product if you have heart disease, high blood pressure, difficulty in urination due to enlargement of the prostate gland or narrow angle glaucoma unless directed by a physician. Accidental oral ingestion in infants and children may lead to coma and marked reduction in body temperature.
To avoid contamination of this product, do not touch tip of container to any surface. Replace cap after using. Do not use if solution changes color or becomes cloudy.
Remove contact lenses before using.
Overuse of this product may produce increased redness of the eye.
Use before the expiration date marked on the carton or bottle.
Keep this and all drugs out of the reach of children.
Store between 15° and 25°C (59° and 77°F).
Parents Note: Before using with children under 6 years of age, consult your physician. Keep this and all drugs out of the reach of children. In case of accidental ingestion, seek professional assistance or contact a Poison Control Center immediately.
Caution: Do not use if Pfizer imprinted neckband on bottle is broken or missing.
Distributed By:
CONSUMER HEALTH CARE GROUP, PFIZER INC, NEW YORK, NEW YORK 10017

Shown in Product Identification Guide, page 107

ADVANCED RELIEF VISINE®
Lubricant/Redness Reliever Eye Drops

Description: Advanced Relief Visine is a sterile, isotonic, buffered ophthalmic solution containing polyethylene glycol 400 1%, povidone 1%, dextran 70 0.1%, tetrahydrozoline hydrochloride 0.05%.
Advanced Relief Visine is an ophthalmic solution combining the effects of the decongestant, tetrahydrozoline hydrochloride, with the demulcent effects of polyethylene glycol, povidone and dextran 70. It provides symptomatic relief of conjunctival edema and hyperemia secondary to minor irritations. Tetrahydrozoline hydrochloride is a sympathomimetic agent, which brings about decongestion by vasoconstriction. Reddened eyes are rapidly whitened by this effective vasoconstrictor, which limits the local vascular response by constricting the small blood vessels. The onset of vasoconstriction becomes apparent within minutes. Additional effects include amelioration of burning, irritation and excessive lacrimation. Relief is afforded by three moisturizers: polyethylene glycol 400, povidone and dextran 70.
Polyethylene glycol 400, povidone and dextran 70 are ophthalmic demulcents which have been shown to be effective for the temporary relief of discomfort of minor irritations of the eye due to exposure to wind or sun. They are effective as protectants and lubricants against further irritation or to relieve dryness of the eye.
The effectiveness of tetrahydrozoline hydrochloride in relieving conjunctival hyperemia and associated symptoms has been demonstrated by numerous clinicals, including several double-blind studies, involving more than 2,000 subjects suffering from acute or chronic hyperemia induced by a variety of conditions.
Advanced Relief Visine is a unique eye drop formulation that combines the redness-relieving effects of a vasoconstrictor and the soothing, moisturizing and protective effects of three demulcents.
Indications: Relieves redness of the eye due to minor eye irritations. For use as a protectant against further irritation or to relieve dryness.
Directions: Instill 1 to 2 drops in the affected eye(s) up to 4 times daily.
Active Ingredients: Polyethylene glycol 400 1%; povidone 1%; dextran 70 0.1%; tetrahydrozoline hydrochloride 0.05%.
Inactive Ingredients: Benzalkonium chloride; boric acid; edetate disodium; purified water; sodium borate; sodium chloride.

Continued on next page

Advanced Relief Visine—Cont.

Warnings: If you experience eye pain, changes in vision, continued redness or irritation of the eye, or if the condition worsens or persists for more than 72 hours, discontinue use and consult a physician. If you have glaucoma, do not use this product except under the advice and supervision of a physician. As with any drug, if you are pregnant or nursing a baby, seek the advice of a health professional before using this product. Overuse of this product may produce increased redness of the eye. If solution changes color or becomes cloudy, do not use. To avoid contamination, do not touch tip of container to any surface. Replace cap after using. Remove contact lenses before using this product.
Parents Note: Before using with children under 6 years of age, consult your physician. Keep this and all drugs out of the reach of children. In case of accidental ingestion, seek professional assistance or contact a Poison Control Center immediately.
Caution: Should not be used if Visine-imprinted neckband on bottle is broken or missing.
Storage: Store between 15° and 30°C (59° and 86°F).
How Supplied: In 0.5 fl. oz. and 1.0 fl. oz. plastic dispenser bottle.

Shown in Product Identification Guide, page 107

VISINE A.C®
Seasonal Relief From Pollen & Dust Astringent/Redness Reliever Eye Drops

Description: Visine A.C. is a sterile, isotonic, buffered ophthalmic solution containing tetrahydrozoline hydrochloride 0.05% and zinc sulfate 0.25%. Visine A.C. is a fast-acting, dual-action ophthalmic solution combining the effects of the vasoconstrictor, tetrahydrozoline hydrochloride, with the astringent effects of zinc sulfate. The vasoconstrictor provides temporary relief of conjunctival edema, hyperemia and discomfort, while zinc sulfate helps to relieve itching and burning discomfort due to airborne irritants such as pollen, dust and ragweed.
Tetrahydrozoline hydrochloride is a sympathomimetic agent, which brings about decongestion by vasoconstriction. Reddened eyes are rapidly whitened by this effective vasoconstrictor which limits the local vascular response by constricting the small blood vessels. The onset of vasoconstriction becomes apparent within minutes. Zinc sulfate is an ocular astringent which, by precipitating protein, helps to clear mucus from the outer surface of the eye. The effectiveness of Visine A.C. in temporarily relieving conjunctival hyperemia and eye discomfort due to pollen, dust and ragweed has been clinically demonstrated. In one double-blind study of subjects who experienced acute episodes of minor eye irritation, Visine A.C. produced statistically significant beneficial results versus a placebo of normal saline solution in relieving irritation of bulbar conjunctivae, irritation of palpebral conjunctivae and mucus buildup. Treatment with Visine A.C. also significantly relieved eye discomfort.
Indications: For temporary relief of discomfort and redness due to minor eye irritations.
Directions: Instill 1 to 2 drops in the affected eye(s) up to 4 times daily.
Note: As drops go to work, some users may notice a brief tingling sensation which will quickly pass.
Active Ingredients: Zinc sulfate 0.25%; tetrahydrozoline hydrochloride 0.05%.
Inactive Ingredients: Benzalkonium chloride; boric acid; edetate disodium; purified water; sodium chloride; sodium citrate.
Warnings: If you experience eye pain, changes in vision, continued redness or irritation of the eye, or if the condition worsens or persists for more than 72 hours, discontinue use and consult a physician. If you have glaucoma, do not use this product except under the advice and supervision of a physician. As with any drug, if you are pregnant or nursing a baby, seek the advice of a health professional before using this product. Overuse of this product may produce increased redness of the eye. If solution changes color or becomes cloudy, do not use. To avoid contamination, do not touch tip of container to any surface. Replace cap after using. Remove contact lenses before using this product.
Parents Note: Before using with children under 6 years of age, consult your physician. Keep this and all drugs out of the reach of children. In case of accidental ingestion, seek professional assistance or contact a Poison Control Center immediately.
Caution: Should not be used if Visine-imprinted neckband on bottle is broken or missing.
Storage: Store between 15° and 30°C (59° and 86°F).
How Supplied: In 0.5 fl. oz. and 1.0 fl. oz. plastic dispenser bottle.

Shown in Product Identification Guide, page 107

VISINE L.R.® Long Lasting
Oxymetazoline Hydrochloride/ Redness Reliever Eye Drops

Description: Visine L.R. is a sterile, isotonic, buffered ophthalmic solution containing the vasoconstrictor, oxymetazoline hydrochloride. Visine L.R. is specially formulated to relieve redness of the eye in minutes with effective relief that lasts up to 6 hours.
Indications: Visine L.R. is a decongestant ophthalmic solution designed for the relief of redness of the eye due to minor eye irritations.
Directions: Adults and children 6 years of age or older: Place 1 or 2 drops in the affected eye(s). This may be repeated as needed every 6 hours or as directed by a physician.
Active Ingredients: Oxymetazoline hydrochloride 0.025%.
Inactive Ingredients: Sodium chloride; boric acid; sodium borate; with benzalkonium chloride 0.01% and edetate disodium 0.1% added as preservatives; purified water.
Warnings: If you experience eye pain, changes in vision, continued redness or irritation of the eye, or if the condition worsens or persists for more than 72 hours, discontinue use and consult a physician. If you have glaucoma, do not use this product except under the advice and supervision of a physician. As with any drug, if you are pregnant or nursing a baby, seek the advice of a health professional before using this product. Overuse of this product may produce increased redness of the eye. If solution changes color or becomes cloudy, do not use. To avoid contamination, do not touch tip of container to any surface. Replace cap after using. Remove contact lenses before using this product.
Parents: Before using with children under 6 years of age, consult your physician. Keep this and all drugs out of the reach of children. In case of accidental ingestion, seek professional assistance or contact a Poison Control Center immediately.
Caution: Should not be used if Visine-imprinted neckband on bottle is broken or missing.
Storage: Store between 15° and 30°C (59° and 86°F).
How Supplied: In 0.5 fl. oz. and 1 fl. oz. plastic dispenser bottle.

Shown in Product Identification Guide, page 107

VISINE® ORIGINAL
Tetrahydrozoline Hydrochloride/ Redness Reliever Eye Drops

Description: Visine is a sterile, isotonic, buffered ophthalmic solution containing tetrahydrozoline hydrochloride 0.05%. Visine is a decongestant ophthalmic solution designed to provide symptomatic relief of conjunctival edema and hyperemia secondary to minor irritations, due to conditions such as smoke, dust, other airborne pollutants and swimming. Relief is afforded by tetrahydrozoline hydrochloride, a sympathomimetic agent, which brings about decongestion by vasoconstriction. Reddened eyes are rapidly whitened by this effective vasoconstrictor, which limits the local vascular response by constricting the small blood vessels. The onset of vasoconstriction becomes apparent within minutes.
The effectiveness of Visine in relieving conjunctival hyperemia has been demonstrated by numerous clinicals, including several double-blind studies, involving more than 2,000 subjects suffering from acute or chronic hyperemia induced by a variety of conditions. Visine was found to be efficacious in providing relief from conjunctival hyperemia.
Indications: Relieves redness of the eye due to minor eye irritations.
Directions: Instill 1 to 2 drops in the affected eye(s) up to four times daily.
Active Ingredient: Tetrahydrozoline hydrochloride 0.05%.
Inactive Ingredients: Benzalkonium chloride; boric acid; edetate disodium; purified water; sodium borate; sodium chloride.
Warnings: If you experience eye pain, changes in vision, continued redness or irritation of the eye, or if the condition worsens or persists for more than 72 hours, discontinue use and consult a physician. If you have glaucoma, do not use this product except under the advice and supervision of a physician. As with any drug, if you are pregnant or nursing a baby, seek the advice of a health professional before using this product. Overuse of this product may produce increased redness of the eye. If solution changes color or becomes cloudy, do not use. To avoid contamination, do not touch tip of container to any surface. Replace cap after using. Remove contact lenses before using this product.
Parents Note: Before using with children under 6 years of age, consult your physician. Keep this and all drugs out of the reach of children. In case of accidental ingestion, seek professional assistance or contact a Poison Control Center immediately.
Caution: Should not be used if Visine-imprinted neckband on bottle is broken or missing.
Storage: Store between 15° and 30°C (59° and 86°F).
How Supplied: In 0.5 fl. oz., and 1.0 fl. oz. plastic dispenser bottle and 0.5 fl. oz. plastic bottle with dropper.

Shown in Product Identification Guide, page 107

VISINE® TEARS™
Lubricant Eye Drops OTC

Description:
Visine® Tears™ Lubricant Eye Drops

Visine Tears is specially formulated to cool and comfort dry, irritated eyes. It relieves the dryness caused by computer use, reading, wind, heat and air conditioning, while it protects your eyes from further irritation. Visine Tears is safe to use as often as needed.
Indications: For the temporary relief of burning and irritation due to dryness of the eye and for use as a protectant against further irritation.
Directions: Instill 1 to 2 drops in the affected eye(s) as needed.
Active Ingredients: Polyethylene glycol 400 1%; glycerin 0.2%; hydroxypropyl methylcellulose 0.2%.
Inactive Ingredients: Ascorbic acid; benzalkonium chloride; boric acid; dextrose; disodium phosphate; glycine; magnesium chloride; potassium chloride; purified water; sodium borate; sodium chloride; sodium citrate; sodium lactate.
Warnings: If you experience eye pain, changes in vision, continued redness or irritation of the eye, or if the condition worsens or persists for more than 72 hours, discontinue use and consult a physician.
As with any drug, if you are pregnant or nursing a baby, seek the advice of a health professional before using this product.
If solution changes color or becomes cloudy, do not use.
To avoid contamination, do not touch tip of container to any surface.
Replace cap after using.
Remove contact lenses before using this product.
Parent's note: Before using with children under 6 years of age, consult your physician.
Keep this and all drugs out of the reach of children.
In case of accidental ingestion, seek professional assistance or contact a Poison Control Center immediately.
Caution: Should not be used if Visine-imprinted neckband on bottle is broken or missing.
Storage: Store between 15° and 30°C (59° and 86°F).
How supplied: In 0.5 fl. oz. and 1 fl. oz. plastic dispenser bottle.

Shown in Product Identification Guide, page 107

VISINE® TEARS™ OTC

Preservative-Free, Single-Use Containers

Lubricant Eye Drops

Description:
Visine® Tears™ Preservative Free Lubricant Eye Drops
Visine Tears Preservative Free cools and comforts your dry, scratchy, irritated eyes, and helps them feel their best. It relieves the dryness caused by computer use, reading, wind, heat and air conditioning, while it actually protects your eyes from further irritation. Visine Tears Preservative Free is specially formulated for people whose eyes are sensitive to preservatives and is safe to use as often as needed. It is also sealed in convenient single-use containers.
Indications: For the temporary relief of burning and irritation due to dryness of the eye and for use as a protectant against further irritation.
Directions: Instill 1 to 2 drops in the affected eye(s) as needed.
How to use:
1. To open, completely twist off tab.
2. Instill 1 to 2 drops in the affected eye(s) as needed.
3. Once opened, discard.

Active Ingredients: Polyethylene glycol 400 1%; glycerin 0.2%; hydroxypropyl methylcellulose 0.2%.
Inactive Ingredients: Ascorbic acid; dextrose; disodium phosphate; glycine; magnesium chloride; potassium chloride; purified water; sodium chloride; sodium citrate; sodium lactate; sodium phosphate.
Warnings: If you experience eye pain, changes in vision, continued redness or irritation of the eye, or if the condition worsens or persists for more than 72 hours, discontinue use and consult a physician. As with any drug, if you are pregnant or nursing a baby, seek the advice of a health professional before using this product.
If solution changes color or becomes cloudy, do not use.
To avoid contamination, do not touch tip of container to any surface.
Do not reuse. Once opened, discard.
Remove contact lenses before using this product.
Parents note:
Before using with children under 6 years of age, consult your physician.
Keep this and all drugs out of the reach of children.
In case of accidental ingestion, seek professional assistance or contact a Poison Control Center immediately.
Caution: Use only if unit dose container is intact.
Storage: Store between 15° and 30° C (59° and 86° F).
How Supplied: 1 box contains 28 single-use containers, 0.01 fl. oz. (0.4 mL) each

Shown in Product Identification Guide, page 107

Pharmacia & Upjohn

**100 ROUTE 206 NORTH
PEAPACK, NEW JERSEY 07977**

For Medical and Pharmaceutical information, including emergencies
616-833-8244 or
Fax: 616-833-8414
For patient information
800-253-8600 ext. 3-6004, or
Fax: 616-833-4551.

HEALON® ℞
(sodium hyaluronate)

Description: Healon® is a sterile, nonpyrogenic, viscoelastic preparation of a highly purified, noninflammatory, high molecular weight fraction of sodium hyaluronate.
Healon® contains 10 mg/ml of sodium hyaluronate, dissolved in physiological sodium chloride phosphate buffer (pH 7.0–7.5). This high molecular weight polymer is made up of repeating disaccharide units of N-acetylglucosamine and sodium glucuronate linked by β 1–3 and β 1–4 glycosidic bonds.
Characteristics: Sodium hyaluronate is a physiological substance that is widely distributed in the extracellular matrix of connective tissues in both animals and man. For example, it is present in the vitreous and aqueous humor of the eye, the synovial fluid, the skin and the umbilical cord. Sodium hyaluronates prepared from various human and animal tissues are not chemically different from each other.
Healon® is a specific fraction of sodium hyaluronate developed as an ophthalmo-surgical aid for use in anterior segment and vitreous procedures. It is specific in that:
1. It has a high molecular weight;
2. It is reported to be nonantigenic[1,6];
3. It does not cause inflammatory[2] or foreign body reactions;
4. It has a high viscosity.

Furthermore, the 1% solution of Healon® is transparent, is reported to remain in the anterior chamber for less than 6 days[3] and protects corneal endothelial cells[4,5] and other ocular structures. Healon® does not interfere with epithelialization and normal wound healing.
Uses: Healon® is indicated for use as a surgical aid in cataract extraction (intra- and extracapsular), IOL implantation, corneal transplant, glaucoma filtration and retinal attachment surgery.
In surgical procedures in the anterior segment of the eye, instillation of Healon® serves to maintain a deep anterior chamber during surgery, allowing for efficient manipulation with less trauma to the corneal endothelium and other surrounding tissues.
Furthermore, its viscoelasticity helps to push back the vitreous face and prevent formation of a post-operative flat chamber.
In posterior segment surgery Healon® serves as a surgical aid to gently separate, maneuver and hold tissues. Healon® creates a clear field of vision thereby facilitating intra- and postoperative inspection of the retina and photocoagulation.
Contraindications: At present there are no known contraindications to the use of Healon® when used as recommended.
Precautions: Those normally associated with the surgical procedure being performed. Overfilling the anterior or posterior segment of the eye with Healon® may cause increased intraocular pressure, glaucoma, or other ocular damage.
Postoperative intraocular pressure may also be elevated as a result of pre-existing glaucoma, compromised outflow, and by operative procedures and sequelae thereto, including enzymatic zonulysis, absence of an iridectomy, trauma to filtration structures, and by blood and lenticular remnants in the anterior chamber. Since the exact role of these factors is difficult to predict in any individual case, the following precautions are recommended:

- Don't overfill the eye chambers with Healon® (except in glaucoma surgery—see Application section).
- In posterior segment procedures in aphakic diabetic patients special care should be exercised to avoid using large amounts of Healon®.
- Remove some of the Healon® by irrigation and/or aspiration at the close of surgery (except in glaucoma surgery—see Application section).
- Carefully monitor intraocular pressure, especially during the immediate postoperative period. If significant rises are observed, treat with appropriate therapy.

Care should be taken to avoid trapping air bubbles behind Healon®.
Because Healon® is a highly purified fraction extracted from avian tissues and is known to contain minute amounts of protein, the physician should be aware of potential risks of the type that can occur with the injection of any biological material.
Because of reports of an occasional release of minute rubber particles, presumably formed when the diaphragm is punctured, the physician should be aware of this potential problem. Express a small amount of Healon® from the syringe prior to use and carefully examine the remainder as it is injected.
Avoid reuse of cannulas. If reuse becomes necessary, rinse cannula thoroughly with sterile distilled water.
Sporadic reports have been received indicating that Healon® may become "cloudy" or form a slight precipitate following instillation into the eye. The clinical significance of these reports, if any, is not known since the majority received to date do not indicate any harmful effects on

Continued on next page

Healon—Cont.

ocular tissues. The physician should be aware of this phenomenon and, should it be observed, remove the cloudy or precipitated material by irrigation and/or aspiration.

In vitro laboratory studies suggest that this phenomenon may be related to interactions with certain concomitantly adminstered ophthalmic medications.

Use only if solution is clear.

Adverse Reactions: Healon® is extremely well tolerated after injection into human eyes. A transient rise of intraocular pressure postoperatively has been reported in some cases.

In posterior segment surgery intraocular pressure rises have been reported in some patients, especially in aphakic diabetics, after injection of large amount of Healon®.

Rarely, postoperative inflammatory reactions (iritis, hypopyon) as well as incidents of corneal edema and corneal decompensation have been reported. Their relationship to Healon® has not been established.

Applications

Cataract surgery—IOL implantation

A sufficient amount of Healon® is slowly, and carefully introduced (using a cannula or needle) into the anterior chamber.

Injection of Healon® can be performed either before or after delivery of the lens. Injection prior to lens delivery will, however, have the additional advantage of protecting the corneal endothelium from possible damage arising from the removal of the cataractous lens[5]. Healon® may also be used to coat surgical instruments and the IOL prior to insertion.

Additional Healon® can be injected during surgery to replace any Healon® lost during surgical manipulation (see Precautions section).

Glaucoma filtration surgery

In conjunction with performing of the trabeculectomy, Healon® is injected slowly and carefully through a corneal paracentesis to reconstitute the anterior chamber. Further injection of Healon® can be continued allowing it to extrude into the subconjunctival filtration site and through and around the sutured outer scleral flap.

Corneal transplant surgery

After removal of the corneal button, the anterior chamber is filled with Healon®. The donor graft can then be placed on top of the bed of Healon® and sutured in place. Additional Healon® may be injected to replace the Healon® lost as a result of surgical manipulation (see Precautions section). Healon® has also been used in the anterior chamber of the donor eye prior to trepanation to protect the corneal endothelial cells of the graft[5].

Retinal attachment surgery

Healon® is slowly introduced into the vitreous cavity. By directing the injection, Healon® can be used to separate membranes (e.g., epiretinal membranes) away from the retina for safe excision and release of traction. Healon® also serves to maneuver tissues into the desired position, e.g., to gently push back a detached retina or unroll a retinal flap, and aids in holding the retina against the sclera for reattachment.

How Supplied: Healon® is a sterile, nonpyrogenic, viscoelastic preparation supplied in disposable glass syringes, delivering 0.85 ml, 0.55 ml or 0.4 ml sodium hyaluronate (10 mg/ml) dissolved in physiological sodium chloride-phosphate buffer (pH 7.0–7.5). Each ml of Healon® contains 10 mg of sodium hyaluronate, 8.5 mg sodium chloride, 0.28 mg of disodium hydrogen phosphate dihydrate, 0.04 mg of sodium dihydrogen phosphate hydrate and q.s. water for injection U.S.P. Healon® syringes are terminally sterilized and aseptically packaged.

A sterile single-use 27 G cannula is enclosed in the 0.4 ml, 0.55 ml and 0.85 ml boxes.

Refrigerated Healon® should be allowed to attain room temperature (approximately 30 minutes) prior to use.

For intraocular use.

Store at 2–8°C.

Protect from freezing.

Protect from light.

Caution: Federal law restricts this device to sale by or on the order of a physician.

References:

1. *Richter, W., Ryde, M. & Zetterström*, O.: Nonimmunogenicity of a purified sodium hyaluronate preparation in man.Int Arch Appl Immun 59:45–48 (1979).
2. *Balazs, E. A.:* Ultrapure hyaluronic acid and the use thereof. U.S. Patent 4,141,973 (1979).
3. *Balazs, E. A., Miller, D. & Stegmann, R.:* Viscosurgery and the use of Na-hyaluronate in intraocular lens implantation.Lecture , Cannes, France (1979).
4. *Miller, D. & Stegmann, R.:* Use of Na-hyaluronate in anterior segment eye surgery. Am Intra-Ocular Implant Soc J 6 (1980b) p 13–15.
5. *Pape, L. G. & Balazs, E. A.:* The use of sodium hyaluronate (Healon®) in human anterior segment surgery.Ophthalmol 87 (1980) p 699–705.
6. Richter, W.: Non-immunogenicity of purified hyaluronic acid preparations tested by passive cutaneous anaphylaxis. Int Arch All 47 (1974) p211–217.

MANUFACTURED BY

Pharmacia & Upjohn Inc.
Uppsala, Sweden
For Pharmacia & Upjohn Inc.
7000 Portage Road
Kalamazoo MI, 49001
Revised: 6/96

Healon is covered by
U.S. patent 4,141,973, 1979

HEALON GV™ ℞

(sodium hyaluronate)

Product Information

Description: Healon GV is a sterile, nonpyrogenic, transparent viscoelastic preparation of a highly purified, noninflammatory, high molecular weight (average = 5 million daltons) fraction of sodium hyaluronate. Healon GV contains 14 mg/ml of sodium hyaluronate 7000, dissolved in a physiological sodium chloride-phosphate buffer (pH 7.0–7.5). This polymer consists of repeating disaccharide units of N-acetylglucosamine and sodium glucuronate linked by glycosidic bonds.

Sodium hyaluronate is a physiological substance that is widely distributed in the extracellular matrix of connective tissues in both animals and man. For example, it is present in the vitreous and aqueous humor of the eye, the synovial fluid, the skin and the umbilical cord. Sodium hyaluronate derived from various human or animal tissues do not differ chemically.

Indications: Healon GV is indicated for use in anterior segment ophthalmic surgical procedures.

Healon GV creates and maintains a deep anterior chamber, to facilitate manipulation inside the eye with reduced trauma to the corneal endothelium and other ocular tissues. Healon GV also can be used to efficiently maneuver, separate and control ocular tissues.

Contraindications: There are no known contraindications to the use of Healon GV when used as recommended.

Precautions: Precautions normally considered during ophthalmic surgical procedure should be taken.

Postoperative intraocular pressure may be increased if Healon GV is left in the eye. Due to the greater viscosity of Healon GV, this increase in postoperative IOP may be higher than that caused by leaving the same amount of other sodium hyaluronate viscoelastic products, with lower zero shear viscosity, in the anterior chamber. Since rises in postoperative intraocular pressure, including cases of significant elevation and subsequent complications, have been reported, the following precautions are strongly recommended.

—Special care should be taken to ensure as complete removal as possible by continuing to irrigate/aspirate after you see displacement of the initial bolus of viscoelastic from the eye; continued irrigation/aspiration should facilitate removal of viscoelastic which may remain in the anterior segment.

—Pre-existing glaucoma, other causes of compromised outflow, higher preoperative intraocular pressure and complications in surgical procedures also may lead to increased intraocular pressure; consequently, extra care should be taken in patients with these conditions.

—Carefully monitor intraocular pressure, particularly during the early postoperative period.

—Treat with appropriate intraocular pressure lowering therapy, if required.

Healon GV is a highly purified fraction extracted from avian tissues which may contain minute amounts of protein. The potential risks associated with the injection of biological material should be considered.

Express a small amount of Healon GV from the syringe prior to use and carefully examine it during use to avoid injecting minute rubber particles which may be released when the syringe diaphragm is punctured.

Sodium hyaluronate solution may appear cloudy or form precipitates when it is injected. Based on *in vitro* laboratory studies, this phenomenon may be related to interactions with concomitantly used ophthalmic medications or detergents which remain in reused cannulas. Avoid reuse of cannulas.

Adverse Events: Increased intraocular pressure has been reported after use of Healon GV:

—Increased intraocular pressure is likely to occur if Healon GV is not removed as completely as possible. Clinical judgment concerning the use of this product should be considered in cases where thorough removal may not be possible. The Precautions noted above should be taken to manage any increased postoperative intraocular pressure and to reduce the likelihood of occurence of related postoperative complications such as optic neuropathy, pupillary atonia and dilation, and iris atrophy.

Rarely, postoperative, inflammatory reactions (iritis, hypopyon, endophthalmitis) following the use of sodium hyaluronate, as well as incidents of corneal edema and corneal decompensation, have been reported. Their relationship to sodium hyaluronate has not been established.

How Supplied: Healon GV is a sterile, nonpyrogenic viscoelastic preparation supplied in disposable 0.85 ml and 0.55 ml glass syringes. Each ml of Healon GV contains:

14mg	sodium hyaluronate 7000
8.5mg	sodium chloride
0.28mg	disodium hydrogen phosphate dihydrate
0.04mg	sodium dihydrogen phosphate monohydrate
q.s.	water for injection USP

Healon GV syringes are terminally sterilized and aseptically packaged. A sterile single-use, 27 gauge cannula is included with each syringe.

Preparation and Storage

Refrigerated Healon GV should be held at room temperature for approximately 30 minutes before use. Protect from freezing and exposure to light.

For intraocular use.

Store between 2–8°C.

References:

1. Balazs, E.A.: Ultrapure hyaluronic acid and the use thereof. U.S. patent 4,141,973 (1979).
2. Fry L.L. & Yee R.W. (1993): Healon GV in extracapsular cataract extraction with intraocular lens implantation. Cataract Refract. Surg, 19:409–412.
3. Gaskel A. & Haining W. (1991): A double blind randomized multicentre clinical trial of "Healon GV," compared with "Healon" in ECCE with IOL implantation. Eur J. Implant Ref. Surg. 3:241.

Caution: Federal (US) law restricts this device to sale by or on the order of a physician.

Manufactured By:
Pharmacia AB
Sweden

Manufactured For:
Pharmacia & Upjohn Inc.
7000 Portage Road
Kalamazoo, MI 49001

U.S. patent 4,141,973, 1979.

 February 1994.

XALATAN® ℞
latanoprost
ophthalmic solution
0.005% (50 µg/mL)

DESCRIPTION

Latanoprost is a prostaglandin $F_{2\alpha}$ analogue. Its chemical name is isopropyl-(Z)-7[(1R,2R,3R,5S)3,5- dihydroxy-2-[(3R)-3- hydroxy- 5 -phenylpentyl] cyclopentyl]- 5 - heptenoate. Its molecular formula is $C_{26}H_{40}O_5$ and its chemical structure is:

M.W. 432.58

Latanoprost is a colorless to slightly yellow oil which is very soluble in acetonitrile and freely soluble in acetone, ethanol, ethyl acetate, isopropanol, methanol and octanol. It is practically insoluble in water.

XALATAN Sterile Ophthalmic Solution is supplied as a sterile, isotonic, buffered aqueous solution of latanoprost with a pH of approximately 6.7 and an osmolality of approximately 267 mOsmol/kg. Each mL of XALATAN contains 50 micrograms of latanoprost. Benzalkonium chloride, 0.02% is added as a preservative. The inactive ingredients are: sodium chloride, sodium dihydrogen phosphate monohydrate, disodium hydrogen phosphate anhydrous and water for injection. One drop contains approximately 1.5 µg of latanoprost.

CLINICAL PHARMACOLOGY

Mechanism of Action

Latanoprost is a prostanoid selective FP receptor agonist which is believed to reduce the intraocular pressure by increasing the outflow of aqueous humor. Studies in animals and man suggest that the main mechanism of action is increased uveoscleral outflow.

Pharmacokinetics/Pharmacodynamics

Absorption: Latanoprost is absorbed through the cornea where the isopropyl ester prodrug is hydrolyzed to the acid form to become biologically active. Studies in man indicate that the peak concentration in the aqueous humor is reached about two hours after topical administration.

Distribution: The distribution volume in humans is 0.16±0.02 L/kg. The acid of latanoprost could be measured in aqueous humor during the first 4 hours, and in plasma only during the first hour after local administration.

Metabolism: Latanoprost, an isopropyl ester prodrug, is hydrolyzed by esterases in the cornea to the biologically active acid. The active acid of latanoprost reaching the systemic circulation is primarily metabolized by the liver to the 1,2-dinor and 1,2,3,4-tetranor metabolites via fatty acid β-oxidation.

Excretion: The elimination of the acid of latanoprost from human plasma was rapid ($t_{1/2}$ =17 min) after both intravenous and topical administration. Systemic clearance is approximately 7 mL/min/kg. Following hepatic β-oxidation, the metabolites are mainly eliminated via the kidneys. Approximately 88% and 98% of the administered dose is recovered in the urine after topical and intravenous dosing, respectively.

Animal studies

In monkeys, latanoprost has been shown to induce increased pigmentation of the iris. The results from the preclinical program demonstrated that the increased pigmentation is unlikely to be associated with proliferation of melanocytes. It appears that the mechanism of increased pigmentation is stimulation of melanin production in melanocytes of the iris stroma.

In ocular toxicity studies, administration of latanoprost at a dose of 6 µg/eye/day (4 times the daily human dose) to cynomolgus monkeys has also been shown to induce increased palpebral fissure. This effect has been reversible and occurred at doses above the standard clinical dose level.

INDICATIONS AND USAGE

XALATAN Sterile Ophthalmic Solution is indicated for the reduction of elevated intraocular pressure in patients with open-angle glaucoma and ocular hypertension who are intolerant of other intraocular pressure lowering medications or insufficiently responsive (failed to achieve target IOP determined after multiple measurements over time) to another intraocular pressure lowering medication.

CLINICAL STUDIES

Patients with mean baseline intraocular pressure of 24–25 mmHg who were treated for 6 months in multicenter, randomized, controlled trials demonstrated 6–8 mmHg reductions in intraocular pressure. This IOP reduction with XALATAN Sterile Ophthalmic Solution 0.005% dosed once daily was equivalent to the effect of timolol 0.5% dosed twice daily.

CONTRAINDICATIONS

Known hypersensitivity to latanoprost, benzalkonium chloride or any other ingredients in this product.

WARNINGS

XALATAN has been reported to cause changes to pigmented tissues. The most frequently reported changes have been increased pigmentation of the iris and periorbital tissue (eyelid) and increased pigmentation and growth of eyelashes. These changes may be permanent.

XALATAN Sterile Ophthalmic Solution may gradually change eye color, increasing the amount of brown pigment in the iris by increasing the number of melanosomes (pigment granules) in melanocytes. The long-term effects on the melanocytes and the consequences of potential injury to the melanocytes and/or deposition of pigment granules to other areas of the eye are currently unknown. The change in iris color occurs slowly and may not be noticeable for several months to years. Patients should be informed of the possibility of iris color change.

Eyelid skin darkening has also been reported in association with the use of XALATAN.

XALATAN may gradually change eyelashes; these changes include increased length, thickness, pigmentation, and number of lashes.

Patients who are expected to receive treatment in only one eye should be informed about the potential for increased brown pigmentation of the iris, periorbital tissue, and eyelashes in the treated eye and thus, heterochromia between the eyes. They should also be advised of the potential for a disparity between the eyes in length, thickness, and/or number of eyelashes. These changes in pigmentation and lash growth may be permanent.

PRECAUTIONS

General: Latanoprost is hydrolyzed in the cornea. The effect of continued administration of XALATAN Sterile Ophthalmic Solution on the corneal endothelium has not been fully evaluated.

There have been reports of bacterial keratitis associated with the use of multiple-dose containers of topical ophthalmic products. These containers had been inadvertently contaminated by patients who, in most cases, had a concurrent corneal disease or a disruption of the ocular epithelial surface (see *Information for Patients*).

Patients may slowly develop increased brown pigmentation of the iris. This change may not be noticeable for several months to years (see **WARNINGS**). Typically the brown pigmentation around the pupil spreads concentrically towards the periphery in affected eyes, but the entire iris or parts of it may also become more brownish. Until more information about increased brown pigmentation is available, patients should be examined regularly and, depending on the clinical situation, treatment may be stopped if increased pigmentation ensues. During clinical trials, the increase in brown iris pigment has not been shown to progress further upon discontinuation of treatment, but the resultant color change may be permanent. Neither nevi nor freckles of the iris have been affected by treatment.

XALATAN should be used with caution in patients with active intraocular inflammation (iritis/uveitis).

Macular edema, including cystoid macular edema, has been reported during treatment with XALATAN. These reports have mainly occurred in aphakic patients, in pseudophakic patients with a torn posterior lens capsule, or in patients with known risk factors for macular edema. XALATAN should be used with caution in these patients.

There is limited experience with XALATAN in the treatment of angle closure, inflammatory or neovascular glaucoma.

XALATAN has not been studied in patients with renal or hepatic impairment and should therefore be used with caution in such patients.

XALATAN should not be administered while wearing contact lenses.

Information for Patients (see **WARNINGS**): Patients should be informed about the possibility of iris color change due to an increase of the brown pigment and resultant cosmetically different eye coloration that may occur when only one eye is treated. Iris pigmentation changes may be more noticeable in patients with green-brown, blue/gray-brown or yellow-brown irides.

Continued on next page

Xalatan—Cont.

Patients should also be informed of the possibility of eyelash changes in the treated eye, which may result in a disparity between eyes in lash length, thickness, pigmentation, and/or number.

Patients should also be informed about the possibility of eyelid skin darkening.

The increased pigmentation to the iris and eyelid, as well as the changes to the eyelashes, may be permanent.

Patients should be instructed to avoid allowing the tip of the dispensing container to contact the eye or surrounding structures because this could cause the tip to become contaminated by common bacteria known to cause ocular infections. Serious damage to the eye and subsequent loss of vision may result from using contaminated solutions.

Patients also should be advised that if they develop an intercurrent ocular condition (e.g., trauma, or infection) or have ocular surgery, they should immediately seek their physician's advice concerning the continued use of the multidose container.

Patients should be advised that if they develop any ocular reactions, particularly conjunctivitis and lid reactions, they should immediately seek their physician's advice.

Patients should also be advised that XALATAN contains benzalkonium chloride which may be absorbed by contact lenses. Contact lenses should be removed prior to administration of the solution. Lenses may be reinserted 15 minutes following administration of XALATAN.

If more than one topical ophthalmic drug is being used, the drugs should be administered at least five (5) minutes apart.

Drug Interactions: In vitro studies have shown that precipitation occurs when eye drops containing thimerosal are mixed with XALATAN. If such drugs are used they should be administered with an interval of at least five (5) minutes between applications.

Carcinogenesis, Mutagenesis, Impairment of Fertility:

Latanoprost was not mutagenic in bacteria, in mouse lymphoma or in mouse micronucleus tests.

Chromosome aberrations were observed *in vitro* with human lymphocytes.

Latanoprost was not carcinogenic in either mice or rats when administered by oral gavage at doses of up to 170 µg/kg/day (approximately 2,800 times the recommended maximum human dose) for up to 20 and 24 months, respectively.

Additional *in vitro* and *in vivo* studies on unscheduled DNA synthesis in rats were negative. Latanoprost has not been found to have any effect on male or female fertility in animal studies.

Pregnancy: Teratogenic Effects: Pregnancy Category C.

Reproduction studies have been performed in rats and rabbits. In rabbits an incidence of 4 of 16 dams had no viable fetuses at a dose that was approximately 80 times the maximum human dose, and the highest nonembryocidal dose in rabbits was approximately 15 times the maximum human dose. There are no adequate and well-controlled studies in pregnant women. XALATAN should be used during pregnancy only if the potential benefit justifies the potential risk to the fetus.

Nursing Mothers: It is not known whether this drug or its metabolites are excreted in human milk. Because many drugs are excreted in human milk, caution should be exercised when XALATAN is administered to a nursing woman.

Pediatric Use: Safety and effectiveness in pediatric patients have not been established.

ADVERSE REACTIONS

Adverse events referred to in other sections of this insert:

Eyelash changes (increased length, thickness, pigmentation, and number of lashes); eyelid skin darkening; intraocular inflammation (iritis/uveitis); iris pigmentation changes; and macular edema, including cystoid macular edema (see **WARNINGS** and **PRECAUTIONS**).

Controlled Clinical Trials:

The ocular adverse events and ocular signs and symptoms reported in 5 to 15% of the patients on XALATAN Sterile Ophthalmic Solution in the 6-month, multi-center, double-masked, active-controlled trials were blurred vision, burning and stinging, conjunctival hyperemia, foreign body sensation, itching, increased pigmentation of the iris, and punctate epithelial keratopathy.

Local conjunctival hyperemia was observed; however, less than 1% of the patients treated with XALATAN required discontinuation of therapy because of intolerance to conjunctival hyperemia.

In addition to the above listed ocular events/signs and symptoms, the following were reported in 1 to 4% of the patients: dry eye, excessive tearing, eye pain, lid crusting, lid discomfort/pain, lid edema, lid erythema, and photophobia.

The following events were reported in less than 1% of the patients: conjunctivitis, diplopia and discharge from the eye.

During clinical studies, there were extremely rare reports of the following: retinal artery embolus, retinal detachment, and vitreous hemorrhage from diabetic retinopathy.

The most common systemic adverse events seen with XALATAN were upper respiratory tract infection/cold/flu which occurred at a rate of approximately 4%. Chest pain/angina pectoris, muscle/joint/back pain, and rash/allergic skin reaction each occurred at a rate of 1 to 2%.

Clinical Practice: The following events have been identified during postmarketing use of XALATAN in clinical practice. Because they are reported voluntarily from a population of unknown size, estimates of frequency cannot be made. The events, which have been chosen for inclusion due to either their seriousness, frequency of reporting, possible causal connection to XALATAN, or a combination of these factors, include: eyelash changes (increased length, thickness, pigmentation, and number of lashes); eyelid skin darkening; intraocular inflammation (iritis/uveitis); macular edema, including cystoid macular edema; toxic epidermal necrolysis; asthma; exacerbation of asthma; and dyspnea.

OVERDOSAGE

Apart from ocular irritation and conjunctival or episcleral hyperemia, the ocular effects of latanoprost administered at high doses are not known. Intravenous administration of large doses of latanoprost in monkeys has been associated with transient bronchoconstriction; however, in 11 patients with bronchial asthma treated with latanoprost, bronchoconstriction was not induced. Intravenous infusion of up to 3 µg/kg in healthy volunteers produced mean plasma concentrations 200 times higher than during clinical treatment and no adverse reactions were observed. Intravenous dosages of 5.5 to 10 µg/kg caused abdominal pain, dizziness, fatigue, hot flushes, nausea and sweating.

If overdosage with XALATAN Sterile Ophthalmic Solution occurs, treatment should be symptomatic.

DOSAGE AND ADMINISTRATION

The recommended dosage is one drop (1.5 µg) in the affected eye(s) once daily in the evening.

The dosage of XALATAN Sterile Ophthalmic Solution should not exceed once daily since it has been shown that more frequent administration may decrease the intraocular pressure lowering effect.

Reduction of the intraocular pressure starts approximately 3 to 4 hours after administration and the maximum effect is reached after 8 to 12 hours.

XALATAN may be used concomitantly with other topical ophthalmic drug products to lower intraocular pressure. If more than one topical ophthalmic drug is being used, the drugs should be administered at least five (5) minutes apart.

HOW SUPPLIED

XALATAN Sterile Ophthalmic Solution is a clear, isotonic, buffered, preserved colorless solution of latanoprost 0.005% (50 µg/mL) supplied in plastic ophthalmic dispenser bottles with a dropper tip and tamper evident overcap.

NDC 0013-8303-04

2.5 mL fill, 0.005% (50 µg/mL), in cartons of 1 & 6.

Storage: Protect from light. Store unopened bottle under refrigeration at 2° to 8°C (36° to 46°F).

Once opened the 2.5 mL container may be stored at room temperature up to 25°C (77°F) for 6 weeks.

℞ only

U.S. Patent Nos. 4,599,353; 5,296,504 and 5,422,368.

Manufactured for:
Pharmacia & Upjohn Company
Kalamazoo, MI 49001, USA
By:
Automatic Liquid Packaging, Inc.
Woodstock, IL 60098, USA
Revised April 1999 124000499

Shown in Product Identification Guide, page 107

Ross Products Division Abbott Laboratories Inc.

COLUMBUS, OHIO 43215-1724

CLEAR EYES® OTC

[*klēr īz*]

Lubricant Eye Redness Reliever Drops

Description: Clear Eyes is a sterile, isotonic buffered solution containing the active ingredients naphazoline hydrochloride (0.012%) and glycerin (0.2%). It also contains boric acid, purified water and sodium borate. Edetate disodium and benzalkonium chloride are added as preservatives. Clear Eyes is a lubricant, decongestant ophthalmic solution specially designed for temporary relief of redness and drying due to minor eye irritation caused by smoke, smog, sun glare or swimming. Clear Eyes contains laboratory-tested and scientifically blended ingredients, including an effective vasoconstrictor which narrows swollen blood vessels and rapidly whitens reddened eyes in a formulation which also contains a lubricant and produces a refreshing, soothing effect. Clear Eyes is a sterile, isotonic solution compatible with the natural fluids of the eye.

Indications: For the temporary relief of redness due to minor eye irritation AND for protection against further irritation or dryness of the eye.

Warnings: To avoid contamination, do not touch tip of container to any surface. Replace cap after using. If you experience eye pain, changes in vision, continued redness or irritation of the eye, or if the condition worsens or persists for more than 72 hours, discontinue use and consult a doctor. If you have glaucoma,

do not use this product except under the advice and supervision of a doctor. Overuse of this product may produce increased redness of the eye. If solution changes color or becomes cloudy, do not use. Keep this and all drugs out of the reach of children. In case of accidental ingestion, seek professional assistance or contact a Poison Control Center immediately.
Dosage and Administration: Instill 1 or 2 drops in the affected eye(s) up to four times daily.
How Supplied: In 0.5-fl-oz (15 mL) and 1.0-fl-oz (30 mL) plastic dropper bottles.
(FAN 3379)

CLEAR EYES® ACR OTC
[*klēr īz*]
Astringent/Lubricant Redness Reliever Eye Drops

Description: Clear Eyes ACR is a sterile, isotonic buffered solution containing the active ingredients naphazoline hydrochloride (0.012%), zinc sulfate (0.25%) and glycerin (0.2%). It also contains boric acid, purified water, sodium chloride and sodium citrate. Edetate disodium and benzalkonium chloride are added as preservatives. Clear Eyes® ACR has three active ingredients: (1) astringent, that acts by helping clear mucus from the outer surface of the eye, (2) vasoconstrictor, that acts by removing redness, and (3) demulcent, that acts by protecting and moisturizing dry irritated eyes. Clear Eyes ACR contains laboratory-tested and scientifically blended ingredients, including an effective vasoconstrictor which narrows swollen blood vessels and rapidly whitens reddened eyes in a formulation which also contains a lubricant and produces a soothing effect. Clear Eyes ACR also contains an ocular astringent (zinc sulfate) that precipitates the sticky mucus buildup on the eye often associated with exposure to pollen, dust and smoke, which helps clear the mucus from the outer surface of the eye. Clear Eyes ACR is a sterile, isotonic solution compatible with the natural fluids of the eye.
Indications: For the temporary relief of redness and discomfort due to minor eye irritation, for protection against further eye irritation, and for temporary relief of burning and irritation due to dryness of the eye.
Warnings: To avoid contamination, do not touch tip of container to any surface. Replace cap after using. If you experience eye pain, changes in vision, contained redness or irritation of the eye, or if the condition worsens or persists for more than 72 hours, discontinue use and consult a doctor. If you have glaucoma, do not use this product expect under the advice and supervision of a doctor. Overuse of this product may produce increased redness of the eye. If solution changes color or becomes cloudy, do not use. Keep this and all drugs out of the reach of children. In case of accidental ingestion, seek professional assistance or contact a Poison Control Center immediately.
Dosage and Administration: Instill 1 or 2 drops in the affected eye(s) up to four times daily.
How Supplied: In 0.5-fl-oz (15 mL) and 1.0-fl-oz (30 mL) plastic dropper bottles.
(FAN 3618)

CLEAR EYES® CLR OTC
[*klēr īz*]
SOOTHING DROPS
Contact Lens Relief

Description: CLEAR EYES CLR Soothing Drops is a sterile, isotonic solution with a borate buffer system, sodium chloride, hydroxypropyl methylcellulose and glycerin, with sorbic acid (0.25%) and edetate disodium (0.1%) as the preservatives.
Indications(Uses): CLEAR EYES CLR Soothing Drops may be used with daily and extended wear soft (hydrophilic) contact lenses for the following:

- Moistening of daily wear soft lenses while on the eyes during the day.
- Moistening of extended wear soft lenses upon awakening and as needed during the day.
- Moistening of extended wear soft lenses prior to retiring at night.

Placing 1 or 2 drops of CLEAR EYES CLR Soothing Drops on the eye followed by blinking 2 or 3 times will relieve minor irritation, discomfort and blurring which may occur while wearing lenses.
Contraindications(Reasons Not To Use): Patients allergic to any ingredient including sorbic acid (preservative) in CLEAR EYES CLR Soothing Drops should not use this product.
Warnings:

- PROBLEMS WITH CONTACT LENSES AND LENS CARE PRODUCTS COULD RESULT IN SERIOUS INJURY TO THE EYE. It is essential that you follow your eye care professional's direction and all labeling instructions for proper use of your lenses and lens care products. EYE PROBLEMS, INCLUDING CORNEAL ULCERS, CAN DEVELOP RAPIDLY AND LEAD TO LOSS OF VISION; THEREFORE, IF YOU EXPERIENCE EYE DISCOMFORT, EXCESSIVE TEARING, VISION CHANGES, REDNESS OF THE EYE, IMMEDIATELY REMOVE YOUR LENSES AND PROMPTLY CONTACT YOUR EYE CARE PROFESSIONAL.

All contact lens wearers must see their eye care professional as directed. If your lenses are for extended wear, your eye care professional may prescribe more frequent visits.

- Never touch the dropper tip of the container to any surface, since this may contaminate the solution. If drops turn yellow, discard and use fresh (colorless) drops.
- Replace cap after every use.

Precautions:

- Always wash and rinse your hands before handling your lenses.
- Store at room temperature.
- Keep container tightly closed when not in use.
- Use before the expiration date marked on the containers and cartons.
- Keep this and all medications out of the reach of children.

Adverse Reactions(Problems and What To Do): The following problems may occur while wearing contact lenses:

- Eyes stinging, burning or itching (irritation)
- Excessive watering (tearing) of the eyes
- Unusual eye secretions
- Redness of the eyes
- Reduced sharpness of vision (visual acuity)
- Blurred vision
- Sensitivity to light (photophobia)
- Dry eyes

If you notice any of the above problems, immediately remove and examine your lenses.
If the problem stops and the lenses appear to be undamaged, thoroughly clean, rinse and disinfect the lenses and reinsert them. If the problem continues or a lens appears to be damaged, IMMEDIATELY remove your lenses and IMMEDIATELY consult your eye care professional. **Do not reinsert a damaged lens.**
If any of the above symptoms occur, a serious condition such as infection, corneal ulcer, neovascularization or iritis may be present. Seek immediate professional identification of the problem and treatment to avoid serious eye damage.
Transient contact urticaria (red wheals or streaks on the skin) may occur from use of this product.
Directions: CLEAR EYES CLR Soothing Drops may be used as needed throughout the day. If minor irritation, discomfort or blurring occur while wearing lenses, place 1 or 2 drops on the eye and blink 2 or 3 times. If discomfort continues, immediately remove lenses and immediately see your eye care professional.
How Supplied: CLEAR EYES CLR Soothing Drops are supplied in sterile 0.5 fl oz (15 mL) and 1.0 fl oz (30 mL) plastic bottles. The containers and cartons are marked with lot number and expiration date.
(FAN 3486)

MURINE TEARS® OTC
[*mur 'ēn*]
Lubricant Eye Drops

Description: Murine Tears eye lubricant is a sterile buffered solution containing the active ingredients 0.5% polyvinyl alcohol and 0.6% povidone. Also contains benzalkonium chloride, dextrose, disodium edetate, potassium chloride, purified water, sodium bicarbonate, sodium chloride, sodium citrate and sodium phosphate (mono- and dibasic). Murine Tears is a sterile, hypotonic solution formulated to more closely match the natural fluid of the eye for gentle, soothing relief from minor eye irritation while moisturizing and relieving dryness. Use as desired to temporarily relieve minor eye irritation, dryness and burning.
Indications: For the temporary relief or prevention of further discomfort due to minor eye irritations and symptoms related to dry eyes.
Warnings: To avoid contamination, do not touch tip of container to any surface. Replace cap after using. If you experience eye pain, changes in vision, continued redness or irritation of the eye, or if the condition worsens or persists for more than 72 hours, discontinue use and consult a doctor. If solution changes color or becomes cloudy, do not use. Keep this and all drugs out of the reach of children. In case of accidental ingestion, seek professional assistance or contact a Poison Control Center immediately.
Dosage and Administration: Instill 1 or 2 drops in the affected eye(s) as needed.
How Supplied: In 0.5-fl-oz (15 mL) and 1.0-fl-oz (30 mL) plastic dropper bottles.
(FAN 3379)

MURINE TEARS® PLUS OTC
[*mur 'ēn*]
Lubricant Redness Reliever Eye Drops

Description: Murine Tears Plus is a sterile, non-staining buffered solution containing the active ingredients 0.5% polyvinyl alcohol, 0.6% povidone and 0.05% tetrahydrozoline hydrochloride. Also contains benzalkonium chloride, dextrose, disodium edetate, potassium chloride, purified water, sodium bicarbonate, sodium chloride, sodium citrate and sodium phosphate (mono- and dibasic). Murine Tears Plus is a sterile, hypotonic, ophthalmic solution formulated to more closely match the natural fluid of the eye. It contains demulcents for

Continued on next page

Murine Tears Plus—Cont.

gentle, soothing relief from minor eye irritation as well as the sympathomimetic agent, tetrahydrozoline hydrochloride, which produces local vasoconstriction in the eye. Thus, the drug effectively narrows swollen blood vessels locally and provides symptomatic relief of edema and hyperemia of conjunctival tissues due to eye allergies, minor local irritations and conjunctivitis. Use up to four times daily, to remove redness due to minor eye irritation. The effect of Murine Tears Plus is prompt (apparent within minutes) and sustained.
Indications: For the temporary relief or prevention of further discomfort due to minor eye irritations and symptoms related to dry eyes PLUS removal of redness.
Warnings: To avoid contamination, do not touch tip of container to any surface. Replace cap after using. If you experience eye pain, changes in vision, continued redness or irritation of the eye, or if the condition worsens or persists for more than 72 hours, discontinue use and consult a doctor. If you have glaucoma, do not use this product except under the advice and supervision of a doctor. Overuse of this product may produce increased redness of the eye. If solution changes color or becomes cloudy, do not use. Keep this and all drugs out of the reach of children. In case of accidental ingestion, seek professional assistance or contact a Poison Control Center immediately.
Dosage and Administration: Instill 1 or 2 drops in the affected eye(s) **up to four times daily.**
How Supplied: In 0.5-fl-oz (15 mL) and 1.0-fl-oz (30 mL) plastic dropper bottles.
(FAN 3379)

Vision Pharmaceuticals, Inc.

1022 N. MAIN STREET
MITCHELL, SD 57301
www.visionpharm.com

VIVA-DROPS® OTC
Lubricant Eye Drops

Description: VIVA-DROPS® is a preservative-free, non-oily, sterile ophthalmic lubricant for relief from irritation due to dryness of the eye or discomfort caused by exposure to wind, sun or dry air. The patented formulation of VIVA-DROPS® includes antioxidants that protect the active ingredient from autooxidation.
Contains: **Active**: polysorbate 80.
Inactives: purified water, sodium chloride, citric acid, edetate disodium, with retinyl palmitate, mannitol, sodium citrate, and pyruvate as antioxidants.

FDA APPROVED USES

Indications: FOR USE AS A LUBRICANT TO PREVENT FURTHER IRRITATION OR TO RELIEVE DRYNESS OF THE EYE.

Warnings: If you experience eye pain, changes in vision, continued redness or irritation of the eye, or if the condition persists for more than 72 hours, discontinue use and consult a doctor. If solution changes color or becomes cloudy, do not use. Keep this and all drugs out of the reach of children.
Directions: Instill 1 or 2 drops in the affected eye(s) as needed.
How Supplied: In 10mL (NDC 54891-001-02) and 15mL (NDC 54891-001-01) bottles.
Store at room temperature.
U.S. Patent No. 5,032,392

Wyeth-Ayerst Pharmaceuticals

Division of American Home Products
P.O. BOX 8299
PHILADELPHIA, PA 19101

PHOSPHOLINE IODIDE® ℞
[fos "fo 'lĭn i "o-dīd]
(echothiophate iodide for ophthalmic solution)

Caution: Federal law prohibits dispensing without prescription.
Description: Chemical name: (2-mercaptoethyl) trimethylammonium iodide O,O-diethyl phosphorothioate.
Phospholine Iodide occurs as a white, crystalline, water-soluble, hygroscopic solid having a slight mercaptan-like odor. When freeze-dried in the presence of potassium acetate, the mixture appears as a white amorphous deposit on the walls of the bottle.
Each package contains materials for dispensing 5 mL of eyedrops: (1) bottle containing sterile Phospholine Iodide in one of four potencies [1.5 mg (0.03%), 3 mg (0.06%), 6.25 mg (0.125%), or 12.5 mg (0.25%)] as indicated on the label, with 40 mg potassium acetate in each case. Sodium hydroxide or acetic acid may have been incorporated to adjust pH during manufacturing. (2) a 5 mL bottle of sterile diluent containing chlorobutanol (chloral derivative), 0.55%; mannitol, 1.2%; boric acid, 0.06%; and exsiccated sodium phosphate, 0.026%. (3) sterilized dropper.
Clinical Pharmacology: Phospholine Iodide is a long-acting cholinesterase inhibitor for topical use which enhances the effect of endogenously liberated acetylcholine in iris, ciliary muscle, and other parasympathetically innervated structures of the eye. It thereby causes miosis, increase in facility of outflow of aqueous humor, fall in intraocular pressure, and potentiation of accommodation.
Phospholine Iodide (echothiophate iodide) will depress both plasma and erythrocyte cholinesterase levels in most patients after a few weeks of eyedrop therapy.
Indications and Usage:
Glaucoma
Chronic open-angle glaucoma. Subacute or chronic angle-closure glaucoma after iridectomy or where surgery is refused or contraindicated. Certain non-uveitic secondary types of glaucoma, especially glaucoma following cataract surgery.
Accommodative Esotropia
Concomitant esotropias with a significant accommodative component.
Contraindications:

1. Active uveal inflammation.
2. Most cases of angle-closure glaucoma, due to the possibility of increasing angle block.
3. Hypersensitivity to the active or inactive ingredients.

Warnings:

1. Succinylcholine should be administered only with great caution, if at all, prior to or during general anesthesia to patients receiving anticholinesterase medication because of possible respiratory or cardiovascular collapse.
2. Caution should be observed in treating glaucoma with Phospholine Iodide (echothiophate iodide) in patients who are at the same time undergoing treatment with systemic anticholinesterase medications for myasthenia gravis, because of possible adverse additive effects.

(See **"Precautions**—Drug Interactions" for further information.)

Precautions:
General

1. Gonioscopy is recommended prior to initiation of therapy. Routine examination to detect lens opacity should accompany clinical use of Phospholine Iodide.
2. Where there is a quiescent uveitis or a history of this condition, anticholinesterase therapy should be avoided or used cautiously because of the intense and persistent miosis and ciliary muscle contraction that may occur.
3. While systemic effects are infrequent, proper use of the drug requires digital compression of the nasolacrimal ducts for a minute or two following instillation to minimize drainage into the nasal chamber with its extensive absorption area. To prevent possible skin absorption, hands should be washed following instillation.
4. Temporary discontinuance of medication is necessary if cardiac irregularities occur.
5. Anticholinesterase drugs should be used with extreme caution, if at all, in patients with marked vagotonia, bronchial asthma, spastic gastrointestinal disturbances, peptic ulcer, pronounced bradycardia and hypotension, recent myocardial infarction, epilepsy, parkinsonism, and other disorders that may respond adversely to vagotonic effects.
6. Anticholinesterase drugs should be employed prior to ophthalmic surgery only as a considered risk because of the possible occurrence of hyphema.
7. Phospholine Iodide (echothiophate iodide) should be used with great caution, if at all, where there is a prior history of retinal detachment.
8. Temporary discontinuance of medication is necessary if salivation, urinary incontinence, diarrhea, profuse sweating, muscle weakness, or respiratory difficulties occur.
9. Patients receiving Phospholine Iodide who are exposed to carbamate- or organophosphate-type insecticides and pesticides (professional gardeners, farmers, workers in plants manufacturing or formulating such products, etc.) should be warned of the additive systemic effects possible from absorption of the pesticide through the respiratory tract or skin. During periods of exposure to such pesticides, the wearing of respiratory masks, and frequent washing and clothing changes may be advisable.

Drug Interactions
Phospholine Iodide potentiates other cholinesterase inhibitors such as succinylcholine or organophosphate and carbamate insecticides. Patients undergoing systemic anticholinesterase treatment should be warned of the possible additive effects of Phospholine Iodide.
Carcinogenesis, Mutagenesis, Impairment of Fertility
No data is available regarding carcinogenesis, mutagenesis, and impairment of fertility.
Pregnancy:
Teratogenic Effects—Pregnancy Category C: Animal reproduction studies have not been conducted with Phospholine Iodide. It is also not known whether Phospholine Iodide can cause fetal harm when administered to a pregnant woman or can affect reproduction capacity. Phospholine Iodide (echothiophate iodide) should be given to a pregnant woman only if clearly needed.
Nursing Mothers
Because of the potential for serious adverse reactions in nursing infants from Phospholine Iodide, a decision should be made whether to discontinue nursing or to discontinue the drug, taking into account the importance of the drug to the mother.

Adverse Reactions:
1. Although the relationship, if any, of retinal detachment to the administration of Phospholine Iodide has not been established, retinal detachment has been reported in a few cases during the use of Phospholine Iodide in adult patients without a previous history of this disorder.
2. Stinging, burning, lacrimation, lid muscle twitching, conjunctival and ciliary redness, browache, induced myopia with visual blurring may occur.
3. Activation of latent iritis or uveitis may occur.
4. Iris cysts may form, and if treatment is continued, may enlarge and obscure vision. This occurrence is more frequent in children. The cysts usually shrink upon discontinuance of the medication, reduction in strength of the drops or frequency of instillation. Rarely, they may rupture or break free into the aqueous. Regular examinations are advisable when the drug is being prescribed for the treatment of accommodative esotropia.
5. Prolonged use may cause conjunctival thickening, obstruction of nasolacrimal canals.
6. Lens opacities occurring in patients under treatment for glaucoma with Phospholine Iodide have been reported and similar changes have been produced experimentally in normal monkeys. Routine examinations should accompany clinical use of the drug.
7. Paradoxical increase in intraocular pressure may follow anticholinesterase instillation. This may be alleviated by prescribing a sympathomimetic mydriatic such as phenylephrine.
8. Cardiac irregularities.

Dosage and Administration:

Directions for Preparing Eyedrops
1. Use aseptic technique.
2. Tear off aluminum seals, and remove and discard rubber plugs from both drug and diluent containers.
3. Pour diluent into drug container.
4. Remove dropper assembly from its sterile wrapping. Holding dropper assembly by the screw cap and, WITHOUT COMPRESSING RUBBER BULB, insert into drug container and screw down tightly.
5. Shake for several seconds to ensure mixing.
6. Do not cover nor obliterate instructions to patient regarding storage of eyedrops.

Glaucoma

Selection of Therapy

The *medication prescribed* should be that which will control the intraocular pressure around-the-clock with the least risk of side effects or adverse reactions. "Tonometric glaucoma" (ocular hypertension without other evidence of the disease) is frequently not treated with any medication, and Phospholine Iodide (echothiophate iodide) is certainly not recommended for this condition. In early chronic simple glaucoma with field loss or disc changes, pilocarpine is generally used for initial therapy and can be recommended so long as control is thereby maintained over the 24 hours of the day.

When this is not the case, Phospholine Iodide 0.03% may be effective and probably has no greater potential for side effects. If this dosage is inadequate, epinephrine and a carbonic anhydrase inhibitor may be added to the regimen. When still more effective medication is required, the higher strengths of Phospholine Iodide may be prescribed with the recognition that the control of the intraocular pressure should have priority regardless of potential side effects. In secondary glaucoma following cataract surgery, the higher strengths of the drug are frequently needed and are ordinarily very well tolerated.

The *dosage regimen* prescribed should call for the lowest concentration that will control the intraocular pressure around-the-clock. Where tonometry around-the-clock is not feasible, it is suggested that appointments for tension-taking be made at different times of the day so that inadequate control may be more readily detected. Two doses a day are preferred to one in order to maintain as smooth a diurnal tension curve as possible, although a single dose per day or every other day has been used with satisfactory results. Because of the long duration of action of the drug, it is never necessary or desirable to exceed a schedule of twice a day. The daily dose or one of the two daily doses should always be instilled just before retiring to avoid inconvenience due to the miosis.

Early Chronic Simple Glaucoma

Phospholine Iodide (echothiophate iodide) 0.03% instilled twice a day, just before retiring and in the morning, may be prescribed advantageously for cases of early chronic simple glaucoma that are not controlled around-the-clock with other less potent agents. Because of prolonged action, control during the night and early morning hours may then sometimes be obtained. A change in therapy is indicated if, at any time, the tension fails to remain at an acceptable level on this regimen.

Advanced Chronic Simple Glaucoma and Glaucoma Secondary to Cataract Surgery

These cases may respond satisfactorily to Phospholine Iodide 0.03% twice a day as above. When the patient is being transferred to Phospholine Iodide (echothiophate iodide) because of unsatisfactory control with pilocarpine, carbachol, epinephrine, etc., one of the higher strengths, 0.06%, 0.125%, or 0.25% will usually be needed. In this case, a brief trial with the 0.03% eyedrops will be advantageous in that the higher strengths will then be more easily tolerated.

Concomitant Therapy

Phospholine Iodide may be used concomitantly with epinephrine, a carbonic anhydrase inhibitor, or both.

Technique

Good technique in the administration of Phospholine Iodide requires that finger pressure at the inner canthus should be exerted for a minute or two following instillation of the eyedrops, to minimize drainage into the nose and throat. Excess solution around the eye should be removed with tissue and any medication on the hands should be rinsed off.

Accommodative Esotropia (Pediatric Use)

In Diagnosis

One drop of 0.125% may be instilled once a day in both eyes on retiring, for a period of two or three weeks. If the esotropia is accommodative, a favorable response will usually be noted which may begin within a few hours.

In Treatment

Phospholine Iodide (echothiophate iodide) is prescribed at the lowest concentration and frequency which gives satisfactory results. After the initial period of treatment for diagnostic purposes, the schedule may be reduced to 0.125% every other day or 0.06% every day. These dosages can often be gradually lowered as treatment progresses. The 0.03% strength has proven to be effective in some cases. The maximum usually recommended dosage is 0.125% once a day, although more intensive therapy has been used for short periods.

Technique

(See **"Dosage and Administration—**Glaucoma.")

Duration of Treatment

In diagnosis, only a short period is required and little time will be lost in instituting other procedures if the esotropia proves to be unresponsive. In therapy, there is no definite limit so long as the drug is well tolerated. However, if the eyedrops, with or without eyeglasses, are gradually withdrawn after about a year or two and deviation recurs, surgery should be considered. As with other miotics, tolerance may occasionally develop after prolonged use. In such cases, a rest period will restore the original activity of the drug.

How Supplied: Each package contains sterile Phospholine Iodide (echothiophate iodide), sterile diluent, and dropper for dispensing 5 mL eyedrops of the strength indicated on the label. Four potencies are available:

NDC 0046-1062-05 .... 1.5 mg package for 0.03%
White amorphous deposit on bottle walls.
Aluminum crimp seal is blue.
NDC 0046-1064-05 ... 3 mg package for 0.06%
White amorphous deposit on bottle walls.
Aluminum crimp seal is red.
NDC 0046-1065-05 .... 6.25 mg package for 0.125%
White amorphous deposit on bottle walls.
Aluminum crimp seal is green.
NDC 0046-1066-05 .... 12.5 mg package for 0.25%
White amorphous deposit on bottle walls.
Aluminum crimp seal is yellow.

Handling and Storage
Store under refrigeration (2°–8°C).
Reconstituted product may be stored at room temperature (approximately 25°C.) for up to four weeks.

Manufactured by:
Ayerst Laboratories
A Wyeth-Ayerst Company
Philadelphia, PA 19101

Shown in Product Identification Guide, page 107

INTRAOCULAR PRODUCT INFORMATION

The information concerning each product in this section has been prepared by the manufacturer, and edited and approved by the manufacturer's medical department, medical director, or medical counsel.

For those products that have official package circulars, the descriptions in *Physicians' Desk Reference For Ophthalmology* must be in full compliance with Food and Drug Administration regulations. For more information, please turn to the Foreword. In presenting the following material, the publisher is not necessarily advocating the use of any product listed.

Bausch & Lomb Surgical

555 WEST ARROW HIGHWAY
CLAREMONT, CA 91711

Direct Inquiries to:
Customer Services (800) 338-2020

Bausch & Lomb Surgical, a division of Bausch & Lomb, manufactures a complete line of ophthalmic products, including refractive surgery systems, foldable and PMMA intraocular lenses, phacoemulsification and vitreoretinal microsurgical equipment, handheld ophthalmic surgical instruments, and viscoelastics.

Bausch & Lomb Surgical manufactures and distributes refractive surgery products including automatic corneal shapers, excimer laser systems and disposable blades. Intraocular lens products include the Chiroflex® one-piece foldable IOL, which can be inserted through incisions of less than 3mm incision.

Bausch & Lomb Surgical also offers Soflex™, a line of three-piece foldable lenses, Chiroflex* plate haptic lenses with single-handed Passport* lens inserters, along with the small incision PMMA lenses, featuring Peripheral Detail Technology and EZVUE™ violet haptics. Bausch & Lomb Surgical also distributes Amvisc® and Amvisc® Plus sodium hyaluronate, Ocucoat* methylcellulose along with a complete line of phacoemulsification systems including the Millennium* and Catalyst Microsurgical systems.

Bausch & Lomb Surgical provides the widest selection of pre-market approved lenses available for posterior and anterior chamber. IOLs are available in many styles, including one-piece designs and special high and low diopter powers. Bausch & Lomb Surgical offers Vitrasert* Sterile intravitreal implant with Cytovene* (ganciclovir 4.5 mg) for the treatment of CMV retinitis.

For information on refractive surgery systems or intraocular lenses or any other products, please contact your Bausch & Lomb Surgical sales representative.

AMVISC® PLUS ℞
(sodium hyaluronate)

Description: AMVISC® PLUS is a sterile nonpyrogenic solution of sodium hyaluronate. AMVISC® PLUS contains 16 mg/mL of sodium hyaluronate adjusted to yield approximately 55,000 centistokes dissolved in physiological saline and exhibits an osmolality of approximately 340 milliosmoles.

Characteristics: Sodium hyaluronate is a high molecular weight polysaccharide composed of sodium glucuronate and N-acetylglucosamine. Sodium hyaluronate is ubiquitously distributed throughout the tissues of the body and is present in high concentrations in such tissues as vitreous humor, synovial fluid, umbilical cord and the dermis of rooster combs. Sodium hyaluronate functions as a tissue lubricant (1,2) and it is thought to play an important role in modulating the interactions between adjacent tissues. It can also act as a viscoelastic support maintaining a separation between tissues. Sodium hyaluronates prepared from different tissues may have different molecular weights but are thought to have the same chemical structure. The sodium hyaluronate in AMVISC® PLUS is prepared from the dermis of rooster combs (3). It has a molecular weight greater than 1,000,000, is reported to be nonantigenic (4,5), does not cause foreign body reactions, is nonpyrogenic and is well tolerated in human eyes (6). AMVISC® PLUS does not interfere with normal wound healing processes.

Indications: AMVISC® PLUS is indicated for use as a surgical aid in ophthalmic anterior (7) and posterior (6) segment procedures including • extraction of cataract • implantation of an intraocular lens (IOL) • corneal transplantation surgery • glaucoma filtering surgery • surgical procedures to reattach the retina.

Due to its lubricating and viscoelastic properties, transparency and ability to protect corneal endothelial cells (8), AMVISC® PLUS helps maintain anterior chamber depth and visibility, minimizes interaction between tissues, and acts as a tamponade and vitreous substitute during retina reattachment surgery. AMVISC® PLUS also preserves tissue integrity and good visibility when used to fill the anterior and posterior segments of the eye following open sky procedures.

Contraindications: At the present time there are no contraindications to the use of AMVISC® PLUS when used as recommended as an intraocular implant.

Applications:

1. Cataract surgery and IOL implantation—The required amount of AMVISC® PLUS is slowly infused through a needle or cannula into the anterior chamber. The protective effect of AMVISC® PLUS as an aid is optimized when the injection is performed prior to cataract extraction and insertion of the IOL and is effective for both intra- and extracapsular cataract procedures. AMVISC® PLUS may be applied to the IOL prior to insertion. Additional AMVISC® PLUS can be injected as required to facilitate surgical procedures (SEE PRECAUTIONS).
2. Corneal transplant surgery—The corneal button is removed and the anterior chamber filled with AMVISC® PLUS until it is level with the surface of the cornea. The donor graft is then placed on top of the AMVISC® PLUS and sutured into place. Additional AMVISC® PLUS can be used as required to aid in surgical procedures (SEE PRECAUTIONS).
3. Glaucoma filtration surgery—AMVISC® PLUS is injected through a corneal paracentesis to restore and maintain anterior chamber volume during the performance of the trabeculectomy. Additional AMVISC® PLUS can be used as required to aid in the surgical procedures (SEE PRECAUTIONS).
4. Intraocular injection in conjunction with scleral buckling procedures for retina reattachment—After release of subretinal fluid and development of buckling by tying the mattress sutures, air is injected into the vitreous cavity and then exchanged with AMVISC® PLUS injected through a needle (22 to 30 gauge) passed via the pars plana epithelium. The volume of AMVISC® PLUS injected (2–4 mL) will vary with the volume of the subretinal fluid released and the space occupied by the buckle.

Precautions: Those precautions normally considered during anterior segment and retina reattachment procedures are recommended.

There may be increased intraocular pressure following surgery (9) caused by preexisting glaucoma or by the surgery itself. For these reasons the following precautions should be considered.

- An excess quantity of AMVISC® PLUS should not be used. • AMVISC® PLUS should be removed from the anterior chamber at the end of surgery. • If the postoperative intraocular pressure increases above expected values, correcting therapy should be administered. • AMVISC® PLUS is prepared from a biological source and the physician should be aware of the possible effects of using any biological materials. • Reuse of cannula should be avoided. Even after cleaning and rinsing, resterilized cannula could release particulate matter as AMVISC® PLUS is injected. It is recommended that disposable cannula be used when administering AMVISC® PLUS. • There have been isolated reports of diffuse particulates or haziness appearing after injection of AMVISC® PLUS into the eye. While such reports are infrequent and seldom associated with any effects on ocular tissues, the physician should be aware of this occurrence. If observed, the particulate matter should be removed by irrigation and/or aspiration.

Adverse Reactions: Sodium hyaluronate is a natural component of the tissues of the body and is extremely well tolerated in human eyes. Transient postoperative inflammatory reactions were reported in clinical trials (6) and oral and topical steroid preparations were administered. AMVISC® PLUS is tested in animals to determine that each batch is essentially noninflammatory. Since sodium hyaluronate molecules are noninflammatory, any phlogistic response is considered to be caused by the surgical procedures. The best index of the degree of phlogistic response is the postoperative clarity of the vitreous cavity. As outlined above a transient postoperative increase in intraocular pressure has been observed following the use of sodium hyaluronate in anterior segment surgery. On rare occasions postoperative reactions including inflammation, corneal edema and corneal decompensation have been reported. The relationship to the use of AMVISC® PLUS has not been established.

How Supplied: AMVISC® PLUS is a sterile viscoelastic preparation supplied in a disposable glass syringe delivering either 0.5 mL or 0.8 mL of sodium hyaluronate dissolved in physiological saline. Each mL of AMVISC® PLUS contains 16 mg of sodium hyaluronate adjusted to yield approximately 55,000 centistokes, 9 mg of Sodium Chloride and q.s. Sterile Water for Injection USP. AMVISC® PLUS exhibits an osmolality of approximately 340 milliosmoles. Sodium hydroxide and/or hydrochloric acid are added to adjust pH (if necessary). AMVISC® PLUS syringes are terminally sterilized and aseptically packaged. Contents of unopened and undamaged pouches are sterile. Refrigerated AMVISC® PLUS should be allowed to reach room temperature (approximately 20 to 45 minutes, depending on volume) prior to use.

For Intraocular Use: Store at 2–8°C. Protect from freezing.

Caution: Federal U.S. law restricts this device to sale by or on the order of a physician.

References:

1. Swann DA, Radin EL, Nazimiec, Weisser PA, Curran N, Lewinneck G. Role of hyaluronic acid in joint lubrication. Ann Rheum Dis 1974; 33:318.
2. Radin EL, Paul IL, Swann DA, Schottstaedt ES. Lubrication of synovial membrane. Ann Rheum Dis 1971; 30:322.
3. Swann DA, Studies of Hyaluronic Acid. I. The preparation and properties of rooster comb hyaluronic acid. Biochim Biophys Acta 1968; 156:17.
4. Richter W. Non-immunogenicity of purified hyaluronic acid preparations tested by passive cutaneous anaphylaxis. Int Arch Allergy 1974; 47:211.
5. Richter, W, Ryde EM, Zetterstrom EO. Non-immunogenicity of a purified sodium hyaluronate preparation in man. Int Arch Appl Immunol 1979; 59:45.
6. Pruett RC, Schepens CL, Swann DA, Hyaluronic acid vitreous substitute. A six-year clinical evaluation. Arch Ophthalmol 1979; 97:2325.
7. Pape LG, Balazs EA. The use of sodium hyaluronate (Healon®) in human anterior segment surgery. Ophthalmol 1980; 87:699.
8. Miller D, Stegmann R. Use of Na-hyaluronate in anterior segment eye surgery. Am Intra-Ocular Implant Soc J 1980; 6:13.
9. Miller D, Stegmann R. The use of Healon® in intraocular lens implantation. Int Ophthalmol Clinics 1982; 22:177.

Size	Reorder #
0.5 mL	60051
0.8 mL	60081

Manufacturer:
Bausch & Lomb Surgical, Inc.
555 West Arrow Highway
Claremont, CA 91711 USA
(800) 338-2020 or (909) 624-2020, ext. 1225
Regulatory Affairs Product Surveillance
Fax (909) 399-1646
Revised December 1996
Made in the U.S.A.

PO11-602-01 PIN 555-200 Rev. 12/96

AMVISC® ℞

Information listed for AMVISC Plus also applies to AMVISC with the following exceptions.

- AMVISC contains 12 mg/mL sodium hyaluronate adjusted to yield approximately 40,000cs dissolved in physiological saline.
- AMVISC is a sterile viscoelastic preparation supplied in a disposable glass syringe delivering either 0.50mL or 0.80mL sodium hyaluronate dissolved in physiological saline. Each mL of AMVISC contains 12mg sodium hyaluronate adjusted to yield approximately 40,000cs, 9.0mg of sodium chloride and sterile water for injection. U.S.P.q.s.

For more information regarding AMVISC Plus or AMVISC viscoelastics contact: Bausch & Lomb Surgical, Inc., 555 West Arrow Highway, Claremont, California 91711. Toll free: 800-423-1871 ext. 1225.

VITRASERT*

Sterile Intravitreal Implant with Cytovene® (ganciclovir, 4.5 mg)

FOR INTRAVITREAL IMPLANTATION ONLY

Description: The Vitrasert Implant contains the antiviral drug ganciclovir. Each Vitrasert implant contains a minimum of 4.5 mg ganciclovir.

Each Vitrasert Implant contains a ganciclovir tablet which contains the inactive ingredient, magnesium stearate, (0.25%). Each tablet is coated with polyvinyl alcohol and ethylene vinyl acetate polymers.

The chemical name of ganciclovir is 9-[[2-hydroxy -1- (hydroxymethyl)ethoxy] methyl]guanine, and has the following structure:

O
HN
N
H_2N
N
N
O
CH_2OH
CH_2OH

Ganciclovir is a white to off-white crystalline powder with a molecular formula of $C_9H_{13}N_5O_4$, and molecular weight of 255.23. Ganciclovir has a solubility of 4.3 mg/mL in water at 25°C.

Clinical Pharmacology: Virology

Ganciclovir is a synthetic nucleoside analogue of 2′-deoxyguanosine that inhibits replication of herpes viruses both in vitro and in vivo. Sensitive human viruses include cytomegalovirus (CMV), herpes simplex virus -1 and -2 (HSV-1, HSV-2), Epstein-Barr virus (EBV) and varicella zoster virus (VZV). Clinical studies have been limited to assessment of efficacy in patients with CMV infection.

Median effective inhibitory doses (ED_{50}) of ganciclovir for human CMV isolates tested in vitro in several cell lines ranged from 0.2 to 3.0 µg/mL. The relationship between in vitro sensitivity of CMV to ganciclovir and clinical response has not been established. Ganciclovir inhibits mammalian cell proliferation in vitro at higher concentrations (10 to 60 µg/mL) with bone marrow colony forming cells being the most sensitive ($ID_{50} \geq 10$ µg/mL) of those cell types tested.

Emergence of viral resistance has been reported based on in vitro sensitivity testing of CMV isolates from patients receiving intravenous ganciclovir treatment. The prevalence of resistant isolates is unknown, and there is a possibility that some patients may be infected with strains of CMV resistant to ganciclovir. Therefore, the possibility of viral resistance should be considered in patients who show poor clinical response.

Pharmacokinetics

In a clinical trial of Vitrasert Implants, 26 patients (30 eyes) received a total of 39 primary implants and 12 exchange implants (performed 32 weeks after the implant was inserted or earlier if progression of CMV retinitis occurred). Because most of the exchanged implants were empty, the time the implant actually ran out of drug was unknown, and a precise in-vivo release rate could not be calculated. However, approximate in-vivo release rates could be determined for the exchanged implants, which ranged from 1.00 µg/h to more than 1.62 µg/h.

In 14 implants (3 exchanged, 11 autopsy) in which the in-vivo release rate could accurately be calculated, the mean release rate was 1.40 µg/h, with a range from 0.5 to 2.88 µg/h. The mean vitreous drug levels in eight eyes (4 collected at the time of retinal detachment surgery; 2 collected from autopsy eyes within 6 hours of death and prior to fixation; 2 collected from implant exchanges) was 4.1 µg/mL.

Indications and Usage: The Vitrasert Implant is indicated for the treatment of CMV retinitis in patients with acquired immunodeficiency syndrome (AIDS).

The diagnosis of CMV retinitis is opthalmologic and should be made by indirect ophthalmoscopy. Other conditions in the differential diagnosis of CMV retinitis include candidiasis, toxoplasmosis, histoplasmosis, retinal scars, and cotton wool spots, any of which may produce a retinal appearance similar to CMV. For this reason, it is essential that the diagnosis of CMV be established by a physician familiar with the retinal presentation of these conditions.

The Vitrasert Implant is for intravitreal implantation only.

Clinical Trials

In a randomized, controlled parallel group trial conducted between May 1993 and December 1994, treatment with the Vitrasert Implant was compared to treatment with intravenous ganciclovir (Cytovene-IV; Roche) in 188 patients with AIDS and newly diagnosed CMV retinitis. Patients randomized to the Cytovene-IV treatment group received Cytovene-IV solution at induction doses (5 mg/kg twice daily) for 14 days, followed by maintenance dosing (5 mg/kg once daily). Based on masked assessment of fundus photographs,

Continued on next page

Vitrasert—Cont.

the median time to progression was approximately 210 days for the Vitrasert Implant treatment group compared to approximately 120 days for the intravenous ganciclovir treatment group.

Contraindications

The Vitrasert Implant is contraindicated in patients with hypersensitivity to ganciclovir or acyclovir, and in patients with any contraindications for intraocular surgery, such as external infection or severe thrombocytopenia.

Warnings: CMV retinitis may be associated with CMV disease elsewhere in the body. The Vitrasert Implant provides localized therapy limited to the implanted eye. The Vitrasert Implant does not provide treatment for systemic CMV disease. Patients should be monitored for extraocular CMV disease.

As with any surgical procedure, there is risk involved. Potential complications accompanying intraocular surgery to place the Vitrasert Implant into the vitreous cavity may include, but are not limited to, the following: vitreous loss, vitreous hemorrhage, cataract formation, retinal detachment, uveitis, endophthalmitis, and decrease in visual acuity.

Following implantation of the Vitrasert Implant, nearly all patients will experience an immediate and temporary decrease in visual acuity in the implanted eye which lasts for approximately two to four weeks post-operatively. This decrease in visual acuity is likely a result of the surgical implant procedure.

Precautions: General

As with all intraocular surgery, sterility of the surgical field and the Vitrasert Implant should be rigorously maintained. The Vitrasert Implant should be handled only by the suture tab in order to avoid damaging the polymer coatings since this could affect release rate of ganciclovir inside the eye. The Vitrasert Implant should not be resterilized by any method.

A high level of surgical skill is required for implantation of the Vitrasert Implant. A surgeon should have observed or assisted in surgical implantation of the Vitrasert Implant prior to attempting the procedure.

Information for Patients

The Vitrasert Implant is not a cure for CMV retinitis, and some immunocompromised patients may continue to experience progression of retinitis with the Vitrasert Implant. Patients should be advised to have ophthalmologic follow-up examinations of both eyes at appropriate intervals following implantation of the Vitrasert Implant.

As with any surgical procedure, there is risk involved. Potential complications accompanying intraocular surgery to place the Vitrasert Implant into the vitreous cavity may include, but are not limited to, the following: intraocular infection or inflammation, detachment of the retina, and formation of cataract in the natural crystalline lens.

Following implantation of the Vitrasert Implant, nearly all patients will experience an immediate and temporary decrease in visual acuity in the implanted eye which lasts for approximately two to four weeks post-operatively. This decrease in visual acuity is likely a result of the surgical implant procedure.

The Vitrasert Implant only treats eyes in which it has been implanted. Additionally, because CMV is a systemic disease, patients should be monitored for extraocular CMV infections (e.g., pneumonitis, colitis) in the body.

Patients should be advised that ganciclovir has caused decreased sperm production in animals and may cause infertility in humans. Women of childbearing potential should be advised that ganciclovir causes birth defects in animals and should not be used during pregnancy.

Patients should be advised that ganciclovir has caused tumors in animals. Although there is no information from human studies, ganciclovir should be considered a potential carcinogen.

Drug Interactions

No drug interactions have been observed with the Vitrasert Implant. There is limited experience with use of retinal tamponades in conjunction with the Vitrasert Implant.

Carcinogenesis, Mutagenesis

Ganciclovir was carcinogenic in the mouse at oral doses of 20 and 1000 mg/kg/day. At the dose of 1000 mg/kg/day there was a significant increase in the incidence of tumors of the preputial gland in males, forestomach (nonglandular mucosa) in males and females, and reproductive tissues (ovaries, uterus, mammary gland, clitoral gland, and vagina) and liver in females. At the dose of 20 mg/kg/day, a slightly increased incidence of tumors was noted in the preputial and harderian glands in males, forestomach in males and females, and liver in females. Except for histiocytic sarcoma of the liver, ganciclovir-induced tumors were generally of epithelial or vascular origin. Although the preputial and clitoral glands, forestomach, and harderian glands of mice do not have human counterparts, ganciclovir should be considered a potential carcinogen in humans.

Ganciclovir increased mutations in mouse lymphoma cells and DNA damage in human lymphocytes in vitro at concentrations between 50–500 and 250–2000 µg/mL, respectively. In the mouse micronucleus assay, ganciclovir was clastogenic at doses of 150 and 500 mg/kg (IV) (2.8 − 10x human exposure based on AUC) but not 50 mg/kg (exposure approximately comparable to the human based on AUC). Ganciclovir was not mutagenic in the Ames Salmonella assay at concentrations of 500–5000 µg/mL.

Impairment of Fertility

Ganciclovir caused decreased mating behavior, decreased fertility, and an increased incidence of embryolethality in female mice following intravenous doses of 90 mg/kg/day. Ganciclovir caused decreased fertility in male mice and hypospermatogenesis in mice and dogs following daily oral or intravenous administration of doses ranging from 0.2–10 mg/kg.

Pregnancy: Teratogenic Effects: Pregnancy Category C

Ganciclovir has been shown to be embryotoxic in rabbits and mice following intravenous administration and teratogenic in rabbits. Fetal resorptions were present in at least 85% of rabbits and mice administered 60 mg/kg/day and 108 mg/kg/day, respectively. Effects observed in rabbits included: fetal growth retardation, embryolethality, teratogenicity, and/or maternal toxicity. Teratogenic changes included cleft palate, anophthalmia/microphthalmia, aplastic organs (kidney and pancreas), hydrocephaly, and brachygnathia. In mice, effects observed were maternal/fetal toxicity and embryolethality.

Daily intravenous doses of 90 mg/kg administered to female mice prior to mating, during gestation, and during lactation caused hypoplasia of the testes and seminal vesicles in the month-old male offspring, as well as pathologic changes in the nonglandular region of the stomach (see Carcinogenesis, Mutagenesis subsection).

Although each Vitrasert Implant contains from 4.5 to 6.4 mg of ganciclovir, which is released locally in the vitreous, there are no adequate and well-controlled studies in pregnant women on the effects of the Vitrasert Implant. Therefore, the Vitrasert Implant should be used during pregnancy only if the potential benefit justifies the potential risk to the fetus.

Nursing Mothers

It is not known whether ganciclovir from the Vitrasert Implant is excreted in human milk. Daily intravenous doses of 90 mg/kg administered to female mice prior to mating, during gestation, and during lactation caused hypoplasia of the testes and seminal vesicles in the month-old male offspring, as well as pathologic changes in the non-glandular region of the stomach. Because many drugs are excreted in human milk and, because carcinogenicity and teratogenicity effects occurred in animals treated with ganciclovir, mothers should be instructed to discontinue nursing if they have a Vitrasert Implant.

Pediatric Use

Safety and effectiveness in pediatric patients below 9 years of age have not been established.

Adverse Reactions: During clinical trials, the most frequent adverse events seen in patients treated with the Vitrasert Implant involved the eye.

During the first two months following implantation, visual acuity loss of 3 lines or more, vitreous hemorrhage, and retinal detachments occurred in approximately 10–20% of patients. Cataract formation/lens opacities, macular abnormalities, intraocular pressure spikes, optic disk/nerve changes, hyphemas and uveitis occurred in approximately 1–5%.

Adverse events with an incidence of less than 1% were: retinopathy, anterior chamber cell and flare, synechia, hemorrhage (other than vitreous), cotton wool spots, keratopathy, astigmatism, endophthalmitis, microangiopathy, sclerosis, choroiditis, chemosis, phthisis bulbi, angle closure glaucoma with anterior chamber shallowing, vitreous detachment, vitreous traction, hypotony, severe post-operative inflammation, retinal tear, retinal hole, corneal dellen, choroidal folds, pellet extrusion from scleral wound, and gliosis.

Dosage and Administration

Each Vitrasert Implant contains a minimum of 4.5 mg of ganciclovir, and is designed to release the drug over a 5 to 8 month period of time. Following depletion of ganciclovir from the Vitrasert Implant, as evidenced by progression of retinitis, the Vitrasert Implant may be removed and replaced.

Handling and Disposal

Caution should be exercised in handling of the Vitrasert Implant in order to avoid damage to the polymer coating on the implant, which may result in an increased rate of drug release from the implant. Thus, the Vitrasert Implant should be handled only by the suture tab. Aseptic technique should be maintained at all times prior to and during the surgical implatation procedure.

Because the Vitrasert Implant contains ganciclovir, which shares some of the properties of anti-tumor agents (i.e., carcinogenicity and mutagenicity), consideration should be given to handling and disposal of the Vitrasert Implant according to guidelines issued for antineoplastic drugs.

How Supplied: The Vitrasert Implant is supplied in individual unit boxes in a sterile Tyvek package (NDC 61772–002–01). Store at room temperature, 15–30°C (59–86°F). Protect from freezing, excessive heat and light.

CAUTION: Federal law prohibits dispensing without prescription.

Manufacutred by: Bausch & Lomb Surgical, Inc.
555 W. Arrow Highway
Claremont, CA 91711
800/338-2020
USA

 U.S. Patent #5,378,475. Foreign Patents pending.
U.S. Patent #4,355,032, #4,507,305 (ganciclovir compound) 130128 Rev. B